# Advanced Principles of Clinical Toxicology

# Advanced Principles of Clinical Toxicology

Editor: Mary Durrant

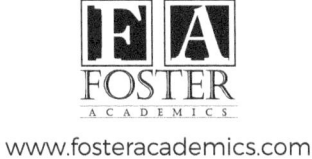

FOSTER
ACADEMICS

www.fosteracademics.com

www.fosteracademics.com

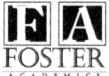

Cataloging-in-Publication Data

Advanced principles of clinical toxicology / edited by Mary Durrant.
    p. cm.
Includes bibliographical references and index.
ISBN 978-1-63242-584-3
1. Clinical toxicology. 2. Toxicology. 3. Clinical medicine. I. Durrant, Mary.
RA1218.5 .A38 2019
615.9--dc23

Foster Academics,
118-35 Queens Blvd., Suite 400,
Forest Hills, NY 11375, USA

ISBN 978-1-63242-584-3 (Hardback)

# Contents

# Preface

Clinical toxicology is a subspecialty of medicine. It studies the toxicology of drugs and provides diagnosis and treatments as well as prevention techniques to counter poisoning and adverse effects of medications, toxicants and biological agents. Clinical toxicology studies also deal with adverse drug reactions, acute or chronic poisoning, drug overdoses, substance abuse, etc. It is practiced by physicians as well as other health professionals, non-physicians and pharmacists. Clinical toxicology has varied applications, such as evaluating the health impacts from exposure to toxic substances, contributing to pharmaceutical research and drug safety, handling the aftermath of critical events of bioterrorism, chemical warfare and biological warfare. It is also significant in analyzing and interpreting diagnostic tests and forensic studies in clinical and forensic laboratories. This book presents researches and studies performed by experts across the globe. It elucidates the concepts and innovative models around prospective developments with respect to this field. This book, with its detailed analyses and data, will prove immensely beneficial to professionals and students involved in this area at various levels.

All of the data presented henceforth, was collaborated in the wake of recent advancements in the field. The aim of this book is to present the diversified developments from across the globe in a comprehensible manner. The opinions expressed in each chapter belong solely to the contributing authors. Their interpretations of the topics are the integral part of this book, which I have carefully compiled for a better understanding of the readers.

At the end, I would like to thank all those who dedicated their time and efforts for the successful completion of this book. I also wish to convey my gratitude towards my friends and family who supported me at every step.

Editor

# Apache II Scoring as an Index of Severity in Organophosphorus Poisoning

**Qaiser Jamal[1], Attiya Sabeen Rahman[1]\*, Muhammad A Siddiqui[2], Mehwish Riaz[1], Maryam Ansari[1] and Saleemullah[1]**

[1]Department of Medicine, Karachi Medical and Dental College and Abbasi Shaheed Hospital, Karachi, Pakistan

[2]School of Health Sciences, Queen Margaret University, Edinburgh, UK

\*Corresponding author: Attiya Sabeen Rahman, Department of Medicine, Karachi Medical and Dental College and Abbasi Shaheed Hospital, Karachi, Pakistan, E-mail: nervousystem.asr@gmail.com

## Abstract

**Objectives:** The purpose of the study was to determine the mortality rate in organophosphate poisoning patients and relationship between the clinical severity of OPP with APACHE II score and serum cholinesterase levels.

**Methodology:** This is a cross sectional study conducted in medical intensive care unit. Baseline variables and clinical characteristics were summarized with frequencies (percentages) for categorical variables and mean (standard deviation) for continuous variables. Receiver operating characteristic (ROC) curves were generated with a 95% CI to assess the relationship between individual APACHE II scores and mortality rates.

**Results:** The patient's average age was 25.16 ± 9.95 years. 56.6% were female and 78.8% patients were suicidal. Patient who had stayed in the hospital >15 days had 33.3% mortality (p=0.13). Total 12 (10.6%) patients required mechanical ventilation out of which only one (8.3%) patient expired (p=0.86). The average APACHE II score was 3.73 ± 3.95. The APACHE II score for predicting death risk had fair discrimination as indicated by ROC curve of 0.67 (CI. 0.512-0.833). There was no significant association (p=0.29) between serum cholinesterase level and APACHE II score regarding the severity of poisoning. However, significant association (p<0.001) was found between outcome and serum cholinesterase levels.

**Conclusion:** The mortality rate reported was 9.7%. There was no significant association between serum cholinesterase level and APACHE II score regarding the severity of poisoning. However, significant association was found between outcome and serum cholinesterase levels.

**Keywords:** Organophosphorus; Poisoning; APACHE II; Serum cholinesterase; Mortality, Complications

## Introduction

Acute poisoning is a major public health issue in many countries around the world [1]. Pesticide self-poisoning is killing an estimated 350,000 people every year [2]. The World Health Organization (WHO) has identified pesticide poisoning as the single most common method of suicide worldwide [3]. Worldwide, an estimated 3,000,000 people are exposed to organophosphate (OP) or carbamate agents each year, with up to 300,000 fatalities [4,5]. In the United States, there were more than 8000 reported exposures to these agents in 2008, resulting in fewer than 15 deaths [5,6]. According to WHO two million people attempt suicide and one million accidental poisoning cases occur each year worldwide. However it is the deliberate self-poisoning that causes the great majority of the deaths and the immense strain the pesticides put on hospital services particularly Asia [7]. In India, rate of suicidal poisoning with OP compounds ranges from 10.3 to 43.8% [8]. OP poisoning is the most common cause (27.64%) and has the highest death rate (13.88%) of poisoning in Bangladesh [9]. The incidence in Sri Lanka is 10,000–20,000 hospital admissions annually [10]. It is estimated that there are 34,000 suicides annually in the Middle East region and 20% of suicides in the Middle East region are the result of pesticide ingestion [11,12]. OP is the commonest suicidal agent in Pakistan. The exact prevalence of OP poisoning is unknown in Pakistan as many cases are un-notified due to religious, social or cultural reasons. However reported incidence of deliberate self-poisoning (DSP) in Pakistan is about 8 per 100,000 in men and women [7,12,13].

OP insecticides are the most important pesticides and act through phosphorylating the active site of cholinesterase's, resulting in acetylcholine build-up. This produces excessive cholinergic stimulation, causing clinical features in both the peripheral and central nervous systems [2]. Toxicity generally results from accidental or intentional ingestion of, or exposure to, agricultural pesticides [4,7].

The Acute Physiology and Chronic Health Evaluation (APACHE II) is a severity score and mortality estimation tool developed from a large sample of ICU patients in the United States by Knaus et al. in 1985 [14]. Twelve physiological variables have been included in the APACHE II model in which the effects of chronic health status and age included in the model, weighted on the basis of their relative effect, to provide a single score along with a maximum of 71 are incorporated. Later admission in the ICU, in the first 24 h worst value was recorded used for each physiological variable [15]. The APACHE-II scoring system was found useful for classifying patients according to their disease severity. There was an inverse relationship between the high score and the length of stay as well higher chances of mortality [14]. The purpose of this study was to assess correlation of APACHE II score with the mortality of patients of organophosphorus poisoning and to determine the association of cholinesterase level and APACHE II score regarding the severity of poisoning.

## Materials and Methods

This is a cross sectional study conducted in medical intensive care unit in Abassi Shaheed Hospital from December 2013 to March 2014. All patients were admitted through the emergency room and diagnosed on the basis of history/exposure to the OP compound. History/exposure to OP compound in any form that is liquid, tablet, powder, and gaseous or direct contact with skin were included. Patients or attendants of patients giving history of ingestion were asked to bring bottle/container of the compound. Some of them were already carrying container with them. While diagnosing these cases clinical signs suggestive of muscarinic involvement like excessive salivation, sweating, miosis, lacrimation, diarrhea was taken in account. The diagnosis of acute OPP in patients was based on the following criteria: (A) ingestion of insecticide, pesticide oral or injectable (B) characteristic clinical sign and symptoms of OPP (C) decreased serum cholinesterase activity.

All patients admitted in intensive care unit aged >15 years (as this study was done in a adult medical intensive care unit) with organophosphorus poisoning within 48 h of taken OP were included in the study. Other argochemical, carbamate, paraquat or drug poisoning were excluded from the study.

## Outcome Measures

Mortality rate of OPP.

Clinical grading of severity by bardin classification.

APACHE 2 scoring.

## Serum cholinesterase levels

Patients were evaluated with regard to demographic information, mode of exposure, frequency of clinical signs and symptoms, duration of hospitalization, complications and outcome of each patient was recorded. All the patients were graded regarding clinical findings in relation to Bardin classification [16,17]. As indicated in the Table 1, patients were graded (grade 0,1,2,3) according to the clinical findings on admission in acute organophosphate intoxication.

| Grade 0: | No Clinical Manifestations |
|----------|----------------------------|
| Grade 1: | Hypersecretion, Fasciculation, Consciousness |
| Grade 2: | Grade 1+Hypotension, Unconsciousness |
| Grade 3: | Grade 2+Stupor, Abnormal Chest X-Ray, PO$_2$ <10 mmHg |

Table 1: The degree of organophosphate poisoning.

## Laboratory parameters

The following labs were done in all patients as per requirement of patient and for APACHE II scoring: complete blood count, urea, creatinine, electrolytes, arterial blood gases, and serum cholinesterase level. APACHE II score was calculated for every patient. Normal cholinesterase levels in our laboratory were 5400-13200 U/l. Severity of OPP was classified into 3 groups [18,19]. According to serum cholinesterase activity severe was <500, moderately severe was

500-1000 and mild was >1000 U/l. All patients were treated under a single treatment protocol.

## Treatment protocol for all patients

**Gastric lavage in emergency room:** Atropine infusion in pediatric chamber @8 micro drops per minute till patient is fully atropinized (that is resolution of bronchorrhea, heart rate of >80 bpm). If these targets were achieved than 150 mg of atropine is diluted in normal saline and given at 8 micro drops per minute. It takes 24-48 h to completely atropinized and thereafter it is slowly tapered off.

**Oximes:** Inj pralidoxime methylsulphate was given to patients with a loading dose of 2 gm. I/V infusion in 0.9% saline and then 1 gm 8 hourly.

**Benzodiazepines:** are used for patients in agitation and/or psychosis (diazepam 0.05-0.3 mg/kg/dose, lorazepam 0.05-0.1 mg/kg/dose or midazolam 0.15-0.2 mg/kg/dose). Decontamination dermal spills-wash the head and body with soap and water and removal of contaminated clothes, shoes and any other material with spills. Complications like aspiration pneumonia, sepsis, and hospital acquired infections were dealt accordingly.

## Statistical analysis

Baseline variables and clinical characteristics were summarized with frequencies (percentages) for categorical variables and mean (standard deviation [SD]) for continuous variables. The chi-squared test was used for comparing the proportions of categorized measurements. Receiver operating characteristic (ROC) curves were generated and the area under the curve (AUC) calculated together with a 95% CI to assess the relationship between individual APACHE II scores and mortality rates [20].

## Results

The patients ranged from 14 to 65 years of age, with an average age of 25.16 ± 9.95 years. More than half of patients were female. About 40% were married and less than one third of the study participants were from poor families and non-educated (Table 2). One hundred and three patients (91.2%) were attempted first time and 10 (8.8%) had history of previous poisoning. With regard to the nature of incidence, 89 patients (78.8%) were suicidal and 24 (21.2%) were accidental. Almost all patients (99%) have taken liquid form of OP. Among the all patients 96 (85%) had no history of psychiatric illness and 17 (15%) were with psychiatric illness in which 3 (2.7%) had family history.

According to Bardin grading of clinical severity 63 (55.8%) were in Grade 0, 33 (29.2%) were in Grade 1, 15 (13.3%) were in Grade 2 and only 2 (1.8%) patients were in Grade 3. Percentage of patients presented with a GCS of 10-15 was 89.4% and 10.6% patients had a GCS ranged 3 to 9. Patients with a low GCS had a mortality of 25% while those with a better GCS had a mortality of 7.9% (P=.06). Only one patient suffered from seizures. The mean duration of stay in the hospital was 7.33+8.6 days. Patient who had stayed in the hospital for <15 days had 8% mortality rate and those stayed >15 days had 33.3% mortality (P=.13). Total 12 (10.6%) patients required mechanical ventilation out of which only one (8.3%) patient died (P=.86). A total 16 (14.1%) patients suffered from complications. Two patients (1.7%) suffered from acute respiratory distress syndrome (ARDS) and both expired, aspiration pneumonia was reported in four (3.5%) patients out of which two passed away, sepsis was seen in five (4.4%) patients in which four deceased, urosepsis was found in two (1.7%) patients both treated successfully, Ventilator acquired pneumonia (VAP) was seen in four (3.5%) patients wherein three failed to survive.

| Variables | Subcategory | n (%) |
|---|---|---|
| Gender | Male | 49 (43.4) |
| | Female | 64 (56.6) |
| Marital Status | Unmarried | 46 (40.7) |
| | Engaged | 15 (13.3) |
| | Married | 47 (41.3) |
| | Divorced | 3 (2.7) |
| | Widow | 1 (0.9) |
| | Multiple Marriages | 1 (0.9) |
| Education | Uneducated | 31 (27.4) |
| | Under Matric | 45 (39.8) |
| | Matric | 24 (21.2) |
| | Inter | 10 (8.8) |
| | Graduate | 3 (2.7) |
| Socioeconomic Status | Poor | 34 (30.1) |
| | Average | 66 (58.4) |
| | Satisfactory | 13 (11.5) |

Table 2: Patients demographics.

The patients' average APACHE II score was 3.73 ± 3.95. Table 3 shows the distribution according to APACHE II score intervals and that 94% of the patients were in the interval between 0 and 10. The receiver operating characteristic curve, based on the sensitivity and complemented specificity of predicted death risk, shows an area under the curve of 0.67 CI: 0.512-0.833 (Figure 1).

| APACHE II Score | Survived | Deceased | Total |
|---|---|---|---|
| 0-5 | 80 (70.8) | 7 (6.2) | 87 (77) |
| 43014 | 16 (14.2) | 3 (2.7) | 19 (16.8) |
| 42309 | 4 (3.5) | 0 | 4 (3.5) |
| >15 | 2 (1.8) | 1 (0.9) | 3 (2.7) |
| Total | 102 (90.3) | 11 (9.7) | 113 (100) |

Table 3: Apache II score ranges and outcomes of treatment.

The mean serum cholinesterase levels were 4390.57 ± 4259. There was no significant association (P=.011) observed between serum cholinesterase level and APACHE II score regarding the severity of poisoning (Table 4). However, significant association (P<.001) was found between patient's outcomes and serum cholinesterase levels. Patients with cholinesterase level >1000 were 77 (68.2%), 500-1000 were 32 (28.3%) and <1000 were 4 (3.5%).

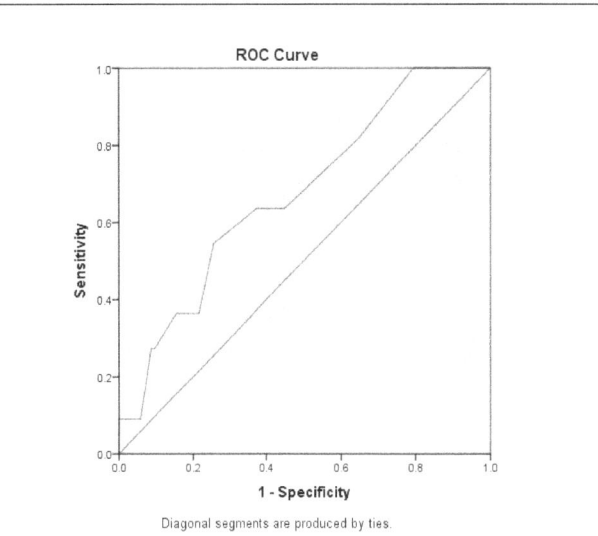

**Figure 1:** Shows discrimination power (Receiver Operating Curve) APACHE Score to predict mortality was 0.67, means out of 100 this score prediction will be correct in 67 patients.

| | APACHE | | | | Total | P Value |
|---|---|---|---|---|---|---|
| | 0-5 | 6-10 | 11-15 | >15 | | |
| Cholinesterase Level | | | | | | 0.011 |
| <500 | 2 (1.8) | 1 (0.9) | 0 | 1 (0.9) | 4 (3.5) | |
| 500-1000 | 22 (19.5) | 5 (4.4) | 3 (2.7) | 2 (1.8) | 32 (28.3) | |
| >1000 | 63 (55.8) | 13 (11.5) | 1 (0.9) | 0 | 77 (68.1) | |
| Total | 87 (77) | 19 (16.8) | 4 (3.5) | 3 (2.7) | 113 (100) | |

Table 4: Apache score and cholinesterase level: Mild to severe poisoning

There was no significant relationship between Apache 2 score and the clinical grading of severity by Bardin criteria (P=0.9). There was also no significant association (P=0.64) of clinical grading of severity and serum cholinesterase levels (Table 5).

| | Bardin Criteria | | | | Total | P Value |
|---|---|---|---|---|---|---|
| | Grade 1 | Grade 2 | Grade 3 | Grade 4 | | |
| APACHE Score | | | | | | 0.9 |
| 0-5 | 48 (42.5) | 24 (21.2) | 13 (11.5) | 2 (1.8) | 87 (77) | |
| 43014 | 11 (9.7) | 6 (5.3) | 2 (1.8) | 0 | 19 (16.8) | |
| 42309 | 3 (2.7) | 1 (0.9) | 0 | 0 | 4 (3.5) | |
| >15 | 1 (0.9) | 2 (1.8) | 0 | 0 | 3 (2.7) | |

| Total | 63 (55.8) | 33 (29.2) | 15 (13.3) | 2 (1.8) | 113 (100) | |
|---|---|---|---|---|---|---|
| Cholinesterase | | | | | | 0.64 |
| <500 | 3 (2.7) | 1 (0.9) | 0 | 0 | 4 (3.5) | |
| 500-1000 | 19 (16.8) | 11 (9.7) | 2 (1.8) | 0 | 32 (28.3) | |
| >1000 | 41 (36.3) | 21 (18.6) | 13 (11.5) | 2 (1.8) | 77 (68.1) | |
| Total | 63 (55.8) | 33 (29.2) | 15 (13.3) | 2 (1.8) | 113 (100) | |

**Table 5:** Apache Score and Cholinesterase level with clinical grading of severity.

## Discussion

Our study found that the mean age of patients was 25.16 ± 9.95 years, with more than half females. Our mortality rate in OPP patients was 9.7%. 89.4% had a GCS of 10-15. Patients with a low (3-9) GCS had 25% mortality while those with a better GCS (10-15) had 7.9% mortality. Only one patient had suffered from seizures. 12 (10.6%) patients' required mechanical ventilation and only one died. A total 16 (14.1%) patients suffered from complications. Two patients (1.7%) suffered from acute respiratory distress syndrome (ARDS) and deceased, aspiration pneumonia was reported in four (3.5%) patients out of which two expired, sepsis was seen in five (4.4%) patients in which four passed away, urosepsis was found in two (1.7%) patients both treated successfully, Ventilator acquired pneumonia was seen in four (3.5%) patients three died. There was no significant association observed between severe cholinesterase level and APACHE-II score in context to the severity of poisoning. Significant association was found between patient's outcome and severe cholinesterase level.

A study conducted in Singapore on 23 OPP cases observed an ICU mortality of 13% [18], while we had a mortality rate of 9.7% they also found that an APACHE-II score of 26 or higher accurately predicated death with 95% sensitivity and 100% specificity. In contrast to our study, they have concluded that APACHE-II score differentiated patients in to 3 severity groups (P=.004) and co-related well with severity of OPP and cholinesterase levels [18]. Mechanical ventilation was required in 74% while in our study only 10.6% required mechanical ventilation another study found that APACHE-II score to be correlated with the severity of OPP, cholinesterase level and mortality (P<.05) [21]. Previous studies have reported mortality in OPP cases between 10% and 89%, [22]. However, with intensive care management, mechanical ventilation for respiratory failure and use of atropine remains at 10-20%, [23,24] whereas our patients mortality rate was 9.7%.

A study conducted retrospectively in 48 patients showed a mean age of 32.5 ± 16.4 years with 34 females [25]. Study results found that 87.5% had attempted suicide while in our study 78.8% were attempted suicide and 21.1% were accidental. Their mean cholinesterase level on admission was 1281.4 ± 4259 (our mean serum cholinesterase levels were 4390.57+4259). Mechanical ventilation was required by 58% of patients, while in this study 10.6% of patient's required mechanical ventilation. The average duration of length of ICU stay was 10.3 ± 9.22 days, [23] whereas the mean duration of stay of our patients was 7.33 ± 8.7 days. The most common complication reported by them in 48 patients was aspiration pneumonia in 12 patients, ARDS in seven patient's sepsis in nine patient's septic shock in in five patients and

renal failure in five patients. While our complication rate was much lower which was two patients had ARDS, aspiration pneumonia in four patients, sepsis in five patients, urosepsis in two patients and four suffered from VAP. They showed that APACHE-II score was inversely correlated with serum cholinesterase level at admission. They significantly correlated mortality with GCS and APACHE-II score. They reported a mortality rate of 22% which was much higher than this study [25].

There are no validated scoring systems for categorizing severity of predicating outcome, although many have been proposed. The highly variable history and the fact to determine the ingested dose make it difficult to predict the outcome for an individual. Thus, early discovery, quick access to medical care careful maintenance of patency of airway, meticulous attention towards presenting aspiration pneumonia and aggressive oxime and atropine therapy may reduce morbidity and mortality.

## Conclusion

The mortality rate reported was 9.7%. There was no significant relationship between the clinical grading of organophosphate poisoning, Apache II score and serum cholinesterase levels. However, significant association was found between patient's outcomes and serum cholinesterase levels.

## References

1. Senarathna L, Jayamanna SF, Kelly PJ, Buckley NA, Dibley MJ, et al. (2012) Changing epidemiologic patterns of deliberate self-poisoning in a rural district of Sri Lanka. BMC Public Health 12: 593-601.

2. Konickx LA, Bingham K, Eddleston M (2014) Is oxygen required before atropine administration in organophosphorus or carbamate pesticide poisoning?-A cohort study. Clin Toxicol 52: 531-537.

3. Bertolote JM, Fleischmann A, Butchart A, Besbelli N (2006) Suicide, suicide attempts and pesticides: a major hidden public health problem. Bull World Health Organ 84: 260.

4. Eddleston M, Phillips MR (2004) Self-poisoning with pesticides. 328: 42-44.

5. Bronstein AC, Spyker DA, Cantilena LR, Green JL, Rumack BH (2009) 2008 Annual Report of the American Association of Poison Control Centers' National Poison Data System (NPDS): 26th Annual Report. Clin Toxicol 47: 911-1084.

6. Bird S (2010) Organophosphate and carbamate poisoning.

7. Ali P, Anwer A, Bashir B, Jabeen R, Haroon H (2012) Clinical outcome of organophosphorus. JLUMHS 11: 15-18.

8. Prasad DRMM, Jirli PS, Mahesh M, Mamatha S (2013) Relevance of Plasma Cholinesterase to Clinical Findings in Acute Organophosphorous Poisoning. Asia Pac J Med Toxicol 2: 23-27.

9. Chowdhury FR, Bari MS, Alam MMJ, Rahman MM, Bhattacharjee B, et al. (2014) Organophosphate poisoning presenting with muscular weakness and abdominal pain - a case report. BMC Res Notes 7: 140.

10. Faiz MS, Mughal S, Memon AQ (2011) Acute and late complications of organophosphate poisoning. J Coll Physicians Surg Pak 21: 288-290.

11. Gunnell D, Eddleston M, Phillips MR, Konradsen F (2007) The global distribution of fatal pesticide self-poisoning: Systematic review. BMC Public Health 7: 357-372.

12. Haider S, Haider I (2001) Deliberate self-harm. Pak J Med Sci 17: 151-155.

13. Khurram M, Mahmood N (2008) Deliberate Self Poisoning, Experience at Medical Unit. J Pak Med Assoc 55: 455-457.

14. Naved SA, Siddiqui S, Khan FH (2011) APACHE-II score correlation with mortality and length of stay in an intensive care unit. J Coll Physicians Surg Pak 21: 4-8.

15. Vincent JL, Moreno RP (2010) Clinical review: scoring systems in the critically ill. Crit Care 14: 207-216.

16. Bardin PG, Van Eeden SF, Moolman JA, Foden AP, Joubert JR (1994) Organophosphate and carbamate poisoning. Arch Intern Med 154:1433-1441.

17. Amanvermez R, Baydin A, Yardan T, Basol N, Gunay M (2010) Emergency laboratory abnormalities in suicidal patients with acute organophosphate poisoning. Turk J Biochem 35: 29-34.

18. Lee P, Tai DYH (2001) Clinical features of patients with acute organophosphate poisoning requiring intensive care. Intensive Care Med 27: 694-699.

19. Tafuri J, Roberts J (1987) Organophosphate poisoning. Ann Emerg Med 16: 193-202.

20. Hanley JA, McNeil BJ (1982) The meaning and use of the area under a receiver operating characteristic (ROC) curve. Radiology 143: 29–36.

21. Brun G, Teixeira E, Barroso C (1992) Severity evaluation of ventilated patients at a respiratory intensive care unit with APACHE-II system. Acta Med Port 5: 75-78.

22. Banday TH, Tathineni B, Desai MS, Naik V (2015) Predictors of Morbidity and Mortality in Organophosphorus Poisoning: A Case Study in Rural Hospital in Karnataka, India. N Am J Med Sci 6: 259-265.

23. Du Toit PW, Muller FO, Van Tonder WM, Ungerer MJ (1981) Experience with the intensive care management of organophosphate insecticide poisoning. S Afr Med J 60: 227-229.

24. Bardin PG, Van Eeden SF, Joubert JR (1987) Intensive care management of acute organophosphate poisoning. S Afr Med J 72: 593-597.

25. Sungurtekin H, Giirses E, Balci C (2006) Evaluation of Several Clinical Scoring tools in Organophosphate poisoned patients. Clin Toxicol 44: 121-126.

# 2

# Atherogenic and Haematologic Indices of Paracetamol-Overdosed Albino Rats Treated with Aqueous Leaf Extracts of *Euphorbia heterophylla* and *Jatropha curcas*

**Chidi Uzoma Igwe\*, Linus Nwaogu, Emmanuel Uche Olunkwa, Martin Otaba and Viola Onwuliri**

*Department of Biochemistry, Federal University of Technology, Owerri, Nigeria*

**\*Corresponding author:** Chidi Uzoma Igwe, Department of Biochemistry, Federal University of Technology, Owerri, Nigeria, E-mail: igwechidi9@gmail.com

## Abstract

**Objective:** The protective effect of aqueous leaf extracts of *Euphorbia heterophylla* and *Jatropha curcas* against paracetamol-induced acute changes in lipid, atherogenic and haematologic parameters of albino rats were studied.

**Methodology:** Twenty-five adult male albino rats weighing 180 to 200 g were randomly assigned into 5 experimental groups (I-V) of five animals each. Group I animals were administered 10 ml of distilled water, while group II rats were given 1000 mg/kg paracetamol. Groups III-V were pretreated with vitamin C (500 mg/kg), *E. heterophylla* (200 mg/kg) and *J. curcas* (1000 mg/kg) respectively, 1 h before administration of 1000 mg/kg paracetamol. The animals were orally administered the extracts/drugs daily for 14 days.

**Result:** Paracetamol administration reduced significantly (p<0.05) the total cholesterol, triglyceride, high density lipoprotein cholesterol (HDL-c), low density lipoprotein cholesterol (LDL-c) and total non HDL-c concentrations as well as white blood cell (WBC) count of the animals when compared with the control. Pre-treatment of the animals with vitamin C non-significantly (p>0.05) countered the observed effects of paracetamol overdose more than the extracts of *E. heterophylla* and *J. curcas*. Acute paracetamol overdose did not significantly (p>0.05) affect most of the atherogenic risk predictor indices and haematological parameters studied.

**Conclusion:** The results indicate that atherogenic and haematologic indices were less responsive than lipid parameters to paracetamol-induced toxicity. Furthermore, aqueous leaf extracts of *E. heterophylla* and *J. curcas* had less protective effect than vitamin C against serum lipidaemic changes induced by paracetamol.

**Keywords:** Acetaminophen; Drug overdose; Lipid profile; Medicinal plants; Vitamin C; Atherogenic indices

## Introduction

Many medicinal plant species contain both important nutrients and phytochemicals that could be pharmacologically essential [1]. The ethnopharmacological importance and application of plants in the treatment of diseases and illments in traditional setting have been an age-long practice [2]. Currently, herbal products are preferred by many people because of less testing time, higher safety, efficacy, cultural acceptability and assumed 'lesser' side effects. Furthermore, the phytochemicals present in plant-based products are thought be compatibility with the human body because they form part of the daily chemicals, humans ingested with food [3]. *Euphorbia heterophylla* and *Jatropha curcas* are among such traditional plants that have been reported to be useful for various purposes.

*E. heterophylla* plants are commonly available in temperate and tropical regions of the world. They occur in nature as herbs, shrubs or trees [1,4]. The plant is commonly called Mexican fire plant, milk weed and Spurge weed [5]. *E. heterophylla* belongs to the family Euphorbiaceae and to the subgenus *Poinsettia*, a group with stipules modified into glands [6]. It has a milky sap that is poisonous. Notwithstanding the poisonous nature of the plant's sap, it has been widely use in the treatment of various tropical diseases such as malaria, asthma, eczema and gonorrhea, as well as wart and respiratory tract infection [5]. In southeastern Nigeria, Igbo traditional doctors use the aqueous leaf extract of *E. heterophylla* for treatment of bacterial and parasitic infections of the blood and skin, and as a purgative [7]. Many pharmacologically important phytochemicals such as 4-hydroxylbenzoic acid, quercetin, beta-amyrin, and stigmasterol were isolated from the leaves. Similarly, essential and non essential amnio acids including, but not limited to, alanine, aspartic acid, cysteine, serine, proline, methionine and glutamic acid were also found to be present in the plant's leaf extract [8]. It was also observed that oral administration of aqueous leaf extract of the plant significantly reduced plasma glucose concentration of experimental induced diabetes in rats [9]. Aqueous leaf extract of *E. heterophylla* has also been reported to have good anticoagulant and preservative effect on human whole blood [10].

Like *E. heterophylla*, *J. curcas* L. is a widely grown flowering plant. It is a perennial plant that belongs to the Euphorbiaceae family [11]. The plant grows into a large shrub or small tree of up to 5 m in height. In the tropics, *J. curcas* is commonly grown as a living fence in fields and settlements [12]. All parts of the plant are very poisonous. The seed of *J. curcas* was reported to contain a purgative, phytotoxic oil called curcin, which causes dehydration and cardiovascular collapse as a result of haemorrhagic gastro-enteritis, and central nervous system depression [13]. However, it is gaining a lot of economic significance because of its several potentials in industrial application and medicinal values. The leaves of *J. curcas* are traditionally used in different forms in West Africa for the treatment of various ailments like fever, guinea worm sores, joint rheumatism, mouth infections and jaundice [3].

Paracetamol, also known as acetaminophen, is a widely used over-the-counter non-steriodal anti-inflammartory drug (NSAID) for treatment of pains and fever [14]. It is not a very strong analgesic, but can be used in conjuction with opioid analgesics in the management of more severe pains such as post-surgical and cancer pains [15]. It is generally safe when used at recommended doses even when taken for a long time. However, when taken in overdose paracetamol can be very toxic and fatal [16]. Paracetamol toxicity has been ascribed to the formation of Nacetylpbenzoquinon eimine (NAPQI), a toxic metabolite by hepatic cytochrome P450 [17]. NAPQI oxidizes the lipids and proteins of tissues, depletes glutathione and alters calcium homeostasis [18]. The oxidation of lipids and damage to liver hepatocytes could lead to derangements in lipid profile. The role of derangement in lipid profile in the progression of cardiovascular diseases (CVD) has been well established, with primary interest in CVD therapy focused on deranged low density lipoprotein cholesterol (LDL-c) levels [19]. High plasma triglyceride and cholesterol levels are both independent and synergistic risk factors for cardiovascular diseases and are often correlated with hypertension, obesity and diabetes mellitus [20]. Significant elevations in plasma low density lipoprotein (LDL) and very low density lipoprotein (VLDL) cholesterol concentrations are known risk factors for cardiovascular disease and are also often seen in hypertension and obesity [21]. Meanwhile, different combinations or ratios of these lipid profile parameters have been reported to be better indices for identification of high risk individuals to CVDs than direct use of the lipid parameters themselves [19]. Atherogenic index of plasma (AIP), atherogenic coefficient (AC) and Castelli's risk indices (CRIs) are the ratios of such lipid profile parameters that have been studied as markers of lipid atherogenic risk [22]. They are calculated lipid fraction ratios which are suggestively gaining attention in clinical setting for assessing the risk of CVD, over and above the routinely used lipid profile parameters [23]. In this study, we investigated the protective effect of the aqueous leaf extracts of *J. curcas* and *E. heterophylla* against paracetamol-induced changes in atherogenic and haematologic indices of albino rats.

## Materials and Methods

### Plants collection and extract preparation

The leaves of *Jatropha curcas* and *Euphorbia hetrophylla* were collected from bushes around Eziobodo in Owerri West Local Government Area of Imo State. They were authenticated by a botanist, Mr Francis Nwanze of the Department of Forestry and Wildlife, Federal University of Technology Owerri, Nigeria.

Apparently healthy leaves of the two plants were separately air-dried for 2 weeks and then oven-dried at a temperature of 50˚C for 8 h to a constant weight. Using pestle and mortar, the dried leaves were ground into powder form. The powders were separately stored in labeled air-tight containers. Five hundred grams (500 g) of each leaf powder was soaked in 1,000 ml of distilled water for 48 h and filtered with whatman filter paper No. 1. The filtrate was evaporated to dryness. Then the dried powder was suspended in 100 ml of 0.5% tween 80 solvent in a 500 ml beaker, allowed to stand for 1 hr and filtered. The filtrate was evaporated in an electric oven at 50˚C to obtain the stock

solutions. Then, respective doses of 200 mg/kg and 1000 mg/kg for *E. heterophylla* and *J. curcas* were prepared from the stocks. Each concentrate was transferred into labeled glassware and refrigerated at 4˚C until needed.

### Drugs used

The paracetamol and vitamin C tablets used were products of Emzor Pharmaceuticals Ltd, Nigeria. They were sourced from Orchad Pharmacy in Owerri, Nigeria. Each tablet containing 1000 mg of paracetamol was dissolved in 10 ml of distilled water, while each tablet of vitamin C containing 100 mg of ascorbic acid was dissolved in 1 ml of distilled water. They were reconstituted and administered as 1000 mg/kg and 500 mg/kg body weight of the animals respectively.

### Laboratory animals

Laboratory animals used were made up of 25 adult male albino rats (*Rattus novergicus*) weighing between 180 g and 200 g, obtained from the Department of Vertinary Medicine, University of Nigeria, Nsukka. The animals were kept in stainless steel cages under good laboratory conditions of humidity (60 ± 0.2 %), temperature (30 ± 1˚C) and a 12 h light/dark cycle. They were kept for 14 days to acclimatize to laboratory conditions in the Animal House Unit of Department of Biochemistry, Federal University of Technology Owerri. During the acclimatization period, they were provided with clean water and standard feed (Growers marsh, Vital Feeds Ltd.) *ad libitum*. Ethical approval was obtained for the study protocol from the University ethical committee. Principles of Laboratory Animal Care (NIH Publication, 1985-1993) were fully adopted in all the experimental procedures involving the use and handling of the laboratory animals.

### Grouping of animals

After acclimatization period, the albino rats were randomly allotted into 5 groups of 5 rats each. Group I served as the negative control and were orally administered daily dose of 10 ml/kg body weight of distilled water only. Group II served as the positive control and were orally administered daily dose of 1000 mg/kg of paracetamol. Group III animals (the standard group) were pretreated with oral dose of 500 mg/kg of vitamin C solution one hour before the oral administration of 1000 mg/kg of paracetamol. Group IV animals were pretreated with single oral dose of 200 mg/kg of *Euphorbia heterophylla* leaf extract one hour before administration of 1000 mg/kg of paracetamol. This served as test group 1. Group V animals were pretreated with daily oral dose of 1000 mg/kg of *Jatropha curcas* leaf extract 1 h before administration of 1000 mg/kg of paracetamol. This served as test group 2. The chosen dose ranges for the paracetamol and aqueous plant extracts used were based on result of earlier toxicity studies [1,24,25]. The oral administration of the drugs and plant extracts were for a period of fourteen days.

### Sample collection

At the end of the 14 days of treatment, the animals were fasted overnight, anaesthetized with diethyl ether and sacrified. Then, 5 mL of whole blood was collected by cardiac puncture. About 3 mL of each blood sample was gently dispensed into a well labeled 10 ml capacity plain sample bottle, while the rest was dispensed into ethylene diamine tetra acetic acid (EDTA) bottle. The blood samples in the plain bottles were allowed to clot and centrifuged at 2000 rpm for 15 minutes to separate sera from the clot. The sera were carefully separated into fresh labeled sample bottles and were used for lipid profile analysis, while the EDTA containing whole blood was used for haematological parameters.

## Lipid profile analyses

Serum triglyceride (TG), total cholesterol (TC) and high density lipoprotein cholesterol (HDL-c) concentrations were determined using enzymatic colorimetric method [26], phosphotungstate precipitation and enzymatic endpoint methods [27] with the aid of commercial reagent kits (Randox Laboratories Ltd, UK). Calculation of the concentration of low density lipoprotein cholesterol (LDL-c) in the serum was as previously described [28].

## Calculations of the atherogenic indices

Serum total non-HDL cholesterol (TnHDL-c) concentration was calculated as TC – HDL-c [29], while Castelli's Risk Index I (CRI-I) and Castelli's Risk Index II (CRI-II) were determined as TC / HDL-c and LDL-c / HDL-c respectively [22,30]. Atherogenic index of plasma (AIP) and atherogenic coefficient (AC) levels were calculated as log (TG / HDL-c) and (TC - HDL-c) / HDL-c respectively [31,32].

## Haematological analyses

Haemoglobin concentration of the anticoagulated blood was determined using Cyan-methaemoglobin method. Heamatocrit method was used in the determination of Packed Cell Volume (PCV), while Romanowsky stains/May-Grunwald-Giemsa Stain Technique

was used in the determination of white and red blood cell counts [33,34].

## Statistical analysis

Data obtained from the analyses were presented as mean ± standard deviation. The data generated were statistically analysed using one way Analysis of Variance (ANOVA) and Tukey Post HOC test with the aid of GraphPad Prism Version 5.3 (GraphPad, USA). Values that gave $p \leq 0.05$ were taken to be statistically significant.

## Results

Table 1 shows the lipid profile and atherogenic predictor indices of the paracetamol overdosed animals. Paracetamol treatment reduced significantly ($p<0.05$) the TG, TC, and HDL-c concentrations, but increased the LDL-c and total non-HDL cholesterol concentrations of the animals in comparism to the control animals. Treatment of the paracetamol overdosed animals with vitamin C and extracts of *E. heterophylla* and *J. curcas* increased non-significantly ($p>0.05$) the concentrations of the lipid and lipoproteins of the treated groups. Paracetamol overdose did not change significantly ($p>0.05$) the Castelli's Risk Index I (TC/HDL-c ratio), Castelli's Risk Index II (LDL-c/HDL-c ratio), atherogenic coefficient [(TC - HDL-c)/HDL-c ratio] and atherogenic index of plasma (Log [TG/HDL-c]) of the animals when compared with the control, vitamin C, *E. heterophylla* and *J. curcas* groups.

| Parameters | Negative Control | Positive Control (Paracetamol) | Standard Group (Vitamin C) | Test Group 1 (E.heterophylla) | Test Group 2 (J. curcas) |
|---|---|---|---|---|---|
| TG (mg/dl) | 150.74 ± 6.90[a] | 137.64 ± 7.5[b] | 145.09 ± 6.30[ab] | 140.80 ± 4.70[ab] | 143.37 ± 4.90[ab] |
| TC (mg/dl) | 198.51 ± 4.60[a] | 182.30 ± 5.50[b] | 189.79 ± 6.80[ab] | 186.80 ± 4.60[b] | 187.56 ± 7.30[ab] |
| HDL-c (mg/dl) | 40.34 ± 0.26[a] | 36.94 ± 0.16[b] | 38.72 ± 0.26[c] | 37.97 ± 0.16[d] | 37.84 ± 0.13[d] |
| LDL-c (mg/dl) | 82.66 ± 0.39[a] | 89.80 ± 0.42[b] | 85.12 ± 0.70[c] | 84.83 ± 0.48[c] | 84.55 ± 0.83[c] |
| CRI-I | 4.92 ± 0.64[a] | 4.94 ± 0.70[a] | 4.90 ± 0.61[a] | 4.92 ± 0.40[a] | 4.96 ± 0.41[a] |
| CRI-II | 2.22 ± 0.09[a] | 2.24 ± 0.06[a] | 2.20 ± 0.02[a] | 2.23 ± 0.01[a] | 2.23 ± 0.03[a] |
| TnHDL-c(mg/dl) | 158.18 ± 4.80[a] | 165.36 ± 5.20[b] | 151.07 ± 6.60[ab] | 148.83 ± 4.80[ab] | 149.72 ± 7.00[ab] |
| AC | 3.92 ± 0.03[a] | 3.94 ± 0.08[a] | 3.90 ± 0.04[a] | 3.92 ± 0.09[a] | 3.96 ± 0.05[a] |
| AIP | 0.57 ± 0.02[a] | 0.57 ± 0.01[a] | 0.57 ± 0.02[a] | 0.57 ± 0.01[a] | 0.58 ± 0.01[a] |

**Table 1**: Lipid Profile and Atherogenic Index Parameters of Paracetamol-overdosed Albino Rats Treated with *E. heterophylla* and *J. curcas*. Values are mean ± standard deviation. Values with different alphabet letters per row are statistically significant ($p<0.05$). TC: Total Cholesterol; TG: Triglyceride; HDL-c: High Density Lipoprotein Cholesterol; LDL-c: Low Density Lipoprotein Cholesterol; TnHDL-c: Total Non-HDL-c; CRI-I: Castelli's Risk Index I; CRI-II: Castelli's Risk Index II; AC: Atherogenic Coefficient; AIP: Atherogenic Index of Plasma.

Table 2 shows the haematologic indices of the paracetamol overdosed animals. Paracetamol treatment did not change significantly ($p>0.05$) the blood haemoglobin (Hb) concentration, packed cell volume (PCV) values and red blood cell (RBC) counts of the animals in comparism with the control and those of the vitamin C, *J. curcas* and *E. heterophylla* treated groups. However, there was a significant

($p<0.05$) reduction in the white blood cell (WBC) count of the animals after treatment with paracetamol overdose in comparism with the control. This was significantly ($p<0.05$) attenuated after treatment of the paracetamol overdosed animals with vitamin C, *E. heterophylla* and *J. curcas*.

| Parameters | Negative Control | Positive Control (Paracetamol) | Standard Group (Vitamin C) | Test Group 1 (*E. heterophylla*) | Test Group 2 (*J. curcas*) |
|---|---|---|---|---|---|
| HB (g/dl) | 11.30 ± 1.59[a] | 11.87 ± 1.60[a] | 12.65 ± 1.11[a] | 11.95 ± 1.00[a] | 12.07 ± 0.90[a] |
| PCV (%) | 33.93 ± 4.71[a] | 35.60 ± 4.81[a] | 37.95 ± 3.34[a] | 35.85 ± 3.00[a] | 36.07 ± 2.90[a] |
| WBC (x10$^{12}$/L) | 5.45 ± 0.10[a] | 4.20 ± 0.17[b] | 6.68 ± 0.23[c] | 6.45 ± 0.30[c] | 4.77 ± 0.25[d] |
| RBC (x10$^{12}$/L) | 35.65 ± 4.37[a] | 37.70 ± 4.86[a] | 40.05 ± 3.41[a] | 37.80 ± 2.93[a] | 38.10 ± 3.05[a] |

**Table 2:** Haematological Parameters of Paracetamol-overdosed Albino Rats Treated with *E. heterophylla* and *J. curcas*. Values are mean ± standard deviation. Values with different alphabet letters are statistically significant (p<0.05). HB: Haemoglobin; PCV: Packed cell volume; WBC: white blood cell count; RBC: Red blood cell count.

## Discussion

Induction of lipid peroxidation via the action of N- acetyl-p-benzoquinone imine (NAPQI), a highly reactive intermediate of paracetamol, is the principal route of paracetamol elicited toxicity. This intermediary metabolite covalently binds to cell's intracellular and membrane macromolecules leading to cell death and consequent liberation of intracellular contents including the cytosolic enzymes [35]. The release and induction of cytochrome based enzymes such as CYP2E1, CYP1A2 and CYP3A4, as well as depletion of intracellular glutathione (GSH) and induction of oxidative stress have been reported to be the most important mechanisms involved in the pathogenesis of paracetamol-induced cell injury [18,36]. Interestingly, such damages have been reportedly prevented or ameliorated by herbal preparations.

Results of our study showed that oral administration of overdose of paracetamol decreased serum triglyceride, total cholesterol, and HDL-c concentrations but increased LDL-c concentration. Paracetamol overdose has been reported to cause impairment in lipid and lipoprotein metabolism [37]. This could be as a result of hepatotoxicity that has been associated with excessive intake of paracetamol. The liver is the major organ for metabolism of lipids especially cholesterol and lipoproteins, and a significant site for re-generation of GSH required for control of lipid peroxidation processes in the body. Meanwhile, administration of vitamin C and extracts of *E. heterophylla* and *J. curcas* non-significantly (p>0.05) attenuated the TC concentrations. Serum low density lipoprotein cholesterol (LDL-c) and TG concentrations were equally attenuated in the extracts-treated groups. The concentrations of TC and LDL-c in blood have been reported to be direct related with mortality and morbidity from coronary artery diseases. Isolated rise in blood triglyceride above normal is not an independent risk factor for coronary disease. However, hypertriglyceridaemia becomes a risk factor for coronary disease when associated with high LDL-c and low HDL-c levels in blood. Impaired catabolism of chylomicron remnant, intermediate density lipoprotein (IDL), and LDL gives rise to increase in serum cholesterol [38]. The attenuation in serum TC concentration observed in the extracts-treated rats may be attributed to increase in the serum HDL-c concentration. HDL-c mobilizes cholesterol into the cells thereby decreasing or reducing the formation of atherosclerotic plaque. Relative or absolute decrease in the cholesterol carried in the HDL-fraction of plasma is seen in atherosclerotic patients [39].

Atherogenic indices are strong indicators of the risk of heart disease. The higher their values, the higher the risk of developing cardiovascular problems and vice versa [21,31]. There was no significant difference (p>0.05) observed in the Castelli's index I and II, atherogenic coefficient and atherogenic index of plasma of the paracetamol-overdosed animals in comparism with those of the groups treated with vitamin C, *E. heterophylla* and *J. curcas*. These indicate no potential risk of cardiovascular disease among the treatment groups. However, total non-HDL cholesterol (TnHDL-c) was significantly (p<0.05) increased in the paracetamol-overdosed group in comparism to the control. Administration of vitamin C, *E. heterophylla* and *J. curcas* to the paracetamol-challenged animals significantly (p<0.05) lowered the TnHDL-c values of the treatment groups.

There were no observed significant (p>0.05) changes in the blood parameters (Hb, PCV and RBC) of both the paracetamol-overdosed and the extracts-treated groups in comparism with the control animals. The absence of significant changes in these haematologic parameters suggests that paracetamol overdose and treatment with the extracts did not elicit anaemia-related conditions in the rats. Decreased haemoglobin and haematocrit levels, indicative of anaemia, are associated with intravascular haemolysis [24]. These observations may be due to the understanding that paracetamol metabolism and toxicity occur mainly in the liver. However, there was observed reduction in white blood cell (WBC) count of the paracetamol-overdosed rats while administration of vitamin C, *E. heterophylla* and *J. curcas* extracts led to a significant (p<0.05) increase in the WBC count of the rats, an observation which corroborates previous report that WBC counts are significantly decreased by paracetamol administration [40].

## Conclusion

In the light of the results obtained in this study, it may be concluded that atherogenic and haematologic indices were less responsive than lipid parameters to paracetamol-induced toxicity. Furthermore, aqueous leaf extracts of *E. heterophylla* and *J. curcas* have protective effect, although less than vitamin C, against serum lipidaemic changes induced by paracetamol toxicity. The observations reported herein may explain the widespread use of the extracts of these plants in ethnotraditional medicine practice.

## References

1. Apiamu A, Evuen UF, Ajaja UI (2013) Biochemical Assessment of the Effect of Aqueous Leaf Extract of Euphorbia heterophylla Linn on Hepatocytes of Rats. J Environ Sci Toxicol Food Technol 3: 37-41.

2. Usman MM, Sule MS (2014) Effect of Oral Administration of Aqueous Leaves Extracts of Euphobia lateriflora (Schum and Thonn) On Liver and Kidney Function in Rats. J Environ Sci Toxicol Food Technol 8: 64-67.

3.  Prasad DMR, Izam A, Maksudur RK (2012) Jatropha curcas: Plant of medical benefits. Journal of Medicinal Plants Research 6: 2691-2699.

4.  Omale J, Emmanuel TF (2010) Phytochemical Composition, Bioactivity and wound healing potential of Euphorbia heterophylla (Euphorbiaceae) leaf extract. International Journal on Pharmaceutical and Biomedical Research 1: 54-63.

5.  Okeniyi SO, Adedoyin BJ, Garba S (2013) Phytochemical Screening, Cytotoxicity, Antioxidant and Antimicrobial Activities of Stem and Leave Extracts of Euphorbia heterophylla. Journal of Biology and Life Science. 4: 24-31.

6.  Mosango DM (2008) Euphorbia heterophylla L. In: PROTA (Plant Resources of Tropical Africa / Ressources végétales de l'Afrique tropicale). Schmelzer GH & Gurib-Fakim A (Editors). Wageningen, Netherlands.

7.  Ughachukwu PO, Ezenyeaku CCT, Ochiogu BC, Ezeagwuna DA, Anahalu IC (2014) Evaluation of antibacterial activities of Euphorbia heterophylla. Journal of Dental and Medical Sciences 1: 69-75.

8.  Fred-Jaiyesimi AA, Abo KA (2010) Phytochemical and Antimicrobial analysis of the crude extract, petroleum ether and chloroform fractions of Euphorbia heterophylla Linn whole plant. Pharmacognosy Journal 2:16

9.  Annapurna A, Hatware K (2014) Effect of aqueous extract of Euphorbia heterophylla on blood glucose levels of alloxan induced diabetic rats. International Journal of Research in Pharmacy and Chemistry (IJRPC) 4: 669-672.

10. Ughachukwu PO, Ezenyeaku CCT, Onwurah WO, Ifediata FE, Ogamba JO, et al. (2013) Effect on some haematological indices of human whole blood when aqueous leaf extract of Euphorbia heterophylla was used as storage anticoagulant. Afr J Biotechnol 12: 4952-4955.

11. Tharyn R, Jéssica FB, Suzana S, Roberta P, Zonetti PD (2013) Allelopathy of leaf extracts of jatropha (Jatropha curcas L.) in the initial development of wheat (Triticum aestivum L.). IDESIA (Chile) 31: 45-52.

12. Bassey IN, Ogbemudia FO, Harold KO, Idung KE (2012) Combined Antifungal Effects of extracts of Jatropha curcas and Chromolaena odorata on Seed Borne Fungi of Solanum gilo Raddi. Bull Env Pharmacol Life Sci 2: 13-17.

13. Esimone CO, Nworu CS, Jackson CL (2008) Cutaneous wound healing activity of a herbal ointment containing the leaf extract of Jatropha curcas L. (Euphorbiaceae). International Journal of Applied Research in Natural Products 1: 1-4.

14. Aghababian RV (2010) Essentials of Emergency Medicine. Jones & Bartlett Publishers, Sudbury, MA.

15. SIGN - Scottish Intercollegiate Guidelines Network (2008) Guideline 106: Control of pain in adults with cancer "6.1 and 7.1.1". National Health Service (NHS), Scotland.

16. FDA (2008) Advisory Committees Meeting Materials on Drugs Safety and Risk Management.

17. Wallace JL (2004) Acetaminophen hepatotoxicity: NO to the rescue. Br J Pharmacol 143: 1-2.

18. Aba PE, Eneasato CP, Onah JA (2016) Effect of Quail Egg Pretreatment on the Lipid Profile and Histomorphology of the Liver of Acetaminophen-Induced Hepatotoxicity in Rats. J Applied Biol & Biotech 4: 034-038

19. Bhardwaj S, Bhattacharjee J, Bhatnagar MK, Tyagi S (2013) Atherogenic Index of Plasma, Castelli Risk Index and Atherogenic Coefficient- New Parameters in Assessing Cardiovascular Risk. Int J Pharm Bio Sci 3: 359-364.

20. McBride PE (2007) Triglycerides and risk for coronary heart disease. JAMA 298: 336-338.

21. Rakib H, Marjana K, Swagata SL, Mahmudur RM, Paritosh C, et al. (2014) Preclinical lipid profile studies of a classical Ayurvedic preparation "Arjunarista" after chronic administration to male Sprague-dawley rats. Int J Pharm 4: 146-150.

22. Igwe CU, Iheme CI, Alisi CS, Nwaogu LA, Ibegbulem CO, et al. (2016) Lipid profile and atherogenic predictor indices of albino rabbits administered coconut water as antidote to paracetamol overdose. Journal of Coastal Life Medicine 4: 974-979.

23. Koleva DI, Andreeva-Gateva PA, Orbetzova MM, Atanassova IB, Nikolova JG (2015) Atherogenic Index of Plasma, Castelli Risk Indexes and Leptin/Adiponectin Ratio in Women with Metabolic Syndrome. International Journal of Pharmaceutical and Medical Research 3: 12-19.

24. Igbinosa OO, Oviasogie EF, Igbinosa EO, Igene O, Igbinos AIH, et al. (2013) Effects of Biochemical Alteration in Animal Model after Short-Term Exposure of Jatropha curcas (Linn) Leaf Extract. The ScientificWorld Journal 798096: 5.

25. Okechukwu PCU, Nzubechukwu E, Ogbansh ME, Ezeani N, Nworie MO, et al. (2015) The Effect of Ethanol Leaf Extract of Jatropha curcas on Chloroform Induced Hepatotoxicity in Albino Rats. Global J Biotech & Biochem 10: 11-15.

26. Bucolo G, David H (1973) Quantitative determination of serum triglycerides by the use of enzymes. Clin Chem 19: 476-482.

27. Allain CC, Poon LS, Chan CS, Richmond W, Fu PC (1974) Enzymatic determination of total serum cholesterol. Clin Chem 20: 470-475.

28. Friedewald WT, Levy RI, Friedrickson DS (1972) Estimation of the concentration of low-density lipoprotein cholesterol in plasma, without use of the preparative ultracentrifuge. Clin Chem 18: 499-502.

29. Brunzell JD, Davidson M, Furberg CD, Goldberg RD, Howard BV, et al. (2008). Lipoprotein management in patients with cardiometabolic risk: consensus conference report from the American Diabetes Association and the American College of Cardiology Foundation. J Am Coll Cardiol 51: 1512-1524.

30. Castelli WP, Abbott RD, McNamara PM (1983) Summary estimates of cholesterol used to predict coronary heart disease. Circulation 67: 730-734.

31. Brehm A, Pfeiler G, Pacini G, Vierhapper H, Roden M (2004) Relationship between serum lipoprotein ratios and insulin resistance in obesity. Clin Chem 50: 2316-2322.

32. Dobiásová M (2004) Atherogenic index of plasma [log(triglycerides/HDL-cholesterol)]: theoretical and practical implications. Clin Chem 50: 1113-1115.

33. Lewis SM, Bain BJ, Bates I (2001) Dacie and Lewis Practical Haematology. 9th Edition. Churchill Livingstone, New York.

34. CBOH- Central Board of Health (2003) Haematology Standard Operating Procedures for Hospital Laboratories Level III. Mipal Printers, Lusaka, Zambia.

35. Adeneye AA, Olagunju JA, Elias SO, Olatunbosun DO, Mustafa AO, et al. (2008) Protective activities of the aqueous root extract of Harungana madagascariensis in acute and repeated acetaminophen hepatotoxic rats. International Journal of Applied Research in Natural Products 1: 29-42.

36. Lebda MA, Taha NM, Korshom MA, Mandour AEA, Goda, RI (2013) Ginger (Zingiber officinale) potentiate paracetamol induced chronic hepatotoxicity in Rats. J Med Plants Res 7: 3164-3170.

37. Kobashigania JA, Kasiska BL (1997) Hyperlipidemia in solid organ transplantation. Transpl 63: 333-338.

38. Okeke CU, Braide SA, Ekezie J, Okwandu BN (2011) The influence of age on lipid profile among women taking hormonalcontraceptives. Int J Biol Chem Sci 5: 840-844.

39. Batista M, Franceschini S (2003) Impact of Nutritional Counseling in Reducing Serum Cholesterol in Public Health Service Patients. Arq Bras Cardiol 80: 167-170.

40. Vidhya MHL, Bai MMS (2012) Beware of Paracetamol Toxicity. J Clinic Toxicol 2: 142.

# 3

# Blood Profiles and Histopathological Changes of Liver and Kidney Tissues from Male Sprague Dawley Rats Treated with Ethanol Extracts of *Clinacanthus nutans* Leaf

Sajjarattul Nurul Nadia Asyura[1], Hazilawati Hamzah[1*], Rosly Mohamad Shaari[2], Shanmugavelu Sithambaram[2] and Noordin Mohamed Mustapha[1]

[1]*Department of Veterinary Pathology and Microbiology, Faculty of Veterinary Medicine, University Putra Malaysia, 43400 Serdang, Selangor, Malaysia*

[2]*Animal Research Centre, Malaysian Agricultural Research and Development Institute, 43400 Serdang, Malaysia*

*Corresponding author: Hazilawati Hamzah, University Putra Malaysia, 43400 Serdang, Selangor, Malaysia, E-mail: hazilawati@upm.edu.my

## Abstract

**Background:** *Clinacanthus nutans* (*C. nutans*) or commonly known as 'Sabah snake grass' or 'Belalai Gajah' is a widely known herb used to treat Herpes simplex virus (HPV), skin rashes and snake bite.

**Objective:** This study aim is to evaluate the toxicity of ethanol extract of *C. nutans* leaf extract on 90-day sub chronic toxicity study in male Sprague Dawley rats.

**Method:** A total of 40, 6-week male Sprague Dawley rats were divided into 5 groups (n=8) namely control, vehicle (10% DMSO), and 3 treatment groups which received a daily oral dose of *C. nutans* leaf extract at 75 (low dose), 125 (medium dose), and 250 (high dose) mg/kg for 90 days via oral gavage. Blood sample were collected at the end of the experiment for evaluation of haematology and serum biochemistry. Selected organs including liver and kidneys were collected for histopathological examination. The toxicity were evaluated by observing and evaluating the changes of body weight, haematology and serum biochemistry parameters and histopathology changes of liver and kidney tissues.

**Results:** There was no mortality sign of sub chronic toxicity observed during the observation period. Body weight, haematology parameters and organ relative weight showed no significant difference in control and treatment groups meanwhile in serum biochemistry parameters, observed a significant difference (P<0.05) in level of LDH and creatinine kinase in high dose group showed significant lower(P<0.05) compared to control. Nevertheless the levels of LDH and creatinine kinase were still in normal range. Significant abnormal histopathological changes (P<0.05) such as centrilobular sinusoid dilatation/centrilobular necrosis, hydropic degeneration/cytoplasmic vacuolation and inflammation were observed in liver tissues in medium and high dose groups. Kidney tissue showed a significant abnormal histopathology changes (P<0.05) such as granular cast and cellular cast were observed in medium and high dose group.

**Conclusion:** It is concluded that 125-250 mg/kg ethanol extract of *C. nutans* leaves induce hepatotoxicity and renal toxicity.

**Keywords:** Sub chronic oral toxicity study; *Clinacanthus nutans*; Haematology; Serum biochemistry; Histopathology changes

## Introduction

*Clincanthus nutans* (*C. nutans*) is a popular local herb belongs to family Acanthaceae that grows in tropical Asian countries [1]. It is locally known as 'Sabah snake grass' or 'rumput belalai gajah' (Malaysia). Meanwhile in Thailand and Indonesia, *C. nutans* is known as 'Phayo yo' and 'Dandang Gendis', respectively. In Thailand, *C. nutans* are traditionally used for skin rashes, snake and insects bites, diabetes mellitus and diarrhoea treatment [1,2]. Apart from that, it is also used as anti-viral against herpes simplex virus (HSV) and varicella-zoster virus (VZV) [3]. The leaves of *C. nutans* are boiled and traditionally used as medicine to treat dysentery in Sukajadi village in West Java, Indonesia [4].

Nowadays, the leaves of *C. nutans* have gained its popularity as supplement and medicine to treat various types of illness especially cancer. It is believed the consumption of *C. nutans* leaves as tea can cure the illness without knowing its side effects. The therapeutic effect of *C. nutans* against cancer has not been clinically tested in laboratory animals although the consumption of *C. nutans* is increasing without knowing its toxicology effects. Only a few toxicity studies of *C. nutans* leaves have been carried out in the laboratory rats to determine its toxicity. Previous studies carried out by P'ng et al. [5] and Peng et al. [6] has shown extract of *C. nutans* leaves did not cause toxicity in laboratory mice. However a study by Chin et al. [7] reported extract of *C. nutans* leaves cause a significant increase in liver weight and serum biochemistry parameters (serum total proteins and albumin/globulin ratios) which suggest hepatotoxicity.

The toxicology evaluations of *C. nutans* leaves are very important in order to know the side effects especially the people who consume it as a supplement and medicine. The health promoting benefits of both herbal plants have been known and being used in many countries especially for its medicinal properties. The increasing use of these herbal plants has resulted in concerns of the safety and effectiveness. Hence, through the toxicity studies in laboratory animal, the toxicology of these plants can be determined as a safeguard to the public health and to raise public awareness on the toxicity of *M. citrifolia* fruits and *C. nutans* leaves. The toxicology studies also provide a pre-clinical safety evaluation before it can be performed and evaluated in human. Thus the objective of this study is to investigate sub chronic oral toxicity of ethanol extract of *C. nutans* leaves in male Sprague Dawley rats.

## Materials and Methods

### Plant preparation and extraction

*Clinacanthus nutans* leaves were obtained from Malaysian Agriculture Research and Development Institute (MARDI) research station located at Muadzam Shah, Pahang. The *C.nutans* leaves were washed and dried under the sun for 48 h. Lastly, the dried samples were ground into powder and were kept in a container at 4°C. The ground samples were extracted with 70% ethanol (Merck, German) at a ratio 1 g of sample to 40 mL of ethanol. Each mixture was placed in an orbital shaker (Heidoph Unimax 1010, German) at 200 rpm at room temperature approximately for 2 h [8]. The mixture was filtered twice through a filter paper (Whatman No. 4). Later, the ethanol was removed by a rotary evaporator (BUCHI Rotavapor R-200, Switzerland). The semisolid extracts were obtained after was freeze-dried in a freeze-dryer (The VIRTIS Company, USA). The semisolid extracts was considered as *C. nutans* leaf extracts and used in this study. Each extracts were dissolved with 10% DMSO and were given to the rats via oral gavage. The dissolved extracts were freshly prepared every week based on the body weight.

### Animal management, routine and experimental design

All animals used in the experiments were subjected to approval by the Animal Care and Use Committee (ACUC) MARDI, Serdang and were conducted at the Animal Metabolism, Toxicology and Reproductive Centre (AMTREC), MARDI, Serdang. A total 40 male Sprague Dawley (SD) rats at age of 5-6 weeks old with an average weight between 160-180 g were used in the studies. The rats were acclimated to the housing conditions in polycarbonate plastic cage with temperature within the range of 22-27°C, humidity at the range 40%-70% and balance of 12 h light/12 h dark cycle. The bedding and water were replaced every day and the cages were cleaned when it is necessary. The rats were divided into five groups (n=8) namely control (group A), vehicle (10% DMSO) (group B), and 3 treatment groups; 75 (low dose) (group C), 125 (medium dose) (group D) and 250 (high dose) (group E) mg/kg of body weight. The extracts of *C. nutans* leaves were dissolved in 10% DMSO before orally given to the rats. In control group, the rats received no treatment, while in vehicle group the rats were given 10% DMSO by oral gavage. All rats had free access to water and commercial chow ad libitum. The rats were observed daily for any mortality and signs of toxicity, and were weighed weekly throughout the study period.

## Haematology Analysis

### Blood sampling

At the end of the experimental period all rats were humanely sacrificed with an overdose of sodium pentobarbital euthanasia solution via intramuscular injection. Blood samples were collected by using 21 gauge needle and 3 mL syringe via posterior vena cava. 1 mL of blood samples were collected into anticoagulant blood collection tube (EDTA tube). The blood was mixed well to prevent from clotting stored on ice.

### Complete blood count

The blood samples were analysed for complete blood count using an automated haematology analyser (Cell Dyn* 3700, Abbott Diagnostics, USA) for the total RBC, WBC, platelet count, haemoglobin (Hb) concentration, mean corpuscular volume (MCV) and mean corpuscular haemoglobin concentration (MCHC) were calculated. Blood smear was stained using Wright stain and examined under a light microscope at 10X, 20X, 40X, 60X and 100X magnifications. Differential WBC count was determined manually by counting 100 WBC on the blood smears. The absolute values of each type of WBC (lymphocytes neutrophils, eosinophils, monocytes and basophils were calculated by multiply the percentage of each WBC type to the total WBC count from the automated analyser.

### Capillary blood preparation

Microhaematocrits were filled up about third quarter of the capillary with blood from the EDTA tubes. The capillary tubes were wiped with tissue until it is cleaned and dried. The end of the capillary tubes was sealed by flame from Bunsen burner with the heated up technique. The capillary tubes were placed in a microhaematocrit centrifuge (Hettich Haematocrit 210, Germany) and centrifuged at 10,000 rpm for 5 minutes. This procedure was run to separate blood and plasma. RBC will be at the bottom of the capillary tubes and the plasma will be at the top of the capillary.

### Packed cell volume

The centrifuged capillary tubes were further analysed for packed cell volume (PCV) using microhaematocrit reader (Hawksley). The base of RBC was intersected with the base line of the reader. Meanwhile the top of plasma was intersected with the top line of the reader by moving the holder left or right, before the middle line of the reader was adjusted to intersect with the top of RBC and the measuring ruler. The PCV percentage was obtained from the middle line and the measuring reader intercept. The values were converted into percentage (L/L).

### Icterus index

The centrifuged capillary tubes were used to determine the icterus index. The plasma separated in the capillary tube was compared with an icteric index standard board colour degree to determine the icteric standard index of the samples.

### Plasma protein determination

The centrifuge capillary tubes were later analysed for plasma protein concentration. The top of the capillary tubes were broken and the plasma liquid was dropped onto a prism refractometer (Atago T2-NE,

Japan). The plasma protein concentration was determined by observing the refractometer and the concentration value were read according to the scale.

## Serum biochemistry analysis

Blood samples were collected into plain tube and were centrifuged (Centrifuge S417R, Eppendorf, CA) for 15 minutes at 3000 rpm to obtain the serum. The serum was further analysed for cholesterol, triglyceride, high-density lipoprotein cholesterol (HDL-cholesterol), creatinine, urea, total bilirubin, total protein (TP), albumin (ALB), globulin, aspartate aminotransferase (AST), alanine aminotransferase (ALT), gamma-glutamyl transpeptidase (GGT), inorganic phosphorus (IP), alkaline phosphatase (ALP), uric acid (UA), lactate dehydrogenase (LDH), creatine kinase (CK), glucose using an automated clinical chemistry analyser (TRX 7010, Biorex Mannheim, Germany).

## Histopathological analysis

At the end of the experimental period, all rats were sacrificed with overdose of xylazine and ketamine. Selected organs of each rat such as were collected in cold [pH 4] normal saline. The organs were cleaned from blood, weighed and examine for gross lesions for gross examination. The organs were then fixed in 10% buffered formalin solution. The process of tissue fixation was in 48 h duration in clean 10% formalin solution. The organs samples were processed at the Serology laboratory, Faculty Veterinary Medicine, UPM, Serdang. All of the samples were trimmed about 0.5 cm thickness and were placed in cassettes. Later the cassettes were placed into a 10% formalin solution overnight, before they were placed and undergone series of dehydrated process for about 16 h in an automated processor (Leica ASP300, Germany). The samples then were embedded with paraffin to form a block and left cool by a processor machine (Leica EG1160, Germany). The samples were trimmed about 3-5 μm thickness using a sectioning rotary microtome (Leica RM2155, Germany), and directly placed the tissue sectioning in 45°C water bath before mounting on slides. All the glass slides were labeled with a diamond pen and continue mounted on a hot plate (54°C) overnight. Later all the slides were undergone a series of steps for Haematoxylin and Eosin (H&E) staining protocol. Lastly, the samples were examined under a light microscope at 10X, 20X, 40X, 60X and 100X magnifications.

## Lesion characteristics

Toxicological lesions such as inflammation, activated kupffer cells, hydropic degeneration, periportal necrosis, midzonal mecrosis, and centrilobular necrosis in the liver were examined and were scored. Meanwhile in kidney tissue, toxicological lesions such as cellular cast, granular cast, protein cast, inflammation, hydropic degeneration/cytoplasmic vacuoaltion and necrosis were examined and were scored. The lesions scoring in both liver and kidney tissues were scored as 0=normal, 1=mild (1%-30%), 2=moderate (31%-70%) and 3=severe (>70%), based on the percentages of tissues affected.

## Statistical analysis

The average body weight, haematology and serum biochemistry data were expressed as Mean ± SEM and analysed by using one-way ANOVA and Tukey test. Meanwhile for histopathology examination, data was expressed as Mean ± SEM and analysed using by using Kruskal Wallis for global comparison of groups of all parameters and on-parametric and Mann-Whitney-U test for comparison between two groups. These data's were analysed using statistical software, IBM SPSS Statistic 21.0.

## Results

### Average body weight

The average body weight of rats in oral toxicity study of *C. nutans* extract that were taken weekly and are presented in Figure 1. Rats in groups A, B, C, D and E continuously gained weight from week 1 to week 12. The body weight (mean ± SEM) of the rats at week 12 were arranged in an ascending order are 390.09 ± 13.38 g (group B), 390.89 ± 16.24 g (group C), 434.56 ± 23.7 g (group E), 445.90 ± 11.09 g (group A) and 464.89 ± 15.59 g (group D). There were no significant differences (P>0.05) in the body weight between all groups throughout the study period.

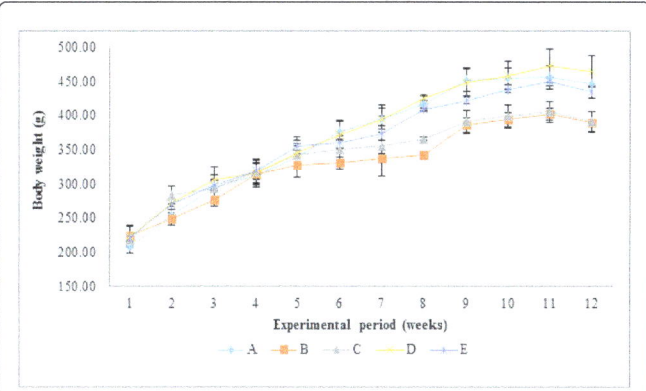

**Figure 1:** Mean (± SEM) body weights of male SD rats received repeated doses of ethanol extract of *C. nutans* leaves by oral gavage in 90-day duration. (**Note:** A: Control; B: Vehicle (10% DMSO); C: Low Dose; D: Medium Dose; E: High Dose).

### Haematology, serum biochemical analyses and organ to body weight ratio

The haematology results of rats in sub chronic oral toxicity study of *C. nutans* leaf extract at week 12 are shown in Table 1 and Table 2. There were no significant differences (P>0.05) observed in the results between all groups compared to control. The serum biochemical results of rats in sub chronic oral toxicity study of *C. nutans* extract at week 12 are shown in Table 3. The results showed significant differences (P<0.05) in some of the results. The LDH level of rats in high dose group (1595.00 ± 164.39 U/L) was significantly (P<0.05) lower compared to control (2659.30 ± 82.13 U/L). The similar trend was seen in the CK value of rats in high dose group (441.71 ± 58.41 U/L) compared to control (941.83 ± 89.78 U/L). However, the values were still within the reference ranges (Patterino and Argentino-Stroino, 2006). The results of liver, kidneys, lungs, heart, thymus, thyroids, brain, adrenals, testes and spleen ratio to the body weight (%) of rats in in sub chronic oral toxicity study of *C. nutans* extract are presented in Table 4. There were no significant differences (P>0.05) in the ratio at week 12 of the study between the groups.

## Histopathological scoring of mean lesion scores

Kruskal Wallis test for the global comparison of organ toxicity among groups showed significant results (P<0.05) for the sinusoidal dilatation, cytoplasmic vacuolation and inflammation in the liver, and granular cast in the kidney (Table 5). Mann-Whitney U test showed significant differences (P<0.05) for the sinusoidal dilatation, cytoplasmic vacuolation and inflammation in the liver of medium and high dose groups compared to control (Table 6). Meanwhile in the kidney, granular cast was significantly different (P<0.05) in medium and high dose groups compared to control (Table 6). Results of sub chronic oral toxicity of *C. nutans* leaf extract showed significant lesions in the liver and kidney of medium and high dose groups compared to low dose group. Lesions observed in the liver and kidney is shown in Figures 2 and 3. It is concluded that administration of *C. nutans* leaves ethanol extract, daily for 90 days at high (250 mg/kg of body weight) and medium (125 mg.kg of body weight) doses induce mild hepatic and renal toxicity in rats. Administration of the extract daily for 90 days at low dose (75 mg/kg of body weight) induces no hepatic and renal toxicity.

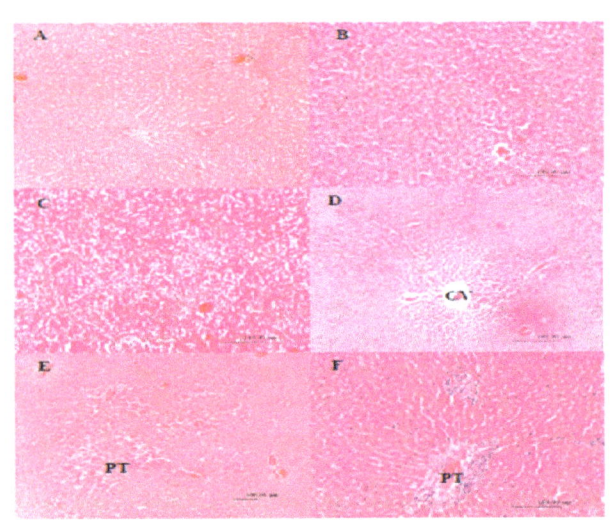

Figure 2: Photomicrographs of rat's liver sections at the end of experimental period (day 90). (A) Normal liver section from a rat in control group (H&E stain, X200). (B) Mild cytoplasmic vacuolation from a rat in high dose *C. nutans* group (H&E stain, X200). (C) Marked cytoplasmic vacuolation (scored as 3) from a rat in high dose *C. nutans* group (H&E stain, X200). (D) Sinusoidal dilatations were observed around the central vein (CV) (centrilobular necrosis). Midzonal necrosis was observed in the areas. The lesions were characterised by presence of necrotic cells with eosinophilic cytoplasm and pyknotic nuclei (scored as 1) from a rat in high dose *C. nutans* group (H&E stain, X200). (E) Periportal and midzonal necrosis characterised by with pyknotic nuclei, eosinophilic cytoplasm and atrophied hepatocytes was observed (scored as 1) from a rat in high dose *C. nutans* group (H&E, X200). (F) Mild hepatitis was observed around the portal triad (PT) and in liver parenchyma (scored as 1) from a rat in high dose *C. nutans* group (H&E, X2000).

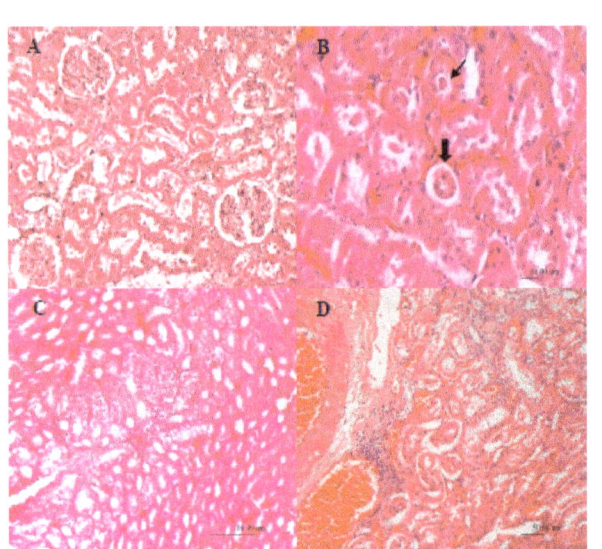

Figure 3: Photomicrographs of rat's kidney sections at the end of experimental period (day 90). (A) Normal renal section from a rat in control group (H&E stain, X200). (B) Granular cast (thin arrow) and cellular cast (thick arrow) were present in the renal tubules (scored as 1) from a rat in high dose *C. nutans* group (H&E stain, X400). (C) Prominent cytoplasmic vacuolation of renal tubular cells indicating or known as hydropic degeneration (scored as 1) from a rat in high dose *C. nutans* group (H&E stain, X200). (D) Infiltration of lymphocytes in the interstitial tissues (scored as 1) from a rat in high dose *C. nutans* group (H&E stain, X200).

## Discussion

The herbal industry is a fast growing industry worldwide. The increment demand in herbal supplements, health functional food, and skin care and herbs functional drinks has led to an increment of growing of herbal industry [9]. High demand in alternative medicine is also a contributing factor to the use of herbal products such as Traditional Chinese Medicine, Ayurveda and Jamu [9]. *Clinacanthus nutans* (rumput belalai gajah) is popular Malaysian herbs that are currently being studied for pharmaceuticals, medicinal and market potential.

*Clinacanthus nutans* either in crude, extract or also its biochemical compound is used in dose-dependent method for multiple purposes. For example, treatment 100 µg/mL of *C. nutans* leaf extract is a good anti-oxidant in several of cancer cell lines [10]. Basically, selected doses of ethanol extract of *C. nutans* administration via oral gavage to the rats were based on the OECD guidelines for testing chemicals version 408 (repeated dose 90-day oral toxicity study). In sub chronic oral toxicity study (90-day) (OECD versions 407 and 408), at least three dose levels are used and the dose level is selected from four fixed levels, 5, 50, 300 and 2000 mg/kg of body weight. Thus dose levels at 75 mg/kg, 125 mg/kg and 125 mg/kg of extract was used in the studies.

Sprague Dawley rats were used as animal model in the toxicity studies of ethanol extract of *Morinda citrifolia* and *Clinacanthus nutans*. The Sprague Dawley rat is an outbred multipurpose breed of albino rat. It was developed by R. Dawley, 1975 with the collaboration of Sprague Dawley Company, Madison, Wisconsin. Sprague Dawley rat extensively used in the medical research and laboratory lab due to its advantages such as easy to breed, short life spans, calmness and easy to handle. The criteria of the Sprague Dawley rats make it an ideal model for this research. The Sprague Dawley rat also has been used to study the toxicity of Malaysia herbal plant such as Mitragyna speciose Korth (MS) (ketum), Carica papaya Linn (betik), and Momordica charantia (peria katak) [11-13].

Body weight is one of parameters used for evaluating health status of experimental animals [14]. Herbal extracts can contribute suppression of animal's appetite which leads to reduction in body weight of animals [15]. Decrease in body weight could also be associated with normal physiological adaptation responses of the body towards plant extracts or compounds [16]. A study conducted by Harizal et al. [17] reported an increased in animal body weight is related to the accumulation of the body fats rather than the toxicity effects after administration of single dose of methanol extract of Mitragyna speciosa Korth (ketum). The weekly body weight of sub chronic toxicity studies of *C. nutans* is shown in the Figure 1. In the current study, repeated administration of the extract for 90 day showed increases in body weight throughout the study period. Apart from that, no significant differences (P>0.05) were observed in the weekly average body weight between the groups of all rats throughout the study period. No physical changes were observed in this study.

Haematology is the study of the morphology and physiology of blood. It is an important toxicology evaluation of any compounds including herbal plant, chemicals and drugs [18]. Blood is a bodily fluid that delivers necessary substance such as oxygen and nutrients (example: glucose, amino acids and fatty acids) to the tissues and cells. It also transports metabolic waste products to the kidneys and liver to be filtered and excreted. The red blood cells (RBCs) or also called erythrocytes is one types of blood cells that delivering oxygen ($O_2$) to the body tissues and cells. Low RBCs is associated with anaemia and sometimes toxicity [19,20]. A study by Waldron [21] and Flora et al. [22] found the number of RBCs in cases of lead poisoning was lower compared to the normal. Meanwhile in plant toxicity, Adedapo et al. [23] reported low RBCs (anaemia) in rodents after crude extract of Euphorbia was orally administrated to the rats. Differ with a study by Okokon et al., an increase of RBCs values were reported after administration of ethanol extract of Croton Zambesicus in rats. This is due to the presence of alkaloids in the root extract that stimulate erythropoiesis. In this present study, the sub chronic oral toxicity study of *C. nutans* extract (Table 1) did not showed any significant differences (P>0.05) in the values of RBCs, PCV, haemoglobin (Hb), mean corpuscular volume (MCV), mean corpuscular haemoglobin concentration (MCHC), icterus index and plasma protein when compared to the control. The normal values of haematology parameters in this study indicate the plant extract did not induce anaemia and jaundice within the 90 days of animal trials.

| Group/Parameter | RBC (10$^{12}$/L) | Hb (g/L) | PCV (L/L) | MCV (fL) | MCHC (g/L) | Icterus index | Plasma protein (g/L) |
|---|---|---|---|---|---|---|---|
| A | 9.42 ± 0.17 | 173.2 ± 0.32 | 0.56 ± 0.02 | 56.56 ± 1.03 | 307.11 ± 7.47 | 2.00 ± 0.00 | 80.00 ± 0.00 |
| B | 10.00 ± 0.44 | 176.1 ± 0.73 | 0.54 ± 0.03 | 54.44 ± 3.66 | 328.00 ± 21.56 | 2.00 ± 0.00 | 78.33 ± 1.67 |
| C | 9.84 ± 0.90 | 172.4 ± 0.44 | 0.53 ± 1.09 | 54.84 ± 0.94 | 317.77 ± 2.58 | 2.00 ± 0.00 | 81.63 ± 2.27 |
| D | 9.55 ± 0.90 | 166.1 ± 0.47 | 0.52 ± 1.03 | 54.42 ± 0.95 | 319.77 ± 2.58 | 2.00 ± 0.00 | 76.25 ± 1.83 |
| E | 9.77 ± 0.14 | 172.1 ± 0.48 | 0.52 ± 0.01 | 53.14 ± 1.16 | 295.73 ± 30.91 | 2.00 ± 0.00 | 77.50 ± 2.50 |

Table 1: The erythron parameters, icterus index and plasma protein values (mean ± SEM) of Sprague Dawley (SD) rats in subchronic oral toxicity study of ethanol extract of *C. nutans* leaves at the end of experimental period (Values in the same column with similar superscripts were not significantly different at P>0.05. Note: A: Control; B: Vehicle (10% DMSO); C: Low Dose; D: Medium Dose; E: High Dose.).

The white blood cells (WBCs) or also called leukocytes are the cells in the immune systems which play a role in body defence from foreign materials and infectious diseases. The leukocytes are produced in the haematopoietic stem cells or also known as bone marrow. Abnormal low count of normal WBCs or neutropenia with low level of RBCs (anaemia) can be characterised as leukaemia. Meanwhile an increase in the number of white cells (leucocytosis) in the blood is a sign of infection [24-26]. A study by Okokon et al. reported leucocytosis in

rats after orally administration of ethanol extract of Croton Zambesicus and might be a sign of infection. The present study showed administration of *C. nutans* leaf extracts for 90-day (Table 2 and Table 3) showed no significant differences (P>0.05) in the leukocytes count. The differential WBCs count such as neutrophil, lymphocytes, monocytes, eosinophils and basophils also showed no significant differences (P>0.05) in these study.

| Parameter/Group | A | B | C | D | E |
|---|---|---|---|---|---|
| WBC (x 10$^9$/L) | 5.74 ± 0.68 | 7.54 ± 0.51 | 7.05 ± 0.85 | 7.15 ± 0.68 | 6.78 ± 0.63 |
| Neutrophils (x 10$^9$/L) | 0.96 ± 0.87 | 2.15 ± 0.49 | 1.53 ± 0.38 | 1.77 ± 0.45 | 0.96 ± 0.20 |
| Lymphocytes (x 10$^9$/L) | 4.43 ± 0.36 | 5.00 ± 0.29 | 4.88 ± 0.50 | 4.85 ± 0.31 | 5.27 ± 0.89 |
| Monocytes (x 10$^9$/L) | 0.34 ± 0.07 | 0.28 ± 0.04 | 0.44 ± 0.09 | 0.36 ± 0.04 | 0.39 ± 0.04 |

| | | | | | |
|---|---|---|---|---|---|
| Eosinophils (x 10$^9$/L) | 0.00 ± 0.00 | 0.12 ± 0.04 | 0.17 ± 0.03 | 0.15 ± 0.01 | 0.18 ± 0.03 |
| Basophils (x 10$^9$/L) | 0.00 ± 0.00 | 0.01 ± 0.00 | 0.01 ± 0.01 | 0.02 ± 0.01 | 0.01 ± 0.01 |

**Table 2:** The total white blood cell (WBC) and WBC differential count (mean ± SEM) of Sprague Dawley (SD) rats in subchronic oral toxicity study of ethanol extract of *C. nutans* leaves at the end of experimental period (Values in the same row with similar superscripts were not significantly different at P>0.05. Note: A: Control; B: Vehicle (10% DMSO); C: Low Dose; D: Medium Dose; E: High Dose).

Serum biochemical analysis provides a valuable tool in evaluating the effects of herbal extracts in tissue [18]. Increased serum enzymes for examples ALP, ALT and GGT are due to cell membrane and tissue damage [27]. Previous study revealed administration of 4000 mg/kg of body weight of Herniaria glabra extract in rodents showed sign of hepatotoxicity with evidence of marked elevation in ALT and AST levels [16]. Increased levels of serum AST and CK together with LDH are an indication of muscle injury or increased muscle activity or myocardial infarction [27,28]. Previous study has shown injection of doxorubicin produces cardio toxicity in rats as indicated by the increment of LDH and CK levels in the serum [29]. Meanwhile decrease in the muscle enzymes are related to decrease in muscle activity [28,30].

| Parameter/Group | A | B | C | D | E |
|---|---|---|---|---|---|
| IP (mmol/L) | 4.24 ± 0.32 | 4.09 ± 0.28 | 3.90 ± 0.31 | 3.89 ± 0.19 | 3.96 ± 0.15 |
| Urea (mmol/L) | 7.93 ± 0.60 | 6.76 ± 0.50 | 7.95 ± 0.53 | 7.51 ± 0.41 | 7.68 ± 0.70 |
| Creatinine (μmol/L) | 85.66 ± 2.88 | 78.50 ± 5.19 | 82.50 ± 2.81 | 92.00 ± 4.31 | 87.50 ± 3.58 |
| Glucose (mmol/L) | 5.68 ± 0.81 | 6.40 ± 2.07 | 7.58 ± 1.87 | 5.32 ± 1.40 | 6.05 ± 1.25 |
| Cholesterol (mmol/L) | 2.47 ± 0.34 | 2.12 ± 0.26 | 2.07 ± 0.16 | 2.38 ± 0.18 | 1.96 ± 0.16 |
| T.Bil (μmol/L) | 1.53 ± 0.10 | 1.35 ± 0.13 | 1.511 ± 0.13 | 1.11 ± 0.09 | 1.08 ± 0.14 |
| ALT (U/L) | 57.91 ± 4.64 | 51.90 ± 4.25 | 45.73 ± 2.76 | 55.06 ± 3.76 | 48.22 ± 4.71 |
| ALP (U/L) | 121.17 ± 10.85 | 111.83 ± 4.93 | 98.12 ± 10.22 | 119.00 ± 6.33 | 110.50 ± 13.73 |
| GGT (U/L) | 0.00 ± 0.00 | 0.00 ± 0.00 | 0.00 ± 0.00 | 0.00 ± 0.00 | 0.00 ± 0.00 |
| AST (U/L) | 180.45 ± 10.49 | 160.52 ± 12.55 | 127.79 ± 8.66 | 153.33 ± 16.09 | 142.05 ± 11.10 |
| CK (U/L) | 941.83 ± 89.78 | 807.00 ± 155.37 | 567.12 ± 100.75 | 644.62 ± 127.66 | 441.71 ± 58.41 |
| LDH (U/L) | 2659.30 ± 82.13 | 2220.00 ± 312.81 | 1688.10 ± 310.42 | 1932.90 ± 343.63 | 1595.00 ± 164.39 |
| TP (g/L) | 91.96 ± 3.76 | 84.50 ± 6.36 | 87.21 ± 3.78 | 92.07 ± 4.25 | 88.35 ± 2.87 |
| ALB (U/L) | 46.58 ± 2.20 | 39.13 ± 3.60 | 41.32 ± 1.55 | 45.30 ± 2.11 | 43.24 ± 1.48 |
| Globulin (g/L) | 45.53 ± 1.56 | 45.37 ± 2.76 | 40.92 ± 1.90 | 47.77 ± 2.14 | 45.11 ± 1.39 |
| TG (μmol/L) | 0.65 ± 0.05 | 0.60 ± 0.07 | 0.46 ± 0.02 | 0.66 ± 0.07 | 0.58 ± 0.05 |
| UA (μmol/L) | 354.93 ± 48.34 | 343.60 ± 45.27 | 229.62 ± 23.18 | 313.05 ± 34.39 | 286.34 ± 15.92 |
| HDL-C (mmol/L) | 0.99 ± 0.04 | 0.84 ± 0.09 | 1.00 ± 0.05 | 1.09 ± 0.07 | 1.02 ± 0.05 |
| LDL-C (mmol/L) | 1.35 ± 0.29 | 1.16 ± 0.15 | 0.97 ± 0.10 | 1.15 ± 0.09 | 0.82 ± 0.10 |

**Table 3:** The serum biochemical parameter (mean ± SEM) of Sprague Dawley (SD) rats in subchronic oral toxicity study of ethanol extract of *C. nutans* leaves at the end of experimental period (Values in the same row with different superscripts were significantly different at P<0.05. Note: A: Control; B: 10% DMSO; C: Low Dose; D: Medium Dose; E: High Dose).

The current study of sub chronic (Table 4) toxicity study of *C. nutans* leaf extract showed decreases in AST, LDH and CK levels in the serum, which suggested decreased muscle activity rather than toxicity. These findings were different from previous study P'ng et al. [5] and Chin et al. [7] who observed no significant differences (P>0.01) in the serum biochemical parameters of rats treated with methanol extract of *C. nutans* leaves up to 900 mg/kg of body weight in both 14-day and 28-day toxicity studies. Decreased serum biochemical values were also reported by [31] that showed a significant decrease in creatinine after ethanol extract of *C. nutans* leaves at 1000 mg/kg of body weight for 90-day was administrated to rats. Although a few serum biochemical values in this study and also study done by Chavalittumrong et al. were decrease, the values were still within normal ranges. However, decrease in those serum biochemistry values might also be related to the body compensatory mechanisms, body utilisation, alterations, or maintaining of the normal conditions. Decrease in LDH level is mainly due to the inhibition or reduction of synthesis of aspartate and alpha-ketoglutarate in the Krebs cycle. The inhibition of the synthesis of aspartate and alpha-ketoglutarate enzymes is due to reduce amount of ADP which causes accumulation of NADH and in turn inhibit synthesis of a number of enzymes [32]. Decrease or normal level of

serum biochemical parameters could also be related to the half-life of the enzymes in the blood. The concentration of previously increased enzymes, for example due to acute injury, will reduce one-half of the increased concentration over a period of time. Another reason for decrease in serum biochemical parameters is the cytoprotective effect of the extracts towards muscle or liver. Histopathological examination of liver tissue is required to support the cytoprotective effect of the herbs.

| Organ/Group | A | B | C | D | E |
|---|---|---|---|---|---|
| Liver | 3.31 ± 0.03 | 3.15 ± 0.23 | 2.99 ± 0.22 | 2.86 ± 0.17 | 2.87 ± 0.10 |
| Kidneys | 0.68 ± 0.02 | 0.68 ± 0.03 | 0.74 ± 0.06 | 0.64 ± 0.04 | 0.67 ± 0.04 |
| Lungs | 0.51 ± 0.03 | 0.61 ± 0.06 | 0.50 ± 0.05 | 0.46 ± 0.03 | 0.47 ± 0.02 |
| Heart | 0.31 ± 0.01 | 0.32 ± 0.02 | 0.37 ± 0.04 | 0.29 ± 0.16 | 0.28 ± 0.01 |
| Thymus | 0.07 ± 0.00 | 0.08 ± 0.01 | 0.10 ± 0.01 | 0.08 ± 0.00 | 0.09 ± 0.01 |
| Thyroids | 0.16 ± 0.01 | 0.19 ± 0.02 | 0.22 ± 0.02 | 0.18 ± 0.01 | 0.18 ± 0.01 |
| Brain | 0.42 ± 0.02 | 0.46 ± 0.01 | 0.53 ± 0.05 | 0.46 ± 0.02 | 0.44 ± 0.03 |
| Adrenals | 0.05 ± 0.01 | 0.05 ± 0.02 | 0.01 ± 0.01 | 0.01 ± 0.00 | 0.01 ± 0.00 |
| Testes | 0.73 ± 0.03 | 0.81 ± 0.05 | 0.94 ± 0.13 | 0.78 ± 0.03 | 0.82 ± 0.03 |
| Spleen | 0.17 ± 0.01 | 0.14 ± 0.01 | 0.18 ± 0.01 | 0.14 ± 0.03 | 0.21 ± 0.06 |

**Table 4:** The ratio of organ to relative body weight (%) (mean ± SEM) of Sprague Dawley (SD) rats in subchronic oral toxicity study of ethanol extract of *C. nutans* leaves at the end of experimental period.

The lesions scoring for liver and kidneys in the toxicity study of *C. nutans* were described with none when no toxicity was observed, one for 1%-30% toxicity was observed, two for 30%-70% toxicity was observed ad three more than 70% toxicity was observed. In the present study, histopathological examination revealed that daily administration of *C. nutans* extracts for 90 days induced toxicity in the liver and kidney tissues for medium (125 mg/kg) and high doses (250 mg/kg). Lesion scoring results of the organs were significantly different (P<0.05) from control. Histopathological lesions of sinusoidal dilatation, cytoplasmic vacuolation, inflammation, cellular cast and granular cast were scored mildly in the liver and kidneys of herbal treated groups. However the findings were not related to the results of

serum biochemical parameters of liver and kidneys where all the values were within the normal ranges. Histopathological findings in this study was comparable to Saganuwan et al. [30] where they reported that aqueous leaf extract of Morinda Lucida at dose of 1626.5 mg/kg administrated to rats causes tubular degeneration of kidney and mild mononuclear cellular infiltration in liver. Similar to our findings, they found serum biochemical parameters particularly AST was not increased, but indeed significantly decreased (P<0.05). Glucose, creatinine, total protein, and bilirubin were also significantly decreased (P<0.05) compared to control. All the values, however, were still within the normal ranges.

| | | Group | | | | | |
|---|---|---|---|---|---|---|---|
| Organ | Mean scores of lesions | A | B | C | D | E | Kruskal Wallis test for global comparisons of organs lesions among groups. (Asymptotic Significant P<0.05) |
| | Inflammation | 0 | 0 | 0 | 1.00 ± 0.00 | 1.12 ± 0.29 | 0.00* |
| | Activated Kupffer cells | 0 | 0 | 0 | 0 | 0 | 1.00 |
| Liver | Hydropic degeneration | 0 | 0 | 0.80 ± 0.20 | 1.00 ± 0.00 | 1.50 ± 0.32 | 0.01* |
| | Periportal necrosis | 0 | 0 | 0 | 0.14 ± 0.14 | 0.75 ± 0.36 | 0.07** |
| | Midzonal necrosis | 0 | 0 | 0 | 0.14 ± 0.14 | 0.75 ± 0.36 | 0.07** |

| | | | | | | | |
|---|---|---|---|---|---|---|---|
| | Centrilobular necrosis | 0 | 0 | 0 | 0.57 ± 0.20 | 1.12 ± 0.29 | 0.03* |
| | Mean score | 0 | 0 | 0.13 ± 0.03 | 0.47 ± 0.08 | 0.87 ± 0.27 | 0.19 |
| Kidney | Inflammation | 0 | 0 | 0.40 ± 0.24 | 0.42 ± 0.20 | 0.50 ± 0.18 | 0.26 |
| | Hydropic degeneration/cytoplasmic vacuolation | 0 | 0 | 0.14 ± 0.14 | 0.14 ± 0.14 | 0.40 ± 0.24 | 0.44 |
| | Necrosis | 0 | 0 | 0 | 0 | 0 | 1.00 |
| | Cellular cast | 0 | 0 | 0 | 0 | 0.12 ± 0.12 | 0.64 |
| | Granular cast | 0 | 0 | 0.40 ± 0.24 | 0.71 ± 0.18 | 0.75 ± 0.16 | 0.02* |
| | Protein cast | 0 | 0 | 0 | 0 | 0 | 1.00 |
| | Mean score | 0 | 0 | 0.15 ± 0.10 | 0.21 ± 0.08 | 0.29 ± 0.07 | 0.56 |

**Table 5:** Result of scoring of lesion of scores in the liver and kidneys of Sprague Dawley (SD) rats in all groups of sub chronic oral toxicity study of ethanol extract of *C. nutans* leaves at the end of the experimental period (Note: A: Control; B: 10% DMSO; C: Low Dose; D: Medium Dose; E: High Dose (n=8 rats in each groups). The symbol * denotes the values were significantly different (P<0.05) between treated groups and control. The symbol ** denotes the values were almost significantly different (P>0.05) between treated groups and control.).

A previous study by Deschpande et al. [33] on the effects of ethanol extract of turmeric in rats and mice for 90 days revealed some abnormalities in the liver tissues. The administration of high dose of turmeric (5%) for 90 days showed a significant difference for focal necrosis with regeneration in the hepatocytes of both mice and rats. A study by Abalaka et al. [34] on the effects of extract of *Adenuim obesum* stem bark in rats revealed vacuolation of hepatocytes and congestion of blood vessels after being administrated with 5000 mg/kg of body weight of ethanol extract of *Adenuim obesum* stem bark. Serum biochemical parameters of the rats and mice particularly AST, ALP and ALT were all normal. Arsad et al. [35] also reported similar lesions in the kidney and liver tissues as observed in our study, although their results of the toxicity of *Rhaphidophora decursiva* (Roxb.) Schott extract were not significantly different (P>0.05) compared to control in both serum and histopathological findings. Chin et al. reported administration of methanol extract of *C. nutans* leaf up to 900 mg/kg of body weight showed significant (P<0.01) increase in total serum protein, albumin to globulin ratio and relative liver weight in rats. Increase in the total serum protein and albumin could be due to dehydration as a result of in appetence. While an increase in liver weight might related to liver injury. However histopathology examination was not conducted in the study. sub chronic toxicity studies conducted by Rosly et al. [36] showed administration of *M. citrifolia* crude fruits up to 5000 mg/kg of body weight and 2000 mg/kg of body weight showed significant (P<0.05)

decrease in total protein, and decreased in total white blood cells and spleen weight in rats, respectively. Nevertheless the values were still within the normal ranges. The histopathology examination of liver and kidneys revealed no significant differences (P>0.05) related to the treatments. There was no toxicity observed by Rosly et al. [36] although they used high concentrations of *M. citrifolia* fruits in their studies. The main reasons for that are the fruits were given to the rats in a crude form, and the crude fruit powder mixed with the ground rat pellet was fed to the rat ad libitum; the rats received the fruits in a small quantity throughout the day compared to oral gavage administration. Hepatic necrosis at the periportal and midzonal was observed in sub chronic oral toxicity of *C. nutans* leaf extract although it was not significant different (P>0.05) compared to control. Meanwhile centrilobular necrosis/centrilobular sinusoidal dilatation was observed in the study and significantly different (P<0.05) in sub chronic toxicity study of *C. nutans* for medium and high doses. Renal granular cast was observed and significant (P<0.05) in oral sub chronic toxicity study of *C. nutans* leaf extract for medium and high doses, respectively. Meanwhile renal cellular cast was observed in sub chronic oral toxicity study of *C. nutans* leaf extracts although it was significant (P<0.05) only in high dose. Hydropic degeneration/cytoplasmic vacuolation was observed in sub chronic study of *C. nutans* leaf extracts although it was not significantly different (P>0.05) compared to control.

| Organ | Groups (Asymptotic significant ([P<0.05]) | | | | | | | | | |
|---|---|---|---|---|---|---|---|---|---|---|
| | | A vs B | A vs C | A vs D | A vs E | B vs C | B vs D | B vs E | C vs D | C vs E | D vs E |
| Liver | Inflammation | 1.00 | 1.00 | 0.01* | 0.01* | 0.04 | 0.00 | 0.02 | 0.23 | 0.32 | 0.56 |
| | Activated Kupffer cells | 1.00 | 1.00 | 1.00 | 1.00 | 1.00 | 1.00 | 1.00 | 1.00 | 1.00 | 1.00 |
| | Hydropic degeneration | 1.00 | 0.10 | 0.00* | 0.01* | 0.04 | 0.00 | 0.02 | 0.23 | 0.32 | 0.56 |
| | Periportal necrosis | 1.00 | 1.00 | 0.39 | 0.13 | 1.00 | 0.51 | 0.51 | 0.39 | 0.07 | 0.14 |
| | Midzonal necrosis | 1.00 | 1.00 | 0.39 | 0.13 | 1.00 | 0.51 | 0.51 | 0.39 | 0.07 | 0.14 |

| | | | | | | | | | | | |
|---|---|---|---|---|---|---|---|---|---|---|---|
| | Centrilobular necrosis | 1.00 | 1.00 | 0.04* | 0.05* | 1.00 | 0.10 | 0.10 | 0.07 | 0.00 | 0.14 |
| | Mean score | 1.00 | 0.85 | 0.30 | 0.23 | 0.68 | 0.35 | 0.36 | 0.38 | 0.29 | 0.42 |
| Kidney | Inflammation | 1.00 | 0.13 | 0.31 | 0.10 | 0.23 | 0.19 | 0.14 | 0.92 | 0.73 | 0.78 |
| | Hydropic degeneration/cytoplasmic vacuolation | 1.00 | 0.39 | 1.00 | 0.39 | 0.51 | 0.51 | 0.23 | 1.00 | 0.33 | 0.33 |
| | Necrosis | 1.00 | 1.00 | 1.00 | 1.00 | 1.00 | 1.00 | 1.00 | 1.00 | 1.00 | 1.00 |
| | Cellular cast | 1.00 | 1.00 | 0.01* | 0.01* | 1.00 | 1.00 | 0.54 | 1.00 | 0.42 | 0.35 |
| | Granular cast | 1.00 | 0.13 | 0.01* | 0.01* | 0.23 | 0.05 | 0.03 | 0.29 | 0.22 | 0.88 |
| | Protein cast | 1.00 | 1.00 | 1.00 | 1.00 | 1.00 | 1.00 | 1.00 | 1.00 | 1.00 | 1.00 |
| | Mean score | 1.00 | 0.60 | 0.55 | 0.55 | 0.66 | 0.62 | 0.49 | 0.86 | 0.61 | 0.72 |

Table 6: Results of Mann-Whitney U test for comparison between groups of the toxicity lesions in liver and kidney of Sprague Dawley (SD) rats in sub chronic oral toxicity study of ethanol extract of *C. nutans* leaves. (Note: A: Control; B: 10% DMSO; C: Low Dose; D: Medium Dose; E: High Dose (n=8 rats in each groups). The symbol * denotes the values were significantly different (P<0.05) between treated groups and control.)

## Conclusion

90 days daily administration of ethanol extract of *C. nutans* leaf induced mild degree of toxicity in liver and kidneys of the rats. High dose (250 mg/kg of body weight) of the extract induced more prominent histopathological lesions. Prolong daily administration (more than 90 days) of the extract will probably induced moderate to severe toxicity in liver and kidney.

## Acknowledgements

The authors would like to thank Ministry of Science, Technology and Innovation (MOSTI), Malaysia for providing Science Fund Research Grant (06-01-04-SF1375) for this project.

## References

1. Sakdarat S, Shuyprom A, Ayudhya TDN, Waterman PG, Karagianis G (2006) Chemical composition investigation of the Clinacanthus nutans Lindau leaves. Thai J Phyto 13: 2459-2551.

2. Uawonggul N, Thammasirirak S, Chaveerach A, Chuachan C, Daduang J, et al. (2011) Plant extract activities against the fibroblast cell lysis by honey bee venom. J Med Plant Res 5: 1978-1986.

3. Yuann, JMP, Wang JS, Jian HL, Lin CC, Liang JY (2012). Effects of Clinacanthus nutans (Burm.f) Lindau leaf extracts on protection of plasmid DNA from riboflavin photoreaction. MC-Transaction of Biotechnology 4: 45-58.

4. Maxwell J (2001) Vegetation in the Siphandone Wetlands. In: Daconto G, editor. Siphandone wetlands. CESVI, Bergamo, Italy. p. 169.

5. P'ng XW, Akowuah GA, Chin JH (2012) Acute oral toxicity study of Clinacanthus nutans in mice. Int J Pharm Pharm Sci 3: 4202-4205.

6. Peng TW, P'ng XW, Chin JH, Akowuah GA (2014) Effect of methanol extract of Clinacanthus nutans on serum biochemical parameters in rats. J App Pharm Sci 6: 77-86.

7. Chin JH, Akowuah GA, Sabu MC, Khalivulla SI (2014) Sub-acute (28 days) toxicity study of methanol leaves extract of Cinacanthus nutans in rats. Int J Pham 4: 61-69.

8. Othman A, Ismail A, Ghani AN, Adenan I (2007) Antioxidant capacity and phenolic content of cocoa beans. Food Chem 100: 1523-1530.

9. Faezah A, Mohd Azlan SZ, Noorasiah S, Fadzilah AAM (2015) Prosiding Persidangan Kebangsaan Ekonomi Malaysia 10: 227-238.

10. Yong YK, Tan JJ, Teh SS, Mah SH, Cheng Lian Ee, et al. (2013) Clinacnathus nutans extracts are antioixidant with antiproliferative effect on cultured human cancer cell lines. Evid Based Complement Alternat Med 2013: 8.

11. Kamal MSA, Ghazali AR, Yahya NA, Wasiman MI, Ismail Z (2012) Acute toxicity study of standardized Mitragyna speciose Korth aqueous extract in Sprague Dawley rats. J Plant Stud 1: 120-129.

12. Nurul Husna R, Noriham A, Noorain A, Aziziah H, Farah Amna O (2013). Acute oral toxicity effects of Momordica Charantia in Sprague Dawley rats. Int J Biosci Biochem Bioinforma 3: 408-410.

13. Ismail Z, Halim SZ, Abdullah NR, Afzan A, Abdul Rashid BA, et al. (2014) Safety evaluation of oral toxicity of Carica papaya Linn. Leaves: A sub chronic toxicity study in Sprague Dawley rats. J Evid Based Complement Altern Med 2014:741470.

14. Teo S, Stirling D, Thomas S, Hoberman A, Kiorpes A, et al. (2002) A 90-day oral gavage toxicity study of D-methylpenidate and D, L-methylpenidate in Sprague-Dawley rats. Toxicology 179: 183-196.

15. Ogbonnia SO, Mbaka GO, Anyika EN, Osegbo OM, Igbokwe NH (2010) Evaluation of acute toxicity of hydro-ethanolic extract of chromolaena odorata (L.) king and robinson (Fam. Asteracea) in rats. Agri Biol J North Am 1: 869-865.

16. Rhiouani HR, Nazari P, Kamli-Nejad M, Lyoussi B (2008) Acute and sub chronic oral toxicity of an aqueous extract of leaves of Herniaria glabra in rodents. J Ethnopharmacol 118: 378-386.

17. Harizal SN, Mansor SM, Hasnan J, Tharakan JK, Abdullah J (2010) Acute toxicity study of standardized methanolic extract of Mitragyna speciosa Korth in rodent. J Enthapharmacol 131: 404-409.

18. Ashafa AOT, Orekoya LO, Yakubu MT (2012) Toxicity profile ethanolic extract of Azadirachta indica stem bark in male Wistar rats. Asian Pac J of Trop Biomed 2: 811-817.

19. Taib IS, Budin SB, Ain SMSN, Mohamed J, Louis SR, et al. (2009) Toxic effects of Litsea elliptica Blume essential oil on red blood cells of Sprague-Dawley rats. J Zhejiang University Sci B 10: 813-819.

20. Mozos I (2015) Mechanisms Linking Red Blood Cell Disorders and Cardiovascular Diseases. BioMed Res Int 2015.

21. Waldron HA (1966) The anemia of lead poisoning: A review. Brit J Ind Med 23: 83-100.

22.  Flora G, Gupta D, Tiwari A (2012) Toxicity of lead: a review with recent updates. Interdiscip Toxicol 5: 47-58.

23.  Adedapo AA, Abatan MO, Olorunsogo OO (2004) Toxic effects of some plants in the genus Euphorbia on haematological and biochemical parameters of rats. Veterinarski arhiv 74: 53-62.

24.  Okokon JE, Nwafor PA, Ekpo MD (2010) Sub chronic toxicity studies of the ethanolic root extract of Croton zambesicus. Pak J Pharm Sci 23: 160-169.

25.  Kelaidi C, Ades L, Fenaux P (2011) Treatment of acute promyelocytic leukemia with high white cell blood counts. Mediterr J of Hematol Infect Dis 3: 3-8.

26.  Coombs CC, Tavakkoli M, Tallman MS (2015) Acute promyelocytic leukemia: where did we start, where are we now, and the future. Blood Cancer J 5: e304.

27.  Morrone FB, Spiller F, Edelwises MIA, Meurer L, Engroff P (2009) Effect of temozolomide treatment on the adenine nucleotide hydrolysis in blood serum of rats with implanted gliomas. Appl Cancer Res 29: 118-124.

28.  Schwane JA, Johnson SR, Vandenakker CB, Armstrong RB (1983) Delayed-onset muscular soreness and plasma CPK and LDH activities after downhill running. Med Sci in Sports and Exerc 15: 51-56.

29.  Abdul-Raheem IT, Abdel-Ghany AA (2009) Hesperidin alleviates doxorubicin-induced cardiotoxicity in rats. J Egypt Nat Canc Inst 21: 175-184.

30.  Saganuwan SA, Aondoaver AD, Roman IT (2014) Reassesment of acute and chronic toxicity effect of aqueous leaf extract of Morinda Lucida in Rattus Norvegicus. J Haematol Res 1: 36-46.

31.  Chavalittumrong P, Attawish A, Rugsamon P, Chuntapet P (2013) Toxicological study of clinacanthus nutans (Burm. f.) Lindau. Bull Dep Med Sci 37: 323-338.

32.  Smolková K, Ježek P (2012) The role of mitochondrial NADPH-dependent isocitrate dehydrogenase in cancer cells. Int J Cell Biol.

33.  Deschpande SS, Lalitha VS, Ingle AD, Raste AS, Gadre SG, et al. (1998) Sub chronic oral toxicity of turmeric and ethanolic turmeric extract in female mice and rats. Toxicol Lett 95: 183-195.

34.  Abalaka SE, Fatihu MY, Ibrahim NDG, Ambali SF (2014) Hepatoxicity of ethanol extract of Adenium Obesum stem bark in Wistar rats. Br J of Pharm Res 4: 1041-1052.

35.  Arsad SS, Esa NM, Hazilawati H (2014) Histopathologic changes in liver and kidneys tissue from male Sprague Dawley rats treated with Rhaphidophora decursiva (Roxb.) schoot extract. J Cytol Histol S4: 001.

36.  Rosly SM, Shanmugavelu S, Murugaiyah M, Hadija H, Ahmad Tarmizi S, et al. (2011) Sub chronic oral toxicity of Morinda citrifolia (mengkudu) in Sprague Dawley rats. Pertanika J Trop Agri Sci 34: 341-349.

# 4

# *Calendula officinalis* Protection Against Cytotoxicity Effects of Personal Care Products on HaCaT Human Skin Cells

**Abdullah M Alnuqaydan**[*] **and Barbara J Sanderson**

*Department of Medical Biotechnology, School of Medicine, Flinders University, Australia*

[*]**Corresponding author:** Abdullah M Alnuqaydan, Department of Medical Biotechnology, School of Medicine, Flinders University, GPO Box 2100, Adelaide, SA 5001, Australia, E-mail: A.alnuqaydan@gmail.com

## Abstract

**Background:** Human skin is normally exposed to ionizing and UV radiations and on occasions it may also be subjected to beauty products or drugs that the host uses; all of which can generate reactive oxygen species (ROS).

**Objective:** In this study, *Calendula officinalis* extract, which contains antioxidant compounds, was examined for its protective effects against the products that generate ROS- induced cytotoxic activity towards human skin cells.

**Methodology:** The protection against cytotoxicity by *Calendula officinalis* extract was investigated *in vitro* using a dose-response on HaCaT human skin cells. The proprietary aqueous calendula extract C from biodynamically grown plant was examined. Protection against cytotoxicity was measured via the methyl tetrazolium cytotoxicity (MTT) assay. Cells were exposed to the calendula extracts for 48h before being exposed to personal care products consisting of two head lice treatments -Lice Breaker (Permethrin 1% w/w) and Organix Pyrethrum treatment (4 g/L Pyrethrins, 16 g/LPiperonyl Butoxide) and two beauty products -Nivea Visage Q10 plus Anti-Wrinkle face moisturizer + $TiO_2$; and Nivea Visage Q10 Plus Anti-Wrinkle face moisturizer (without $TiO_2$) for 1h.

**Results:** The effect of different concentrations of calendula extract on HaCaT human skin cells *in vitro* was explored. Doses of 1% (v/v) [1.4 mg dry weight equiv/ml] or less showed no toxicity. Cells were also exposed to the calendula extract for 48 hours before being exposed to the four personal care products for 1h. using the MTT cytotoxicity assay; it was observed that extract of *Calendula officinalis* gave time-dependent and concentration-dependent protection against harmful products that induce cell killing. Pre-incubation with the calendula extract for 48 hours significantly increased survival relative to the population without the extract by 30% and 47.4%, respectively, following treatment with personal care products.

**Conclusion:** This study demonstrates that calendula extract contains bioactive and free radical scavenging compounds that significantly protect against personal care products that generate oxidative stress cytotoxicity in a human skin cell culture model.

**Keywords:** Toxicity; *Calendula officinalis*; Beauty products; Lice treatments; Cell culture

## Introduction

Human skin exposed to ionizing and UV radiations or drugs and/or personal care products such as head lice treatments or beauty products that could generate reactive oxygen species (ROS) in vast quantities, could oxidize degrading pathways [1]. Uncontrolled ROS can be implicated in many aspects of pathogenesis such as human skin disorders, for example cutaneous neoplasia [1,2]. In human skin there are many agents that can produce oxidative stress including industrial sources, UV radiation, food contaminants, additives, drugs or cosmetic products [1,3]. Also, reactive nitrogen species (RNS) can be formed from exposure to environmental agents like xenobiotics [1]. Oxidative stress interacts with the process of variety of skin diseases [1]. Calendula flower has been shown to protect against cells being killed and chromosomal damage induced by hydrogen peroxide ($H_2O_2$) in HaCaT human skin cells [4,5]. It was shown that *Calendula officinalis* contains a number of compounds with antioxidants and free radicals with scavenging potential. Also, Calendula plant was used as a skin conditioning agent in cosmetics because of its anti-inflammatory properties [6]. The other use of the Calendula plant includes treatment for first degree burns and rashes [6]. However, chemical head lice treatments and chemical beauty products can induce toxicity and genotoxicity in human skin cells [7]. The hypothesis is that personal care products such as chemical head lice treatments and beauty products induce toxicity effects by producing oxidative stress in human skin cells.

In this study, we examine two head lice treatments (Lice Breaker treatment (Permethrin 1% w/w) and Organix Pyrethrum treatment (4 g/L Pyrethrins plus 16 g/L Piperonyl Butoxide)) and two beauty products (Nivea Visage Q10 plus Anti-Wrinkle face moisturizer (contains mixture of chemicals ingredients) + $TiO_2$; and Nivea Visage Q10 Plus Anti-Wrinkle face moisturizer (contains mixture of chemicals ingredients) (without $TiO_2$). The objective of this study is that to determine the ability of the calendula flower extract to protect human skin cells against any detrimental effects of these personal care products on human skin cells *in vitro*.

## Material and Methods

### Materials

1640 RPMI medium, foetal bovine serum (FBS) and penicillin/ streptomycin were purchased from Gibco, Invitrogen, Barcelona. Phosphate buffered saline (PBS) and 3-(4, 5-dimethylthiazol-2-yl)-2, 5-diphenyltetrazolium bromide (MTT) were purchased from (Sigma™). Media for growth and treatment were 1640 RPMI medium with 10% FBS. All the reagents used in this study were purchased from Sigma-Aldrich unless otherwise stated.

### Plant extract and characterization

The characterization of calendula extract C and its ability to protect human skin cells HaCaT against hydrogen peroxide ($H_2O_2$) induced oxidative stress cell killing and genetic damage was published previously [4,5]. Briefly, dried flowers of *Calendula officinalis* were supplied by an industry partner (Jurlique International, Mount Barker, South Australia) from biodynamically grown plants. Calendula extract C was prepared as a proprietary aqueous extract. It was diluted in RPMI media to make the treatment solution. The determination of density for extract C (1.036) was carried out at 20°C from the average of 10 independent measurements. The dry weight of extract C was 1.4 mg/ml as determined after extracts samples were freeze dried at -56°C at 3.4 Pa for 24h. The Folin–Ciocalteu assay was used to estimate polyphenol composition and the gallic acid equivalent of extract C was 10.83 mg GAE/g dry weight. Also, DPPH assay was used in previously published work to perform the free radical inhibition of extract C. Extract C showed 47.7% radical inhibitions at concentration 2.5% (3.5 mg/ml dry weight equivalent).

### Cell culture

A human non-cancer keratinocytes cell line HaCaT was like a gift from the Department of Haematology & Genetic Pathology - Flinders Medical Centre, School of Medicine at Flinders University, Adelaide, South Australia. It was maintained in RPMI 1640 medium, with 10% fetal bovine serum (FBS) and 1% penicillin/streptomycin (Thermo Scientific, Australia). Cells were seeded in tissue culture flasks and incubated at 37°C in a 5% $CO_2$ fully humidified incubator. HaCaT cells were subcultured when they reached 60–80% confluence.

### Cell treatment

HaCaT cells were treated to allow toxicity exposure before the protection assay being conducted. Microplates 96 wells -flat bottom were seeded with 104 cells/well and incubated for 19 h to allow cells to adhere at a temperature of 37°C in 5% $CO_2$. The media were aspirated and replaced with 200 µl of the treatment solution which was 0.125, 0.5, 1.0, 2.0 and 5% (v/v) extract C per well for 48 h. Then follow up with 100 µl products treatments (head lice treatments or titanium dioxide or beauty products) for 1 h before MTT assay analysis. The negative or zero control was media.

### MTT cell survival assay

To measure cell viability of HaCaT human skin, the methyl tetrazolium cytotoxicity assay was performed as published [4,8,9]. Briefly, the treatment solution was aspirated, and wells washed twice with PBS, cells were incubated with 200 µl MTT (0.5 mg/ml)/well for 4 h at 37°C. Formazan crystals were then dissolved in SDS (20% sodium dodecyl sulphate in 0.02 M HCL) for overnight. The absorbance was measured on an ELISA plate reader with the background reference wavelength of 630 nm and a test wavelength of 570 nm.

### Statistical analysis

The experiments were done in triplicate and data is presented as the mean ± S.E.M. One-way ANOVA with Tukey's posthoc test was carried out using SPSS software, version 22. Also, one-tailed t-test was also used. Differences were considered to be statistically significant when the P-value was less than 0.05.

## Results

The toxicity of Calendula extract C on HaCaT cells *in vitro* was explored by incubating cells with extract for 48 h. Figure 1 showed the toxicity of extract *C. calendulas* extract C showed toxicity only at a high dose (5%) for the 48h treatment time. At the lowest doses, the extract (0.125, 0.5, 1.0 and 2.0 % (v/v)) was not toxic on HaCaT skin cells for any of the treatment periods. This effect could involve a period of contact between these components and the cells, such that these toxic components would be taken up by cells, thus reducing the cellular viability. Therefore, in contrast, lower concentrations of such extracts would not be toxic if incorporated into products at a safe dose, which is difficult to ascertain on human skin. The toxicity at the higher doses of calendula extracts that has been found in this study needs to be translated into a recommendation for use of calendula extract on human skin.

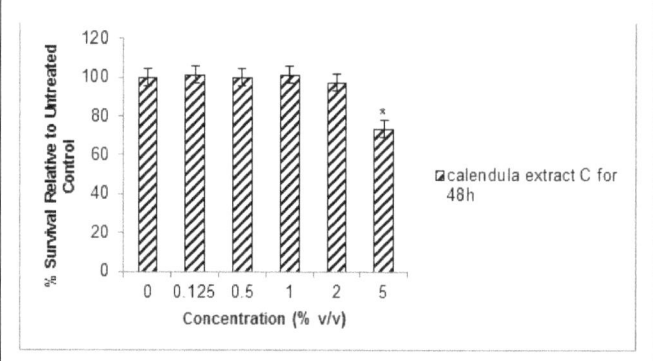

Figure 1: Relative survival at 48 h for calendula extract. HaCaT cells were treated for the time indicated then assayed by MTT assay (see section 2.4). Data are shown as mean survival relative to the untreated control ± SEM; n=3. * = treatments are significantly different from the 0 untreated controls at p<0.05.

Head lice treatments can induce cell killing act as apoptosis or necrosis [7]. Figure 2 showed the toxicity results of personal care products on HaCaT human skin cells. HaCaT human skin cells were pre-treated for 48h with 1% calendula extract C then followed by 1 h treatment with personal care products (beauty products or head lice treatments). Permethrin doses of 10% and 100%, Pyrethrum doses of 10% and 50% and Nivea visage at doses 0.3% and 3% with or without $TiO_2$ proved to be significantly toxic in HaCaT cells when measured by MTT assay.

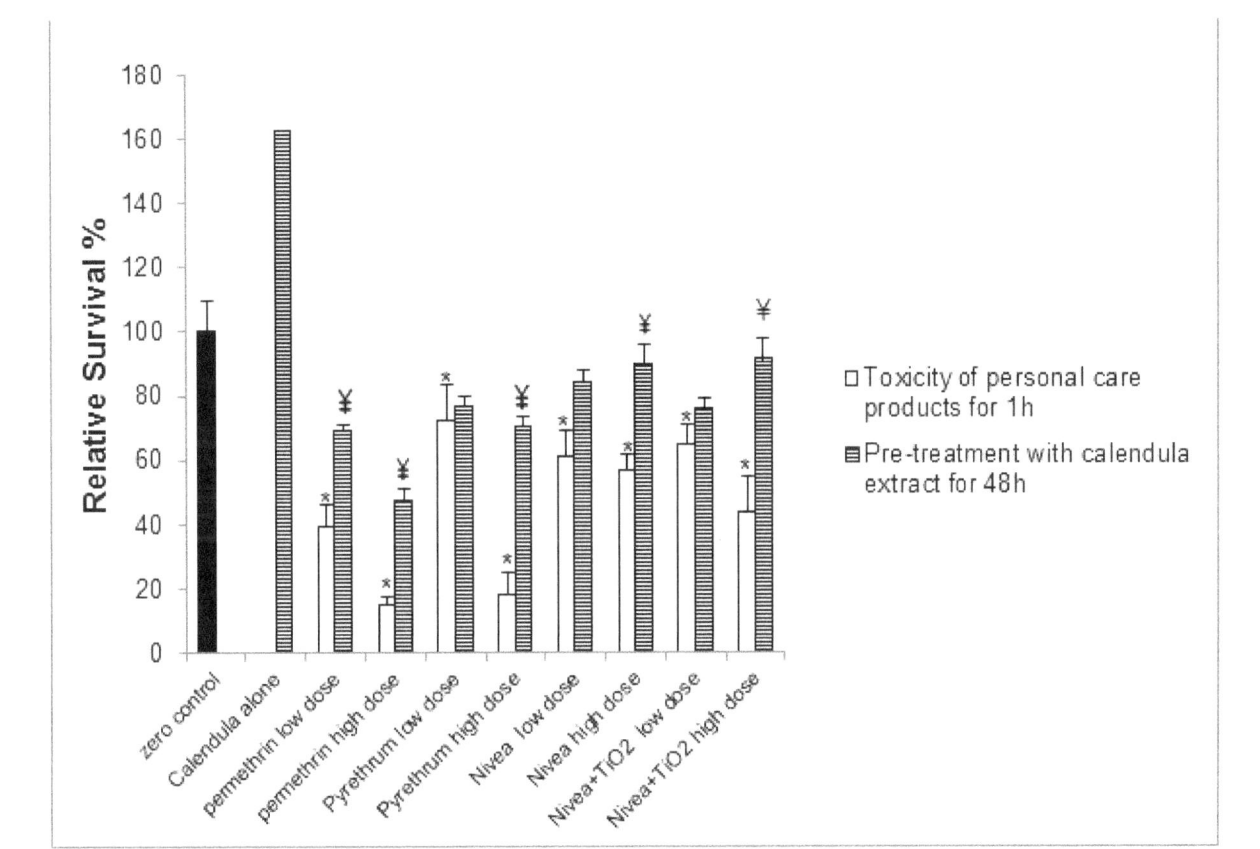

**Figure 2:** Toxicity and Calendula protection of personal care products on HaCaT human skin cells measured by MTT assay. Permethrin (low dose; 10%, high dose; 100%), Pyrethrum (low dose; 10%, high dose; 50%), Nivea visage without $TiO_2$ (low dose; 0.3%; high dose; 3%) and Nivea visage with $TiO_2$ (low dose; 0.3%; high dose 3%). Data shown as mean ± SEM, n=3. * = treatments are significantly different from the 0 untreated control at p<0.05. ¥= pre-treatment with calendula extract significantly different from products toxicity (protection).

The lower concentration of Calendula extract C 1% chosen as pre-treatment for HaCaT cells due to its safety treatment for HaCaT cells for all treatments period. *Calendula officinalis* extract showed the ability to protect significantly against toxicity effects of personal care products including $TiO_2$ treatment after treated HaCaT cells with Calendula extract C for 48h as illustrated in Figure 2. Calendula treatment for 48h offers more protection than 24h treatment time (Data not shown).

| Sample | Toxicity for 1 h | Pre-treatment with calendula extract for 48 h |
|---|---|---|
| Medium control | 100 ± 1.3 | 100 ± 1.5 |
| $TiO_2$ low dose (150 µg/ml) | *67.8 + 1.4 | 73.6 ± 10.9 |
| $TiO_2$ high dose (200 µg/ml) | *58.2+3.2 | **73.3 ± 5.2 |

**Table 1:** Untreated control and Titanium Dioxide ($TiO_2$) the positive control of beauty products. Data shown as mean ± SEM, n=3. * = treatments are significantly different from the 0 untreated control at

p<0.05. **= treatment is significantly different from $TiO_2$ dose at p<0.03 carried out using one- tailed T-Test.

Table 1 shows the untreated and positive controls of Titanium dioxide $TiO_2$ in the experiments. Cells were incubated for 48 h with calendula extract C alone there was a mean increase of 62% in relative survival. This is likely due to some cell growth during the incubation period.

It is important that the protection observed for the personal care products is real. The reason is that the positive control $TiO_2$ challenge still results in cells being killed and only a small level of protection. Of note, the treatment of calendula alone lead to an increase in cell number. This was not used as the untreated control as the correct control was the untreated cells.

## Discussion

The human body is exposed to variety of pro-oxidants in the environment including drugs, chemicals, mixtures, radiation, pollutants or cosmetics. These agents can target lipid-rich membranes, cellular DNA or proteins to produce toxicity. Personal care products such as beauty products can generate oxidative stress in human skin cells [1]. The increases in ROS play a role in a variety of skin diseases and carcinogenesis [1,10]. Beauty products and head lice treatments examined in this study induced significant toxicity in HaCaT human skin cells. The hypothesis was that personal care products such as beauty products or head lice treatments could generate oxidative stress in human skin cells. As a result, there was significant toxicity induced after treating HaCat cells with these products for 1h. The toxicity results of personal care products on HaCaT cells were measured by MTT assay which is a relative survival assay. *Calendula officinalis* showed protection activity against hydrogen peroxide ($H_2O_2$) induced oxidative stress cell killing and chromosomal damage [4,5]. Therefore, HaCaT cells treated with Calendula extract C to produce bioactivity antioxidant compounds did protect against toxicity of personal care products (beauty products and head lice treatments) that caused oxidative stress cell killing. The protection offered by Calendula extract C was time-dependent as explored early [4,5]. It was noted that there was significantly higher protection after pre-treatment with calendula extract with compounds that displayed higher toxicity when induced by the treatment of compounds alone. This was seen in the protection with the high of Pyrethrum, Nivea visage and Nivea visage with $TiO_2$. Further work needs to be done to understand the mechanism of action of calendula plant components and how they work to protect human skin cells. $TiO_2$ was classified as a carcinogenic nanoparticle used in cosmetics. Titanium dioxide ($TiO_2$) plays a role in the induction of apoptosis as well as oxidative stress [11-13]. One study indicated that Titanium dioxide $TiO_2$ can affect the mitochondria [14].

Calendula extract contains bioactives and free radical scavenging compounds that can interact with ROS to either eliminate them or minimise their deleterious effects [1]. These antioxidants or bioactive compounds including ascorbic acid, vitamin E, Vitamin C, alpha-tocopherol, quercetin, beta-carotene and amino acid [1,4]. Oxidative stress also drives the production of oxidation products, e.g. 4-hydroxy-2-nonenal or malonaldehyde that can denature proteins and alter apoptosis or influence the release of pro-inflammatory mediators such as cytokines in inflammatory skin diseases [1]. Moreover, ROS in the induction of many biological responses can act as second messengers such as in the generation of cytokines [15]. The alterations in cellular proteins or peroxidation of lipid-rich membranes caused by ROS can contribute to a range of skin diseases or cancer [1]. Experimental evidence supports the role played by ROS in the cancer process [1,10].

The increases of ROS in the cell, through either endogenous or exogenous factors, contribute to the carcinogenesis process. This could occur via genotoxic effects resulting in oxidative DNA adducts or via modification of gene expression [10]. MTT assay was employed in this study as a colorimetric assay for mammalian cell growth and survival, and it depends on the ability of viable cells to metabolize the yellow and water-soluble tetrazolium salt in the mitochondria of living cells. It can be used for mitochondrial dysfunction [9,16]. Mitochondrial damage is linked to the induction of mutations [17]. Moreover, mitochondrial DNA mutation and alteration in gene expression (mutation in the gene encoding for complexes I, II, IV and V) has been identified in many types of cancers and human tumours [17]. The mutation rate in mitochondrial is reported to be greater than in nuclear DNA [18].

In conclusion, it is evident that beauty products and head lice treatments examined in this study induced significant toxicity on HaCaT human skin cells, and that could be due to generating oxidative stress in skin cells. This process contributes to skin disorders such as inflammation and carcinogenesis or cancer. Also, the positive control of $TiO_2$ beauty product which is a carcinogen nanoparticle does play a

role in the oxidative stress by damaging the mitochondria in the cell [11-14]. Finally, this study indicated that *Calendula officinalis* extract C does protect HaCaT human skin cells against the toxicity caused by beauty products and head lice treatments. Further work could be done to determine the potential protection of calendula extract against the chromosome damage induced by personal care products also fluorescent cell viability dyes to specify the damaged chromosome and cancer type on Human skin cells.

## Acknowledgments

We thank the Ministry of Education, Saudi Arabia, for partial support of this project. Also, thanks to Professor Christopher Franco, Head of Medical Biotechnology, School of Medicine, Flinders University for reviewing the manuscript.

## References

1.  Bickers DR, Athar M (2006) Oxidative stress in the pathogenesis of skin disease. J Invest Dermatol 126: 2565-2575.

2.  Black HS (2004) ROS: a step closer to elucidating their role in the etiology of light-induced skin disorders. J Invest Dermatol 122: xiii-xiv.

3.  Athar M (2002) Oxidative stress and experimental carcinogenesis. Indian J Exp Biol 40: 656-667.

4.  Alnuqaydan AM, Lenehan CE, Hughes RR, Sanderson BJ (2015) Extracts from *Calendula officinalis* Offer *in Vitro* Protection Against H2O2 Induced Oxidative Stress Cell Killing of Human Skin Cells. Phytother Res 29: 120-124.

5.  Alnuqaydan AM, Lenehan CE, Hughes RR, Sanderson BJ (2015) Extracts from *Calendula officinalis* offer *in vitro* protection against H2 O2 induced oxidative stress cell killing of human skin cells. Phytother Res 29: 120-124.

6.  Re TA, Mooney D, Antignac E, Dufour E, Bark I, et al. (2009) Application of the threshold of toxicological concern approach for the safety evaluation of calendula flower (*Calendula officinalis*) petals and extracts used in cosmetic and personal care products. Food Chem Toxicol 47: 1246-1254.

7.  Alnuqaydan AM, Sanderson B (2016) Genetic damage and celll killing induction by five head lice treatments on HaCaT human skin cells. J Carcinog Mutagen 7.

8.  Young FM, Phungtamdet W, Sanderson BJ (2005) Modification of MTT assay conditions to examine the cytotoxic effects of amitraz on the human lymphoblastoid cell line, WIL2NS. Toxicology *in Vitro* 19: 1051-1059.

9.  Mosmann T (1983) Rapid colorimetric assay for cellular growth and survival: application to proliferation and cytotoxicity assays. J Immunol Method 65: 55-63.

10. Klaunig JE, Kamendulis LM (2004) The role of oxidative stress in carcinogenesis. Annu Rev Pharmacol Toxicol 44: 239-267.

11. Bhattacharya K, Davoren M, Boertz J, Schins R, Hoffmann E, et al. (2009) Titanium dioxide nanoparticles induce oxidative stress and DNA-adduct formation but not DNA-breakage in human lung cells. Part Fibre Toxicol 6: 8977-8976.

12. Park EJ, Yi J, Chung KH, Ryu DY, Choi J, et al. (2008) Oxidative stress and apoptosis induced by titanium dioxide nanoparticles in cultured BEAS-2B cells. Toxicol Lett 180: 222-229.

13. Reeves JF, Davies SJ, Dodd NJF, Jha AN (2008) Hydroxyl radicals (OH) are associated with titanium dioxide (TiO2) nanoparticle-induced cytotoxicity and oxidative DNA damage in fish cells. Mutat Res 640: 113-122.

14. Tucci P, Porta G, Agostini M, Dinsdale D, Iavicoli I, et al. (2013) Metabolic effects of TiO2 nanoparticles, a common component of sunscreens and cosmetics, on human keratinocytes. Cell Death Dis 4: e549.

15. Briganti S, Picardo M (2003) Antioxidant activity, lipid peroxidation and skin diseases. What's new. J Eur Acad Dermatol Venereol 17: 663-669.

16. Brand MD, Nicholls DG (2011) Assessing mitochondrial dysfunction in cells. Biochem J 435: 297-312.

17. Tamura G, Nishizuka S, Maesawa C, Suzuki Y, Iwaya T, et al. (1999) Mutations in mitochondrial control region DNA in gastric tumours of Japanese patients. Eur J Cancer 35: 316-319.

18. Wang E, Wong A, Cortopassi G (1997) The rate of mitochondrial mutagenesis is faster in mice than humans. Mutat Res 377: 157-166.

19. Satran D, Henry CR, Adkinson C, Nicholson CI, Bracha Y, et al. (2005) Cardiovascular manifestations of moderate to severe carbon monoxide poisoning. J Am Coll Cardiol 45: 1513-1516.

20. Henry CR, Satran D, Lindgren B, Adkinson C, Nicholson CI, et al. (2006) Myocardial injury and long-term mortality following moderate to severe carbon monoxide poisoning. JAMA 295: 398-402.

# 5

# Toxicology and Safety Determination for a Novel Therapeutic Dual Carbon Monoxide and Oxygen Delivery Agent

**Hemant Misra**[1*], **Friedericke Kazo**[1] and **Judith A. Newmark**[2]

[1]*Prolong Pharmaceuticals LLC, 300B Corporate Court, South Plainfield, NJ 07080, USA*

[2]*Toxikon Corporation, 15 Wiggins Avenue, Bedford, MA 01730, USA*

[*]**Corresponding Author**: Hemant Misra, Ph.D, Prolong Pharmaceuticals LLC, 300B Corporate Court, South Plainfield, NJ 07080, USA, E-mail: hmisra@prolongpharma.com

## Abstract

Conditions in patients with hemoglobinopathies are far more complex and variable than in healthy humans due to the cascade of injury from hypoxia. Resulting complications can lead to tissue death, organ dysfunction and even death. Multi-faceted treatment is needed to address the array of complications. SANGUINATE™ (PEGylated, bovine carboxyhemoglobin) has multiple mechanisms of action that may prove effective. It acts both as a carbon monoxide-releasing molecule and as an oxygen transfer agent and is designed to safely perfuse the microvasculature to oxygenate tissue. Designing toxicology studies must not only deal with ensuring the safety of its mechanisms but deal with the potential safety issues of using bovine hemoglobin for both acute and chronic administration. Similar products have previously been shown to have effects on inflammation, vasoactivity, cardiac toxicity and nephrotoxicity as well as pro-coagulant activity. Therefore, studies were designed to thoroughly address the potential of these effects in conjunction with the traditional toxicology and safety pharmacology studies.

These toxicology and safety studies were designed to address the FDA's particular concerns of this novel drug candidate. There were several unique features to this preclinical program including a renal functional study, immunohistochemical and special staining of tissues, measurement of hemoglobin in the urine, measurement of troponin in the serum, inclusion of high dose/high volume groups, and analysis of interference for clinical pathology parameters. To address toxicity and safety concerns of its use as a single or repeating dose therapeutic, SANGUINATE was tested in pivotal studies using three species in repeating doses. There were no adverse effects identified for any doses and therefore, a no observed adverse effect level (NOAEL) was not determined even at dosage levels of 1200 mg/kg (monkey), 1600 mg/kg (pig) and 2400 mg/kg (rat). The completion of these studies permitted SANGUINATE to move into clinical trials.

**Keywords** PEGylation; Toxicology; Safety; SANGUINATE; Hemoglobin; Preclinical

## Introduction

SANGUINATE (PEGylated bovine carboxyhemoglobin) is a dual action carbon monoxide (CO) releasing/oxygen ($O_2$) transfer agent whose functional components (CO, bovine hemoglobin and polyethylene glycol) contribute to its unique mechanisms of action. Due to the unique properties of its components, SANGUINATE has the potential to reduce or prevent the effects of hypoxia and protect the vasculature thereby preventing or reducing the extent of tissue damage.

While SANGUINATE is not traditional hemoglobin (Hb)-based oxygen carrier (HBOC), the Guidance for Industry: Criteria for Safety and Efficacy Evaluation of Oxygen Therapeutics as Red Blood Cell Substitute [1] provides a basis for the preclinical program design. Cell-free Hb has well-known effects on the vasculature. It readily extravagates and scavenges vascular endothelial nitric oxide (NO). NO is an important endogenous intercellular messenger that modulates blood flow, thrombosis and neural activity. Scavenging of NO by free Hb can result in systemic vasoconstriction, decreased blood flow, increased release of proinflammatory mediators and potent vasoconstrictors, and a loss of platelet inactivation. Free Hb also rapidly oxidizes to methemoglobin, which through its reactive iron moiety, causes oxidative damage to the blood vasculature and organs. Cell free Hb is known to cause iron deposition in tissue. The toxicity associated with iron is due to its role in catalyzing the generation of radicals which in turn damage cellular macromolecules and cause cell death and tissue injury.

In the 1990s, HBOCs were under development and then discontinued as a number of safety-related problems arose resulting in effects such as inflammation, vasoactivity, cardiac toxicity and nephrotoxicity as well as pro-coagulant activity [2-7]. Although not a conventional HBOC, SANGUINATE is designed to address these issues through the use of PEGylation [8,9] and carboxylation [10]. The modification of Hb with polyethylene glycol increases the effective molecular size, thereby preventing extravasation and the scavenging of NO. The release of CO may have therapeutic activity through the inhibition of vasoconstriction as well as by its anti-inflammatory activity.

Although this is a standard toxicology program in many ways, there are several unique features that were incorporated based on the novelty of the product. For this type of product, it was necessary to carefully design the studies to address traditional toxicology and safety concerns, pharmacokinetic (PK) and pharmacological effects, as well as to specifically address the theoretical concerns of inflammation, vasoactivity, cardiac toxicity and nephrotoxicity, and pro-coagulant activity. Therefore, the toxicology and safety study design incorporated assessments to address issues that are unique to this class of products (Table 1). Unique features to this program included a renal glomerular filtration rate and renal blood flow study, immunohistochemical staining for tumor necrosis factor alpha (TNF-α, inflammatory marker), malondialdehyde (MDA, oxidative marker), and Prussian Blue iron staining for kidneys, myocardium, vasculature, and brain (cerebrum and cerebellum). Additional clinical pathology assessments included measurement of the cardiac diagnostic marker, troponin, in the serum. Elimination of SANGUINATE was assessed by measuring the levels of hemoglobin in the urine. High dose/high volume groups were included to further increase the dosing levels of SANGUINATE and to provide an increased safety margin. The cardiovascular safety study in monkey included additional clinical pathology and histopathology toxicity assessments. Interference studies were used to identify and correct for the interference of hemoglobin with the proper assessment of clinical pathology parameters that are based on colorimetric methods, and is a complex analysis that will be elaborated upon in a separate manuscript. This paper will focus on the toxicology and safety aspects of this program and the unique designs that enabled FDA approval of SANGUINATE for clinical trials.

| Challenge | Testing Approach |
| --- | --- |
| Inflammation and oxidative stress | Immunohistochemistry for TNF-α and MDA in kidneys, myocardium, vasculature, and brain |
| Cardiac Toxicity | Electrocardiograms, clinical chemistry including Troponin, histopathology, and full cardiovascular and pulmonary assessment in telemetered monkeys |
| Nephrotoxicity | Renal glomerular filtration rate and renal blood flow study; clinical chemistry; urinalysis; histopathology; measured presence of hemoglobin in urine |
| Safety Margin | High dose/high volume groups included to maximize dosing levels |
| Clinical Pathology Interference | Interference assessment and correction for affected parameters |

Table 1: Challenges and Unique Features in the SANGUINATE Toxicity and Safety Program.

## Methodology

The SANGUINATE preclinical program consisted minimally of PK, genotoxicity, and toxicity and safety studies (several other studies were conducted during drug development). PK studies were performed in both rat and pig species. Animals were dosed with 40 mg/ml SANGUINATE by IV with a single dose at 2, 4, and 8 ml/kg. Blood was collected at timepoints out to 144 hours post dosing, and samples were analyzed for SANGUINATE concentration.

Genotoxicity was performed per OECD guidelines. SANGUINATE was evaluated for its ability to induce chromosomal aberrations (mitotic index evaluation and definitive chromosomal aberration assay) in cultured human peripheral blood lymphocytes *in vitro* in the presence and absence of metabolic activation. The *Salmonella typhimurium* and *Escherichia coli* Reverse Mutation Assay (Ames Assay) was conducted to evaluate the potential of SANGUINATE to induce reverse mutations in histidine (his⁻ to his⁺) and tryptophan (tryp⁻ to tryp⁺) genes in *S. typhimurium* and *E. coli*. The Rodent Bone Marrow Micronucleus Assay was evaluated for induction of a statistically significant increase in the frequency of micronuclei in the bone marrow erythrocytes of mice.

The *in vivo* toxicity and safety program for SANGUINATE included toxicity and safety studies across 3 different species: Sprague Dawley Rats, Gottingen Minipigs, and Cynomolgus Monkeys (Table 2). Parameters evaluated for the assessment of toxicity included clinical observations, body weights, ophthalmic observations, food consumption, hematology, clinical chemistry, coagulation, urinalysis (Table 3), and organ weights and histopathology (Table 4). Additional assessments included in some of the studies were special histopathology staining, toxicokinetics, functional observational battery, immunogenicity, and cardiovascular measurements (Table 4).

| Study | Animals | SANGUINATE Dose Levels / Regimen | Parameters | Observations |
| --- | --- | --- | --- | --- |
| Determination of Glomerular Filtration Rate and Renal Blood Flow Following Single Intravenous Administration of SANGUINATE in Rats | Rat (n=222) | 160, 280, 400 mg/kg<br><br>Single dose IV | Glomerular Filtration Rate (GFR) and Renal Blood Flow (RBF) | There were no abnormal clinical observations within the study time period to suggest any acute toxic effect of treatment with the test article. Within 24 hours of SANGUINATE single-dose intravenous administration, no changes were observed in glomerular filtration rate (GFR) or renal blood flow (RBF) measured clearance. |
| Five–Day Repeat Dose Toxicity Study of SANGUINATE (PEGylated Bovine Hemoglobin) in Rats with a 14–Day Recovery Period | Rat (n=294) | 100, 200, 400 mg/kg<br><br>5-day repeat dose; 5 min iv infusion | Food consumption, body and organ weight measurements, clinical observations, functional observational battery, hematology, blood chemistry, coagulation, urinalysis, immunogenicity, | No test article related effects on standard parameters. Significant differences for clinical chemistry parameters including increased creatinine, decreased albumin, and decreased alkaline phosphatase activity. Histopathological results revealed no macroscopic and/or microscopic treatment related findings, and no target organs and /or treatment related findings. Iron staining |

|  |  |  | and histopathology including special staining. | was exclusively in the brain (minimal to mild) and in the kidneys (minimal to moderate), but was not considered biologically relevant. SANGUINATE was well tolerated up to and including 400 mg/kg after single and after 5 days intravenous administration. No NOAEL. |
|---|---|---|---|---|
| Maximum Feasible Dose Study of SANGUINATE in Rats | Rat (n=20) | 2400 mg/kg<br><br>5-day repeat dose (MFD); slow iv push | Body weights and clinical observations, blood and urine collected for clinical pathology, gross necropsy and select target organs for histopathology. | Treatment related findings were noted in clinical observations, and in the evaluation of clinical pathology and histopathology. No adverse effects on body weights. Urine discolored and slight increase in the WBC and RBC. Clinical signs included excretion of red/brown fluid from the urogenital area and red fluid/staining around eyes, and piloerection. There were changes in the percentage of lymphocytes, and an increase in the percentage of neutrophils in both sexes and monocytes in males. A decrease in hemoglobin was also seen. The values of total bilirubin and creatinine were increased, and albumin and total protein were significantly decreased. Microscopic evaluation showed treatment related findings that were limited to the kidneys and heart in both sexes. The evaluations showed overt signs of systemic toxicity. |
| Six Months Repeat Dose Toxicity Study of SANGUINATE<br><br>(PEGylated Bovine Hemoglobin) in Rats<br><br>With a 30-Day Recovery Period | Rat (n=506) | 100, 200, 400, 2400 mg/k<br><br>6-mo monthly, repeat dose; 5 min iv infusion | Food consumption, body and organ weight measurements, clinical and ophthalmic observations, clinical signs of neurotoxicity, hematology, serum chemistry, coagulation, urinalysis, immunogenicity, and histopathology including special staining. | Prolonged bleeding was noted in groups receiving SANGUINATE, and the negative controls DPH and Hextend, following intravenous dosing and/or retro-orbital blood sample collection. This procedure-related bleeding was not seen in the NaCl control groups. Significant, dose-dependent, albumin, total protein, total bilirubin, AST, ALP, amylase, calcium, creatinine and BUN effects were seen, not on all days. Recovery groups presented no significant abnormalities, indicating recovery from any treatment-related effects. Microscopic evaluation of liver and kidneys did not confirm any test article related effects on these or other organs compared to the controls. |
| Nine Months Repeat Dose Toxicity Study of SANGUINATE<br><br>(PEGylated Bovine Hemoglobin) in Minipigs<br><br>with a 30-Day Recovery Period | Pig (n=86) | 100, 200, 400, 1600 mg/kg<br><br>9-mo monthly; 10-15 min iv infusion | Food consumption, body and organ weight measurements, clinical and ophthalmic observations, electrocardiographic exams, hematology, serum chemistry, coagulation, urinalysis, immunogenicity, and histopathology including special staining. | Majority of assessments showed no specific effects including body weights, ophthalmic exams, the amount of oxy- and deoxy-hemoglobin in whole blood, electrocardiographic exams, and immunogenicity. Some differences in organ weights (heart, liver, adrenal, and brain) were observed, but were not considered biologically relevant. Iron staining was observed in the brain and kidney and in one animal in the carotid aortas and jugular vein, but was not considered biologically relevant. TNF-α and MDA staining had no clear dose trend. The only clinical sign considered related was diarrhea, observed in 25% of the animals assigned to the 1600 mg/kg SANGUINATE group. Some differences in hematology and clinical chemistry parameters were observed. A significant increase in prothrombin time and activated partial thromboplastin time was observed but not clinically relevant. A NOAEL could not be determined. |
| Evaluation of Cardiovascular (Hemodynamic) and Pulmonary Function Following Intravenous Administration of SANGUINATE™ (PEGylated Bovine Hemoglobin) in Conscious Telemetered Male Cynomolgus Monkeys | Monkey (n=4) | 100, 200, 400, 1200 mg/kg<br><br>5-day repeat dose; 5-10 min iv injection | Clinical observations, clinical pathology, histopathology, toxicokinetics, ECG, hemodynamics, and pulmonary parameters | Observations included loose or soft feces, delayed/ prolonged bleeding times, facial and inguinal erythema, pink skin color, petichiae on the leg, decreased activity and white foamy/frothy feces, small red areas on the abdomen and extremities. Clinical chemistry showed no Troponin, increased creatinine, increased BUN, decreased amylase , decreased ALK, and slightly decreased ALT. There were no microscopic findings that indicated direct test article toxicity. 100 and 200 mg/kg were not associated with changes in heart rate, blood pressure, ECG or pulmonary parameters. 400 mg/kg was associated with minimal increases in arterial pressure after the first dose and slight increases in heart rate and arterial pressure following the fifth dose. 1200 mg/kg/day was associated with decreased heart rate and increased arterial pressure. Following the fifth day of dosing at 1200 mg/kg/day, increases in heart rate, arterial pressure and QTc were noted as well as decreases in respiratory rate. |

**Table 2:** Summary of SANGUINATE Toxicity and Safety Program.

| Hematology | Clinical Chemistry | Coagulation |
|---|---|---|
| Differential White Blood Cell Count | Alanine Aminotransferase (ALT) | Activated Partial Thromboplastin Time (APTT |
| Hematocrit (HCT) | Albumin (ALB) | Prothrombin Time (PT) |
| Hemoglobin (HGB) | Albumin/Globulin Ratio (A/G) | |
| Mean Corpuscular Hemoglobin (MCH) | Alkaline Phosphatase (ALK) | Urinalysis |
| Mean Corpuscular Hemoglobin Concentration (MCHC) | Amylase | Appearance – color, clarity, volume |
| Mean Corpuscular Volume (MCV | Aspartate Aminotransferase (AST) | Bilirubin |
| Oxy-Carboxy and Met-hemoglobin | Blood Urea Nitrogen (BUN) | Glucose |
| Platelet Count (PLA) | Calcium (Ca) | Ketones |
| Red Blood Cell (Erythrocyte) Count (RBC) | Chloride (Cl) | Leucocytes |
| White Blood Cell (Leukocyte) Count (WBC) | Cholesterol (CHOL) | Microscopic examination of sediment |
| | Creatinine (CREAT) | Nitrites |
| | Gamma Glutamyltransferase (GGT) | Occult Blood |
| | Globulin | pH |
| | Glucose | Specific Gravity |
| | Inorganic Phosphorus (PHOS) | Total Protein |
| | Lipase | Urinary hemoglobin |
| | Potassium (K) | Urobilinogen |
| | Sodium (Na) | Volume |
| | Total Bilirubin | |
| | Total Protein (TP) | |
| | Triglycerides (TRIG) | |

**Table 3:** General Clinical Pathology Parameters: Hematology, Clinical Chemistry, Coagulation, and Urinalysis.

| | | |
|---|---|---|
| Adrenal gland | Small intestine, duodenum | Small intestine, ileum |
| Aorta | Lung (with mainstem bronchi) | Small intestine, jejunum |
| Bone marrow | Lymph node, mesenteric | Spinal cord (cervical, mid-thoracic, lumbar) |
| Bone with articular surface, femur | Lymph nodes, submandibular (L/R) | Spleen |
| Brain (cerebrum, cerebellum, medulla/pons) | Mammary gland | Stomach |
| Epididymis (males) | Nasal turbinate | Testes (males, paired) |
| Esophagus | Nerve, sciatic | Thymus |
| Eyes (w/optic nerve) | Ovaries (females, paired) | Thyroid (with parathyroid) |
| Heart | Pancreas | Tongue |
| Injection Site | Pituitary gland | Trachea |
| Kidney | Prostate gland (males) | Ureter (paired) |
| Large intestine, cecum | Salivary gland, mandibular (L/R) | Urinary bladder |

| Large intestine, colon | Seminal Vesicles | Uterus (females) |
|---|---|---|
| Large intestine, rectum | Skeletal muscle | Cervix |
| Liver | Skin | Vagina (females) |

Table 4: General Tissues Used in Histopathology Study.

A study was performed to analyze the effects of SANGUINATE (160, 280, and 400 mg/kg) on renal glomerular filtration rate (GFR) and renal blood flow (RBF) following single intravenous administration to Sprague Dawley rats, based on the plasma clearance of surrogate markers. Inulin, [Carboxyl-$^{14}$C], was utilized in the measurement of GFR and Aminohippuric Acid, P-[Glycyl-1-$^{14}$C], was used in the measurement of RBF. The control article was USP 0.9% Sodium Chloride for Injection (NaCl). Animals were administered inulin or aminohippuric acid as tracers. There were a total of 7 groups. In each group, a subset of animals was administered inulin, and another subset received p-aminohippuric acid. The animals were intravenously administered the specified dose of test or control article on study Day 1. Before tracer administration, animals were weighed and hydrated by oral administration of NaCl at a dose level of 25 mL/kg. The urinary bladder was expressed by induced micturition through manual pressure applied above the pubic area. Radiolabeled inulin or aminohippuric acid tracer was given intravenously at a dose level of 500 mg/kg within 24 ± 2 hours following treatment with the test or control article. Animals were placed into metabolic cages with food and water withheld for the remaining duration of the study. Samples of arterial blood and urine (as available) were collected from each animal at 30 ± 5 and 60 ± 5 minutes. The time and volume of urine collection were recorded for the determination of urine output. Animals were humanely sacrificed following the final sample collection. Levels of radioactivity were determined through sample analysis in duplicate on a scintillation counter. Blood samples were solubilized to produce a solution compatible with the liquid scintillation cocktail in the determination of radioactivity. Urine samples were measured directly on the scintillation counter. Renal glomerular filtration rate (GFR) and renal blood flow (RBF) were calculated based on the clearance of inulin or p-aminohippuric acid, respectively.

An evaluation was performed of the potential toxicity and the toxicokinetic profile of the test article, SANGUINATE, after single dose and after five days repeated IV administration to Sprague Dawley rats at the doses of 0, 100, 200 and 400 mg/kg, and the reversibility of any toxic effect after a 14–day recovery period. One group was treated with 200 mg/kg of Purified Bovine Hemoglobin (positive control group). Two additional groups (negative controls) were treated with 200 mg/kg of deoxy-PEGylated bovine hemoglobin (DPH) or 5.0 mL/kg Hextend (Hospira). There were 15 male and 15 female animals per group. On Days 2, 6 and 20, ten animals in each group (5 males and 5 females) were sacrificed. To study the toxicokinetic profile of SANGUINATE, an additional 6 males and 6 females per group were used. Parameters evaluated for the assessment of toxicity included food consumption, body and organ weight measurements, clinical observations, clinical signs of neurotoxicity, hematology, blood chemistry, coagulation, urinalysis, immunogenicity, and histopathology. Histopathological analysis included special staining to indicate TNF-α expression, oxidative damage (MDA staining) or iron accumulation (Prussian Blue staining).

The potential toxicity using repeat dosing with a maximum feasible high dose 2400 mg/kg of SANGUINATE at a dose volume of 60 mL/kg/day was assessed for 5 consecutive days. Twenty (20) rats were used in the study and were placed into 5 dose groups each with 2 males and 2 females. Each animal received 30 mL/kg via an intravenous injection twice a day of the following test or control articles: NaCl, SANGUINATE, PEGylated bovine hemoglobin (PBH), DPH, or Hextend. Body weights were taken daily and animals were observed for clinical signs of toxicity prior to the initial dose and following the last dose of the day. Blood and urine were collected for clinical pathology evaluation at the end of the study. A gross necropsy was performed on all animals and select target organs were collected for microscopic examination. Parameters evaluated included food consumption, body and organ weight measurements, clinical and ophthalmic observations, clinical signs of neurotoxicity, hematology, serum chemistry, coagulation, urinalysis, immunogenicity, and histopathology.

A six month study was performed in Sprague Dawley Rats to evaluate the potential toxicity and the toxicokinetic profile of Sanguinate after once a month IV administration, and the reversibility of any toxic effect after a 30-day recovery period. Animals received doses of 0, 100, 200 and 400 mg/kg. One group was treated with 200 mg/kg of PBH (positive control), and two groups (negative controls) were treated with 200 mg/kg of DPH or 5.0 mL/kg Hextend. Two additional groups received a high volume dose of 60 mL/kg of the vehicle control or 2400 mg/kg of Sanguinate. Some animals per sex receiving the high volume control or 2400 mg/kg of Sanguinate were sacrificed on Day 61 and some animals per sex receiving 2400 mg/kg were sacrificed on Day 74. To study the toxicokinetic profile of Sanguinate, 6 or 9 animals/group/sex were used with groups surviving 60 days or 180 days, respectively. Parameters evaluated for the assessment of toxicity included food consumption, body and organ weight measurements, clinical and ophthalmic observations, functional observational battery (FOB) exams, hematology, serum chemistry, coagulation, urinalysis, immunogenicity, and histopathology. Interference for clinical pathology parameters was characterized and corrections were applied.

A nine month study in Gottingen Minipigs was performed to evaluate the potential toxicity and the toxicokinetic profile of the test article, Sanguinate, after once a month IV administration, and the reversibility of any toxic effect after a 30–day recovery period. Animals received doses of 0, 100, 200, and 400 mg/kg. One group was treated with 200 mg/kg of PBH (positive control) and two groups (negative controls) were treated with 200 mg/kg of DPH or 5.0 mL/kg Hextend. Two additional groups received a high volume dose of 40 mL/kg of the vehicle control or 1600 mg/kg of Sanguinate. On Day 276, some animals per sex in each group receiving 0, 100, 200, or 400 mg/kg of Sanguinate, PBH, DPH, or Hextend were sacrificed. On Day 300, some animals per sex receiving 0 or 400 mg/kg of Sanguinate were sacrificed. Some animals per sex receiving the high volume control or 1600 mg/kg of Sanguinate were sacrificed on Day 91 and some animals per sex receiving 1600 mg/kg were sacrificed on Day 105. To study the toxicokinetic profile of Sanguinate, blood samples from 4 animals per sex per group were obtained on Days 1, 90 and 270 (0, 100, 200, and 400 mg/kg Sanguinate, PBH, DPH and Hextend groups) and from 3 animals per sex assigned to 1600 mg/kg Sanguinate on Days 1 and 90. Parameters evaluated for the assessment of toxicity included food consumption, body and organ weight measurements, clinical and ophthalmic observations, electrocardiographic exams, hematology, serum chemistry, coagulation, urinalysis, immunogenicity, and histopathology. Interference for clinical pathology parameters was characterized and corrections were applied.

A study was performed to determine the potential acute and repeat dose, intermittent dose effects of SANGUINATE on cardiac, circulatory and pulmonary functions and electrocardiograms (ECG) of conscious telemetered male Cynomogus monkeys (Table 5).

| Cardiovascular Parameters |
| --- |
| Systolic arterial pressure |
| Diastolic arterial pressure |
| Mean arterial pressure |
| Heart rate |
| P duration |
| PR interval |
| QRS interval |
| R amplitude |
| QT interval |
| **Pulmonary Parameters** |
| Respiration rate |
| Minimum |
| Maximum |
| Inspiration time |
| Expiration time |
| Depth |

Table 5: Cardiovascular and Pulmonary Parameters.

There was one treatment group of 4 Cynomolgus monkeys each receiving the PBH (positive control), DPH (negative control), Hextend (negative control) the vehicle and four doses of SANGUINATE (100 mg/kg/day, 200 mg/kg/day, 400 mg/kg/day and 600 mg/kg/2x per day) with a washout period in between dosing regimens. Treatments were administered once per day for 5 days except for the vehicle control #2 and the 1200 mg/kg/day total dose which were administered twice daily approximately 6 hours apart. The 1200 mg/kg/day total high dose was also administered on Day 114, for toxicokinetic purposes, and again on Day 127. One-minute means of hemodynamic, pulmonary and ECG parameters were measured on the first and last dosing day of each 5-day treatment arm as well as on Day 127. One minute tracings of the ECGs were printed at 15 minutes prior to dosing and at 30 minutes, 1, 2, 4, 8, 12 and 22 hours post-dose on each recording day for review by a veterinary cardiologist. Blood for evaluation of serum

chemistry was collected from all animals prior to treatment initiation and on each dosing day prior to dosing and on Day 128 prior to terminal sacrifice. Blood for toxicokinetic evaluation was collected on Day 114 at selected timepoints. Selected tissues were harvested at necropsy on Day 128 from all animals and were evaluated microscopically. Interference for clinical pathology parameters was characterized and corrections were applied.

## Results

### Pharmacokinetic Studies

In both rat and pig species, a dose-dependent pattern in terms of $C_{max}$ and AUC was observed. When adjusted for dose, there appeared to be a solid linear response in both $C_{max}$ and AUC. In the rat, the estimated half-life was 12 hr in all groups. In the pig, the estimated half-life was 12 hours in the low and mid-dose groups and 22 hours in the high dose group.

### Genotoxicity Studies

In the Chromosomal Aberration assay the results showed that the SANGUINATE at concentrations of 5, 1.66, and 0.55 mg/mL did not induce statistically significant chromosomal aberrations (does not include chromatid gaps or polyploidy cells) as compared to the negative control group both in the presence and absence of metabolic activation. The confirmatory assay, involving extended exposure of cells to the test substance for 23 hours in the absence of metabolic activation, also showed lack of induction of chromosomal aberrations by the test substance. SANGUINATE was considered non-clastogenic in human peripheral blood lymphocytes. The results of the definitive Ames assay showed that the SANGUINATE did not increase the frequency of revertants at any of the test concentrations in any of the strains tested both in the presence and absence of metabolic activation. The results of the confirmatory assay were consistent with the negative results from the definitive assay. Under the test conditions, the test substance was non-mutagenic in the test species. In the Micronucleus assay there was no statistically significant increase in the frequency of micronucleated PCEs in the test substance dose group as compared to the negative control group. SANGUINATE was considered non-clastogenic, under the experimental conditions.

### Renal Glomerular Filtration Rate

There were no abnormal clinical observations within the study time period to suggest any acute toxic effect of treatment with the test article. Calculated GFR and RBF values were evaluated by ANOVA followed by post hoc group comparison. There were no statistically significant differences in the RBF among groups in males and females at 30 and 60 minutes. For GFR analysis, data from males and females were combined. In general, no statistically significant differences were observed at 30 minutes when groups were compared. Analysis at 60 minutes was not possible due to the small number of samples. Therefore, the SANGUINATE was not observed to produce changes in the inulin and p-aminohippuric acid clearance at the analyzed time points, within 24 hours of single dose intravenous administration in rats.

### Repeat dose toxicity and safety studies

The five-day repeat dose study in rats had no test article related effects on body and organ weight, clinical observations, functional observational battery assessments, food consumption, hematology, coagulation, urinalysis, histopathology, or immunogenicity. Statistically significant differences were observed for several clinical chemistry parameters including increased creatinine (Days 3, 4, 5, 6 and 7), decreased albumin (Days 4 and 5), and decreased alkaline phosphatase activity (Days 6 and 7). No dose trend was recognized on Days 14 and 20. Histopathological results revealed that there were no macroscopic and/or microscopic treatment related findings, and no target organs and /or treatment related findings were determined. Iron staining was observed exclusively in the brain and in the kidneys. The staining intensity detected was minimal to mild in the brain and minimal to moderate in the kidneys. Given the absence of meaningful findings during the functional observational battery assessments and the absence of any test article related microscopic findings, the iron staining observed in the kidney and brain was not considered biologically relevant. The toxicokinetics demonstrated a dose dependent increase in $C_{min}$ values in both males and females, particularly in the Day 5 animals, suggesting a minor risk of accumulation following 5 consecutive days of intravenous dosing of SANGUINATE to rats. Based upon evaluation criteria used for the study, SANGUINATE was considered to be well tolerated up to and including 400 mg/kg after single and after 5 days intravenous administration to Sprague Dawley rats. The NOAEL of SANGUINATE in this study could not be determined as there were no adverse effects at the highest dose level.

In the maximum feasible dose study, treatment related findings were noted in clinical observations, and in the evaluation of clinical pathology and histopathology. There were no adverse effects on body weights. Urine was discolored and there was a slight increase in the WBC and RBC in animals receiving SANGUINATE, PBH, and DPH relative to those receiving NaCl. Clinical signs attributed to treatment within their respective groups included excretion of red/brown fluid from the urogenital area and red fluid/staining around eyes of animals receiving SANGUINATE, PBH and DPH; piloerection in those receiving SANGUINATE and DPH; and abnormal breathing, lethargy, and dehydration were observed in animals receiving DPH. There were changes in hematology parameters considered biologically meaningful and attributed to treatment. When compared to historical values by sex and to the NaCl treated control group, animals treated with SANGUINATE and DPH had changes in the percentage of lymphocytes, an increase in the percentage of neutrophils in both sexes and monocytes in males. A decrease in hemoglobin was also seen after treatment with SANGUINATE, DPH and Hextend. Changes in clinical chemistry parameters and coagulation factors that were significantly different from the NaCl group and did not fall within historical ranges were considered biologically meaningful and attributed to treatment with SANGUINATE, DPH or Hextend. The values of total bilirubin and creatinine were increased and were above ranges for both sexes. Albumin and total protein were significantly decreased in groups treated with SANGUINATE, DPH, and Hextend and cholesterol levels were decreased in Hextend treated females. Microscopic evaluation showed treatment related findings that were limited to the kidneys and heart in both sexes in groups receiving SANGUINATE and DPH. The evaluations defined in the procedure showed that there were overt signs of systemic toxicity following treatment of a 2.4 g/kg dose of SANGUINATE, PBH, and DPH and 60 mL/kg of Hextend.

The majority of assessments evaluated in the six month study in rat showed no specific effects related to Sanguinate. These included body weights, functional observational battery assessments, ophthalmic

exams, food consumption, the amount of oxy- and deoxy-hemoglobin in whole blood, Troponin I, and immunogenicity. Significant adverse clinical observations included prolonged bleeding, which was dose dependent and considered related to treatment with Sanguinate and DPH. Clinical observations in the moribund animals correlated to the prolonged bleeding and may have contributed to the morbidity seen and clinical chemistry findings. Morbidity was considered test article related. Toxicokinetic analysis (Figures 1 and 2) showed a dose dependent pattern in terms of $C_{max}$ and AUC with both reaching peaks in the 2400 mg/kg dose group on Day 1 and in the 400 mg/kg dose group on Days 90 and 180. When adjusted for dose, there appeared to be a linear response in both $C_{max}$ and AUC. The detection of measurable plasma concentrations of PEG-Hemoglobin at the 144 hour time points in the 2400 mg/kg dose groups suggested the possibility of a minor risk of accumulation following a 5 minute intravenous infusion of very high dose Sanguinate to rats. Females of the high volume/high dose test article groups had significant change in clotting parameters while males had a strong trend toward increased clotting times. Urine was brown and contained significant levels of hemoglobin in the high dose/ high volume test article treated groups. Urine volume showed a significant decrease in male animals, however only was significant on Days 121 and 181 in the high dose female group. In the high volume/high dose groups, urine volume decrease was significantly different from the control for both sexes and was attributed to treatment with Sanguinate. This effect was fully recoverable in all groups tested. Statistically significant differences in clinical chemistry included many parameters. Given the moderate and transient effect of some observations, most of these differences were not considered biologically significant. Significant, dose dependent albumin, total protein, total bilirubin, AST, ALP, amylase, calcium, creatinine and BUN effects were seen in both sexes. Recovery groups presented no significant clinical chemistry parameter abnormalities. Liver and kidneys had significant increases in organ weights in relationship to dose. TNF-α findings were not considered specific to treatment, and MDA staining was similarly inconclusive. Iron staining was observed in the brain and kidneys of study animals. Staining in the brain was not considered biologically relevant, but staining of the kidney was much higher for the high volume/high dose Group. Microscopic evaluation of liver and kidneys did not confirm any test article related effects on these or other organs. The immunogenicity data indicated that Sanguinate did not induce an immunogenic response, which was consistent with other PEGylated proteins that have been long approved by the FDA [11]. To summarize, test article related effects were seen with bleeding, early deaths, monocytes, urine volume, clinical chemistry, organ weights, and iron staining. The identification of a NOAEL dose level and target organs for toxicity was inconclusive.

The majority of assessments evaluated in the nine month study in pig showed no specific effects related to SANGUINATE. These included body weights, ophthalmic exams, and the amount of oxy- and deoxy-hemoglobin in whole blood, electrocardiographic exams, and immunogenicity. Some differences in organ weights (heart, liver, adrenal, and brain) were observed, but those differences were not considered biologically relevant. Iron staining was observed in the brain and kidney and in one animal in the carotid aortas and jugular vein, but it was not considered biologically relevant. Immunostaining for TNF-α and MDA in all examined tissues had no clear dose trend and scattered positivity was interpreted as non-test article related. The only clinical sign considered related to treatment with SANGUINATE was diarrhea, observed in 25% of the animals assigned to the 1600 mg/kg SANGUINATE group. The toxicokinetics data (Figures 1 and 2) showed a dose dependent pattern in terms of $C_{max}$ and AUC with both reaching peaks in the 1600 mg/kg dose group on Day 1 and 90 and in the 400 mg/kg dose group on Day 270. When adjusted for dose, there appeared to be a solid linear response in both $C_{max}$ and AUC. Measurable plasma concentrations of PEG-Hb at the 144 hour time points in the 1600 mg/kg dose group were detected on Days 1 and 90. Although slightly elevated plasma concentrations were observed in SANGUINATE (200 mg/kg) treated animals compared to DPH treated animals on Days 90 and 270, there was no remarkable difference observed between the $t_{1/2}$, Tmax, dose adjusted $C_{max}$, and $AUC_{0-\infty}$ between SANGUINATE and DPH treated animals. Selected hematology and clinical chemistry parameters were corrected to account for SANGUINATE interference. Some differences in hematology and clinical chemistry parameters were observed. In addition, a significant increase in prothrombin time and activated partial thromboplastin time was observed in all the test article treated groups compared to their respective controls. None of these differences were considered clinically relevant, given the absence of abnormal clinical observations and histopathological correlates. The immunogenicity data indicated that Sanguinate did not induce an immunogenic response, which was consistent with other PEGylated proteins that have been long approved by the FDA [11]. According with the parameters for the study, there were no adverse effects identified for any dose in this study; therefore, a no observed adverse effects level (NOAEL) could not be determined.

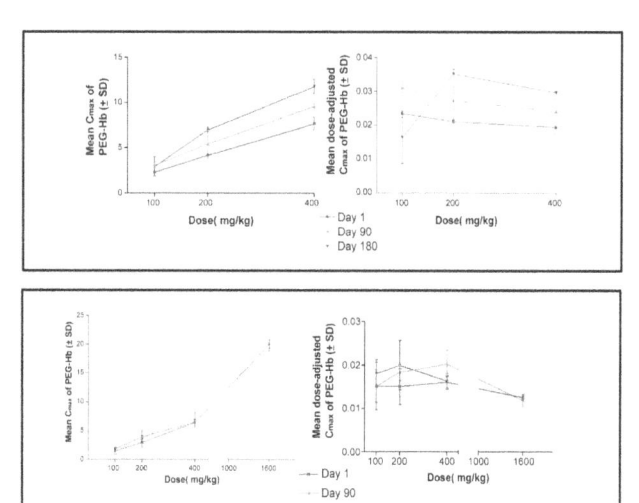

**Figure 2:** Mean $C_{max}$ of SANGUINATE in Rats (6 month study) and Pigs (9 month study).

The acute and repeat dose, intermittent dose effects of SANGUINATE on cardiac, circulatory and pulmonary functions and electrocardiograms (ECG) of conscious telemetered male Cynomogus monkeys were examined. Loose or soft feces were noted in two of four animals on Day 44 24-hours following the first administration of the high dose SANGUINATE at 400 mg/kg. Following the twice a day administration of the total high dose of SANGUINATE (1200 mg/kg/day), observations included delayed/prolonged bleeding times, facial and inguinal erythema, pink skin color, petichiae on the leg, decreased activity and white foamy/frothy feces. Following the additional total high dose of 1200 mg/kg/day on Day 114, clinical observations were limited to small red areas on the abdomen and extremities. Further, no clinical observations were noted on Day 127 with the exception of loose feces for one animal. Clinical chemistry showed no detectable levels of Troponin, increased creatinine, increased BUN, decreased amylase, decreased ALK, and slightly decreased ALT. There were no microscopic findings that indicated direct test article toxicity. Some of the findings may be considered an indication of toxicity in dosed animals from non-instrumentation studies, but there were no untreated or sham control study specific animals to compare microscopic findings against. Administration of 100 and 200 mg/kg SANGUINATE as either single doses or 5 daily doses were not associated with any definitive changes in heart rate, blood pressure, ECG or pulmonary parameters. Administration of 400 mg/kg SANGUINATE was associated with minimal increases in arterial pressure following the first dose and slight increases in heart rate and arterial pressure following the fifth dose. No definitive changes in ECG or pulmonary parameters were noted at the 400 mg/kg dose level. The first day of dosing of the total high dose of SANGUINATE (1200 mg/kg/day) was associated with decreased heart rate and increased arterial pressure but no biologically relevant changes in ECG or pulmonary pressures. Following the fifth day of dosing at 1200 mg/kg/day, increases in heart rate, arterial pressure and QTc were noted as well as decreases in respiratory rate. The additional doses of 1200 mg/kg/day on Day 127 were associated with increased heart rate and pressure but no definitive changes in ECG or pulmonary parameters (Figure 3).

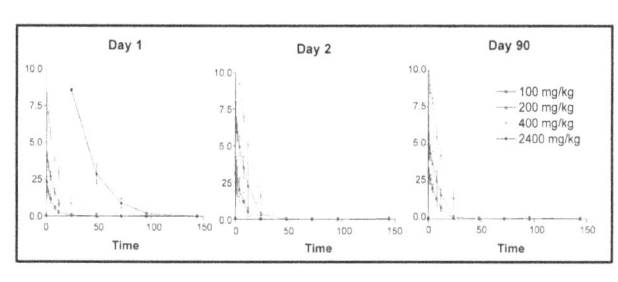

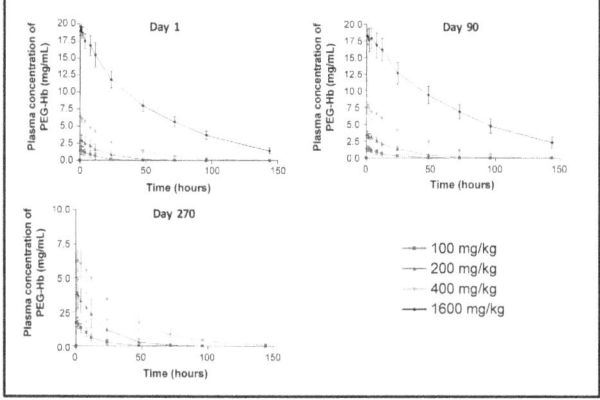

**Figure 1:** Mean Plasma Concentration of SANGUINATE in Rats (6 month study) and Pigs (9 month study).

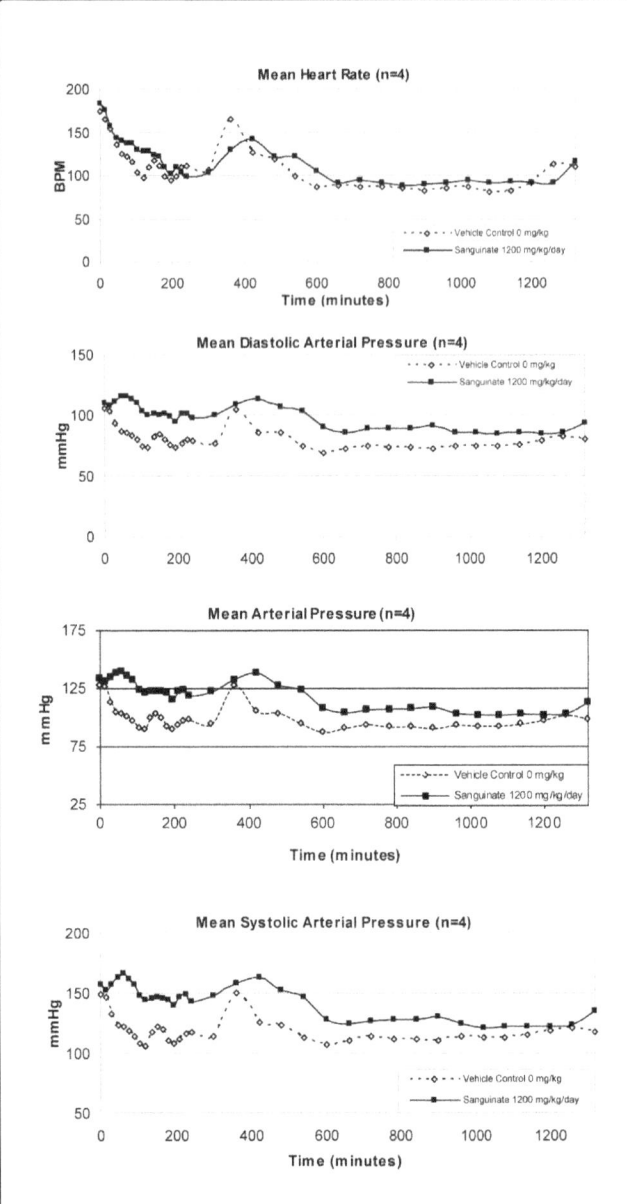

**Figure 3:** Effects of Intravenous Administration of 1200 mg/kg/day SANGUINATE™ Upon Cardiovascular Parameters (Day 127).

## Discussion

Unlike HBOCs, SANGUINATE is both a CO and oxygen delivery agent. Historically, oxygen carriers were under development primarily as blood substitutes for trauma indications. However due to SANGUINATE's unique mechanisms of action, it is under development as an acute and chronic therapeutic for specific indications. As such, the preclinical development program not only had to incorporate the theoretical toxicity concerns of PEG-Hb but address both toxicity concerns of repeat and chronic dosing. Critical to the success of this testing program was not only addressing the concerns that arose from the experiences of HBOC development but establishing a collaborative effort with feedback from the FDA to design a program that would move the program into clinical trials.

Unique features to this program included a renal glomerular filtration rate and blood flow study; immunohistochemical staining for TNF-α (inflammatory marker), malondialdehyde (oxidative marker), and Prussian Blue iron staining in kidneys, myocardium, vasculature, and brain (cerebrum and cerebellum); troponin in the serum; hemoglobin in the urine; high dose/high volume groups; inclusion of toxicity parameters within the cardiovascular safety study in monkey; and interference characterization and correction.

To address the issue as to whether the Hb moiety of SANGUINATE induced inflammation or oxidative stress, two well-characterized markers, TNF-α (an inflammatory marker) and MDA (an oxidative marker) were assessed in the 6 and 9 month rat and pig studies. TNF-α and MDA staining had no dose trend and was not considered to be significant in either the rat or pig, indicating that SANGUINATE is not causing inflammation or oxidative effects in these tissues. To determine whether SANGUINATE contributed to iron deposition, tissue sections from kidneys, myocardium, vasculature, and brain were stained using Prussian blue techniques. Iron staining was present in the brain and kidneys of both rat and pig, particularly in the high dose/high volume group. However, these findings were not considered biologically relevant as further microscopic evaluation of liver and kidneys did not confirm any test article related effects.

The colloidal nature of PEGylated proteins allows SANGUINATE to act as a plasma expander, and dosing levels of SANGUINATE are limited by the volume administered. Therefore, high dose/high volume groups were added to both the 6 and 9 month rat and pig toxicity studies in an attempt to increase the exposure and produce some signs of toxicity. The potential for cardiotoxicity was specifically addressed through the use of clinical chemistry including Troponin, histopathology, ECGs, and a cardiovascular and pulmonary safety study in monkeys. Clinical chemistry or histopathological findings were reversible or were not considered biologically relevant. Although there were some changes in heart rate and blood pressure, there were no definitive changes in ECG or pulmonary parameters. The potential for nephrotoxicity was specifically addressed through a renal glomerular filtration rate and blood flow study, clinical chemistry, urinalysis, measurement of hemoglobin in the urine, the high dose/high volume group, and histopathology. There were no changes in renal glomerular filtration rate or blood flow. Clinical chemistry or histopathological findings were reversible or were not considered biologically relevant. Although urine contained hemoglobin and there were some changes in urine volume, these changes were reversible. Overall, cardiotoxic and nephrotoxic signs were not significant. It is also relevant to note that SANGUINATE was non-immunogenic in both rat and pig.

Despite the history of adverse effects seen with HBOCs, SANGUINATE was well tolerated and safe at doses anticipated for human clinical trials. At dosages up to 400 mg/kg, no significant renal, cardiovascular or pulmonary toxicity was observed nor were there any abnormal body and organ weight measurements, clinical and ophthalmic observations, hematology, serum chemistry, coagulation, urinalysis and histopathology results. At doses of 1200 and 1600 mg/kg, changes in heart rate, arterial pressure and respiration were noted. Although no NOAEL could be determined for SANGUINATE within a study, it is likely to fall between 1200 and 2400 mg/kg. While there were signs of toxicity following dosing at the highest levels, the highest intended dose level for humans is 320 mg/kg infused over 2 hours which is 7 times lower than highest doses provided to animals. Recently three compassionate use eINDs were approved by US-FDA for the treatment of patients with hemoglobin levels below 4 g/dL. These patients received multiple infusions of SANGUINATE and no adverse effects attributable to SANGUINATE were observed. Following infusion of SANGUIANTE, improved cerebral oximetry and status (i.e. ability to responds to commands, reports of "feeling better", discharge from ICU) were observed.

## Conclusion

Chronic toxicology studies used the highest doses and the largest volumes that were permitted by the governing Animal Ethics Committee. As can be seen from the listed reports, Prolong has performed a comprehensive array of short-term and longer-term nonclinical toxicology studies, as well as pharmacology/toxicokinetics studies. Due to its lack of toxicity, a NOAEL could not be determined from these studies, even at doses up to 2400 mg/kg. Toxicity-related findings from the studies, including doses and method of administration, are provided in Table 2. A summary report of histopathology findings from the three long-term preclinical studies (in rat, mini-pig, and non-human primate) explained that, "…no direct toxic test article related macroscopic or microscopic findings were found in the protocol-specified blinded tissues [brain, kidneys, lungs] from these three studies. As no specific test article related dose effect was noted, no NOAEL could be determined for these studies".

As such, the program outlined above was successful. Based on the safety profile, the US FDA as well as other regulatory agencies have approved clinical testing of SANGUINATE in human patients for multiple indications. A phase I study has been completed and is consistent with the preclinical studies. SANGUINATE was found to be safe and well-tolerated in healthy human volunteers at doses of 80 mg/kg, 120 mg/kg, and 160 mg/kg [12]. Multiple doses of SANGUINATE have been used in Sickle Cell patients as well [13,14]. By using rational study design and including additional features to address specific concerns a comprehensive preclinical toxicity and safety program enabled the approval of SANGUINATE for Phase II clinical use worldwide for multiple indications.

## References

1. Guidance for Industry: Criteria for Safety and Efficacy Evaluation of Oxygen Therapeutics as Red Blood Cell Substitutes (2004) FDA.

2. Cabrales P, Friedman JM (2013) HBOC vasoactivity: interplay between nitric oxide scavenging and capacity to generate bioactive nitric oxide species. Antioxid Redox Signal 18: 2284-2297.

3. Natanson C, Kern SJ and Lurie P, Banks SM, Wolfe SM (2008) Cell-free hemoglobin-based blood substitutes and risk of myocardial infarction and death- a meta-analysis. JAMA 299:2304-2312.

4. Gladwin MT, Kanias T, Kim-Shapiro DB (2012) Hemolysis and cell-free hemoglobin drive an intrinsic mechanism for human disease. J Clin Invest 122: 1205-1208.

5. Buehler PW, Baek JH, Lisk C, Connor I, Sullivan T, et al. (2012) Free hemoglobin induction of pulmonary vascular disease: evidence for an inflammatory mechanism. Am J Physiol Lung Cell Mol Physiol 303: L312-326.

6. Tsai AG, Cabrales P, Manjula BN, Acharya SA, Winslow RM, et al. (2006) Dissociation of local nitric oxide concentration and vasoconstriction in the presence of cell-free hemoglobin oxygen carriers. Blood 108: 3603-3610.

7. Chan WL, Tang NL, Yim CC, Lai FM, Tam MS (2000) New features of renal lesion induced by stroma free hemoglobin. Toxicol Pathol 28: 635-642.

8. Zhao T, Yang Y, Zong A, Tan H, Song X, et al. (2012) N-terminal PEGylation of human serum albumin and investigation of its pharmacokinetics and pulmonary microvascular retention. Biosci Trends 6: 81-88.

9. Veronese FM, Pasut G (2005) PEGylation, successful approach to drug delivery. Drug Discov Today 10: 1451-1458.

10. Kanu A, Whitfield J, Leffler CW (2006) Carbon monoxide contributes to hypotension-induced cerebrovascular vasodilation in piglets. Am J Physiol Heart Circ Physiol 291: H2409-2414.

11. Veronese FM, Mero A (2008) The impact of PEGylation on biological therapies. BioDrugs 22: 315-329.

12. Misra H, Lickliter J, Kazo F, Abuchowski A (2014) PEGylated Carboxyhemoglobin Bovine (SANGUINATE™): Results of a Phase I Clinical Trial. Artif Organs.

13. Parmar D (2014) A Case Study of SANGUINATE™ in a Patient with a Comorbidity due to An Underlying Hemoglobinopathy. (2014) J Sickle Cell Dis Hemoglobinopathies.

14. Alaali, Y. Use of Sanguinate in Acute Chest Syndrome. (2014) J Sickle Cell Dis Hemoglobinopathies.

# 6

# Carbon Monoxide Exposure Associated with High-Risk Features and Intentional Exposure are Infrequently Treated with Hyperbaric Oxygen

**Renee L Riggs**[1], **Frederick W Fiesseler**[2*], **Neeraja Kairam**[3], **Lisa Reedman**[3], **Dave Salo**[3] and **Richard Shih**[3]

[1]*Department of Emergency Medicine, UMDNJ-Robert Wood Johnson Medical School at New Brunswick, USA*

[2]*Atlantic Hyperbaric Associates, Morristown New Jersey, USA*

[3]*Department of Emergency Medicine, Morristown Medical Center, USA*

*\*Corresponding author:* Frederick Fiesseler, DO, Department of Emergency Medicine Morristown Medical Center, 100 Madison Avenue, Morristown, NJ 07960, USA, E-mail: ffiesseler@yahoo.com

## Abstract

Data is conflicting regarding the management of carbon monoxide (CO) poisoned patients.

**Objective:** To determine the emergency department management (ED) of intentional CO poisoned patients regarding hyperbaric oxygen therapy (HBO2), compared to those who are unintentionally exposed.

**Methodology**

**Design:** A multi-center retrospective emergency department cohort study.

**Population:** Consecutive patients presenting to 23 Northeastern United States hospital emergency departments, comprising academic, non-academic, urban, suburban, and rural hospitals with the International Classification of Disease primary diagnosis of "toxic effects CO". Patients were "a priori" divided into intentional/unintentional and "high-risk" (syncope, serum carboxyhemoglobin level ≥ 20%, change in mental status, cardiac arrest, and/or seizures) or "low-risk" (without the above).

**Results:** "Toxic effects of CO" was diagnosed in 1136 patients, 1026 charts were available for analysis and 52 (4.8%) met inclusion criteria as intentional.Mean age was 40 years (standard deviation (SD) ± 13), for intentional patients. Overall, high risk intoxication was reported in 12% (N = 124/1026) of patients, compared to 50% (N= 26/52) of the intentional patients (p ≤ 0.0001). Mean overall CO level was 7%, compared to an intentional rate of 17% (p ≤ 0.0001). Fifty percent of intentionally exposed high-risk patients received HBO2, while only 36% (N = 45/124) of high-risk patients overall did (p = 0.27).

**Conclusions:** Carbon monoxide poisoned patients with intentional exposures and high-risk clinical features are not more likely to receive HBO2.

## Introduction

Carbon monoxide (CO) poisoning is the most common cause of toxicological related death in America and worldwide. Between 2000-2009, the National Poison Data System, reported 68,316 CO exposures representing 0.29% of all poison exposure cases [1]. Carbon monoxide exposures comprise 0.02-0.05% of emergency department (ED) visits [2,3]. An important subset of CO exposure patients are those that are intentional. This patient population is speculated to have more co-ingestants, have a greater likelihood of high-risk exposures, have psychiatric illness obscuring subtle CO effects, and have a delayed presentation. Historical data in such patients is often inaccurate, also [4]. All these factors contribute to the complexity of assessing and managing such patients.

Neurological sequela is one of the most dreaded complications related to this toxin [5-7]. A multi-center randomized blinded study reported hyperbaric oxygen therapy to be beneficial in preventing persistent neurological sequelae following carbon monoxide exposure, with a number needed to treat of six [8]. Carbon monoxide's toxic effects are thought to be related to: decreased carrying capacity of oxygen with a leftward shift in the oxyhemoglobin disassociation curve, lipid peroxidation, inhibition of oxidative phosphorylation, and direct myoglobin injury.

Our null hypothesis is that intentional CO poisoned patients receive hyperbaric oxygen therapy more frequently, than those who are not. This study also sought to determine if differences in management of unintentional versus intentional exposures occurred. Specifically, a comparison of the high-risk patient subgroup treatments was analyzed.

## Methodology

### Design

This was a multi-center retrospective ED cohort study.

## Population

It comprised of twenty-three emergency departments in Northeastern United States including academic, non-academic, urban, suburban, and rural hospitals. Six of the contributing hospitals perform hyperbaric oxygen therapy (HBO2). Consecutive patients with the International Classification of Disease (ICD-9) primary diagnosis of intentional "toxic effects of CO," from January 2000 to December 2006 were enrolled.

## Protocol

Patient demographic data was compiled in an Excel (Microsoft, Redmond, WA) spreadsheet. "A priori" patients were divided into four groups: "high-risk" (syncope, serum carboxyhemoglobin level ≥ 20%, changes in mental status, cardiac arrest, and/or seizures), "low-risk" (without the above), intentional exposure and unintentional exposure. The above criteria have previously been shown to be markers of disease severity [9].

## Statistics

Statistical data was performed utilizing a two-tailed Fisher Exact Test and Mann-Whitney, with a preset alpha of 0.05 for significance where appropriate.

A board certified/eligible Emergency Physician or Pediatric Emergency Physician participated in the care of all participants. Medical evaluations were performed as per the discretion of the treating physician. All charts with ICD-9 diagnosis of "carbon monoxide" were extracted using an electronic charting system via web Emergency Medicine Analysis and Reporting System Data Services (eMARS). A manual chart review was then performed by two independent physicians after charts were blinded for personal identifiers. Exclusion criteria included: incorrect ICD9 diagnosis, primary treatment by non-emergency medicine physicians, and chart unavailability. If a disagreement existed regarding mechanism, a third physician made the final determination. The institutional review board approved this study.

## Results

Toxic effects of CO were diagnosed in 1136 patients. Of these 1026 (90.3%) charts were available for analysis. Fifty-two patients (5%) met inclusion criteria as intentional exposures. Fifty-one of the patient exposures occurred from auto exhaust, the remaining one via a charcoal briquette fire. Mean age of intentional exposures was 40 years (standard deviation (SD) ± 13), compared with an overall mean age of 30 years (SD ± 20). Sixty-six percent of intentional exposures were male, and compared with an overall female predominance of 59% (Table 1).

| Characteristics of intoxicated patients | Types of intoxication | | | |
|---|---|---|---|---|
| | Intentional | Overall1 | Intentional high risk | Overall high risk |
| Total number of males and females | 52 | 1026 | 26 | 124 |
| Mean age (years) | 40 | 30 | 41 | 40 |
| Number of females (%) | 18 (34) | 603 (59) | 8 (31) | 40 (32) |
| Number of patients admitted/ transferred (%) | 28/10 (73) | 91/33 (12) | 18 (69) | 76 (61) |
| Number of "High risk" patients[2] (%) | 26 (50) | 124 (12) | 26 | 124 |
| Number of HBO2 therapy (%) | 12 (23) | 56 (5) | 13 (50) | 45 (36) |
| Number of EKG recorded (%) | 29 (56) | 182 (18) | 16 (62) | 76 (61) |
| Number of arterial blood draw (%) | 26 (48) | 241 (23) | 16 (62) | 58 (47) |
| Number of use of serum cardiac markers (%) | 10 (19) | 61 (6) | 6 (23) | 26 (21) |
| Number of patients with repeat COHb (%) | 10 (19) | 74 (7) | 6 (23) | 32 (26) |
| Mean COHb | 17% | 7% | 26% | 22% |

**Table 1:** Characteristics of intentional and unintentional carbon monoxide intoxicated patients.

[1]Intentional and unintentional (i.e. accidental) intoxications.

[2]Carboxyhemoglobin level higher than 20%, syncope, change in mental status, cardiac arrest, and/or seizures.

COHb: Serum Carboxyhemoglobin level; HBO2: Hyperbaric Oxygen Therapy; EKG: Electrocardiogram; N: Number of individuals.

Mean CO level was 7% (95% CI = 0-20) overall, compared to the intentional exposure level of 17% (95% CI = 1-33%) (p ≤ 0.0001). With regard to intentional exposures: admission occurred in 73% of patients with 61% being admitted to a psychiatric floor. Of admitted intentional patients, those with medical admissions had a mean CO level of 13% (95% CI = 2-24%) compared to a level of 18% (95% CI = 10-26%) in those admitted to psychiatry.

High-risk intoxication was reported in 12% (N = 124/1026) of patients, and comprised 50% (N = 26/52) of the intentional patients (p ≤ 0.0001). Etiology for intentional high-risk stratification included: elevated CO level (N = 14), syncope (N = 17), cardiac arrest (N = 3), change in mental status (N = 4) and seizures (N = 2). Intentional high-risk patients had a co-ingestion rate of 25%, which was identical to the low-risk intentional group. Three patients died while in the ED overall, all within the intentional high-risk group, with a mean CO level of 52%.

Overall, high-risk patients, had an electrocardiogram (EKG) assessed 61% (N = 76/124) of the time, versus 62% (N = 16/26) in the intentionally exposed group (p = 1).Overall, twenty-one percent (N = 26/124) of high-risk patients had cardiac serum markers reported, compared to an intentional rate of 24% (p = 0.80).

Of intentional patients, oxygen therapy was initiated in 91%, with 16% requiring intubation. Overall, 36% (N = 45/124) of high risk patients received HBO2 compared with an intentional rate of 50% (p = 0.27) (Table 2).

| Baseline characteristics in intoxicated patients | Mean age (years) | Male gender (%) | Mean COHb (%) | Intubation (%) |
|---|---|---|---|---|
| Intentional HBO2 therapy | 38 | 70 | 22 | 4 |
| Unintentional HBO2 therapy | 40 | 68 | 22 | 6 |
| Intentional NMBO2 therapy | 40 | 56 | 14 | 12 (50% died) |
| Unintentional NMBO2 therapy | 32 | 44 | 7 | 1 |
| Intentional, no O2 | 35 | 70 | 5 | 0 |
| Unintentional, no O2 | 24 | 42 | 2.5 | 0 |

**Table 2:** Baseline characteristics based on treatment in carbon monoxide intoxicated patients.

$HBO_2$: Hyperbaric Oxygen Therpay; $NMBO_2$: Normobaric Oxygen Therapy; $O_2$: Oxygen; COHb: Serum Carboxyhemoglobin Level

## Discussion

Utilization of HBO2 in CO poisoned patients while remaining controversial is thought to be most beneficial in high-risk patients. In fact, the latest "Cochrane Collaboration" authors conclusion states, "Existing randomized trials do not establish whether the administration of HBO2 to patients with carbon monoxide poisoning reduces the incidence of adverse neurologic outcomes. Additional research is needed to better define the role, if any, of HBO2 in the treatment of patients with carbon monoxide poisoning" [10]. Conversely, Weaver gave HBO2 therapy for CO poisoning a level of evidence of "A" (Meta-analysis of randomized controlled trials) and a class recommendation of IIa (weight of evidence/opinion is in favor of usefulness/efficacy) in his review of the subject [11]. This study found that only 36% of high risk patients received HBO2 therapy compared to 50% (not statistically significant) of high risk intentional exposure cases.

Intentional CO exposed patients may have subtle neurological deficits overlooked because of underlying psychiatric confounding factors (attention, concentration, and affect disorders), and poor cooperation. In these patients the threshold for treatment may need to be lowered. Conversely, one could intuit that if co-ingestions are present causing clinical symptoms such as alteration in mental status, a higher threshold for treatment may be utilized. Unfortunately, little information is available regarding this issue and more research is required to determine which intentionally overdosed patients would benefit most from this therapy and the effects of co-ingestions on treatment protocols.

A significant number of patients that are seen in the emergency department comprise CO exposure. Our intentional CO exposure rate of 4.8 percent was far less than that of Weaver 31% and Scheinkestel 69% [8,12]. This study depicts the incidence of patients presenting to the ED, while most prior studies represent subjects referred from other institutions for HBO2, a different patient population. Hampson also demonstrated an intentional source of CO poisoning of 35% in those

patients treated at their facility, again this depicts a different subset from our ED population [13]. Most prior studies regarding intentional CO exposure and treatment depict those referred for HBO2 therapy and not those presenting to the ED.

HBO2 while thought to be beneficial is not without potential deleterious consequences. Confounding factors such as: availability, oxygen toxicity, barotrauma, risk of transport, and cost need to be tabulated. Each individual patient needs to be evaluated uniquely as to his/her risk stratification regarding these factors. Data remains conflicted regarding the management of carbon monoxide (CO) poisoned patients [8,12,14-18].

The cardiovascular system, a primary organ system susceptible to injury, was examined with EKG or cardiac serum enzymes in only 61% of high-risk patients. Historically, thirty percent of severely exposed patients demonstrate abnormal EKG's and 35% have abnormal cardiac markers [19]. Henry also demonstrated an incidence of abnormal cardiac markers/kg of 37% in HBO2 treated patients. Importantly, patients with elevated cardiac serum markers had a hazard ratio of 2.1 of dying (p=0.009) [20].Patients with high-risk CO intoxication should have EKG and cardiac marker testing. Our data suggests that less than adequate cardiac assessment is occurring in these patients.

Three patients in our study had cardiac arrest in the ED. All three patients ultimately died. Short-term mortality is only one concern regarding this disease process. Long-term increased mortality rates among survivors of CO poisoning has also recently been appreciated. Hampson reported on 162 subject deaths in long-term follow-up, while the expected number was only 87. Most of the excess mortality was in the group treated for intentional poisoning. Both short and long-term mortality is a concern in intentionally intoxicated patients [13].

Lastly, our study is not without limitations. Weaver demonstrated that greater than half of those patients with severe CO intoxication develop symptoms of persistent neurological sequelae [8]. Unfortunately, our study was unable to assess neurological sequelae. Physicians need to be more cognizant of the potential for persistent/delayed neurological sequelae and the utility of HBO2. As with all retrospective studies, important information is often not collected or recorded. Inaccuracy of data secondary to patient/ physician inaccuracies can also occur. One could speculate that our large study population limits these effects. In addition, patient morbidity and mortality outcomes data was not available. Further studies are needed to determine why some patients are referred for HBO2 therapy while others are not. Standardized evidence based treatment and referral protocols might be beneficial. It is possible that patients who would likely benefit from this treatment are not being referred for such care.

## Conclusion

Carbon monoxide poisoned patients with intentional exposures and high-risk clinical features are not significantly more likely to receive HBO2 therapy.

## References

1. Centers for Disease Control and Prevention (CDC) (2011) Carbon monoxide exposures--United States, 2000-2009. MMWR Morb Mortal Wkly Rep 60: 1014-1017.

2. Partrick M, Fiesseler F, Shih R, Riggs R, Hung O (2009) Monthly variations in the diagnosis of carbon monoxide exposures in the emergency department. Undersea Hyperb Med 36: 161-167.

3. Hampson NB (1998) Emergency department visits for carbon monoxide poisoning in the Pacific Northwest. J Emerg Med 16: 695-698.

4. ApterA, Horesh N, Gothelf D, Graffi H, Lepkifker E (2001) Relationship between self-disclosure and serious suicidal behavior. Compr Psychiatry 42: 70-75.

5. Ernst A, Zibrak JD (1998) Carbon monoxide poisoning. N Engl J Med 339: 1603-1608.

6. Weaver LK (2009) Clinical practice. Carbon monoxide poisoning. N Engl J Med 360: 1217-1225.

7. Choi IS (1983) Delayed neurologic sequelae in carbon monoxide intoxication. Arch Neurol 40: 433-435.

8. Weaver LK, Hopkins RO, Chan KJ, Churchill S, Elliott CG, et al. (2002) Hyperbaric oxygen for acute carbon monoxide poisoning. N Engl J Med 347: 1057-1067.

9. KK Jain (2004) Textbook of Hyperbaric Medicine. Hogrefe & Huber Publishers, Cambridge MA, USA.

10. Buckley NA, Juurlink DJ, Isbister G, et al. (2011) Hyperbaric oxygen for carbon monoxide poisoing. Cochrane Database Syst Rev. 4.

11. Weaver LK (2011) Hyperbaric oxygen in the critically ill. Crit Care Med 39: 1784-1791.

12. Scheinkestel CD, Bailey M, Myles PS, Jones K, Cooper DJ, et al. (1999) Hyperbaric or normobaric oxygen for acute carbon monoxide poisoning: a randomised controlled clinical trial. Med J Aust 170: 203-210.

13. Hampson NB, Rudd RA, Hauff NM (2009) Increased long-term mortality among survivors of acute carbon monoxide poisoning. Crit Care Med 37: 1941-1947.

14. Tibbles PM, Perrotta PL (1994) Treatment of carbon monoxide poisoning: a critical review of human outcome studies comparing normobaric oxygen with hyperbaric oxygen. Ann Emerg Med 24: 269-276.

15. Mathieu D, Wattel F, Mathieu-Nolf M, et al. (1996) Randomized prospective study comparing the effect of HBO vs. 12 hours NBO in non-comatose CO-poisoned patients: results of the preliminary analysis. Undersea Hyperb Med 7.

16. Raphael JC, Elkharrat D, Jars-Guincestre MC, Chastang C, Chasles V, et al. (1989) Trial of normobaric and hyperbaric oxygen for acute carbon monoxide intoxication. Lancet 2: 414-419.

17. Raphael JC, Chevret S, Driheme A, et al. (2004) Managing carbon monoxide poisoning with hyperbaric oxygen (Abstract) J ToxicolClinToxicol. 42: 455-456.

18. Thom SR, Taber RL, Mendiguren II, Clark JM, Hardy KR, et al. (1995) Delayed neuropsychologic sequelae after carbon monoxide poisoning: prevention by treatment with hyperbaric oxygen. Ann Emerg Med 25: 474-480.

19. Satran D, Henry CR, Adkinson C, Nicholson CI, Bracha Y, et al. (2005) Cardiovascular manifestations of moderate to severe carbon monoxide poisoning. J Am Coll Cardiol 45: 1513-1516.

20. Henry CR, Satran D, Lindgren B, Adkinson C, Nicholson CI, et al. (2006) Myocardial injury and long-term mortality following moderate to severe carbon monoxide poisoning. JAMA 295: 398-402.

# 7

# Case Series of Overdosed Patients Managed in an Observation Unit

Kristen Rizzo[1*], Paul Dominici[1], Adam Rowden[1], Jonathan Abraham[1], Kathryn T Kopec[2], Henry Swoboda[3], Milciades A Mirre-Gonzalez[1], Abdullah Khalid[4], Kathia Damiron[1] and Chris Villaflor[1]

[1]Department of Emergency Medicine, Albert Einstein Medical Center, Philadelphia, PA, United States

[2]Department of Emergency Medicine, Duke University Hospital, PA, United States

[3]Department of Emergency Medicine, Rush University Medical Center, PA, United States

[4]Department of Emergency Medicine, UPMC Mercy, PA, United States

*Corresponding author: Rizzo k, Albert Einstein Medical Center, Philadelphia, PA, United States, E-mail: kristen.lasher@gmail.com

## Abstract

**Background:** Observation units (OU) are an increasing aspect of hospitals in the United States. OU provide more efficient use of resources in an increasingly taxed healthcare system. The majority of poisoned patients' medical issues resolve within 24 hours, making them ideal candidates for an OU. The purpose of this study was to examine the types and safety of overdoses placed in our OU at Einstein Medical Center Philadelphia, an urban, level one trauma center with 100,000 emergency department (ED) visits annually in Philadelphia, Pennsylvania. We hypothesized that the majority of patients admitted to the OU do not require further medical intervention or upgrading to a higher level of care.

**Methods:** The study is a retrospective chart review of patients with ICD-9 codes associated with overdose or poisoning admitted to our OU between 7/1/10 and 12/31/12. A total of 137 patients were identified, 112 were included. Exclusions were: admission to the hospital prior to transfer to OU (17); transfer to psychiatry (4); miscoded (2); and seen at another site (2). Research associates, reviewed medical charts using a structured data collection form to record disposition, age, gender, etnicity, ingested substances, mental status, medical interventions and any upgrades in disposition.

**Results:** Between 7/1/10 and 12/31/12 there were 112 patients admitted to the OU. Patient's age ranged from 17 to 76 years old (mean 38), with 46 males (41%) and 66 females (59%). Ethnicity was mostly African American 73 (65%). A total of 230 different substances were recorded with 61 (26.5%) patients taking more than one intoxicant. The most common overdoses were sedative- hypnotics 66 (28.7%) and antipsychotics 22 (9.6%). Initial OU mental status recorded was: alert and oriented to person, place and time 60 (54%); 46 (41%) sedated, and 6 (5%) confused. The most common medical interventions in the ED were sedatives 18 (16%) and naloxone 12 (10.7%). The most common medical interventions in the OU were: sedatives 24 (21.4%); oxygen 10 (8.9%); and naloxone 5 (4.5%). No intubations or cardiac arrests occurred in the ED or OU. No patients were upgraded to a higher level of care. Seven patients were transferred to psychiatry.

**Conclusions:** The disposition of stable patients to an OU who present to the ED after overdoses appears to be safe. Understanding the types of overdoses that are safe to be managed in an OU can assist in disposition, patient flow, use of resources, and provide appropriate level of care.

**Keywords:** Observation unit; Overdose; Poisoning

## Introduction

Observation units (OU) have become more prevalent in hospitals across the United States (US). Observation units provide a monitored setting for patients with a medical condition that is likely to improve within 24 hours and that do not require an inpatient setting. Cooke et al. suggested that the development of observation units has helped emergency department (ED) flow and time management as well as potentially improving the bed flow throughout the hospital by concentrating resources [1-3]. Even with the increasing number of observation units across the US, healthcare is still trying to determine how to best utilize them. Poisoned or overdosed patients tend to have acute medical issues that often improve within 24 hours of presentation [2,4-6]. Although there are multiple types of overdoses

and poisonings with varying clinical presentations, these patients may be ideal candidates for an observational unit setting. Few studies have been done to evaluate these patients and their clinical course during an observation unit stay.

Hodgkinson et al. evaluated the types of patients that had been poisoned or overdosed on various medications and were monitored in the observation unit attached to the emergency department. The study demonstrated very infrequent upgrading of patients to a full admission status and a likely resolution of clinical symptoms within 24 hours [4]. Sztajnkycer et al. attempted to create an observation unit protocol for overdose patients who showed early success in their study, however they noted the need for further studies with increased patient numbers to validate their findings [7]. Calello et al. examined the use of the observation unit at a pediatric tertiary care center for overdosed or poisoned children, the majority of whom were exposed to cardiovascular and psychoactive drugs. It was found that only 5% of those patients were changed to full admission status, including two unexpected admissions for charcoal aspiration pneumonitis [2].

Beauchamp et al. launched a protocol for the treatment of low-risk APAP overdoses in the OU with 20-hour IV N-acetylcysteine. Patients in his protocol had shorter length of stays than admitted patients with the same diagnosis. Patients who were considered low risk were admitted to the OU if they had normal initial liver enzymes, and elevated APAP levels (above Rumack-Matthew nomogram treatment line). Of these, 65% were discharged from the OU without incident following repeat lab values; 35% were subsequently admitted for elevated LFTs [1].

These studies help support that an observation unit may be an ideal and safe clinical management location for selected overdose patients. However, further studies are needed to help define the specific types of overdoses that are safe to be managed in the observation unit. Understanding the types of overdoses that are safe to be managed in an observation unit can assist in better disposition determination and improved patient flow for a hospital, more efficient use of hospital resources, in addition to providing improved care for the patient. The purpose of this study was to examine the types and safety of overdoses placed in our OU. We hypothesized that the majority of patients admitted to the OU would not require further medical intervention or upgrading to a higher level of care.

## Methods

We performed a retrospective chart review of patients with ICD-9 codes associated with overdose or poisoning admitted to our OU between 7/1/10 and 12/31/12. These patients were admitted through the ED at Einstein Medical Center Philadelphia, an urban, level one trauma center with 100,000 ED visits per year. The OU is an 18 bed unit capable of centralized cardiac monitoring staffed 24 hours daily by mid-level providers with supervision provided by board certified medical toxicologists. There is a toxicology service provided by emergency medicine residents, toxicology fellows and toxicology attending physicians available for consultation as needed in the ED, the OU, as well as throughout the hospital.

The primary endpoint was to determine if those patients placed in the OU were appropriate for management in the OU as opposed to needing full admission to the hospital. Patients deemed safe for observation level management included those with stable vital signs, no significant mental status or respiratory depression requiring intervention and clinical determination by the physician involved with the case. The type of substance involved with the overdose or poisoning was also evaluated.

The following information was collected from the chart: age, gender, ethnicity, past medical history, allergies, home medications, substance used in that visit's overdose or poisoning, vital signs, neurologic status (GCS), clinical signs of intoxication, if medical interventions were needed (including antidote administration, oxygen administration, dialysis or intubation), accu-check, urine drug screen (UDS), lactate, and renal function. It was noted if patients required transition to a higher level of care after their arrival in the OU.

A total of 137 patients were identified, 112 were included. Exclusions were: admission to the hospital prior to transfer to the OU (17); transfer to psychiatry (4); miscoded (2); and seen at other site within the hospital system (2). Research associates reviewed medical charts using a structured data collection form. A second reviewer confirmed the collection of the data obtained from the medical record.

## Results

Between 7/1/10 and 12/31/12 there were a total of 566 patients admitted to the hospital for selected ICD-9 codes. 20% or 112 patients in total were admitted to the OU. Patients' ages ranged from 17 to 76 years old, demographics details are displayed in Table 1.

| Age (years) | |
|---|---|
| Mean | 38.07 |
| Range | 17 to 76 |
| **Sex** | |
| Male | 46 (41.1%) |
| Female | 66 (58.9%) |
| **Race** | |
| AA | 73 (65.2%) |
| White | 21 (18.8%) |
| Hispanic | 13 (11.6%) |
| Asian | 4 (3.6%) |
| Other | 1 (0.9%) |

**Table 1:** Demographics.

Patients reported 230 agents, the most common of which were sedatives. Sixty-one of the 112 patients (54%) admitted to taking more than one agent as detailed on Figure 1.

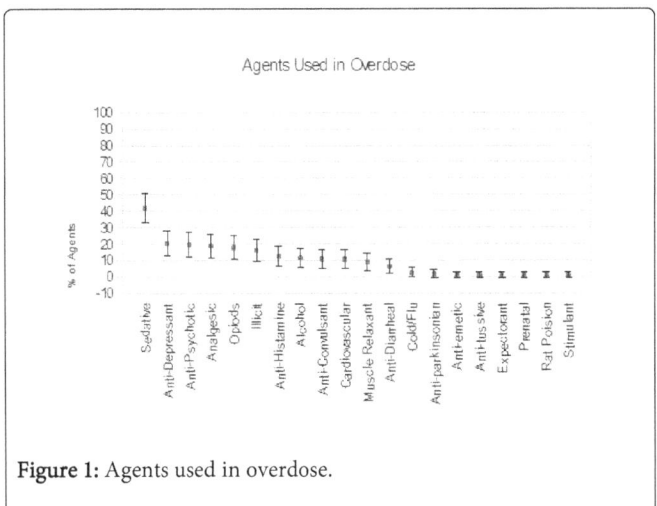

**Figure 1:** Agents used in overdose.

Patients presented with a wide variety of past medical histories; four of the top five most common diagnoses are psychiatric in nature, including depression, suicide attempts, substance abuse and bipolar disorder (Table 2).

| Agent | Frequency | % | CI (95%) | Range |
|---|---|---|---|---|
| Sedative | 47 | 41.96 | 9.14 | 32.82%-51.1% |
| Anti-depressant | 23 | 20.54 | 7.48 | 13.06%-28.02% |
| Anti-psychotic | 22 | 19.64 | 7.36 | 12.28%-27% |
| Analgesic | 21 | 18.75 | 7.23 | 11.52%-25.98% |
| Opoid | 20 | 17.86 | 7.09 | 10.77%-24.95% |
| Illicit | 18 | 16.07 | 6.8 | 9.27%-22.87% |
| Anti-histamine | 14 | 12.5 | 6.12 | 6.38%-18.62% |
| Alcohol | 13 | 11.61 | 5.93 | 5.68%-17.54% |
| Anti-convulsant | 12 | 10.71 | 5.73 | 4.98%-16.44% |
| Cardiovascular | 12 | 10.71 | 5.73 | 4.98%-16.44% |
| Muscle Relaxant | 10 | 8.93 | 5.28 | 3.65%-14.21% |
| Anti-diarrheal | 7 | 6.25 | 4.48 | 1.77%-10.73% |
| Cold/Flu | 3 | 2.68 | 2.99 | -0.31%-5.67% |
| Anti-parkinsonian | 2 | 1.79 | 2.46 | -0.67%-4.25% |
| Antiemetic | 1 | 0.89 | 1.74 | -0.85%-2.63% |
| Antitussive | 1 | 0.89 | 1.74 | -0.85%-2.63% |
| Expectorant | 1 | 0.89 | 1.74 | -0.85%-2.63% |
| Prenatal | 1 | 0.89 | 1.74 | -0.85%-2.63% |
| Rat Poison | 1 | 0.89 | 1.74 | -0.85%-2.63% |
| Stimulant | 1 | 0.89 | 1.74 | -0.85%-2.63% |
| Total | 230 | | | |

**Table 2:** Agents used in overdose.

The most common medical interventions in the OU were: sedatives (21%); oxygen (9%); and naloxone (4%). No intubations or cardiac arrests occurred in the ED or OU. No patients were upgraded to a higher level of care after arrival to the OU. Seven patients were transferred to psychiatry. The frequency of observation unit interventions is noted in Figure 2 and Table 3.

Patients who received OU care had initial GCS scores of 12-15 with low scores throughout their hospital stay ranging from 6-15. The majority of scores (57%) were 15, however 12% of GCS scores were less than 13, suggesting a significant level of altered mental status at some point during the clinical course. Based on the 112 patients, 45% did have altered mental status and 46% were noted to have an abnormal vital sign at some point during their course of treatment. The most common interventions in the OU included monitoring, including telemetry, EKG and repeat laboratory evaluations. Suicidal or assault precautions, which included 1 to 1 monitoring and restraints were also common as self-harm was a common etiology for adult poisonings and overdoses. Other common interventions included

sedatives, most commonly benzodiazepines, and haloperidol less frequently (Table 4).

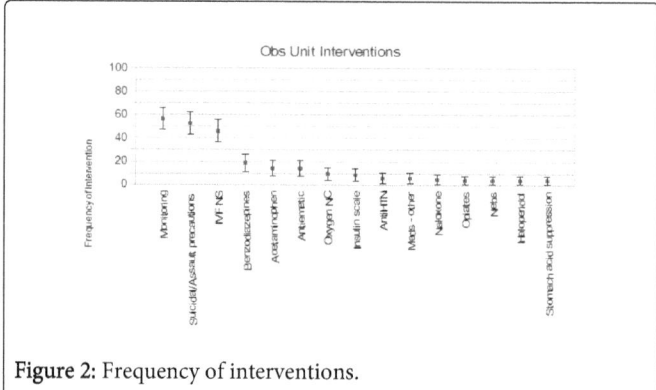

**Figure 2:** Frequency of interventions.

| | Frequency | Percent | CI 95% | Range* |
|---|---|---|---|---|
| Depression | 55 | 49.1 | ± 9.26 | 39.84% to 58.36% |
| Suicidal Attempt | 39 | 34.8 | ± 8.82 | 25.98% to 43.62% |
| HTN | 35 | 31.3 | ± 8.58 | 22.62% to 39.78% |
| Substance Abuse | 33 | 29.5 | ± 8.45 | 21.05% to 37.95% |
| Bipolar Disorder | 24 | 21.4 | ± 7.6 | 13.8% to 29% |
| COPD/Asthma | 20 | 17.9 | ± 7.1 | 10.8% to 25% |
| Diabetes | 19 | 17.0 | ± 6.96 | 10.04% to 23.96% |
| Schizophrenia | 13 | 11.61 | ± 5.93 | 5.68% to 17.54% |
| Anxiety | 11 | 9.82 | ± 5.51 | 4.31% to 15.33% |
| HCV | 9 | 8.04 | ± 5.04 | 3% to 13.08% |
| Seizures | 8 | 7.1 | ± 4.76 | 2.34% to 11.86% |
| HIV | 6 | 5.36 | ± 4.17 | 1.19% to 9.53% |

Table 3: Past medical history.

| Interventions | Frequency | % | CI | Range |
|---|---|---|---|---|
| Monitoring | 60 | 56.6 | 9.44 | 47.16%-66.04% |
| Suicide/Assault Precautions | 56 | 52.83 | 9.5 | 43.33%-62.33% |
| IV Fluids (Normal saline) | 49 | 46.23 | 9.49 | 36.74%-55.72% |
| Benzodiazepines | 20 | 18.87 | 7.45 | 11.42%-26.32% |
| Acetaminophen | 15 | 14.15 | 6.64 | 7.51%-20.79% |
| Antiemetic | 15 | 14.15 | 6.64 | 7.51%-20.79% |
| Oxygen (Nasal cannula) | 10 | 9.43 | 5.56 | 3.87%-14.99% |
| Insulin (scale) | 9 | 8.49 | 5.31 | 3.18%-13.8% |
| Anti-HTN | 6 | 5.66 | 4.4 | 1.26%-10.06% |
| Meds-other | 6 | 5.66 | 4.4 | 1.26%-10.06% |
| Naloxone | 5 | 4.72 | 4.04 | 0.68%-8.76% |
| Opiates | 4 | 3.77 | 3.63 | 0.14%-7.4% |
| Nebulizations | 4 | 3.77 | 3.63 | 0.14%-7.4% |
| Haloperidol | 4 | 3.77 | 3.63 | 0.14%-7.4% |
| Stomach acid suppression | 4 | 3.77 | 3.63 | 0.14%-7.4% |

Table 4: Interventions.

## Discussion

Acutely poisoned patients often require care for a limited period of time, often less than 24 hours, as the intoxicant is metabolized. While co-ingestants or unclear histories may lead to longer periods of care, most ingestion requires only supportive care for a finite length of time that is well suited to an OU. Furthermore, an OU provides an opportunity for consultations, including toxicology, psychiatry and social work to evaluate and provide disposition assistance separate from the pressures of a chaotic emergency department.

Three antidotes were utilized in the OU, but their use was continued from the emergency department. Four patients were started on n-acetyl cysteine (NAC), three of whom continued this in the OU; two patients received bicarbonate in the ED, one of whom continued this in the OU; 12 patients required naloxone in the ED and five patients required additional doses in the OU. The cardiac monitoring of the OU allows the provider to be vigilant for the need for additional antidote medication. While no antidotes were initiated in the OU, the availability of toxicology consultants allows for discussion and possible initiation for appropriate patients. One patient did require dialysis for an aspirin overdose in the OU, under the guidance of the toxicology service.

The direct supervision of the OU by medical toxicologists and the availability of toxicology consultation may have played a direct role in the severity and number of cases managed successfully by the OU. No patient required airway intervention or was upgraded to a higher level of care. The individual comfort level of the observation unit staff will depend on resources and experience. Conceivably, not every OU will be comfortable with a patient requiring first-time dialysis for toxic ingestion. Still others will not want to manage or initiate antidote medication.

## Limitations

This is a retrospective chart review and data collectors were not blinded to the purpose of the project. The OU at this academic center was supervised by medical toxicologists and the results may not be generalizable to other OUs.

## Conclusions

The disposition of stable patients to an OU who present to the ED after undifferentiated OD appears to be safe. Additionally, observation units may be appropriate settings for patients who are not recovered enough to be discharged to home after the standard 4-6 observation period and do not require admission to the hospital. Understanding the types of overdoses that are safe to be managed in an OU can assist in appropriate disposition, patient flow, efficient use of resources, and provide the best level of care for the patient.

## References

1. Beauchamp GA, Hart KW, Lindsell CJ, et al. (2013) Performance of a multi-disciplinary emergency department observation protocol for acetaminophen overdose. J Med Toxicol 9: 235-241.

2. Calello DP, Alperm ER, McDaniel-Yakscoe M, et al. (2009) Observation unit experience for pediatric poison exposures. J Med Toxicol 5: 15-19.

3. Cooke MW, Higgins J, Kidd P (2003) Use of emergency department observation and assessment wards: a systematic literature review. Emerg Med J 20: 138-142.

4. Hodgkinson DW, Jellett LB, Ashby RH (1991) A review of the management of oral drug overdose in the Accident and Emergency Department of the Royal Brisbane Hospital. Arch of Emerg Med 8: 8-16.

5. Hollander JE, McCracken G, Johnson S, et al. (1999) Emergency department observation of poisoned patients: how long is necessary? Acad Emerg Med 6: 887-894.

6. Koylu R, Dundar ZD, Koylu O, et al. (2014) The experience in a toxicology unit: a review of 623 cases. J Clin Med Res 6: 59-65.

7. Sztajnkrycer MD, Mell HK, Melin GJ (2007) Development and implementation of an emergency department observation unit protocol for deliberate drug ingestion in adults – preliminary results. Clin Tox45: 499-504.

# 8

# Detection of Retinal Changes in Patients on Long Term Chloroquine/Hydroxy Chloroquine Therapy using Optical Coherence Tomography

Pratyusha G, Shashi Ahuja* and VS Negi

*Department of Ophthalmology, JIPMER, Puducherry, India*

*Corresponding author: Shashi Ahuja Associate Professor, Department of Ophthalmology, JIPMER, Puducherry, India, E-mail: drshashiahuja@gmail.com

## Abstract

**Background:** The best technique to diagnose chloroquine/ hydroxychloroquine-induced retinopathy changes at the earliest remains ambiguous at present. In this study, we evaluated the time-domain optical coherence tomography (OCT) to identify retinal changes associated with chloroquine and hydroxychloroquine.

**Methods:** One hundred patients with immunological diseases were included in the study. Fifty of them had been on chloroquine and/or hydroxychloroquine therapy for at least five years and the other 50 patients as controls. Detailed ophthalmic examination including Amsler grid , colour vision , automated threshold white perimetry using 10-2 protocol on Humphrey field analyzer, fluorescein angiography when indicated and time domain Optical Coherence Tomography was done.

**Results:** A statistically significant thinning was noted in the superior and inferior quadrants of the parafoveal area. Six patients had changes in fundus. When cases with normal and abnormal fundus were analyzed individually, a statistically significant thinning was noted in the inferior parafoveal region in patients on chloroquine/ hydroxychloroquine having normal fundus when compared to the controls Amsler grid, colour vision, central 10-2 perimetry, FFA were all normal in these patients. There was no significant retinal nerve fiber layer thinning in the peripapillary region Temporal macular thickness was significantly thinner in patients who received the drugs for more than 8 years.

**Conclusions:** Time domain OCT can be used to detect pre- clinical changes of chloroquine/ hydroxychloroquine -induced retinopathy. All patients on long term use of these drugs must undergo regular examinations to diagnose early toxicity.

**Keywords:** Retinopathy; Chloroquine Toxicity; Hydroxychloroquine toxicity; Optical coherence tomography

## Introduction

Chloroquine, a 4-amino quinoline compound has long been used in the treatment and prevention of malaria. Hydroxy chloroquine is a hydroxylated analogue of chloroquine. Of late, these drugs are being used as disease modifying antirheumatic agents (DMARD) in diseases like rheumatoid arthritis and systemic lupus erythematosis [1].

Savarino et al. [2] showed that both chloroquine and hydroxychloroquine can cause retinal toxicity, but the potential seems to be lesser with hydroxy chloroquine. This has been supported by experimental studies which have shown that hydroxy chloroquine is a less potent enhancer of lipofuscinogenesis compared to chloroquine in the retinal pigment epithelial cells [3]. It has also been documented that both the drugs block activation of Toll like receptors (TLR) on dendritic cells and inhibit the TLR signaling [4-6]. HCQ retinopathy has been reported in more than 1% of patients after 5-7 years of usage of the drug and its incidence did not correlate with the age, daily dose or the weight of the patient [7].

Over years, several tests have been used to diagnose chloroquine retinopathy, which include Amsler grid testing, colour vision testing, and central visual field charting [2-10]. Recent studies with spectral domain Optical Coherence Tomography (SD-OCT), multifocal Electro-retinogram (mf ERG), fundus auto fluorescence show promising results in the early detection of chloroquine toxicity [8,9]. The role of time-domain OCT in establishing the diagnosis remains inconclusive, though, in a recent case report , there were suggestions of early chloroquine toxicity even on time Domain OCT [10].

The current study is designed to evaluate changes in macular and peripapillary retinal nerve fiber layers in using time-domain OCT in patients on chloroquine/hydroxy chloroquine therapy for at least 5 years.

## Materials and Methods

The present case-control study was conducted in a tertiary care hospital in south India. The study protocol was approved by the Institutional Ethics Committee and an informed consent was taken from all the patients.

Fifty patients with immunological diseases receiving chloroquine or hydroxy-chloroquine and another 50 age and sex-matched controls having similar immunological diseases but not receiving chloroquine or hydroxy-chloroquine were included in the study. The inclusion criteria were: age above 18 years and chloroquine/hydroxychloroquine therapy given for at least 5 years. The exclusion criteria were: patients with clinical evidence of any other known macular disease, presence of glaucoma or with obscurities in the visual axis, previous retinal surgery, known neurological illness and diabetics.

The data collected included demographic details such as age, sex, primary diagnosis, duration of the illness, medication history (chloroquine or hydroxychloroquine or other drugs; dosage (mg/kg/day) and duration of treatment with each drug), presence of visual complaints like diminution of vision, metamorphopsia, scotomas.

Both cases and control patients underwent the following tests sequentially: 1. Best corrected Snellen's visual acuity test, 2. Amsler grid test, 3. Colour vision test using the Ishihara's pseudo isochromatic plates, 4. Automated threshold white perimetry using 10-2 protocol using Humphrey field analyzer (Zeiss Humphrey Systems, Dublin, CA), 5. Slit lamp biomicroscopic examination to study the fundus, 6. Fluorescein angiography in patients with suspicious lesions to identify subtle retinal pigment epithelial defects and 7. Optical Coherence Tomography.

The details of OCT are as follows: The examination was carried out by using a Stratus OCT (Carl Zeiss, Meditec, Dublin, CA) equipment. The patient was positioned comfortably. The chin was placed on the chin rest and forehead against the forehead strap. One eye was occluded. The patient was instructed to fix on the green target throughout the procedure.

- A fast macular thickness protocol was used to measure the macular thickness. It consisted of six radial line scans which covered a diameter of 6 mm and generated thickness reports for quantitative analysis. The thickness of the macula in the parafoveal region (1-3 mm; inner ring) was noted in the 4 quadrants (superior, inferior, nasal and inferior)
- A fast Retinal Nerve Fibre Layer (RNFL) scan protocol was used for the peripapillary measurements. It consisted of 3 consecutive 360° scans with a diameter of 3.4 mm centered on the optic nerve head, each composed of 256 A-scans taken in a single session. The RNFL thickness parameters calculated by the Stratus-OCT software (version 4.0.1) were average thickness in the temporal, superior, inferior and nasal quadrants.

A signal strength of more than or equal to 6 was taken for an acceptable scan. Average of 3 scans was taken per eye.

## Statistical methods

Age of the cases and controls was compared using an independent-samples t test. Gender distribution was compared using a Chi square test. Thicknesses in the four quadrants in the macular and peripapillary areas were compared using an independent-samples t test. Macular thicknesses in the four quadrants, across the three groups – namely, patients on chloroquine with and without abnormal fundus and the controls – was compared by using a one-way analysis of variance (ANOVA) with posthoc least significant difference (LSD) testing. Pearson's test was used to correlate the duration of therapy vs macular thickness and also the dose of chloroquine/hydroxychloroquine vs retinal thickness. An independent samples t test was used to compare the retinal thickness between patients on therapy for up to 8 years vs more than 8 years. All data were expressed as mean ± SD. A p value of <0.05 was considered statistically significant. SPSS version 16.0 statistical package was used for analysis of the data.

## Results

A total of 50 patients 50 controls were included in the study. The demographic characteristics of these subjects are shown in Table 1. The two groups were age and sex matched to eliminate the effect of age and gender on the retinal thickness on OCT. The distribution of the primary diagnoses between the cases and controls was also comparable. Twenty seven patients received only hydroxychloroquine, while 23 received chloroquine to begin with and were later changed to hydroxy chloroquine. The median duration of therapy with chloroquine was 3.0 years, while that of hydroxychloroquine was 6.0 years.

| | | Controls | Cases | Significance |
|---|---|---|---|---|
| Age (Years) | | 40.1 ± 9.3 | 40.4 ± 8.3 | P=0.89 |
| Sex | Male | 16 | 13 | $X^2$=0.355; df 1; p=0.551 |
| | Female | 34 | 37 | |
| Diagnosis | Rheumatoid arthritis | 30 | 29 | |
| | Systemic Lupus Erythematosis | 13 | 13 | |
| | Sjogrens Syndrome | 4 | 6 | NS |
| | Systemic Sclerosis | - | 1 | |
| | UCTD/ MCTD | 3 | 1 | |
| Duration of treatment in years Median (IQR) | Chloroquine | - | 3.0 (2.00-5.00) | |
| | Hydroxy-chloroquine | - | 6.0 (5.00-7.00) | |
| Dosage (mg.kg$^{-1}$.d$^{-1}$) | Chloroquine | - | 3.7 ± 0.7 | |
| | Hydroxy-chloroquine | - | 5.6 ± 1.1 | |

Table 1: Demographic characteristics of the patients.

## Visual acuity

There was no statistically significant difference between the cases and controls except for one patient with bull' s eye maculopathy in the study group, who had a Snellen's visual acuity of 5/60 in his right eye and 4/60 in his left.

## Dilated fundus examination

Six patients had fundus changes. One patient had a typical bull's eye maculopathy in both eyes. Four others showed pigmentary stippling at the macula in both the eyes. One patient had a pigment epithelial detachment in the right eye.

## Amsler grid testing

The two patients with pigmentary changes at macula had metamorphopsia on Amsler grid testing. The patient with bull's eye maculopathy had a central scotoma. In the rest of the patients, the test was normal.

## Colour vision

Colour vision was normal in all the patients other the patient with bull's eye maculopathy. In this patient, colour vision could not be recorded due to the poor vision.

## Automated visual fields

Visual fields were normal in all the patients. In the patient with bull's eye maculopathy, central visual fields could not be charted due to the poor vision.

## Fluorescein angiography

In those patients with pigmentary stippling, fluorescein angiography was inconclusive.

## Optical Coherence Tomography findings

The macular findings on OCT are shown in table 2. In the cases, a statistically significant thinning was noted in the superior and inferior quadrants of the parafoveal macula (inner ring) compared to the controls (superior: $252 \pm 34$ in the chloroquine group vs. $261 \pm 23$ in the control group; p value 0.033 & inferior: $252 \pm 32$ in the chloroquine group vs. $262\pm26$ in the control group; p value of 0.016). The measures in the temporal and nasal quadrants were not significantly different between the study and control groups.

|  | S(superior) | T (temporal) | I (inferior) | N (nasal) |
|---|---|---|---|---|
| Chloroquine Group | 252 ± 34 | 242 ± 32 | 252 ± 36 | 255 ± 32 |
| Normal Group | 261 ± 23 | 248 ± 24 | 262 ± 26 | 260 ± 26 |
| Significance (p value) | 0.033 | 0.157 | 0.016 | 0.219 |

Table 2: Macular changes associated with chloroquine therapy.

Six cases had changes in their fundus. Further analysis on macular changes was carried out to compare the cases with and without abnormalities of fundus with control patients. The results are shown in Table 3.

| Study Group | Fundus | Superior | Temporal | Inferior | Nasal |
|---|---|---|---|---|---|
| Chloroquine Group | Abnormal Fundus N=10 eyes | 254 ± 24$ | 249 ± 21 | 251 ± 24$ | 253 ± 18 |
| Chloroquine Group | Normal fundus N=88eyes | 253 ± 34* | 243 ± 32 | 253 ± 37* | 257 ± 32$ |
| Control Group | N=100 eyes | 261 ± 22 | 248 ± 23 | 262 ± 26* | 260 ± 24* |
|  |  | $p=0.456 vs. control *p=0.074 vs. control | NS | $p=0.282 vs. control *p=0.048 vs. control | $p=0.700 vs.Chloroquine abnormal fundus *p=0.473 vs. Chloroquine-abnormal fundus |

Table 3: Comparison of macular thickness in cases with or without fundus changes and control group.

One patient had a bull's eye maculopathy; OCT in this patient revealed an atrophic macula (OD: superior: 199, temporal: 186, inferior: 209, nasal: 195 with a Total Macular Volume {TMV} of 5.51 and a foveal thickness of 110. OS: superior: 189, temporal: 178, inferior: 198 and nasal: 195, TMV: 5.31 and foveal thickness of 112). Since this patient had already an advanced disease, he was excluded from the rest of the analysis, the results of which are as follows: The average macular thickness in all quadrants in the parafoveal (inner ring) region in patients with abnormal fundus on chloroquine/ hydroxychloroquine was lesser than in the controls. However it did not reach statistically significant levels probably due to the small sample size (N=10). A statistically significant thinning was noted in the inferior parafoveal region in patients on chloroquine but having normal fundus when compared to the controls ($253 \pm 37$ vs. $262 \pm 26$; p=0.048). A trend towards the same was observed in the superior parafoveal region ($253 \pm 34$ vs $261 \pm 22$; p=0.074).

Changes in peripapillary retinal nerve fibre layer are shown in table 4.

|  | Superior | Temporal | Inferior | Nasal |
|---|---|---|---|---|
| Chloroquine Group | 130 ± 27 | 68.4 ± 19 | 131 ± 26 | 85.4 ± 27 |
| Control Group | 124 ± 23 | 66.3 ± 14 | 133 ± 14 | 89.4 ± 21 |
| Significance (p value) | 0.124 | 0.262 | 0.523 | 0.249 |

Table 4: Changes in peripapillary retinal nerve fibre layer.

There was no significant retinal nerve fiber layer thinning in the peripapillary region in patients on the drug as compared to the controls. There was no significant correlation between the dose of chloroquine or hydroxychloroquine (in mg/kg) and the thickness of retina when analyzed by a Pearson's correlation test (Table 5).

|  | Superior | Temporal | Inferior | Nasal |
|---|---|---|---|---|
| Dose of Chloroquine therapy |  |  |  |  |
| r value | 0.23 | 0.203 | 0.179 | 0.202 |
| p value | 0.109 | 0.157 | 0.213 | 0.159 |
| Dose of Hydroxychloroquine therapy |  |  |  |  |
| r value | 0.008 | 0.046 | 0.035 | 0.021 |
| p value | 0.941 | 0.65 | 0.733 | 0.836 |

Table 5: Correlation of the drug-dose with macular thickenss.

A correlation was attempted between the retinal thickness and the total duration of chloroquine or hydroxychloroquine therapy. The patients were divided into two groups (patients on therapy for 8 years or more vs. therapy for <8 years); temporal macular thickness was significantly different between the two groups ($235 \pm 31$ vs. $249 \pm 31$ respectively; p<0.022) (One-way ANOVA with posthoc LSD test).

## Discussion

Hydroxychloroquine is a commonly used medication in the management of various immunological disorders. The American academy of ophthalmology is concerned that retinal toxicity, although rare, may be more common than previously recognized, based on a study by Wolfe et al which found that the risk exceeded 1% after 5 years [7]. Early chloroquine retinopathy is still inadequately described.

There are numerous tests used for screening but the sensitivity and specificity of each of these objective tests for retinal toxicity is still being debated. Early detection and discontinuation of the drugs can halt further visual loss.

Chloroquine/ hydroxy chloroquine accumulate in the retinal pigment epithelium and disrupts its function [11].

It has been shown that ganglion cell loss occurs in long term chloroquine users using scanning laser polarimetry [12]. Ganglion cell density is highest in the disc. Retinal thickness measurements in this region may reveal early toxicity before functional defects occur which are irreversible.

A recent study using high-speed ultra-high-resolution OCT showed discontinuity or loss of perifoveal photoreceptor inner segment/outer segment junctions and thinning of the outer nuclear layer in patients receiving hydroxychloroquine with normal fundus [9].

A recent report showed significant thinning in the perifoveal and outer macula especially in inferior and temporal quadrants in a patient on chloroquine therapy using time domain OCT [10].

In our patients there was a statistically significant thinning in the parafoveal macula (inner ring) especially in the inferior and superior quadrants among cases. It is important to note that these patients had a normal fundus, red Amsler grid test, perimetry and colour vision test. Since an acquired paracentral scotoma on automated field charting has been described as an early manifestation of retinopathy [13], it is evident that OCT can detect changes even before automated fields can.

Although previous studies have shown peripapillary thinning in patients on the drug [14], our study also found such changes.

When our patients were divided into two groups (patients on therapy for 8 years or more vs. therapy for <8 years), temporal macular thickness was significantly different between the two ($235 \pm 31$ vs. $249 \pm 31$ respectively; $p < 0.022$). This finding reinforces the recommendations of AAO that patients on chloroquine/hydroxy chloroquine should be evaluated for retinopathy after 5 years of usage of the drug [15].

The current study is the largest case series so far in the literature.

Optical coherence tomography could detect the retinopathic changes at the pre-clinical stage of maculopathy when all other tests like Amsler grid, colour vision, automated visual fields, fundus fluorescein angiography were normal.

In conclusion, macular thickness in patients receiving chloroquine/ hydroxychloroquine therapy was significantly thinner than in control group patients. Thinning was more evident if the patient was on the therapy for more than 8 years. Optical coherence tomography could

identify the retinopathy even before changes are evidenced in the automated visual fields. Peripapillary nerve fiber layer thickness is not significantly different between chloroquine users and controls. Routine screening for toxicity should be emphasized for patients on long term chloroquine/ hydroxychloroquine therapy. Our study suggests that OCT should be a part of routine screening for retinopathy. Longitudinal studies will be helpful to further establish the role of time domain OCT in early diagnosis of chloroquine retinopathy.

## References

1.  Rynes RI (1997) Antimalarial Drugs. In: Textbook of Rheumatology (5th edn), Kelly WN, Harris ED Jr, Ruddy S, Sledge CB (Eds), WB Saunders, Philadelphia.

2.  Savarino A, Lucia MB, Giordano F, Cauda R (2006) Risks and benefits of chloroquine use in anticancer strategies. Lancet Oncol 7: 792-793.

3.  Sundelin SP, Terman A (2002) Different effects of chloroquine and hydroxychloroquine on lysosomal function in cultured retinal pigment epithelial cells. APMIS 110: 481-489.

4.  Green NM, Marshak-Rothstein A (2011) Toll-like receptor driven B cell activation in the induction of systemic autoimmunity. Semin Immunol 23: 106-112.

5.  Lenert P (2005) Inhibitory oligodeoxynucleotides - therapeutic promise for systemic autoimmune diseases? Clin Exp Immunol 140: 1-10.

6.  Hennessy EJ, Parker AE, O'Neill LA (2010) Targeting Toll-like receptors: emerging therapeutics? Nat Rev Drug Discov 9: 293-307.

7.  Wolfe F, Marmor MF (2010) Rates and predictors of hydroxychloroquine retinal toxicity in patients with rheumatoid arthritis and systemic lupus erythematosus. Arthritis Care Res (Hoboken) 62: 775-784.

8.  Lyons JS, Severns ML (2007) Detection of early hydroxychloroquine retinal toxicity enhanced by ring ratio analysis of multifocal electroretinography. Am J Ophthalmol 143: 801-809.

9.  Rodriguez-Padilla JA, Hedges TR 3rd, Monson B, Srinivasan V, Wojtkowski M, et al. (2007) High-speed ultra-high-resolution optical coherence tomography findings in hydroxychloroquine retinopathy. Arch Ophthalmol 125: 775-780.

10. Korah S, Kuriakose T (2008) Optical coherence tomography in a patient with chloroquine-induced maculopathy. Indian J Ophthalmol 56: 511-513.

11. Mahon GJ, Anderson HR, Gardiner TA, McFarlane S, Archer DB, et al. (2004) Chloroquine causes lysosomal dysfunction in neural retina and RPE: implications for retinopathy. Curr Eye Res 28: 277-284.

12. Bonanomi MT, Dantas NC, Medeiros FA (2006) Retinal nerve fibre layer thickness measurements in patients using chloroquine. Clinical & Experimental Ophthalmology 34: 130–136.

13. Browning DJ (2002) Hydroxychloroquine and chloroquine retinopathy: screening for drug toxicity. Am J Ophthalmol 133: 649-656.

14. Arana LA, Arana J, Hasimoto AR, Schirr G, Arana E, et al. (2010) Optical coherence tomography to evaluate peripapillary retinal nerve fiber layer in chloroquine patients. Arq Bras Oftalmol 73: 28-32.

15. Marmor MF, Kellner U, Lai TY, Lyons JS, Mieler WF; American Academy of Ophthalmology (2011) Revised recommendations on screening for chloroquine and hydroxychloroquine retinopathy. Ophthalmology 118: 415-422.

# 9

# Aqueous Extract of *Prosopis strombulifera* (LAM) BENTH Induces Cytotoxic Effects against Tumor Cell Lines without Systemic Alterations in BALB/c Mice

Hapon MB[1,2], Hapon MV[3,4], Persia FA[1], Pochettino A[5], Lucero GS[3,4] and Gamarra-Luques C[1,6]

[1]*Laboratorio de Reproducción y Lactancia, IMBECU-CONICET, Mendoza, Argentina*

[2]*Facultad de Ciencias Exactas y Naturales, Universidad Nacional de Cuyo, Mendoza, Argentina*

[3]*Laboratorio de Fitopatología, IBAM-CONICET, Mendoza, Argentina*

[4]*Facultad de Ciencias Agrarias, Universidad Nacional de Cuyo, Mendoza, Argentina*

[5]*Laboratorio de Toxicología Experimental, Facultad de Ciencias Bioquímicas y Farmacéuticas, Universidad Nacional de Rosario, Rosario, Argentina*

[6]*Facultad de Ciencias Médicas, Universidad Nacional de Cuyo, Mendoza, Argentina*

[*]**Corresponding author:** Carlos Gamarra Luques, Instituto de Medicina y Biología Experimental de Cuyo (IMBECU), CCT Mendoza. Av Ruiz Leal s/n. Casilla de Correo 0855. CP 5500, Mendoza Capital, Provincia de Mendoza, Argentina, E-mail: cgamarra@mendoza-conicet.gob.ar

## Abstract

*Prosopis strombulifera* (Lam.) Benth. is a rhizomatous shrub native to the northern and central zones of Argentina. The analgesic and antibiotic properties of this plant had been demonstrated but there are no previous reports of its cytotoxic activity. The goal of this work was to analyze the cytotoxic activity of P. strombulifera against HCT-116 and MCF-7 cell lines, and to evaluate toxic systemic effects in BALB/c mice. Changes induced by the aqueous extract from leaves on tumoral cell lines were studied by MTT (3-(4,5-dimethylthiazol-2-yl)-2,5-diphenyltetrazolium bromide) tetrazolium reduction assay, Trypan blue dye exclusion assay, optical microscopy, Western Blot analysis of PCNA and cPARP, LDH activity, Ames´ test and clonogenic survival. Oral sub-chronic toxicity was assessed on BALB/c mice at concentrations up to 150 mg/animal/day. Analyses included animal/organs weight; erythrocytes, leukocytes and platelets number; and serological determinations of glucose, ASAT, ALAT, urea and creatinine. Extract has induced cytotoxicity, affecting proliferation and viability in both cell lines in a dose and time-response manner. $IC_{50}$ was 2.25 µg/ml and $LC_{50}$ 5.05 µg/ml in HCT-116, while values were 3.01 µg/ml and 7.52 µg/ml, respectively, in MCF-7. In both cell lines, the antiproliferative effect was confirmed by reduction of PCNA protein expression. When $LC_{50}$ concentrations were used, extract-induced necrosis (evidenced by the increase in extracellular LDH activity), apoptosis (increased cPARP protein expression) and clonogenic survival diminution. Mutagenic activity of extract was caused at concentrations of 500 µg/ml (99 and 64-fold higher than HCT-116 and MCF-7 $LC_{50}$ concentrations). Animal studies demonstrated that no significant toxicity was induced. In conclusion, this is the first report of *P. strombulifera* cytotoxic activity against tumoral cell lines. Sub-chronic extract administration did not cause deleterious effects *in vivo*. Altogether, the presented results make *P. strombulifera* a promising natural product for cancer research and treatment.

**Keywords:** *Prosopis strombulifera*; Natural products; Cytotoxicity; Antiproliferative; Lethality; Mutagenicity

## Introduction

At present, more than twelve million people worldwide are diagnosed annually with some type of cancer. At least one third of them will not survive the disease. The progressively aging population, late diagnosis, and poor response to current treatments make cancer the second cause of death around the world [1]. The search for new chemotherapeutic agents is therefore a priority in order to find new therapeutic approaches to improve cancer prognosis and treatment.

Many drugs used in oncology have been provided by nature. Antitumor agent research among natural sources has been a successful strategy. The contribution of plants to cancer treatment is evidenced by the success of drugs like vinblastine, vincristine, irinotecan, topotecan, paclitaxel and docetaxel, as well as a number of other compounds that are currently being evaluated in clinical trials [2,3].

In the Eastern hemisphere, ancestral medicine had been greatly developed and the description of natural bioactive compounds is considerable. In contrast, in Argentina, the study of compounds obtained from regional plants is emerging. There are more than five hundred species of plants in Mendoza province, central west Argentina for which "folkloric medicine" has described several uses to preserve and aid health [4]. Only a small number of them have recently been studied to confirm their phytopharmaceutical properties.

*Prosopis strombulifera* (Lam.) Benth. is a rhizomatous shrub up to 1.5 m in height that grows in the northern and central zones of Argentina [5]. In Mendoza, it is mainly native to the northern part of the province [6]. This species is locally known as "retortuño", "retortón" or "mastuerzo". The plant has been used by the Huarpe pre-Columbian tribe as astringent, anti-inflammatory, odontalgic and anti-diarrheic agent [4,7]. Recent scientific studies have confirmed part of its ethnopharmacological uses, describing the molecular mechanism involved in the analgesic effect of this plant [8] and its biological activity against microorganisms such as *Escherichia coli*, *Staphylococcus aureus* and *Salmonella typhi* [9-11]. The chemical compounds described in the species include flavonoids, tannins, carbohydrates and a small amount of saponins and steroids [8]. The chemical groups described more precisely are the polyamines (putrescine, spermidine and cadaverine) and jasmonic acid derivatives [12]. To our knowledge, there are no reports of cytotoxic actions of *P. strombulifera* related to antiproliferative or lethal activity against tumor cells.

The goal of this work was to analyze the cytotoxic activity of the crude aqueous extract obtained from leaves of *P. strombulifera*. More specifically, the present study was conducted to evaluate antiproliferative, lethal and mutagenic actions of the plant extract *in vitro* against human tumor cell lines HCT-116 and MCF-7 (colorectal cancer and breast adenocarcinoma, respectively), and to evaluate the toxic systemic effects on BALB/c mice.

## Materials and Methods

### Crude extracts preparation

*Prosopis strombulifera* was collected in December 2012 in Lavalle county, Mendoza, Argentina (33° 44'10" S, 68° 21' 30.5" W). The botanical identifications were performed by two of the authors (C Gamarra-Luques and MV Hapon). A voucher specimen (MERL 61824) was deposited in the Mendoza Ruiz Leal herbarium. The crude extract was obtained according to the protocol described by Widmer and Laurent [13]. Briefly, 20 g of leaves were autoclaved in 200 ml distilled water for 1 hour. The solids were then separated by paper filtration and the volume was boiled down to 20 ml. Final extract concentration was representative of 1 g of leaves by milliliter (1 g/ml). Before use, crude extract was sterilized by passing through a 0.22 μm pore size filter.

### Drugs and reagents

DMEM, (Dulbecco´s Modified Eagle Medium), penicillin and streptomycin were obtained from GIBCO, USA. Fetal bovine serum was obtained from Internegocios, Argentina. Primary antibodies against for the following proteins were used at the designated dilutions: cleaved poly (ADP-ribose) polymerase (cPARP, 1:5,000, BD Signal Transduction); proliferating cell nuclear antigen (PCNA, 1:1,000 Novus Biologicals, USA). Alpha-tubulin (1:20,000) and Protease Inhibitor Cocktail were purchased from Sigma-Aldrich, USA. Secondary antibodies conjugated to horseradish peroxidase and rose in rabbit and mouse were obtained from Santa Cruz Biotechnology, USA and Cell Signaling Technology, USA, respectively.

### Cell culture and *in vitro* treatment

The colorectal carcinoma (HCT-116) and mammary adenocarcinoma (MCF-7) cell lines were cultured in DMEM, supplemented with 10% fetal bovine serum, 100 IU of penicillin and 100 μg/ml streptomycin. Culture conditions were fixed at 37°C, in a humidified atmosphere enriched by 5% $CO_2$. 24 hs after cell plating, treatments were dissolved directly in the culture media. Treatment time was different in both cell lines: 48 hs in HCT-116 and 72 hs in MCF-7. The selected treatment times were based on each cell line doubling time (DT) to let the control cells complete, at least, two entire cell cycles. In our culture conditions the DT calculated for HCT-116 was $20.05 \pm 0.1$h and for MCF-7 was $34.53 \pm 0.1$h.

To culture *Salmonella typhimurium*, 2.5% Bacto-Difco nutrient broth was prepared in distilled water. Glucose minimal agar plate (MA plate) contained 1.5% agar, 0.02% $MgSO_4 \cdot 7H_2O$, 0.2% citric acid, 1% $K_2HPO_4$, 0.35% $NaHNH_4PO_4 \cdot 4H_2O$ and 2% glucose. Top agar contained 0.75% agar and 0.5% NaCl.

### Cytotoxicity assay by MTT

A colorimetric assay using MTT was performed [14]. MCF-7 and HCT-116 cells were seeded in 96-well microplates (2,500 and 7,500 cells/well/100 μl, respectively). 24 hrs later, the medium was aspirated and replaced by medium containing *P. strombulifera* extract at concentrations ranging from 0 to 10 μg/ml in both cell lines. HCT-116 cells were then incubated for 48 hrs and MCF-7 for 72 hrs. After the indicated times, medium was replaced by 100 μl of MTT solution (0.5 mg/ml in DMEM, without phenol red or FBS). Cells were incubated for an additional 4 hrs. MTT solution was then removed and 100 μl of DMSO added; the plates were shaken for 10 min to dissolve the formazan crystals. The optical density was measured using a Thermo Scientific Multiscan Elisa reader at 570 nm. The optical density obtained in untreated control cells was taken as 100% viability. Percent cytotoxicity was calculated as 100% viability. The assay was performed three times in triplicate.

### Dye exclusion assay

Dose and time-response experimental designs were performed to quantify cell number and viability by trypan blue exclusion assay. Briefly, $7.5 \times 10^4$ cells were seeded into 6-well plates. When dose-response was analyzed, extract concentration used was in a range of 0 to 14 μg/ml for 48 hrs in HCT-116 and 72 hrs in MCF-7. In a time-response approach, cells were harvested at 0, 12, 24, 36, 48 and 72 hrs after treatment started. Trypsinized cells were resuspended in 1ml of phosphate buffered saline (PBS). Equal volumes of cell suspension and trypan blue (0.3% in PBS) were mixed and incubated for 5 min. Cells were then counted in a Neubauer haemocytometer chamber using a clear-field microscopy. Concentration of extract needed to achieve 50% of growth inhibition is indicated as $IC_{50}$, while extract concentration where 50% cell death was observed is indicated as $LC_{50}$ [15,16]. Assays were performed three times in triplicate.

### Morphological assessment of cell changes

Cells were seeded on cover-slides placed on the bottom of 6 well plates. After 24 hrs, control cells were fixed and stained. Culture medium containing treatment was replaced in the other cell groups. After 48 hrs in HCT-116 and 72 hrs in MCF-7, the remaining cells were fixed with methanol and stained with GIEMSA solution. Cover-slides were then mounted, evaluated and photographed with a Nikon Eclipse 200 microscope.

### Western Blot analysis

After the treatment cells were scraped, pelleted, washed with PBS and lysed by the addition of two volumes of lysis buffer (50 mM Tris–HCl pH 7.4, 150 mM NaCl, 0.5% IGEPAL, 1X Protease Inhibitors Cocktail and 1 mM NaF). Cells were disrupted by passing them through 21 gauge needles and gently rocked on ice for 30 min. Lysates were centrifuged at 16,000 g for 15 min at 4°C, and the supernatant was considered the whole cell extract. Protein content was assessed in the supernatant by the bicinchonic acid method (BCA; Pierce, Rockford, IL). Protein aliquots of 30 μg were separated in a 12% (w/v) acrylamide gel by SDS-PAGE and transferred to PVDF membranes. The blots were blocked in 5% (w/v) non-fat milk in TBS containing 0.1% (v/v) Tween-20. Blots were probed overnight with the appropriate dilution in 2.5% BSA of each of the primary antibodies, and incubated with 1:5,000 dilution of peroxidase conjugate secondary antibody for 1 h at room temperature. The blots were washed, developed by chemiluminescence, using a ChemiDoc XRS + System (Bio-Rad, Laboratories). Band densitometric analysis was performed using Image Lab Software version 4.0 from Bio-Rad Laboratories.

## Lactate dehydrogenase activity determination

LDH enzyme activity was measured in the culture media using a diagnostic LDH-L kit (Wiener lab, Rosario, Argentina) according to the instructions provided by the manufacturer. In brief, the supernatant of each well was collected after treatment. A substrate provided by the kit was then incubated at 37°C for 5 min, followed by the addition of NAD to the mixture. Spectrophotometric absorbance at 340 nm was registered for 2 min. Finally, LDH concentration measured in units/liter (U/l) was obtained by the equation [LDH]=($\Delta$A/min) × factor, where $\Delta$A indicates absorbance difference between second 120 and 1, and factor represents $\varepsilon_{NAD/NADH}$ = 6230 $M^{-1}$ $cm^{-1}$.

## Clonogenic survival assay

To determine whether there is an added long-term lethal imprinting, we subjected pretreated cells to a clonogenic survival assay as previously described [17-20]. Briefly, 500 control and treated viable cells were placed in 6-well plates and cultured in fresh media without treatment until colonies were large enough to be clearly discerned. At this point, medium was removed and dishes were washed with PBS. Colonies were fixed with methanol and stained with crystal violet. The wells were then washed with tap water and dried at room temperature. The colonies, defined as groups of ≥ 30 cells, were scored manually with the aid of an inverted microscope. Clonogenic survival was expressed as the percent number of colonies quantified in the different treatment concentrations, considering the colonies formed by control cells as 100%.

## Mutagenicity assay (Ames' test)

Mutagenicity activity was evaluated in a bacterial reverse mutation assay by the standard plate incorporation assay (Ames´ test) [21]. The *S. typhimurium* histidine-requiring test strains TA98 and TA100 were used. Bacteria were aerobically grown at 37°C in Nutrient Broth Bacto-Difco. The test was carried out by adding 0.2 ml of sterile 0.5 mM histidine-biotin and 0.1 ml of the overnight bacterial culture (approximately 1 × 108 bacteria/ml) to 2.0 ml of molten top agar (45ºC). Concentrations from 0.5 to 500 µl/ml of the *P. strombulifera* crude extract were added to top agar tubes, which were then gently vortexed and subsequently transferred to plates with minimal glucose agar (30 ml/plate). Duplicate plates were poured for each concentration of reaction mixture in at least two independent experiments. After incubation at 37ºC for 48 h in darkness, the His+ revertant colonies were manually counted.

## Animals and *in vivo* treatment

Adult male BALB/c mice bred in our laboratory, 6 weeks old at the onset of treatment, were used. They were kept in a light (lights on 6:00 AM to 10:00 PM) and temperature (22-24°C) room. Mice chow (Cargill, Córdoba, Argentina) and tap water were available *ad libitum*.

Treatments were performed by diluting aqueous extract in the drinking water. Aqueous extract concentrations were in a range of 0-150 mg/animal/day for 28 days. A toxicity study was performed in accordance to "repeated dose 28 day-oral toxicity study in rodents", TG 407-OECD Guidelines for the Testing of Chemicals [22]; when nontoxic compounds are tested, no effects would be expected at a concentration of 1000 mg/kg/day (30 mg for 30 g animal). We tested increased concentrations until extract concentration affected animal water consumption. Animal water consumption and body weight were determined three times a week.

All animals were cared in accordance with the Guiding Principles in the Care and Use of Animals of the US National Institute of Health. All procedures were approved by the Institutional Animal Care and Use Committee of School of Medical Science, Universidad Nacional de Cuyo (Protocol approval N° 30/2014).

## Organ weight, blood cells and serological determinations

After treatment, animals were sacrificed by decapitation and troncal blood was collected. One aliquot was obtained with 10% EDTA to avoid clotting, and used for blood cell quantification. The other aliquot was used to obtain serum after coagulation and centrifugation, and used for biochemical characterization. Animals were necropsied, and liver, kidneys and spleen dissected for macroscopical analysis and weight determination.

Blood cell count was performed according to the Manual Prático de Hematología [23]. To determine hematocrit percentage, blood was centrifuged in heparinized capillaries and the length of fractions measured with a caliper. Erythrocyte, leukocyte and platelet counts were obtained using a, Neubauer hemocytometer chamber, and final concentrations calculated.

Glucose, aspartate aminotransferase (ASAT/GOT), alanine aminotransferase (ALAT/GPT), urea and creatinine serum levels were determined using specific Wienner Lab kits (Wienner Lab, Argentina), according to the manufacturer´s instructions. Briefly, commercial standards and samples were incubated with specific enzymes/substrates and formed products quantified by spectrophotometric absorbance. Final concentrations of products were calculated using mathematical formulas provided with the kit.

## Statistical analysis

Data are expressed as mean ± standard error (SEM). Data were analyzed using GraphPad Prism 5.0 software. To assess $IC_{50}$ and $LC_{50}$, a sigmoidal dose-response analysis was performed and values were considered acceptable when goodness of fit showed $R^2$ ≥ 0.90. Comparisons between two groups were done using Student's T test. When more than two groups were compared, one-way ANOVA followed by Dunnett's multiple comparison test was used. Curve slopes in the study of mice body weight change were compared using linear regressions. In all cases, statistical significance was considered when $p < 0.05$.

## Results

### Cytotoxicity effects of *P. strombulifera* on cancer cell lines.

In this study, we evaluated the aqueous extract activity in a dose and time-response experimental design.

The standard MTT assay was performed to demonstrate cytotoxicity in HCT-116 and MCF-7 cell lines. In both cases, *P. strombulifera* was able to induce cell toxicity in a dose-response manner, and 100% cytotoxicity was reached at concentrations close to 10 µg/ml (Figure 1).

We then quantified proliferation and viability by dye exclusion assay with trypan blue. The $IC_{50}$ and $LC_{50}$ were calculated to determine extract potency (Figure 1). The extract showed the highest potency in HCT-116 cells, the calculated $IC_{50}$ was 2.25 ± 0.1 µg/ml and $LC_{50}$ was 5.05 ± 0.1 µg/ml (Figure 1). In MCF-7, $IC_{50}$ was 3.01 ± 0.1 µg/ml, while $LC_{50}$ was 7.52 ± 0.1 µg/ml. In both cell lines, $IC_{50}$ concentrations were able to reduce proliferation with limited lethal effects. The notorious reduction in cell proliferation at this concentration, without a significant lethality induction, was considered a cytostatic effect. The remaining viable cells at 10 µg/ml were not metabolically active, as shown by MTT cytotoxicity at this concentration.

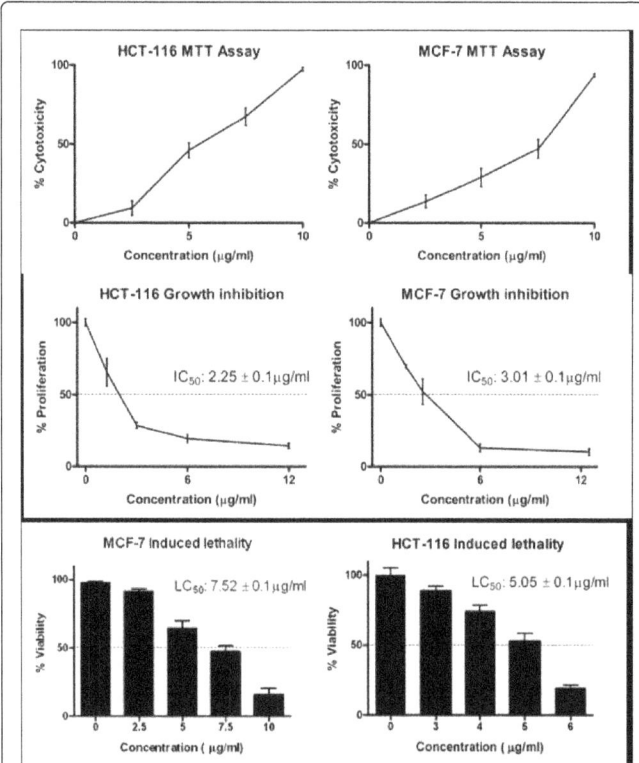

Figure 1: Dose-response effect of *P. strombulifera* crude extract on HCT-116 and MCF-7 cell lines. Cytotoxicity by MTT colorimetric assay, proliferation and viability by trypan blue dye exclusion assay are shown. Results are given as mean ± SEM of three different assays performed in triplicate.

Evaluation of the time-dependent proliferation and viability response revealed that cell damage increased along with the treatment time course (Figure 2). HCT-116 and MCF-7 (Figure 2) morphology changes were observed after treatment with $IC_{50}$ and $LC_{50}$ concentrations. Cell number, nuclear and cytoplasm alterations were more evident at higher concentrations than at the beginning of the treatment.

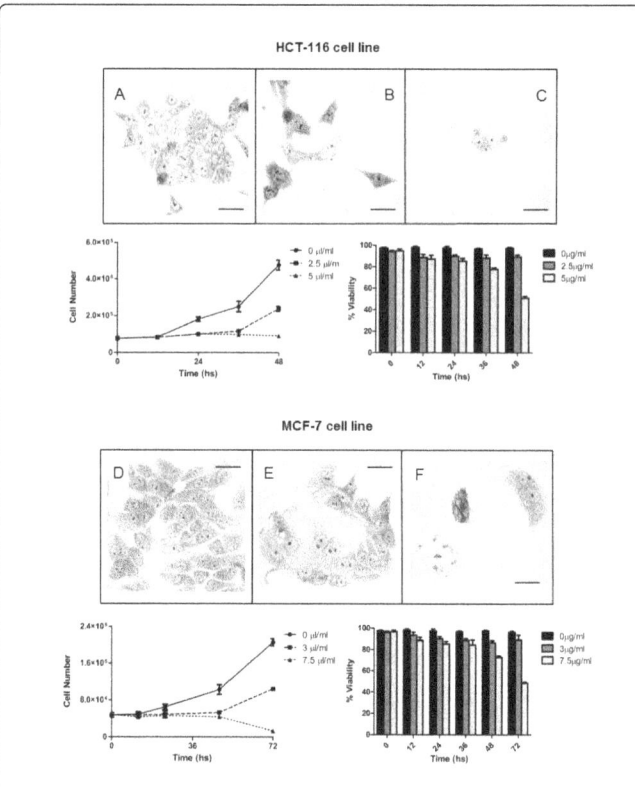

Figure 2: Time-response effect of *P. strombulifera* crude extract on HCT-116 and MCF-7 cell lines. A, B and C show optical microscopy of HCT-116 cells before and after treatment with the respective $IC_{50}$ and $LC_{50}$ concentrations of extract. D, E and F show the same conditions in MCF-7. Cell number and viability is presented at 0, 12, 24, 36 and 48 hrs in HCT-116; and 0, 12, 24, 36, 48 and 72 hrs in MCF-7. Time course of 0 µg/ml, $IC_{50}$ and $LC_{50}$ concentrations are presented for both cell lines. Proliferation and viability results are shown as mean ± SEM of three different assays performed in triplicate.

In both cell lines, cell number response to $IC_{50}$ treatments showed an evident reduction in the proliferation curve slope. On the other hand, $LC_{50}$ concentrations considerably affected cell number; final cell count showed no proliferation in HCT-116 and a lower cell number than at time 0 in MCF-7.

Time course viability was slightly reduced with $IC_{50}$ treatments after 12 hrs in both cell lines. $LC_{50}$ concentrations produced a similar reduction at 12 hrs, accompanied by a notorious reduction in viability during the last 24 hrs of treatment.

The molecular confirmation of cell cycle progression arrest was demonstrated by Western Blot analysis. Figure 3 shows a dose-dependent reduction in the expression of proliferating cell nuclear antigen (PCNA) in both cell lines.

Altogether, the cytotoxic assay, cell number and viability, morphological features, and molecular changes demonstrated a cytotoxic effect of *P. strombulifera* aqueous extract on human tumor cell lines in a dose and time-dependent manner.

## Determination of mode of cell death

After having observed lethal activity of the extract, we performed a new set of assays in order to evidence the mode of cell death related to viability reduction. Western Blot analysis was carried out to reveal apoptosis by detection of cleavage in poly ADP ribose polymerase (PARP) protein. The biochemical determination of extracellular activity of lactactate deshidrogenase enzyme (LDH) was selected to determine necrosis (Figure 3).

Apoptosis, determined by cleaved PARP (cPARP) protein expression increase, was evident in both cell lines when the extract treatment reached $LC_{50}$ concentration (5 µg/ml in HCT-116 and 7.5 µg/ml in MCF-7).

LDH is an intracellular enzyme that leaks into the medium when cells die in association with cytoplasmic membrane disruption. Consequently, determination of LDH activity in medium is a valid method to determine necrosis [24]. Enzyme activity determination showed increased values of LDH starting at $IC_{50}$ concentrations in both cell lines. In HCT-116 cells, LDH values were significantly higher than in the untreated group at concentrations above $IC_{50}$. In both cell lines, LDH activity was statistically different between treatments and control cells at $LC_{50}$.

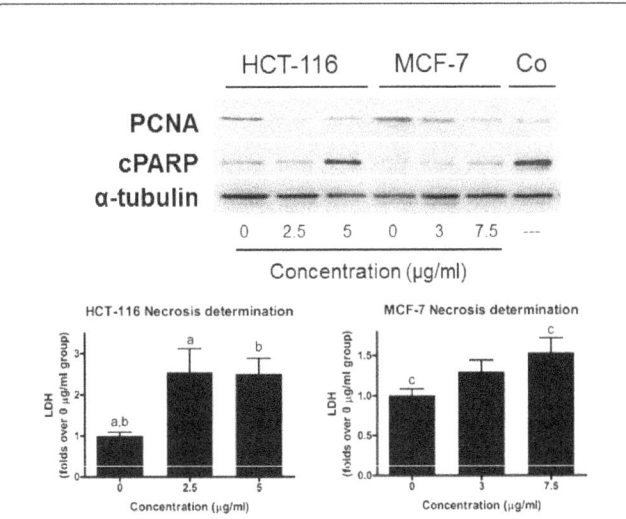

**Figure 3:** Proliferating cell nuclear antigen (PCNA) and cleaved poly ADP ribose polymerase (cPARP) protein expression, and extracellular lactate dehydrogenase activity (LDH) after *P. strombulifera* treatment on HCT-116 and MCF-7 cell lines. Treatment concentrations presented are 0 µg/ml, $IC_{50}$ and $LC_{50}$ in both cell lines. α-tubulin was used as protein loading control. Western Blot positive control group (Co) was obtained from proteins of harvested MCF-7 culture cells. LDH results are shown as mean ± SEM of three different assays performed in triplicate. Statistical difference between treatments and control group (a, b and c) was determined using one-way ANOVA and Dunnett's post-test for multiple comparisons, p<0.05.

Our results indicate that the lethality induced by *P. strombulifera* is not related to an exclusive mode of cell death. Increased expression of cPARP protein, together with an increase in extracellular LDH activity, indicated the coexistence of apoptosis and necrosis.

## Long-term clonogenic survival

We sought to determine whether the cells that had not died in the experimental time period were able to recover from damage and regain the ability to form colonies. Both cell lines assayed were able to recover from the cytostatic effect induced by $IC_{50}$ concentrations (2.25 µg/ml for HCT-116 and 3 µg/ml for MCF-7). When the treatment increased to $LC_{50}$ concentrations (5 µg/ml for HCT-116 and 7.5 µg/ml for MCF-7), we observed a statistically significant reduction in the number of positive colonies, indicating that the cells were not able to recover their reproductive capacity once treatment was ended (Figure 4).

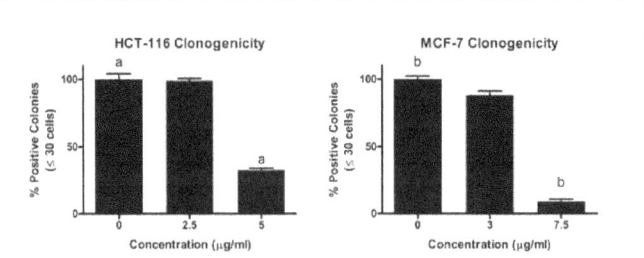

**Figure 4:** Clonogenic survival assay of *P. strombulifera* treated HCT-116 and MCF-7 cell lines. Positive colonies (≥ 30 cells) after 2 weeks are presented. HCT-116 and MCF-7 cells were previously treated at 0 µg/ml, $IC_{50}$ and $LC_{50}$; for 48 and 72 hrs, respectively. Clonogenicity of the control cells was considered 100%. Results are shown as mean ± SEM of three different assays performed in triplicate. Statistical difference between treatments and control group (a and b) was determined by one-way ANOVA and Dunnett's post-test for multiple comparisons, p<0.05.

Changes observed in clonogenicity are interesting because they indicate a long-term reproductive damage when concentrations reach $LC_{50}$ levels. Changes induced by the extract in cell homeostasis affect long-time survival even when the treatment does not kill the cells during initial exposure. In terms of compound efficacy, the reduction in long-term clonogenic survival, in combination with the acute cytotoxic action, suggest the presence of a very effective pharmacological compound.

## Mutagenic activity of *P. strombulifera* crude extract

The *Salmonella* mutagenicity test has been extensively used to measure the mutagenic potential of many compounds [25-27]. The strains TA98 and TA100 have point mutations in the histidine biosynthetic operon that render them unable to grow in the absence of histidine. Cultures of bacterial strains in the presence of mutagenic compounds drive mutations that make microorganisms able to grow and form detectable colonies without adding histidine to the culture agar. Consequently, increased capability to grow and form colonies is indicative of mutagenic activity.

Addition of aqueous *Prosopis* extract to the bacteria culture media did not induce significant mutations until concentrations reached 500 µg/ml. The mutagenic value obtained represents 99 and 64 times the concentrations measured as $LC_{50}$ in HCT-116 and MCF-7, respectively (Figure 5). In accordance with these results, DNA damage is not the mechanism that mediates biological activity of the crude extract at the concentrations that induce cytotoxicity in tumoral cell lines.

## Study of *P. strombulifera* toxic effects on Balb/c mice

After *in vitro* determination of the *P. strombulifera* crude extract activity, we considered it relevant to establish how treatment could affect homeostasis *in vivo*. We performed anatomical, hematological and serological studies to examine possible alterations induced by treatment.

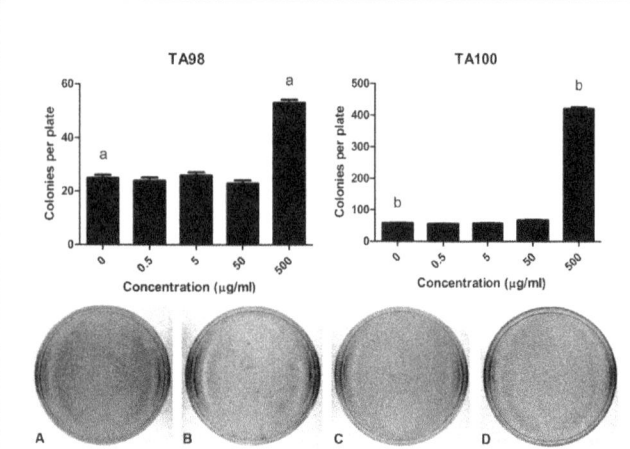

Figure 5: Mutagenicity of *P. strombulifera* crude extract. Revertant colonies of TA98 and TA100 strains of S. typhimurium at different concentrations of extract are presented. Mutagenic capability is evident by bacterial colony growth in agar. Results are shown as mean ± SEM of the absolute number of colonies per plate using one-way ANOVA and Dunnett's post-test for multiple comparisons, (*) p<0.05. Pictures A and B show positive colonies at 0 and 500 µg/ml extract concentration in TA98, while C and D show same concentrations in T100.

Water consumption was calculated as 4.5 ± 0.5 ml/mouse/day. Aqueous extract was then diluted at 30, 90 and 150 mg/mouse/day. Because there were no significant differences between treatments, only the results at the highest concentration used are shown.

Animal body weight change during treatment was recorded. Only a small, not statistically significant reduction in the final weight was induced by extract administration (Figure 6).

We studied the macroscopic appearance of organs and their weight, as well as the number of blood cells, to analyze whether treatment induced toxicity in detoxifying organs, such as liver or kidneys, or a rapidly proliferating fraction of cells, such as spleen and circulating blood cells (Table 1). Organs did not show differences in weight, color or structure. No macroscopical signs of ischemia, bleeding, fibrosis or degenerative proliferation were observed.

Hematocrit and the number of circulating blood cells were similar after treatment. Extract toxicity on rapidly proliferating cells or organs related to the hematological system can therefore be excluded.

Serum values of glucose and urea were determined to evaluate integrity in carbohydrate and protein metabolism, respectively. In addition, hepatic enzymes (ASAT/GOT and ALAT/GPT) and creatinine levels in serum were measured to study the functional status of liver and kidneys, respectively. None of the assessed biochemical parameters showed statistical differences between groups.

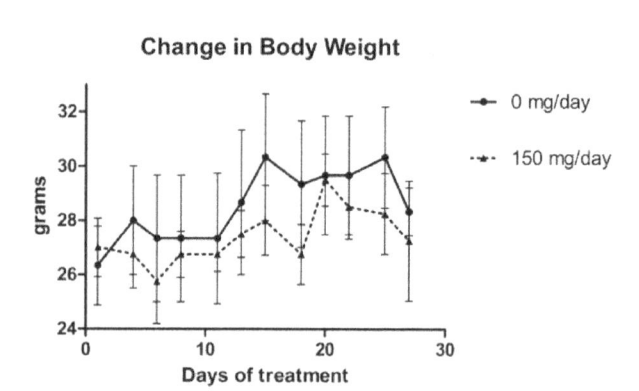

Figure 5: BALB/c change in body weight along sub-chronic toxicity assay (28 days of treatment). Curves of 0 mg/animal/day and 150 mg/animal/day are presented. Mean ± SEM of n=5 animals per group are used. Linear regression analysis (p<0.05) to compare curve slopes did not show significant differences.

| Mouse and organ weight | | |
|---|---|---|
| Detail | 0 mg/day | 150 mg/day |
| Body (g) | 30.67 ± 1.76 | 27.25 ± 2.21 |
| Liver (g) | 1.59 ± 0.30 | 1.32 ± 0.17 |
| Kidneys (g) | 0.43 ± 0.11 | 0.45 ± 0.06 |
| Spleen (g) | 0.15 ± 0.01 | 0.11 ± 0.02 |
| **Blood cell determination** | | |
| Hematocrit (%) | 30.11 ± 0.72 | 32.14 ± 2.85 |
| Erythrocytes ($10^6$ cells/µl) | 3.37 ± 0.67 | 3.32 ± 0.41 |
| Leukocytes ($10^3$ cells/µl) | 3.72 ± 0.41 | 3.41 ± 0.21 |
| Platelets ($10^5$ cells/µl) | 4.87 ± 0.27 | 5.29 ± 0.12 |
| **Serum biochemistry** | | |
| Glucose (mg/dl) | 79.72 ± 12.10 | 99.56 ± 12.81 |
| ASAT/GOT (U/l) | 21.90 ± 3.77 | 30.14 ± 6.45 |
| ALAT/GPT (U/l) | 46.23 ± 16.67 | 33.47 ± 9.60 |
| Urea (g/l) | 0.67 ± 0.07 | 0.82 ± 0.16 |
| Creatinine (mg/l) | 4.93 ± 0.16 | 5.47 ± 0.16 |

Data presented are mean ± SEM of n=5 animals per group. Comparisons by Student's T test (p<0.05) did not show significant differences between 0 mg/animal/day and 150 mg/animal/day.

Table 1: BALB/c anatomical, hematological and serum biochemistry after 28 days of *P. strombulifera* treatment.

## Discussion

Because of their widespread structural and biological diversity, natural products are an important source of new drugs and new chemical entities. Plant-based drug discoveries have mainly led to the development of anticancer and anti-infectious agents, and continue to contribute to the new leads in clinical trials [28]. It is remarkable that approximately 50% of chemotherapeutic agents currently used are natural products, their analogs or derived compounds [29]. The discovery of new drug leads from medicinal plants may be aided by ethnopharmacology, which is a mode of scientific investigation related to the indigenous medicinal uses of a particular species [30]. The main goal of the present work was to describe the *in vitro* cytotoxic effects of *P. strombulifera* and its possible in vivo toxicity. The plant was selected from several native plants in Mendoza, Argentina for which folkloric medicine describes many uses in health preservation.

In the current study, antiproliferative, lethal and mutagenic effects of *P. strombulifera* crude extract was analyzed on colorectal (HCT-116) and breast adenocarcinoma (MCF-7) cell lines, and sub-chronic toxicity was studied in a BALB/c mouse model.

*In vitro* results demonstrate that *P. strombulifera* induces cytotoxicity in HCT-116 and MCF-7 cell lines. The experimental design used in the present work allows discriminating how proliferation and cell death contributes to cytotoxicity. Anti-proliferative and lethal actions increase in a dose and time-dependent manner. *P. strombulifera* activity on cell lines can be compared with 5-fluorouracil (5-FU), an antitumoral agent that is currently used worldwide. While aqueous extract of *P. strombulifera* has $IC_{50}$ and $LC_{50}$ values ranging between 2.5 -7.5 μg/ml, $IC_{50}$ reported values for 5-FU are 18.92 μg/ml in HCT-116 [31] and 7.5 μg/ml in MCF-7 [32]. In terms of compound potency, *P. strombulifera* extract is similar to 5-FU.

Necrosis and apoptosis are the modes of cell death triggered by the extract in both cell lines. Coexistence of both mechanisms is not a new report, even when considering natural derivatives. The same has been reported for the action of the venom of Cuban scorpions *Rhupalurus junceous* on human tumor cell lines of epithelial and hematopoietic origin, as well as on normal cells [33]. The polyamine derivative putrescine-1,4-dicinnamide isolated from the mushroom *Pholiota spumosa* also shows this particularity [34]. It is possible that induction of necrosis and apoptosis by *P. strombulifera* treatment depends on extract concentration and cell line molecular targets. Nevertheless, the dual mechanisms of cell death activated by *P. strombulifera* aqueous extract represent an interesting attribute that increases its biological efficacy.

The clonogenic cell survival assay determines the ability of a cell to proliferate indefinitely, preserving its reproductive capacity to form a large colony or a clone. A cell survival response denotes the relationship between the concentration of the agent used to produce an insult and the fraction of cells that retain their ability to reproduce [17]. The clonogenic survival reduction induced by *P. strombulifera* indicates a long-term reproductive damage. In an oncological context, diminished clonogenicity represents a powerful treatment trait related to the reduction in cell repopulation, a decrease in metastatic potential and a lower emergence of secondary drug resistance [18,35,36].

After having demonstrated *P. strombulifera* cytotoxicity, we considered it relevant to analyze the mutagenic potential of the extract. Actually, in oncology, there are compounds that act by inducing DNA damage. A typical example is the group of platinum derivatives, which mainly form different types of DNA adducts. Despite their confirmed efficacy, platinated drugs act as mutagenic agents by themselves, leading to many undesirable effects. Some of these effects collaborate

to by-pass drug actions and allow the acquisition of harmful biological properties, such as collateral effects, secondary resistance and regrowth capacity. The achievement of these capabilities may increase post-treatment malignancy [37,38]. We performed mutagenicity studies in order to determine whether our extract induces DNA alterations. The results presented herein demonstrate that the extract concentrations used to induce cytotoxic effects did not lead to DNA mutations. Consequently, the extract can be used without risking the unexpected effects observed as a consequence of DNA injuries.

An important contribution of this work is related to the study of in vivo sub-chronic toxic effects. Even though there are several reports of human consumption [4,7,39], there are no detailed toxicological studies related to *P. strombulifera*. Using a healthy model of BALB/c mice, our study excludes any deleterious effects on animal homeostatic balance.

In conclusion, this is the first report of the cytotoxic effect of *P. strombulifera* aqueous extract on *in vitro* cell lines. The outcome of the treatment involves cytostasis at lower concentrations and lethal effects at higher concentrations. The mechanisms associated to cell death are apoptosis and necrosis. Regarding the long-term outcome of treatment, lethal concentrations were able to induce persistent cell damage, as was evidenced by a significant reduction in clonogenic survival assay. Mutagenic activity of the extract was not induced by effective concentrations used on cell lines. Lastly, sub-chronic administration of the extract did not induce toxicity *in vivo*. Altogether, these results make *P. strombulifera* aqueous extract a promising natural product for cancer research and treatment.

## Acknowledgements

The authors are grateful to Dr. Mariella Superina and Tiffany Weidner for the editing of the manuscript. We thank Drs. Fanelli and Nadin for the generous gift of the cell lines and Dr. Ezquer for the reagents provided. This work was supported by 06/J372 and 06/J437 grants, from Secretaría de Ciencia, Técnica y Postgrado (SeCTyP) - Universidad Nacional of Cuyo - Argentina.

## References

1.	Ferlay J, Shin HR, Bray F, Forman D, Mathers C, et al. (2010) Estimates of worldwide burden of cancer in 2008: GLOBOCAN 2008. Int J Cancer 127: 2893-2917.

2.	Pereira DM, Valentao P, Correia-da-Silva G, Teixeira N, Andrade PB (2012) Plant secondary metabolites in cancer chemotherapy: where are we? Curr Pharm Biotechnol 13: 632-650.

3.	Ruffa MJ, Ferraro G, Wagner ML, Calcagno ML, Campos RH, et al. (2002) Cytotoxic effect of Argentine medicinal plant extracts on human hepatocellular carcinoma cell line. J Ethnopharmacol 79: 335-339.

4.	Roig F (2002) Flora medicinal mendocina. Las plantas medicinales y aromáticas de la provincia de Mendoza (Argentina) (1st edn), EDIUNC Serie Manuales Nº 33, Mendoza, Argentina.

5.	Ariza Espinar L, Barboza GE, Bonzani NE, Cantero JJ, Filippa EM, et al. (2006) Flora medicinal de la provincia de Córdoba. Pteridófitas y antófitas silvestres o naturalizadas (1st edn) Museo Botánico, Córdoba, Argentina.

6.	González Loyarte M, Gaviola S, Rodeghiero A, Buk E, Menenti M (2007) Methodological proposal for assessing peripheral lands to the Lavalle irrigated oasis, Mendoza (Argentina). Rev FCA UNCuyo 38: 109-126.

7.	Hadad MA, Ribas YA (2010) Raíces Huarpes: Uso medicinal de plantas en la comunidad de Lagunas del Rosario, Mendoza, Argentina. (1stedn) Eds María Cecilia Montani y Cecilia Vega Riveros, San Juan, Argentina.

8. Saragusti AC, Bustos PS, Pierosan L, Cabrera JL, Chiabrando GA, et al. (2012) Involvement of the L-arginine-nitric oxide pathway in the antinociception caused by fruits of Prosopis strombulifera (Lam.) Benth. J Ethnopharmacol 140: 117-122.

9. Anesini C, Perez C (1993) Screening of plants used in Argentine folk medicine for antimicrobial activity. J Ethnopharmacol 39: 119-128.

10. Pérez C, Anesini C (1994) Antibacterial activity of alimentary plants against Staphylococcus aureus growth. Am J Chin Med 22: 169-174.

11. Pérez C, Anesini C (1994) In vitro antibacterial activity of Argentine folk medicinal plants against Salmonella typhi. J Ethnopharmacol 44: 41-46.

12. Reginato MA, Abdala GI, Miersch O, Ruiz OA, Moschetti E, et al. (2012) Changes in the levels of jasmonates and free polyamines induced by Na2SO4 and NaCl in roots and leaves of the halophyte Prosopis strombulifera. Biologia 67: 689-697.

13. Widmer TL, Laurent N (2006) Plant extracts containing caffeic acid and rosmarinic acid inhibit zoospore germination of Phytophthora spp. pathogenic to Theabroma cacao. European Journal of Plant Pathology 115: 377-388.

14. Mosmann T (1983) Rapid colorimetric assay for cellular growth and survival: application to proliferation and cytotoxicity assays. J Immunol Methods 65: 55-63.

15. Freeburg EM, Goyeneche AA, Seidel EE, Telleria CM (2009) Resistance to cisplatin does not affect sensitivity of human ovarian cancer cell lines to mifepristone cytotoxicity. Cancer Cell Int 9: 4.

16. Musa MA, Badisa VL, Latinwo LM, Cooperwood J, Sinclair A, et al. (2011) Cytotoxic activity of new acetoxycoumarin derivatives in cancer cell lines. Anticancer Res 31: 2017-2022.

17. Munshi A, Hobbs M, Meyn RE (2005) Clonogenic cell survival assay. Methods Mol Med 110: 21-28.

18. Franken NA, Rodermond HM, Stap J, Haveman J, van Bree C (2006) Clonogenic assay of cells in vitro. Nat Protoc 1: 2315-2319.

19. Rafehi H, Orlowski C, Georgiadis GT, Ververis K, El-Osta A, et al. (2011) Clonogenic assay: adherent cells. J Vis Exp.

20. Gamarra-Luques CD, Goyeneche AA, Hapon MB, Telleria CM (2012) Mifepristone prevents repopulation of ovarian cancer cells escaping cisplatin-paclitaxel therapy. BMC Cancer 12: 200.

21. Maron DM, Ames BN (1983) Revised methods for the Salmonella mutagenicity test. Mutat Res 113: 173-215.

22. http://www.oecd-ilibrary.org/environment/oecd-guidelines-for-thetesting-of-chemicals-section-4-health effects

23. http://www.slideshare.net/priscilaoliveira3975/manual-de-hematologia-18585125

24. Tang YQ, Jaganath IB, Sekaran SD (2010) Phyllanthus spp. induces selective growth inhibition of PC-3 and MeWo human cancer cells through modulation of cell cycle and induction of apoptosis. PLoS One 5: e12644.

25. McDaniels AE, Reyes AL, Wymer LJ, Rankin CC, Stelma GN Jr (1993) Genotoxic activity detected in soils from a hazardous waste site by the Ames test and an SOS colorimetric test. Environ Mol Mutagen 22: 115-122.

26. Vargas VM, Motta VE, Henriques JA (1993) Mutagenic activity detected by the Ames test in river water under the influence of petrochemical industries. Mutat Res 319: 31-45.

27. Negi PS, Jayaprakasha GK, Jena BS (2003) Antioxidant and antimutagenic activities of pomegranate peel extracts. Food Chemistry 80: 393–397.

28. Saklani A, Kutty SK (2008) Plant-derived compounds in clinical trials. Drug Discov Today 13: 161-171.

29. Pfisterer PH, Wolber G, Efferth T, Rollinger JM, Stuppner H (2010) Natural products in structure-assisted design of molecular cancer therapeutics. Curr Pharm Des 16: 1718-1741.

30. Heinrich M, Gibbons S (2001) Ethnopharmacology in drug discovery: an analysis of its role and potential contribution. J Pharm Pharmacol 53: 425-432.

31. Xu DB, Wang YL, Yue Y, Wu SC, Ding H (2013) [Inhibitory effect of a novel histone deacetylases inhibitor FK228 on human colon cancer HCT-116 cells in vitro and in vivo]. Zhonghua Zhong Liu Za Zhi 35: 814-818.

32. Gao J, Yan Q, Liu S, Yang X (2014) Knockdown of EpCAM enhances the chemosensitivity of breast cancer cells to 5-fluorouracil by downregulating the antiapoptotic factor Bcl-2. PLoS One 9: e102590.

33. Díaz-García A, Morier-Díaz L, Frión-Herrera Y, Rodríguez-Sánchez H, Caballero-Lorenzo Y (2013) In vitro anticancer effect of venom from Cuban scorpion Rhopalurus junceus against a panel of human cancer cell lines. J Venom Res 4: 5-12.

34. Russo A, Piovano M, Clericuzio M, Lombardo L, Tabasso S, et al. (2007) Putrescine-1,4-dicinnamide from Pholiota spumosa (Basidiomycetes) inhibits cell growth of human prostate cancer cells. Phytomedicine 14: 185-191.

35. Creton G, Benassi M, Di Staso M, Ingrosso G, Giubilei C, et al. (2006) The time factor in oncology: consequences on tumour volume and therapeutic planning. J Exp Clin Cancer Res 25: 557-573.

36. Facompre N, Nakagawa H, Herlyn M, Basu D (2012) Stem-like cells and therapy resistance in squamous cell carcinomas. Adv Pharmacol 65: 235-265.

37. Sedletska Y, Giraud-Panis MJ, Malinge JM (2005) Cisplatin is a DNA-damaging antitumour compound triggering multifactorial biochemical responses in cancer cells: importance of apoptotic pathways. Curr Med Chem Anticancer Agents 5: 251-265.

38. Chaney SG, Campbell SL, Bassett E, Wu Y (2005) Recognition and processing of cisplatin- and oxaliplatin-DNA adducts. Crit Rev Oncol Hematol 53: 3-11.

39. Hurrell JA, Ulibarri EA, Puentes JP, Buet Costantino F, Arenas PM, et al. (2011) Leguminosas medicinales y alimenticias utilizadas en la conurbación Buenos Aires-La Plata, Argentina. Boletín latinoamericano y del caribe de plantas medicinales y aromáticas 10: 443-455.

# 10

# Effect of Ethanol Leaf Extract of *Moringa oleifera* on Oxidative Stress and Atherogenic Indices of Otapiapia-Exposed Albino Rats

**Chidi Uzoma Igwe**[1*], **Linus A. Nwaogu**[1], **Emeka E. Ezeokeke**[1], **Callistus I. Iheme**[1], and **Love Nma Alison**[2]

[1]*Department of Biochemistry, Federal University of Technology Owerri, Owerri, Imo State, Nigeria*

[2]*Department of Biology, Federal University of Technology Owerri, Owerri, Imo State, Nigeria*

[*]**Corresponding author:** Chidi Uzoma Igwe, Department of Biochemistry, Federeal University of Technology Owerri, Owerri, Imo State, Nigeria, E-mail: igwechidi9@gmail.com

## Abstract

**Objective:** Otapiapia is a locally produced, easily accessible, non-regulated household pesticide, which could easily contaminate human food. The ameliorative effect of ethanol leaf extract of *Moringa oliefera* on otapiapia-induced changes in oxidative stress, lipid profile and atherogenic indices of albino rats was investigated using standard methods.

**Methodology:** Twenty-four apparently healthy Wister male albino rats (150-180 g) were divided into 4 groups (I-IV) of 6 animals each. Group I served as the control, while group II animals were given otapiapia contaminated feed and distilled water. Group III were fed uncontaminated diet and *M. oleifera* extract drink. Group IV animals were also given the contaminated diet and *M. oliefera* extract. The feed and drinks were provided *ad libitum* for a period of 14 days.

**Result:** The results show that intake of otapiapia significantly ($p < 0.05$) reduced serum superoxide dismutase and catalase activities and HDL-c concentration but increased significantly ($p < 0.05$) the concentrations of malondialdehyde, total cholesterol, triacylglycerol, LDL-c and VLDL-c. The derangements were significantly more pronounced in the atherogenic predictor indices than with lipid profile values. The observed effects of otapiapia were significantly ($p < 0.05$) countered by administration of *M. oliefera* leaf extract.

**Conclusion:** The results indicate that *M. oleifera* is a potent anti-poison with ameliorative effect against otapiapia-induced changes in biomarkers of oxidative and atherogenic damages in animals.

**Keywords:** Drum stick; Anti-poison; Lipid profile; Pesticides; Drug antidote

## Introduction

Otapiapia is a vernacular name of Eastern Nigeria origin. It is a household name for pesticides, which translates to 'that which completely consumes/devours'. Local pesticide producers emphasize the potency of their products with the name "otapiapia" indicating that such products will completely eradicate all pest problems at homes [1]. Its acceptance and widespread use in Nigeria could be attributed to its cheapness, efficacy, accessibility and affordability. Reports assert that otapiapia is an unspecified pesticide, whose application is regarded as dangerous practice since its chemical constituents are unknown [2]. However, some evidence indicates that dichlorvos is the major active pesticide ingredient of otapiapia formulations. Other chemical constituents reported to be contained in this locally formulated pesticide include toluene, (1-methylethyl)-benzene, 1,2,3-trimethyl benzene, decane, undecane, dodecane and 11,12-dibromo-tetradecan-1-ol acetate [3]. Some may also contain a homemade cocktail of kerosene, oil, alcohol or any other suitable solvent.

For pesticides to be effective against the pests intended for control, they must be biologically active. Thus, they are potentially hazardous to humans, animals, other organisms and the environment. Pesticide toxicity can result from ingestion, inhalation or dermal absorption. People who use pesticides or regularly come in contact with them must understand the relative toxicity, potential health effects, and preventive measures needed to reduce exposure to the products they use [4]. Locally produced pesticides have led to many morbidity and mortality in Nigeria and the world at large [5,6]. Their effects being mainly via contamination of food [2]. Children are more prone to accidental poisoning by such products [7,8].

*Moringa oleifera* is the most widely cultivated species of the family, Moringaceae [9]. It is a slender, softwood small tree that branches freely and can be extensively fast growing. All parts of moringa tree are edible. Moringa-based food has been attributed to have a high protein, amino acids, micronutrients antioxidants, flavonoids and glucosinolate contents. It provides an important supplement to low-nutrition foods such as cereals and bulb crops. Moringa is known in the developing world as a vegetable, a medicinal plant and a source of vegetable oil [10]. It was employed for the treatment of different ailments in the indigenous system of medicine [11]. It has also been found scientifically to have various medicinal effects, as well as blood and water purifying potentials [12].

The present study is aimed at assessing the anti-poison potential of *Moringa oleifera* leaves. The study determined the ameliorative effects of the intake of ethanol extract of *M. oleifera* leaves on oxidative stress, lipid profile and atherogenic indices of albino rats exposed to otapiapia contaminated feed.

## Materials and Methods

### Collection of otapiapia

The locally formulated pesticide, otapiapia was randomly purchased from Eke-onunwa Market in Owerri Municipal Area of Imo State. The pesticides bought were in 10 ml bottles. Examination of the bottles showed that product registration number and chemical contents were not displayed on any of the bottles.

### Preparation of otapiapia contaminated feed

The content of ten bottles of the otapiapia were emptied into a conical flask and mixed. Then, 20 ml was measured out with a calibrated syringe, mixed with 20 ml of distilled water and evenly dispersed on 1000 g of growers' chicken feed (Guinea Feed Nigeria Ltd.). The contaminated feed was air-dried to a constant weight and stored in an air-tight bag at room temperature ready for use.

### Collection of *Moringa* leaves

Healthy leaves of *M. oleifera* were obtained from an Agriculturist, Mr. Patrick Ezegbudo at Umuawulu, Anambra State, Nigeria. The leaves were authenticated at the Department of Forestry and Wildlife, Federal University of Technology, Owerri. The leaves were air-dried to a constant weight and milled to powder form.

### Preparation of plant extract

The dried powdered leaves (500 g) were dissolved in 1200 ml of ethanol and the flask allowed to stand for 4 days with intermittent shaking. The solution was filtered with Whatman No. 1 filter paper into another glass jar of known weight and the filtrate was completely extracted with a soxhlet extractor. The ethanol extract obtained was concentrated to 140 g on a hot plate at 50°C. Suspensions of the extract were prepared in distilled water at 10 g per litre of water.

### Experimental animals

Twenty-four male Swiss albino rats weighing 150-180 g used for the study were purchased from Animal Friend Ltd., Owerri, Imo State.

| Treatment | Groups | | | |
|---|---|---|---|---|
| | Control | CFG | MOG | CF+MOG |
| Uncontaminated feed (100g/day) | √ | - | √ | - |
| Contaminated feed (100g/day) | - | √ | - | √ |
| Distilled water (15 ml/day) | √ | √ | - | - |
| Moringa oleifera | - | - | √ | √ |

Table 1: Animal grouping and treatments. CFG: Contaminated Feed Group; MOG: Moringa oleifera Group; CF+MOG: Contaminated Feed +M. oleifera Group.

The animals were acclimatized to standard laboratory conditions of 12 h light/dark cycle for 14 days at the small animal House of the Department of Biochemistry, Federal University of Technology,

Owerri. They were provided with water and standard uncontaminated feed *ad libitum*. Later, the animals were weighed and randomly allotted into 4 groups of 6 animals each with similar average weight ranges per group. The animals were treated as shown in Table 1.

The contaminated and uncontaminated feed, distilled water and *M. oleifera* extract were freshly provided for each group every morning *ad libitum*. Ethical approval for all stages of the study was obtained from the Federal University of Technology Owerri ethical committee. The animals were humanely handled in accordance with the Principles of Laboratory Animal Care as described in NIH publication of 1985-1993.

### Blood sample collection and processing

At the end of 14 days of treatment, the animals were fasted overnight, anaesthetized with diethyl ether vapour and whole blood was quickly collected by cardiac puncture. About 5 ml of blood collected was dispensed carefully into heparin bottle and thoroughly but gently mixed. The anticoagulated blood was centrifuged at 3000 rpm for 5 minutes and the plasma separated into freshly labeled bottle for determination of the biochemical parameters.

### Analyses of biochemical parameters

The plasma samples were analyzed for the activities of catalase and superoxide dismutase using previously described methods [13,14], while the concentration of malondialdehyde was determined using Gutteridge and Wilkins method [15]. Total cholesterol (TC) and high density lipoprotein cholesterol (HDL-c) concentrations were respectively determined by enzymatic [16] and HDL-c precipitant [17] methods. Triacylglycerol (TG) concentration was assessed as earlier described [18]. The concentrations of plasma LDL-c and VLDL-c were calculated using previously published formulae [19,20].

The atherogenic predictor indices were estimated using the following formulae as earlier described [21,22].

Atherogenic Index of Plasma (AIP)=log TG/HDL-c;

Castelli's Risk Index I (CRI-I)=TC/HDL-c;

Castelli's Risk Index II (CRI-II)=LDL-c/HDL-c; and

Atherogenic Coefficient (AC)=(TC-HDL-c)/HDL-c.

### Statistical analysis

One-way analysis of variance (ANOVA) and Turkey's post-hoc tests were carried out with the aid of GraphPad Prism version 5.3 software (GraphPad Inc., USA) to determine statistical differences between means of the animal groups. Values were adjudged statistically significant at $p \leq 0.05$.

## Results and Discussion

Figure 1 shows that intake of the otapiapia contaminated feed significantly ($p < 0.05$) reduced serum activities of superoxide dismutase (SOD) and catalase (CAT), but significantly ($p < 0.05$) increased the malondialdehyde (MDA) concentration of the animals. SOD and CAT are the key antioxidant enzymes for cellular defense system against oxidative stress. SOD catalyzes the conversion of superoxides ($O_2^-$) to hydrogen peroxide ($H_2O_2$) and thus it is a major defense system for aerobic cells in combating the toxic effects of superoxide radicals. Meanwhile, the product of SOD catalysis is a harmful by-product of many normal metabolic processes. To prevent $H_2O_2$ based damage to cells and tissues, it must be quickly converted into other less toxic substances. CAT is used by cells to rapidly catalyze the decomposition of $H_2O_2$ into less reactive gaseous oxygen and water molecules [23]. The SOD and CAT activities of the animals fed otapiapia contaminated feed were significantly lower than that of the control and *M. oleifera* groups. Toxicants induce disturbances in the physiological state of animals, which could affect enzyme activity. These may cause distortions in cell organelles, which may lead to either elevation or reduction in activity of enzymes, depending on whether there was a cellular damage releasing such enzymes into blood or disruption in the biosynthetic pathway of the enzyme protein [24].

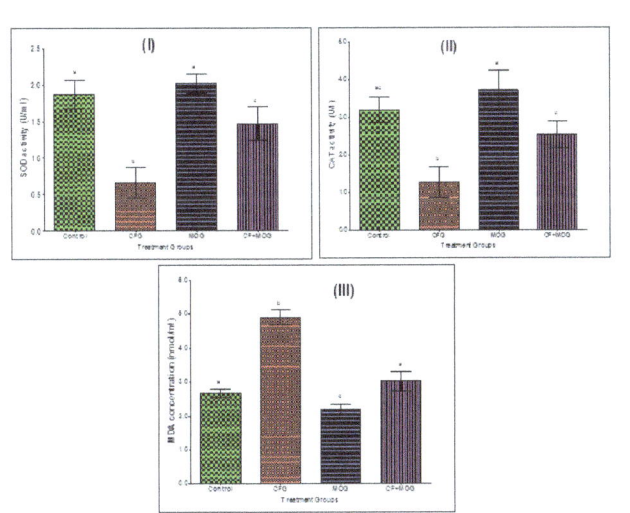

Figure 1: Oxidative stress parameters of albino rats fed otapiapia contaminated diet and *Moringa oleifera* leaf extract. Bars are mean ± standard deviation. Bars with different superscripts per graph are statistically significant (p ≤ 0.05). (I): superoxide dismutase (SOD); (II): catalase (CAT); (III): malondialdehyde (MDA); CFG: contaminated feed group; MOG: M. oleifera group; CF+MOG: contaminated feed+M. oleifera group.

MDA is a product that results from lipid peroxidation of polyunsaturated fatty acids and thus has been applied in the estimation of degree of peroxidation in tissues [25]. The observed significant increase in MDA of the toxicant's exposed animals buttresses the presence of oxidative stress in the exposed animals as indicated by the increased serum activities of SOD and CAT.

*Moringa oleifera* administration to intoxicated animals significantly (p<0.05) ameliorated the observed oxidative toxicity induced by otapiapia. The Figure shows that *M. oleifera* significantly improved CAT and SOD activities but reduced MDA concentrations to values comparable with those of the control animals. The result collaborates an earlier report that *M. oleifera* prevents acetaminophen induced liver injury through restoration of declined glutathione level [26]. The observation could be attributed to the presence in the plant of rich combination of antioxidant phytochemicals that have been reported to possess antioxidant, antitumour and antiinflammatory activities [11,12].

Intake of otapiapia intoxicated feed significantly (p<0.05) increased the plasma concentrations of TC, TG, LDL-c and VLDL-c as shown in

Table 2. On the other hand, the HDL-c concentration of the intoxicated animals reduced significantly. Administration of *M. oleifera*, which had opposite effects to those of otapiapia, significantly ameliorated the observed dyslipidaemia elicited by intake of the contaminated diet. The observed increases in the plasma TC, TG and LDL-c concentrations of otapiapia exposed animals is in agreement with the reported findings of hypercholesterolaemia and hypertriglyceridaemia after induction of organ injury such as in hepatotoxicity with common toxicants [27]. Organophosphate-based pesticides have been reported to cause an increase in total cholesterol and lipid levels [28]. The observed dyslipidaemia may be attributed to the effects of pesticide toxicants on the permeability of liver cell membranes or the blockage of liver bile ducts, causing a reduction or cessation of cholesterol secretion into the duodenum [29].

| Parameters (mmol/l) | Groups | | | |
|---|---|---|---|---|
| | Control | CFG | MOG | CF+MOG |
| TC | 3.73 ± 0.13[ac] | 3.94 ± 0.11[a] | 2.57 ± 0.20[b] | 3.59 ± 0.23[c] |
| TG | 1.56 ± 0.05[a] | 2.45 ± 0.04[b] | 1.52 ± 0.08[a] | 1.66 ± 0.07[a] |
| HDL-c | 0.94 ± 0.06[a] | 0.46 ± 0.05[b] | 1.47 ± 0.07[c] | 0.82 ± 0.08[a] |
| LDL-c | 0.72 ± 0.07[a] | 1.61 ± 0.03[b] | 0.67 ± 0.10[a] | 0.96 ± 0.06[c] |
| VLDL-c | 0.26 ± 0.02[ac] | 0.32 ± 0.01[b] | 0.23 ± 0.03[a] | 0.28 ± 0.03[c] |

Values are mean ± standard deviation. Values with different superscripts per row are statistically significant (p ≤ 0.05). TC: Total Cholesterol; TG: Triacylglycerol; HDL-c: High Density Lipoprotein Cholesterol; LDL-c: Low Density Lipoprotein Cholesterol; VLDL-c: Very Low Density Lipoprotein Cholesterol; CFG: Contaminated Feed Group; MOG: *M. oleifera* Group; CF+MOG: Contaminated Feed+*M. oleifera* Group.

**Table 2:** Lipid and lipoprotein profile parameters of albino rats fed Otapiapia contaminated diet and *Moringa oleifera* leaf extract.

The observed cholesterol lowering ability of *M. oleifera* could be attributed to its saponin content [30]. Saponins prevent excessive intestinal absorption of cholesterol and thus have been associated with the risk reduction for cardiovascular diseases [31]. The observed significant elevation of HDL-c concentration in animals administered *M. oleifera* further indicates its beneficial effect against cardiovascular diseases. HDL-c is synthesized and secreted by liver cells.

It removes excess cholesterol from circulation and carries them back to the liver for degradation or conversion to bile acids [32]. Table 3 shows the effect of intake of otapiapia contaminated diet on atherogenic predictor indices of the animals. The results showed that the intoxicated diet significantly (p<0.05) increased the serum total non-HDL cholesterol concentration with concomitant significant increases in Castelli's risk index I (TC/HDL-c) and II (LDL-c/HDL-c). The diet also significantly increased atherogenic coefficient (TC - HDL-c)/HDL-c) and atherogenic index of plasma (log TG/HDL-c) levels of the treated animals. These are as expected since they are calculated based on the use of HDL-c value as the denominator. Thus, reduction in HDL-c concentration as elicited by the intake of otapiapia led to significantly high values for the atherogenic indices.

Interestingly, administration of *M. oleifera* significantly (p<0.05) ameliorated the observed effects of otapiapia intoxication.

| Parameters | Groups | | | |
|---|---|---|---|---|
| | Control | CFG | MOG | CF+MOG |
| TC/HDL-c | 3.97 ± 0.16 [a] | 8.56 ± 0.27 [b] | 1.75 ± 0.32 [c] | 4.38 ± 0.23 [a] |
| LDL-c/HDL-c | 0.77 ± 0.13 [a] | 3.50 ± 0.19 [b] | 0.46 ± 0.17 [c] | 1.17 ± 0.10 [d] |
| Total non-HDL-c (mmol/l) | 2.79 ± 0.07 [a] | 3.48 ± 0.15 [b] | 1.10 ± 0.09 [c] | 2.77 ± 0.18 [a] |
| (TC-HDL-c) / HDL-c | 2.97 ± 0.10 [a] | 7.56 ± 0.23 [b] | 0.75 ± 0.18 [c] | 3.38 ± 0.26 [d] |
| Log TG/HDL-c | 0.22 ± 0.01 [a] | 0.73 ± 0.05 [b] | 0.12 ± 0.01 [c] | 0.31 ± 0.04 [d] |

**Table 3:** Atherogenic predictor indices of albino rats fed otapiapia contaminated diet and *Moringa oleifera* leaf extract.

These observations were significantly more pronounced in the atherogenic predictor indices than with the exact lipid profile values as reported in Table 2. This further buttresses the link between derangements in lipid profile and the atherogenic predictor indices. However, it also indicatess that the calculated atherogenic predictor indices may be better indicators than lipid profile parameters in monitoring of diseases associated with dyslipidaemia. These findings agree with the earlier reports that determination of the relative proportions of cholesterol in proatherogenic (TC, TG, and LDL-c) and antiatherogenic (HDL-c) lipoproteins are more valuable than the individual lipid measurements in cardiovascular disease (CVD) risk assessment [33].

## Conclusion

Intake of feed contaminated with otapiapia, an organophosphate based pesticide, caused significant decreases in plasma activities of antioxidant enzymes and HDL-c concentrations but increased concentrations of MDA, TC, TG, LDL-c and VLDL-c. It also led to increases in atherogenic predictor indices suggesting possible induction of oxidative stress, dyslipidaemia and associated cardiovascular risk in exposed subjects. Administration of *M. oleifera* extract significantly ameliorated the effects of the otapiapia exposure. The results indicate that *M. oleifera* could be an effective antidote to pesticide-induced oxidative damage, lipid abnormality and other possible atherogenic complications thereof in animals. Further studies are needed to explain the mechanism of pesticide-induced oxidative and lipid abnormality and to ascertain the component(s) of *M. oliefera* extract with the observed potentials.

## References

1. Mortui C (2006) Igbo lesson. Niajaryders.

2. Akunyili D (2007) Otapiapia' not registered with NAFDAC. Daily Triumph Newspaper.

3. Ofordile CP, Okoye PAC, Raphael P (2014) Determination of actual chemical composition of a locally formulated pesticide product in a Nigerian market. Int J Sci Technol 3:264-268.

4. Lorenz ES (2009) "Potential Health Effects of Pesticides". Ag Communications and Marketing 1-8.

5. USEPA (2007) Dichlorvos TEACH Chemical Summary U.S. EPA. Toxicity and Exposure Assessment for Children.

6. Olebunne CE (2009) Social Entrepreneurship; The Nigerian Perspective.

7. Okeniyi SO, Adedoyin BJ, Garba S (2013) Phytochemical Screening, Cytotoxicity, Antioxidant and Antimicrobial Activities of Stem and Leave Extracts of Euphorbia heterophylla. J Biol Lif Sci 4: 24-31.

8. Gilden RC, Huffling K, Sattler B (2010) Pesticides and health risks. J Obstet Gynecol Neonatal Nurs 39: 103-110.

9. Mahmood KT, Mugal T, Haq IU (2010) Moringa oleifera: A natural gift-A review. J Pharmacy 2: 775- 781.

10. Paliwal R, Sharma V, Pracheta SS (2011) A review of Horse Radish Tree (*Moringa oleifera*): A Multipurpose Tree with High Economic and Commercial Importance. As J Biotechnol 3: 317-328.

11. Anwar F, Latif S, Ashraf M, Gilani AH (2007) Moringa oleifera: a food plant with multiple medicinal uses. Phytother Res 21: 17-25.

12. Kumar V, Pandey N, Mohan V, Singh RP (2012) Antibacterial and antioxidant activity of extract of Moringa oleifera leaves-An in vitro study. Int J Pharm Scis Rev Res 12: 89-94

13. Sinha AK (1972) Colorimetric assay of catalase. Anal Biochem 47: 389-394.

14. Olatosin TM, Akinduko DS, Uche CZ, Bardi J (2014) Effects of Moringa oleifera seed oil on acetaminophen-induced oxidative stress and liver damage in Wistar albino rats. IOSR J Pharm Biolo Scis 9: 53-59.

15. Gutteridge JMC, Wilkins S (1982) Copper-dependent hydroxyl radical damage to ascorbic acid: formation of a thiobarbituric acid reactive product. Federation of European Biomedical Societies Letters 327-330.

16. Allain CC, Poon LS, Chan CSG, Richmond W, Fu PC (1974) Enzymatic Determination of total serum cholesterol. Clin Chem 20: 470-475.

17. Lopes-Virella MF, Stone P, Ellis S, Colwell JA (1977) Cholesterol determination in high-density lipoproteins separated by three different methods. Clin Chem 23: 882-884.

18. Bucolo G, David H (1973) Quantitative determination of serum triglycerides by the use of enzymes. Clin Chem 19: 476-482.

19. Friedewald WT, Levy RL, Fredrickson DS (1972) Estimation of the concentration of low density lipoprotein cholesterol in plasma without use of the preparative ultracentrifuge. Clin Chem 18: 499-502.

20. Crook MA (2006) Plasma lipids and Lipoproteins. In: Clinical Chemistry and Metabolic Medicine, 7th edn, Edwalrd Arnold publishers Ltd., UK.

21. Bhardwaj S, Bhattacharjee J, Bhatnagar MK, Tyagi S (2013) Atherogenic index of plasma, Castelli Risk Index and Atherogenic coefficient-New parameters in assessing Cardiovascular Risk. Int J Pharm Biol Sci 3: 359-364.

22. Castelli WP, Abbott RD, McNamara PM (1983) Summary estimates of cholesterol used to predict coronary heart disease. Circulation 67: 730-734.

23. Chelikani P, Fita I, Loewen PC (2004) Diversity of structures and properties among catalases. Cell Mol Life Sci 61: 192-208.

24. Mahmoud K, Shalahmetove T, Deraz SH (2011) Effect of crude oil intoxication on antioxidant and marker enzymes of tissue damage in liver of rats. Inter J Biol Veteri Agric Food Enginer. 5: 93-96.

25. Davey M, Stals E, Panis B, Keulemans J, Swennen R (2005) High-throughput determination of malondialdehyde in plant tissues. Anal. Biochem. 347: 201-207.

26. Fakurazi S, Hairuszah I, Nanthini U (2008) Moringa oleifera Lam prevents acetaminophen induced liver injury through restoration of glutathione level. Food Chem Toxicol 46: 2611-2615.

27. Aba PE, Eneasato CP, Onah JA (2016) Effect of Quail Egg Pretreatment on the Lipid Profile and Histomorphology of the Liver of Acetaminophen-Induced Hepatotoxicity in Rats. J Applied Biol Biotech 4: 034-038.

28. Kalender S, Ogutcu A, Uzunhisarcikli M, Açikgoz F, Durak D, et al. (2005) Diazinon-induced hepatotoxicity and protective effect of vitamin E on some biochemical indices and ultrastructural changes. Toxicology 211: 197-206.

29. Zaahkouk SM, Helal EE, Abd-Rado TI, Rashed SA (2000) Carbamate toxicity and protective effect of Vit A and Vit E on some biochemical aspects of male albino rats. Egyptian J Hosp Medici 1: 60-77.

30. Adesina SK (2005) The Nigerian Zanthoxylum: Chemical and Biological Values African. Compl Alter Med 2: 282-381.

31. Olaleye MT (2007) Cytotoxicity and antibacterial activity of methanolic extract of Hibiscus sabdariffa. J Med Plant Res 1: 009-013.

32. Rahilly Tierney CR, Spiro A, Vokonas P, Gaziano JM (2011) Relation between high-density lipoprotein cholesterol and survival to age 85 years in men (from the VA normative aging study). Am J Cardiol 107: 1173-1177.

33. Ranjit PM, Guntuku G, Pothineni RB (2015) New atherogenic indices: Assessment of cardiovascular risk in postmenopausal dyslipidemia. Asian J Med Sci 6: 25-32.

# 11

# Effect of Sub-Acute Exposure to Nickel on Hematological and Biochemical Indices in Gold Fish (*Carassius auratus*)

**Mahsa Javadi Moosavi[1]\* and Vali-Allah Jafari Shamushaki[2]**

[1]*Gorgan University of Agricultural Science and Natural Resources, Faculty of Fishery and Environmental Science, Golestan, I.R. Iran*

[2]*Department of Fisheries, Gorgan University of Agricultural Sciences and Natural Resources, Gorgan, Iran*

**\*Correspondence author:** Moosavi MJ, Gorgan University of Agricultural Science and Natural Resources, Faculty of Fishery and Environmental Science, Golestan, I.R. Iran, E-mail: javadimoosavi@gmail.com

## Abstract

The increasing use of heavy metals in industry in the modern world unfavorably affects the aquatic environment. Acute toxicity of nickel to the fresh water fish carassius auratus was determined using Probite analyze, Fish were exposed to selected concentration of nickel and the mortality data were determined after 24, 48, 72 and 96 hours. LC50 values for 24,48,72 and 96 hours were calculated with the 95% fiducially limits. The 24,48,72 and 96 hours LC50 values of nickel to the fish were 161.78 ± 3.05, 130.58 ± 2.32, 110.19 ± 1.57, 100.39 ± 0.54 ppm respectively. White blood cell (WBC) count, hemoglobin (Hb) and hematocrit (Hct) level were significantly reduced at experimental concentrations ($p < 0.05$). Red blood cell (RBC) count, mean corpuscular hemoglobin (MCH), cortisol and glucose levels in nickel treated groups were significantly higher than the controlled group at experimental periods ($p < 0.05$) but significant differences were not found in mean corpuscular hemoglobin concentration (MCHC) and mean corpuscular volume (MCV) ($p > 0.05$). In summary, nickel intoxication resulted indicated that hematological and biochemical parameters can be used as an indicator of nickel related stress in fish on exposure to elevated nickel status.

**Keywords:** Heavy metal; Nickel; Contamination; Toxicity

## Introduction

One of the most prominent natural resources is water that its regular supply is extremely much essential for the survival of all living animals. The variations impurities display in water sources are expressed through water quality changeful which are broadly classified as biological and Physicochemical. In the different industries greatly used heavy metals in some industries of the new world adversely affect the aquatic animals after eject of the waste material into water [1]. The improvement coefficient of this metal in the food chain arrived extreme. Once it's absorbed by the animals and people through food chain in the form of fish, shrimp shell fish and plants, it would collect in the corresponding functional organs of the animals and human body. The important action of the environmental toxicologist is to assess impartially the endanger obtained from the presence of such materials. These materials may also alter the quality of water and thus desecrate the fisheries management [2,3].

Nickel is greatly utilized in industry and is a common aquatic pollutant. In natural waters $Ni^{+2}$ is the important chemical species. In aquatic ecosystems nickel interacts with very many inorganic and organic compounds and occurs as soluble salts adsorbed onto materials of various chemical origin [4] many of these interactions are additive or synergistic in producing adverse effects, and some are antagonistic. The toxicity of nickel to aquatic life was intensively investigated during previous decades, and a considerable amount of experimental data has been compiled and reviewed [5]. Fish are used as test organisms in aquatic toxicology because of their top position in the trophic chain and their role as food for humans.

Hematological values are progressively used in fish as indicators of the physiological or sub-lethal stress response to endogenous or exogenous alterations and are more quickly reflected in the poor condition of fish than in other commonly measured [6].

## Material and Method

### Experimental fish and laboratory condition

Acute toxicity tests were conducted on goldfish (10.5 ± 1.0 g and 8.7 ± 1.2 cm) obtained from commercial fish farms, Gorgan, Iran. Only healthy fish, as obtained by their activity and external appearance, were maintained alive on board in a fiberglass tank. Samples were transferred to a 400 L aerated tank with 200 L of test medium. All samples were acclimated for 10 days in 10 aerated fiberglass tanks at 19°C under a constant 12:12 L:D photo period. Acclimatized fish were fed daily a formulated feed. Dead fish were immediately removed with special plastic forceps to avoid possible deterioration of water quality. The average values for aerated and dechlorinated tap water used during the both acclimation period and experiments were pH 8.17 ± 0.40, dissolved oxygen 8.23 + 0.17 mg/L, temperature of 22.26 ± 1°C and total hardness 274+1.57 mg/L as $CaCO_3$. Water was renewed daily, and the water quality parameters mentioned above were measured twice a week during the acclimation period and sub-acute toxicity test.

### Acute toxicity test

Only healthy fish, as indicated by their activity and external appearance, were maintained alive on board in a fiberglass tank. Fish were transferred to a 400 L-aerated tank equipped with aeration with 200 L of test solution. The acute toxicity test was conducted following the Organization for Economic Cooperation and Development guideline under static renewable test conditions. Groups of 21 fish were exposed to various concentrations of nickel for 96 h. Values of mortalities were measured at 24, 48, 72 and 96 h, and dead fish were immediately removed by dip net to avoid possible deterioration of the water quality. The LC50 values were calculated by EPA Probit Analysis V. 1.5 for 24, 48, 72 and 96 h [7].

## Sub chronic test

Following the toxicity test, in order to investigate the effect of nickel on hematological and biochemical parameters of the three fish, two concentrations (40% and 80% of 96-h LC50) were considered. In this stage, 120 randomly selected Carasius auratus from acclimation tanks and randomly graded into several experimental 400-L tanks expose to concentrations of 40% and 80% of 96-h LC50 for a period of seven days to hematological, plasma glucose and cortisol analysis. For sub-acute toxicity assay, the exposure water in the tank was changed daily and freshly prepared solution was added to maintain the concentration of nickel at a constant level. Moreover, during the experiment, water was continuously monitored. A control test without nickel was conducted under the same conditions.

## Biochemistry and hematology

Blood samples were collected from both the control and experimental fishes that survived the 7 Days sub-acute exposure period. The blood samples were taken by cutting posterior caudal vein using ethylenediaminetetraacetate (EDTA) as anticoagulant [8]. Blood, 2.0 ml, was decanted in heparinzed bottles for determination of blood parameters. The microhaematocrit method of Snieszko (31) was used to determine the hematocrit (Ht). Hemoglobin (Hb) concentration was measured with Hb test kit using the cyanmethemoglobin method [9]. Determinations of the number of white blood cell (WBC) and red blood cell (RBC) tests were performed immediately on fresh blood. The number of blood leukocytes and erythrocytes was counted by diluting heparinized blood with Gimsa stain at 1:30 dilution, and cells

were counted using a hemocytometer Neubauer under the light microscope [10]. The derived hematological indices of mean corpuscular volume (MCV), mean corpuscular hemoglobin (MCH) and mean corpuscular hemoglobin concentration (MCHC) were calculated using standard formulae as described by Jain (29): MCV was calculated in femtoliters=Ht/RBC x 10; MCH was calculated in picograms=Hb/RBC x 10; and MCHC=(Hb in 100 mg blood/Hct) x 100. For the biochemical tests, the blood was placed in tubes and allowed to clot at room temperature (approximately 22°C) for 30 min. Serum was removed from the clotted sample after centrifugation at 2795 g for 5 min and frozen at 80°C until analysis. The determination of plasma glucose were carried out using diagnostic kits (Pars Azmoon Co., Iran) at 546 nm and 38°C by the glucose oxidase method [11]. Glucose were measured photometrically according to a method modified based on the quantification of NADH after a glucose oxidation catalyzed by glucose dehydrogenase also cortisol was determined directly from serum using an ELISA kit (DRG Diagnostics, Mountainside, NJ, USA) as described by Shaluei et al.[7].

## Statistical analyses

For each index, Experimental data and those of control were tested by means of analysis of variance (ANOVA). Standard deviation (SD). Significance was set at P=0.05. All analysis was performed using SPSS software (version 18.0).

## Results

The results of the acute toxicity test for the nickel on gold fish are presented in Table 1. No mortality was observed in the control group during the experiment. Fish mortality increased significantly when the concentration and the time of exposure were increased. As expected, the 96-h LC 50 values decreased with increase in exposure time. This indicates an increase in toxicity with exposure duration. Prior to death, fish exhibited rapid gill movement, nervous manifestations, erratic swimming, loss of equilibrium and inability to remain upright.

| | Concentration (ppm) (95% of confidence limits) | | | |
|---|---|---|---|---|
| point | 24 h | 48 h | 72 h | 96 h |
| LC1 | 43.32 ± 3.05 | 32.74 ± 2.32 | 25.13 ± 1.57 | 21.49 ± 0.54 |
| LC10 | 68.54 ± 3.05 | 49.28 ± 2.32 | 35.33 ± 1.57 | 30.83 ± 0.54 |
| LC30 | 114.49 ± 3.05 | 99.44 ± 2.32 | 52.21 ± 1.57 | 65.59 ± 0.54 |
| LC50 | 161.78 ± 3.05 | 130.58 ± 2.32 | 110.19 ± 1.57 | 100.39 ± 0.54 |
| LC70 | 180.35 ± 3.05 | 154.43 ± 2.32 | 132.11 ± 1.57 | 120.19 ± 0.54 |
| LC90 | 199.78 ± 3.05 | 171.59 ± 2.32 | 153.42 ± 1.57 | 150.95 ± 0.54 |
| LC99 | 211.45 ± 3.05 | 199.57 ± 2.32 | 171.13 ± 1.57 | 161.53 ± 0.54 |

Table 1: Lethal Concentrations (LC1-99) of nickel (mean ± Standard Error) depending on time (24-96 h) for goldfish.

## Hematological parameters

Results of hematological parameters (RBC, WBC, Hb, Hct, MCH, MCHC and MCV) of the test and control Goldfish expose to 40% and 80% of LC50 are shown in Table 2.

## Glucose and cortisol

The average plasma glucose levels and cortisol in the unexposed control group of Goldfish was 45 ± 1.19 mg/dl and 27 ± 1.04 ng/ml respectively. As it is obvious from Figures 1 and 2, there was a significant increase in the glucose levels of the treated groups when compared with their respective controls (P<0.05). Glucose plasma levels in gold fish exposed to 40 and 80% of 96 h-LC50 were 57 ± 1.02 and 68 ± 1.08 and also cortisol plasma levels in gold fish exposed to 40 and 80% of 96 h-LC50 were 34 ± 1.02 and 41 ± 1.06, respectively.

There was a significant increase in gold fish exposing 80% of 96 h-LC50 than those exposed to 40% of 96 h-LC50. In fact, the value of glucose decreased with increasing the concentration.

| Fish | Treatments | RBC(106 cells/l) | Hb(g/l-1) | Hct(%) | WBC(cells/l) | MCH (pg/cell) | MCHC(g/l-1) | MCV(µm³/cell) |
|------|-----------|------------------|-----------|--------|--------------|---------------|-------------|---------------|
| Goldfish | Control | 0.68 ± 0.10 a | 7.41 ± 0.04 a | 17.24 ± 0.03 a | 8656.13 ± 217.15 a | 117.1 ± 0.19 a | 47.31 ± 0.14 a | 297 ± 2.31 a |
| | 40% of LC50 | 0.75 ± 0.02 b | 6.00 ± 0.05 b | 14.30 ± 0.05 b | 7533.33 ± 88.19 b | 95.33 ± 0.05 b | 45.91 ± 0.03 a | 295 ± 1.19 a |
| | 80% LC50 | 0.80 ± 0.03 c | 4.90 ± 0.10 c | 11.86 ± 0.05 c | 6400.27 ± 88.19 c | 90.74 ± 0.10 b | 45.62 ± 0.04 a | 294 ± 1.35 a |

**Table 2:** Some hematological parameters values of exposed to nickel in rows and Significant differences from control values (P<0.05). Each value expresses the means ± standard error of three observations. Letters show different compare to control group (n=21).

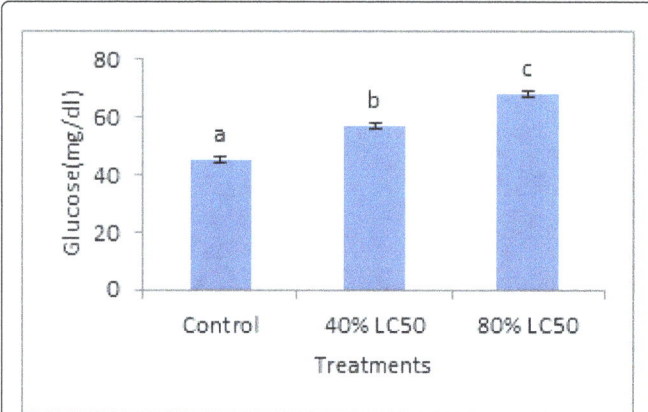

**Figure 1:** Serum cortisol levels in goldfish exposed to sub lethal concentrations of nickel for 7 days.

in the both concentration (40 and 80% LC50), also increased plasma glucose levels were observed on 7 day exposure. The coalition of elevated plasma cortisol and glucose levels is frequently observed following exposure of fish to water pollutants or other stressors, and the relationship very likely is causal: the primary response leads to the secondary via stimulation by cortisol of gluconeogenesis [16-18].

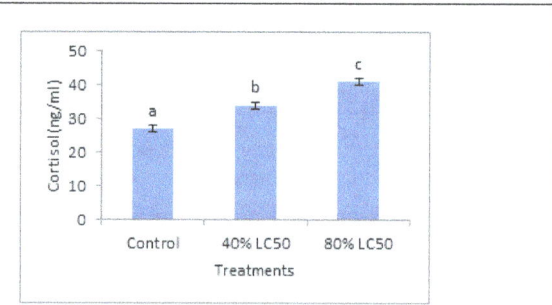

**Figure 2:** Cortisol levels in goldfish exposed to sub lethal concentrations of nickel for 7 days.

## Discussion

It is apparent from the outcome that the heavy metal concentration has a direct effect on the LC50 values of the respective fish. LC50 acquired in the recent study correspond to assess that have been published in the literature for other species of fish. The distinction in acute toxicity may be due to alters in water quality and trial species [12]. The impressionability of fish species to a particular heavy metal is a very main factor for LC50 stages. Fish that are very sensitive to the toxicity of one material may be less or even not sensitive to the toxicity of another metal at the many level of that metal in the ecosystem. Unlike, a metal which is very toxic to a fish species at low concentrations may be less or even non-toxic to other species at the same or even higher concentrations [12].

Serum glucose levels of gold fish exposed to sub-lethal concentrations of nickel for 7 days increased with enlarging concentrations (80% LC50) of nickel in the water. Vinodhini et al. [13] in common carp with exposing of fish to heavy metals showed that the concentrations of serum glucose were significantly elevated. Serum glucose levels also increased with increasing concentrations of Cd in Mugil cephalus [14]. It was indicated that serum glucose stages in fish were affected by many stress parameter, including heavy metals [15]. Exposure to nickel indicates to draw out a temporary stress reply in gold fish. Significantly increased plasma cortisol were evident on 7 day

In sub efficient or stressful situation the chromaffin cells release catecholamine hormones, adrenaline and noradrenaline toward blood circulation [19] Those stress hormones in connection with cortisol circulate and exalt glucose production in fish through glucogenesis and glycogenolysis pathways to cope with the energy demand produced by the stressor for the "fight of flight" reaction. Glucose is then released toward blood circulation and enters into cells through the insulin action [20]

The Ht, Hb, RBC, WBC, MCV, MCH and MCHC of the fishes exposed to nickel are indicated in Table 2. Significant different were watched between the different blood indices with various concentrations of toxicants. The results indicate that changes in hematological parameters of fish may be owed to nickel and are predestine both by the concentrations of the heavy metals in the water and time of exposure and both these factors can cause inverted and non-inverted changes in the homeostatic system of fish [21].

Our results in the hematological indices shown that no significant change was recorded in the mean corpuscular volume (MCV) and mean corpuscular hemoglobin content (MCHC) but there was significant change in the mean corpuscular hemoglobin (MCH) especially at higher concentrations (80% LC50). However, small vacillation was recorded in the MCV and MCHC when compared with the control. Cells released from the spleen, which is an erythropoietic organ would have the lower MCV values when compared with the control. A similar observation was made for Cyprinus carpio after cadmium exposure (30). The significant different in the MCH of the trial fish when compared with the control may be resulted to the decrease in cellular blood iron, resulting in reduced oxygen carrying capacity of blood and eventually stimulating erythropoiesis [22].

Results of the hematological part, indicated that the mean WBC, Ht, and Hb of fish in the control trial were 17.24 ± 0.03 (%), 8656.13 ± 217.15 (cells/l) and 7.41 ± 0.04 g/dl respectively. Decrease in these factors was observed in the trial fish as the concentration increases as a reply to the 7 day exposure to nickel. The sunset were significant at higher concentration (80% LC50) (P<0.05). The decrease in WBC count of the treatment groups may be due to the release of epinephrine during stress which is capable of causing the contraction of spleen [23]. Our results demonstrate that hemoglobin and hematocrit counts could be ascribed to the dissolve of erythrocytes. Similar reductions given by Vinodhini et al. [13]. When exposed fish to polluted environment under in vitro conditions. Therefore, the significant decrease in these factors is an indication of severe anemia caused by exposure of the experimental fish to nickel in the water. Vinodhini et al. [13] observed that various fish species after zinc exposure increased hematocrit levels. They ascribed such an increase in hematocrit values to increase in the size of the erythrocytes as being exhibited for chromium and zinc treated rainbow trout. Observed depression in hematocrit and hemoglobin count linked with decreased and deformed erythrocytes are obvious signs of anemia [24]. Unlike our results Srivastava and Mishra [25] reported that in *Cotisa fasciatus* after acute exposure to sublethal concentration (15 ppm) of lead RBC count were decreased, also reported results similar to ours haematocrit values and haemoglobin content were decreased. However, they recognized haemolytic anaemia on the basis of RBC lysis. The number of leukocytes in fish can also vary between individuals of a single species, depending on the conditions under which the sample of blood is taken or on the physiological conditions of the fish. This individual variation within a species is thought to be too great as to render impractical the use of white blood cell count as a diagnostic tool in fish diseases [26]. The lessen number of WBC may be the result of bio concentration of the checked metal in the kidney and liver. Other authors have associated the cause to hindering of granulopoiesis or lymphpoiesis, induced by primary or secondary changes in haematopoietic organs [23]. Similar our study Annune et al. [27-30] reported a significant increase in RBC count of *C. gariepinus* when exposed to Zinc treatment. They indicated the RBC elevation to blood cell reserve integrated with cell shrinkage as a result of osmotic alterations of blood by the action of the metal. Results of the present investigation indicated that the sub-acute nickel concentrations tested is a toxic substance in goldfish and may cause several changes in the serum biochemical parameters [31,32].

## Acknowledgments

The authors thank the aquaculture research center and Fishery group for the supply of research material. This work was supported by the Gorgan University of Agricultural Sciences and Natural resources.

## References

1.  Hedayati A, Safahieh A, Savari A, Ghofleh Marammazi J (2010) Assessment of aminotransferase enzymes in Yellowfin sea bream under experimental condition as biomarkers of mercury pollution. World Journal of Fish and Marine Science 2: 186-192.

2.  Al-Akel MJK, Shamsi HF (2000) Effect of Cadmium on the cichlid fish Orechromis niloticus: Behavioural and Physiological responces. J. Uni. w: 341-346.

3.  Nath K, Kumar N (1988) Hexavalent chromium: toxicity and its impact on certain aspects of carbohydrate metabolism of the freshwater teleost, Colisa fasciatus. Sci Total Environ 72: 175-181.

4.  Us epa (1980) Ambient water quality criteria for nickel. EPA-440/5-80-060. Office of Water Regulations and Standards. Washington, DC.

5.  Eisler R (1998) Nickel hazards to fish, wildlife and invertebrates: a synoptic review. Biological Science Report USGS/BRD/BSR-1998-0001, Laurel, MD,

6.  Cataldi E, Di Marco P, Mandich A, Cataudella S. Serumparameters (1998) Adriatic sturgeon Acipenser naccarii (Pisces: Acipenseriformes): effects of temperature and stress. Comp Biochem Physiol 121A: 351-354.

7.  Shaluei F, Hedayati A, Jahanbakhshi A, Kolangi H, Fotovat M (2013) Effect of subacute exposure to silver nanoparticle on some hematological and plasma biochemical indices in silver carp (Hypophthalmichthys molitrix). Hum Exp Toxicol 32: 1270-1277.

8.  Schmitt CJ, Blazer VS, Dethloff GM, Tillitt DE, Gross TS, et al. (1999) Biomonitoring of environmental status and trends (BEST) program: Field procedures for assessing the exposure of fish to environmental contaminants. Information and Technology Report USGS/BRD-1999-0007. U.S. Geological Survey, Biological Resources Division, Columbia 68p.

9.  Larsen HN, Snieszko SF (1961) Comparison of various methods of determination of haemoglobin in trout blood. Prog. Fish Cult. 23: 8-17.

10. Stevens ML (1997) Fundamentals of Clinical Hematology. WB Saunders, Philadelphia

11. Jahanbakhshi A, Imanpoor M, Taghizadeh V, Shabani A (2012) Hematological and serum biochemical indices changes induced by replacing fish meal with plant protein (sesame oil cake and corn gluten) in the Great sturgeon (Huso huso) Comp Clin Pathol.

12. Hedayat A, Jahanbakhshi A, shaluei F, Malekpour Kolbadinezhad S (2012) Acute Toxicity Test of Mercuric Chloride (Hgcl2), Lead Chloride (Pbcl2) and Zinc Sulphate (Znso4) in Common Carp (Cyprinus carpio), J Clinic Toxicol. 3: 1.

13. Vinodhini R, Narayanan M (2009) The impact of toxic heavy metals on the hematological parameters in common CARP (Cyprinus carpio l.): Iran. J Environ Health Sci Eng V 6: 23-28.

14. Hilmy AM, Shabana MB, Daabees AY (1985) Effects of cadmium toxicity upon the in vivo and in vitro activity of proteins and five enzymes in blood serum and tissue homogenates of Mugil cephalus. Comp Biochem Physiol C 81: 145-153.

15. Canlo M (1995) Effects of mercury, chromium and nickel on some blood parameters in the carp Cyprinus carpio. Tr. J of Zoology 19: 305-311.

16. Leach GJ, Taylor MH (1982) The effects of cortisol treatment on carbohydrate and protein metabolism in Fundulus heteroclitus. Gen Comp Endocrinol 48: 76-83.

17. Leach GJ, Taylor MH (1980) The role of cortisol in stress-induced metabolic changes in Fundulus heteroclitus. Gen Comp Endocrinol 42: 219-227.

18. Pickering AD, Pottinger TG (1983) Seasonal and diel changes in plasma cortisol levels of the brown trout, Salmo trutta L Gen Comp Endocrinol 49: 232-239.

19. Reid SG, Bernier NJ, Perry SF (1998) The adrenergic stress response in fish: control of catecholamine storage and release. Comp Biochem Physiol C Pharmacol Toxicol Endocrinol 120: 1-27.

20. Iwama GK, Vijayan MM, Forsyth RB, Ackerman PA (1999) Heat shock proteins and physiological stress in fish. American Zoologist, 39: 901-909.

21. Farkas A, Salánki J, Specziár A (2002) Relation between growth and the heavy metal concentration in organs of bream Abramis brama L. populating Lake Balaton. Arch Environ Contam Toxicol 43: 236-243.

22. Hodson PV, Blunt BR, Spray DJ (1978) Chronic toxicity of water borne lead and dietary lead to rainbow trout. (Balmo garnderi) in lake Ontario water. Water Res. 12: 869-878.

23. Svoboda M (2001) Stress in fishes (a review). Bull. VURH Vodnany 4: 169-191.

24. Maheswaran R, Devapanl A, Muralidharan S, Velmurugan B, Ignaeimuthu S (2008) Haematological studies of fresh water fish, Clarias batradrus (L) exposed to mercuric chloride. IJIB 2: 49-54.

25. Srivastava AK, Agrawal SJ (1979) Haematological anomalies in a fresh water teleost, Colisa fasciatus, on acute exposure to cobalt. Acta Pharmacol Toxicol (Copenh) 44: 197-199.

26. Ellis AE (1977) The leucocytes of fish: A review. J Fish Biol 11: 453-491.

27. Annune PA, Ebele SO, Olademeji AA (1994) Acute toxicity of cadmium to juveniles of Clarias gariepinus (Teugels) and Oreochromis niloticus (Trewawas) J Environ Sci Health A29: 1357-1365.

28. Shaluei F, Hedayati A, Jahanbakhshi A, Baghfalaki M (2012) Physiological responses of great sturgeon (Huso huso) to different concentrations of 2-phenoxyethanol as an anesthetic. Fish Physiol Biochem 38: 1627-1634.

29. Jain NC (1986) Schalm's Veterinary Heamatology (4thedn.) Lea and Febiger, Philadelphia: 1221.

30. Koyama J, Ozaki H (1984) Hematological changes of fish exposed to low concentrations of cadmium in the water. Bull. Japan Soc. Sci. Fish 50: 199-203.

31. Snieszko SF (1960) Microhaematocrit as a tool in fishery research and management. U. S. Wildl Serv Sci Rep Fish. 314: 15-23

32. Besten PJ, Munawar M (2005) Ecotoxicological Testing of Marine and Freshwater Ecosystems. Taylor and Francis: 293.

# 12

# Epidemic Self-Poisoning with Seeds of *Cerbera manghas* in Eastern Sri Lanka: An Analysis of Admissions and Outcome

**Pirasath Selladurai[1*], Sundaresan Thadsanamoorthy[2] and Gnanathasan Ariaranee C[3]**

[1]*Teaching Hospital, Jaffna, University of Colombo, Sri Lanka*

[2]*Batticaloa, University of Colombo, Sri Lanka*

[3]*Department of Clinical Medicine, Faculty of Medicine, University of Colombo, Sri Lanka*

[*]**Corresponding author:** Dr. Pirasath Selladurai, Teaching Hospital, Ilavalai North, Ilavalai, Jaffna, University of Colombo, Sri Lanka, E-mail: selladuraipirasath81@gmail.com

## Abstract

The use of plant fruits and seeds as a method of self-poisoning is common in South Asia, with most deaths being due to ingestion of (yellow oleander) seeds. Self-poisoning with the locally common *Cerbera manghas* (CM) fruit is prevalent in the Eastern Province of Sri Lanka. We carried out a retrospective study to determine the clinical manifestations, treatment and outcome of patients with *cerbera manghas* self-poisoning in Batticaloa teaching hospital. Data were collected retrospectively on all cases with *Cerbera manghas* self-poisoning from 1st January 2011 to 31st October 2013.There were 48 patients [mean age: 21(± 0.43) yrs], (male: female=35:13). Twenty four had ingested half of a seed (25 g). Most of the patients were symptomatic with vomiting (48), dizziness (24) and abdominal pain (20). Forty (83.3%) had cardiac arrhythmias that required transfer to the poisoning unit for specialized management. Severe cardiac toxicity was observed among patients (18) with fewer amount of seeds (25 g) compared to patients (8) with large amount of seeds (50 g). The 1st degree heart block (10, 20.8%), 2nd degree heart block (Type I:5, 10.4%, type II:12, 25.0%), complete heart block (10, 20.8%) and sinus bradycardia (5, 10.4%) were ECG findings. Fourteen (29.16%) had high serum potassium concentrations between 6.0 and 6.9 mmol/L; ten had life threatening hyperkalemia (>7.0 mmol/L). All patients were treated with multiple doses of activated charcoal. Temporary cardiac pacing was required in nine (18.7%) cases. There were eight deaths (16.7%), due to third-degree heart block and life threatening hyperkalemia. *Cerbera manghas* self-poisoning was common among young males in Batticaloa district of Sri Lanka's Eastern Province. Cardiac toxicity was observed in patients with fewer amounts of seeds. Patients presenting with complete heart block and severe hyperkalemia had great risk of mortality.

## Key Words:

Plant poisoning; Suicide; Cardiac toxicity; *Cerbera manghas*

## Introduction

While self-poisoning with Pesticides is the most common method of self-harm in Asia, self-poisoning with plant seeds or fruits is also common, especially in the South Asian region [1]. While most deaths follow ingestion of *Thevitia peruviana (*yellow oleander) seeds, other locally common plants are also implicated [2]. We noted that cases of self-poisoning with *Cerbera manghas* (sea mango, pink eyed cerbera, odollam tree) fruits, while being most commonly reported in Tamil Nadu and Kerala [3,4] are seen in the Eastern Province of Sri Lanka.

*Cerbera manghas* is a poisonous plant belonging to the Apocynaceae family notorious for its cardiac glycoside cardiotoxicity. *C. manghasis* called *diyakaduru*in Sinhala, *kattuarali* in Indian Tamil; *natchuchukkaii*in Sri Lankan Tamil. *Cerbera manghas* Linn (previously also *Cerberaodollam Gaertn*) is common along the coasts of south Asia and south East Asia, Northern Australia, and Polynesia. In Sri Lanka, especially along coastal regions, sea mango (*Cerbera manghas*) is a very common plant and readily accessible. It grows to a height of 5 to 10 metres and bears whorled branchlets with terminal lanceolate leaves. The fruit of the sea mango turns bright red at maturity and appear very much like the edible mango (*Mangifera* spp.) fruit. The latex present throughout the plant contains cardenolides (such as cerberin, neriifolin, and cerberoside) (Figure 1) that cause vomiting, cardiac dysrhythmias, and hyperkalemia via inhibition of the Na$^+$/K$^+$ATPase.

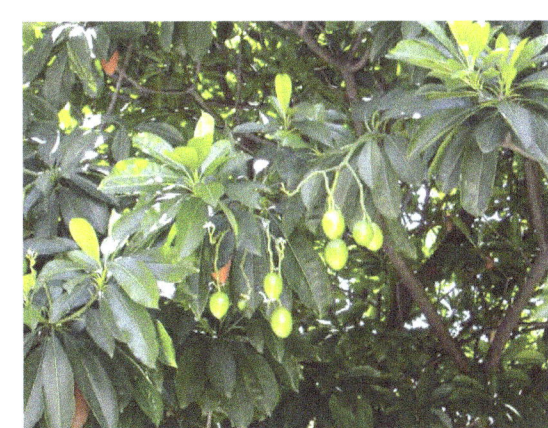

**Figure 1:** Cerbera odollam tree leaves and seeds.

Although widespread in Sri Lanka [5], and well known to be poisonous [6], only a one report has been published from the island.

However, there have been no publications reporting clinical data from poisoned patients.

The aim of this study was to evaluate the clinical manifestations, biochemical findings and outcome of management using currently available treatment in the poisoning unit of a tertiary care hospital in Eastern Sri Lanka.

## Materials and Methods

### Study population

Patients with *Cerbera manghas* poisoning admitted to tertiary care hospital in Eastern Sri Lanka from 1st January 2011 to 31st October, 2013 by were included using predesigned questionnaires, retrospectively.

### Treatment of patients

Patients with *Cerbera manghas* poisoning were treated in medical wards and poisoning unit, tertiary care hospital in Eastern Sri Lanka with different treatment modalities such as activated charcoal, intravenous boluses of atropine/isoprenaline, temporary pacing and supportive measures depending on the clinical manifestations.

### Electrocardiographic monitoring

12-lead standard electrocardiography (INNOMED Medical ECG machine) and 2-lead ECG monitoring were taken during the standard work up of each patient in this unit.

### Blood samples

Five milliliters (5 ml) venous blood was collected from each patient. Serum was separated by centrifuging in a laboratory centrifuge at for three minutes after blood clotting and retraction at room temperature. Serum potassium ($K^+$) and Sodium ($Na^+$) were analyzed at the Department of Chemical Laboratory. Renal function including blood urea nitrogen [BUN], creatinine and liver function indices including SGOT, SGPT, PT and serum protein were analyzed in the clinical laboratory of Batticaloa teaching hospital using standard automated techniques.

### Statistical analysis

Differences between the two groups (patients with significant arrhythmia vs. patients with insignificant arrhythmia) were analyzed with pair-wise comparisons. Baseline results are presented as counts and percentages and as mean ± SD for continuous variables. A P value <0.05 was considered significant.

## Results

We noted 583 cases of poisoning from 1st January, 2011 to 31st October, 2013. Among these, 192 (32.93%) cases were due to Yellow Oleander poisoning, while 48 (8.23%) cases were due to *Cerbera manghas* poisoning. There were 48 patients [Mean age: 21 (± 0.43) yrs], (Male: Female=35:13) with *Cerbera manghas* self-poisoning. The great majority were in the 16-30 year age group (40, 83.3%). The ethnicity of the majority of patients was Tamil (42, 87.5) (Table 1). Twenty four (50%) of them had ingested half a seed (one seed weighted about 20 g) (Table 2).

| Personal Characteristics | | Number of cases (%) |
|---|---|---|
| Sex | Male | 35 (72.9%) |
| | Female | 13 (27.1%) |
| Ethnicity | Tamil | 42, 87.5%), |
| | Muslims | 6 (12.5%) |
| Age | <16yrs | 1 (2.0%) |
| | 16-30 years | 40 (83.3%) |
| | 31-45years | 3 (6.25%) |
| | 4-60years | 3 (6.25%) |
| | >60years | 1 (2.0%) |

Table 1: Personal characteristics of patients.

| Amount of seeds | No of cases (%) |
|---|---|
| 10 g | 24 (50%) |
| 20 g | 10 (20.8%) |
| 40 g | 8 (16.7%) |
| >40 g | 6 (12.5%) |

Table 2: Number of seeds ingested by patients.

Most of the patients were symptomatic with symptoms of cardiac glycoside toxicity including vomiting (48, 100%), dizziness (24, 50%) and abdominal pain (20, 41.6%). Abdominal pain and diarrhea alone was rare presentations. Neurological manifestations such as drowsiness and restless (8, 16.6%) were also associated. Cardiac dysrhythmias such as bradycardia or an irregular pulse were the examination findings. ECG findings showed 1st, 2nd, 3rd degree heart block and sinus bradycardia (Table 3). A normal ECG was found only in 6 patients. Atrial fibrillation was the tachyarrythmias. Mean serum potassium concentration was significantly higher in patients with significant cardiac arrhythmias that required specific management transfer to CCU and temporary pacemaker insertion.

| ECG findings | | No of cases (%) |
|---|---|---|
| 1st degree heart block | | 10 (20.8%) |
| 2nd degree heart block | Type I | 5 (10.4%) |
| | Type II | 12 (2%) |
| 3rd degree heart block | | 10 (20.8%) |
| Sinus bradycardia | | 5 (10.4%) |
| Normal ECG | | 6 (12.5%) |

Table 3: ECG findings of Patients.

Fourteen of them had higher serum potassium concentrations (6.4 (± 0.97) mmol/L). Ten patients had life threatening hyperkalemia [7.4 (± 0.17)]. All patients developed cardiac toxicity and hyperkalemia within 24 hrs of ingestion of seeds. These severe cardiac toxicity and hyperkalemia were observed among patients (16, 33.3%) having half seed of ingestion. All other blood investigations including renal and liver markers are within normal range (Table 4).

| Blood investigations | | Range | No of cases (%) |
|---|---|---|---|
| Serum Electrolytes | Sodium | 13-145 mEg/L | 48 (100%) |
| | Potasium | <5 mEq/L | 6 (12.5%) |
| | | 5-5.5 mEq/L | 15 (31.25%) |
| | | 5.6-6.0 mEq/L | 5 (10.4%) |
| | | 6.1-6.5 mEq/L | 8 (29.16%) |
| | | 6.6-7.0 mEq/L | 4 (8.33%) |
| | | >7.0 mEq/L | 10 (20.8%) |
| | SGPT | <40 U/L | 48 (100%) |
| Liver enzymes | SGOT | 12-20 U/L | 48 (100%) |
| Blood urea | | <30 mg | 48 (100%) |
| Serum Creatinine | | 0.6-1.0 mg/dL | 48 (100%) |
| PT/INR | | 1-1.3 | 48 (100%) |

**Table 4:** Blood Investigations of patients.

All patients were treated with multiple doses of activated charcoal. Patients with bradyarrhythmias were treated with intravenous atropine (18, 37.5%) and intravenous infusions of isoprenaline (4, 12.5%). Temporary cardiac pacing was required in nine of them who had not responded to drug therapy. There were eight deaths who had both 3rd heart block and high serum potassium concentrations (>7.0), (Figure 2; ECG tracings). Three died before definitive treatment could be instituted. The majority of patients with cardiac toxicity had an uneventful recovery. Multiple doses of activated charcoal alone were safe and adequate in most cases in our study. However it was not statistically proven. All patients with hyperkalemia were managed only with insulin-dextrose (10 units Insulin with 50 ml 50% Dextrose regime).

Features of severe toxicity such as persistent vomiting, severe abdominal pain, neurological signs and persistent hyperkalemia were significantly associated with high risk of mortality and morbidity (P<0.05). The risk of cardiac toxicity was observed with patients with ingestion of less amount of seeds (half seed).

## Discussion

A previous study in 2000/2001 showed that *Cerebera manghas* is the cause for 20% deaths from plant poisoning and 4.4% of all self-harm deaths in this hospital on the eastern coast of Sri Lanka [7]. It was the second commonest plant poisoning in Eastern Sri Lanka next to Yellow Oleander Poisoning in our study period. Review of our study confirmed that *Cerbera manghas* plant poisoning produces clinical features typical of cardenolide poisoning [8]: in particularly; vomiting, cardiac dysrrhythmias and hyperkalemia. Electrocardiographic changes are the most obvious marker of *Cerbera manghas* toxicity [9]. The most common ECG abnormality is bradycardia, which may be

sinus bradycardia, sinus arrest or exit block, or AV nodal dissociation (third degree heart block).

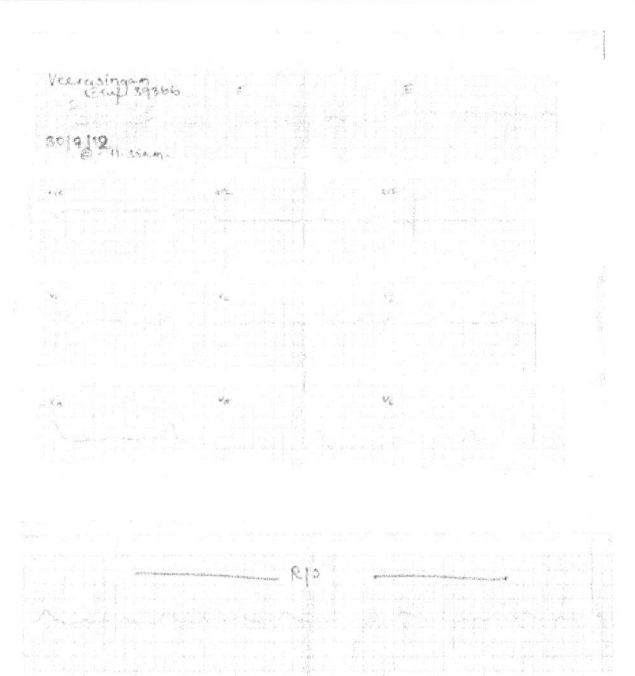

**Figure 2:** ECG tracing of a patient; 54 year old man presented with severe vomiting, abdominal pain and restless following ingestion of half seed of *cerbers manghas* after 8hrs of ingestion. His ECG showed complete heart block. His serum Potassium was 7.9 mmol/dL. He died within 2 hrs of hospital admission even before pacing was instituted.

Management involved gastric lavage, multiple doses of activated charcoal, administration of atropine to counter bradycardia and Insulin-Dextrose to treat hyperkalemia. The effect of atropine on outcomes in cases of bradyarrhythmia has not been formally assessed. However a study from Trivandrum reported a poor outcome if bradycardia did not respond to atropine and atropine was not effective [10].

Cardic arrhythmias and persistent hyperkalemia are important predictable mortality risk for *Cerbera manghas* plant poisoning. There were eight deaths (16.67%) due to third-degree heart block and life threatening hyperkalemia in our study. These deaths were observed among patients having half seed of ingestion. These severe cardiac toxicity and hyperkalemia were observed among patients having half seed of ingestion and not vomiting seeds immediately. This may be due to rapid absorption of seeds in gastrointestinal tract following ingestion. The patients taking more seeds vomited immediately within 2 hrs. As a result, they have less cardiac toxicity compared those having lees amount of ingestion of seeds.

Despite its relative uncommon prevalence compared to Yellow Oleander poisoning, it is much feared by the medical staff due to high case fatality and the lack of pacemakers or anti-digoxin Fab for therapy [11].

A limitation of our study is also same as in previous study [7] that neither blood nor gastric contents were tested for *Cerbera manghas* cardenolides to prove ingestion. The responsible fruit ingestion was identified only from history from patient and relatives. However, *Cerbera manghas* is very well known in the region and easily recognized, increasingly the like hood that the ingested fruit would be accurately identified.

## Conclusion

*Cerbera manghas* self-poisoning was common among young males in Batticaloa district of the Eastern Province. The cardiac toxicity observed within 24 hrs of ingestion of seeds. The severe toxicity was associated with less amount of seeds. Most patients had specific symptoms of *Cerbera manghas* poisoning. AV conduction defects are common. Patients presenting with features of severe toxicity such as persistent vomiting, severe abdominal pain, neurological signs and persistent hyperkalemia has higher risk of mortality.

## Recommendations

*Cerbera manghas* poisoning is the second commonest plant poisoning in Eastern Sri Lanka but lack of resources can significantly impair the successful management in the hospital setting. We would like to emphasize the importance of equipping these hospitals with adequate resources, e.g: pacemakers for therapy *Cerbera manghas* poisoning to prevent adverse outcomes.

## Acknowledgements

We thank the staffs of Department of Emergency, Cardiology and Poisoning Units, Teaching Hospital, Batticaloa for the help during the course of these studies. We also thank Prof. M. Eddleston for his data from his previous paper published in 2008.

## References

1.  Eddleston M, Phillips MR (2004) Self poisoning with pesticides. BMJ 328: 42-44.

2.  Roberts DM, Eddleston M (2004) Yellow Oleander poisoning. In Critical Care update Jaypee, 189-200.

3.  Gaillard Y, Krishnamoorthy A, Bevalot F (2004) Cerbera odollam: a 'suicide tree' and cause of death in the state of Kerala, India. J Ethnopharmacol 95: 123-126.

4.  Modi NS (1988) Modi's Textook of Medical Jurisprudence and Toxicology, (21st ed) Bombay, N.M.Tripathi Private Limited.

5.  National Poisons Information Centre (2004) Poisonous plants of Sri Lanka. National Poisons Information Centre.

6.  Jayatissa LP, Dahdouh-Gueba F, Koedam N (2002) A review of the floral composition and distribution of mangroves in Sri Lanka. Botan Journal Linn Society 138: 29-43.

7.  Eddleston M, Haggalla S (2008) Fatal injury in eastern Sri Lanka, with special reference to cardenolide self-poisoning with Cerbera manghas fruits. Clin Toxicol (Phila) 46: 745-748.

8.  Iyer GV, Narendranath M (1975) A preliminary report on the neurological manifestations of Cerbera odollam poisoning. Indian J Med Res 63: 312-314.

9.  Guruswami MN, Ganapathy MN, Thampai CK (1970) A preliminary study of the pharmacological actions and toxicity of "Cerbera Odollam". Indian J Med Sci 24: 82-87.

10. Narendranathan M, Das KV, Vijayaraghavan G (1975) Prognostic factors in Cerbera Odollum poisoning. Indian Heart J 27: 283-286.

11. Eddleston M, Persson H (2003) Acute plant poisoning and antitoxin antibodies. J Toxicol Clin Toxicol 41: 309-315.

# 13

# Evaluations of Biochemical, Hematological and Histopathological Parameters of Subchronic Administration of Ethanol Extract of Albizia Gummifera Seed in Albino Wistar Rat

Mokennon Debebe[1], Mekbeb Afework[2], Eyasu Makonnen[3], Asfaw Debella[4], Bekesho Geleta[4] and Negero Gemeda[4*]

[1]College of Health Science, Arsi University, Oromia, Ethiopia

[2]Department of Anatomy, College of Health Science, Addis Ababa University, Addis Ababa, Ethiopia

[3]Department of Pharmacology, College of Health Science, Addis Ababa University, Addis Ababa, Ethiopia

[4]Traditional and Modern Medicine Research, Ethiopian Public Health Institute, Addis Ababa, Ethiopia

*Corresponding author: Negero Gemeda, Traditional and Modern Medicine Research, Ethiopian Public Health Institute Addis Ababa, Ethiopia, E-mail: negerof@yahoo.com

## Abstract

Albizia gummifera are plants found in Ethiopia that have different medicinal values. The objective of the present study was to evaluate the toxicological effects of sub-chronic administered hydro-ethanolic (70%) seeds extract of Albizia gummiferain albino Wistar rats. The seeds of these plants were collected from different areas of Ethiopia. They were dried and crushed to powder and macerated with hydro-alcohol and placed in orbital shaker. The extract was then filtered through Whatman filter paper No.1 and the filtrate was evaporated to dryness by Rota vapor and further concentrated by water bath at 40°C. The extract was packed in air tight brown glass bottles and kept in a refrigerator at 4°C. The extract was then administered to rats at different doses to determine the LD 50 of the extract and at doses of 125 mg/kg/day and 250 mg/kg/day for the sub-chronic toxicity study. The LD 50 of Albizzia gummifera were found as 4000 mg/kg and 3500 mg/kg, respectively. Statistically significant difference in body weight was observed in female rats in the 10$^{th}$ week at 250 mg/kg body weight of seeds extract of Albizia gummifera administered group and in the male rats at lowest dose during the 9$^{th}$ and 10$^{th}$ weeks of administration period for seeds extract of Millettia ferruginea. The seeds extract of Albizia gummifera statistically decreased ($p \leq 0.05$) MCHin the male rats at both doses; MCHC at both 125 mg/kg and 250 mg/kg in the female rats; and MCH in the female rats at higher dose and increased RDW-CV in the male rats at both doses. It increased NEUT at the highest dose in both females and males. The seeds extract of Millettia ferruginea decreased ($p \leq 0.05$) in the MCHC and MONO of female rats at the highest doses. ALP, ALT and urea were found significant in the female rats administered with 250 mg/kg of seeds extract. While, seeds extract of Albizia gummifera increased only urea in male rats at 250 mg/kg. Some histopathological changes in liver and kidney were also observed for both plants extracts. There were inflammations, congestions and focal hepatocellular necrosis of the liver tissue. The extracts also produced atrophyof the glomeruli of the kidney. The observed changes in both of the plant seeds extract might have resulted because of the presence of some bioactive ingredients in the extract. Therefore, the active ingredients which might be responsible for toxic insult should be researched with their mechanisms of actions.

**Keywords:** Albizia gummifera; Seeds; Hydroethanolic extract; Toxicity; Wistar Albino Rats

## Introduction

Traditional use of medicinal plants alone or in combination with Western drugs to treat a wide variety of diseases including diarrheal diseases, malaria and liesmaniasis is widely practiced in the Ethiopian communities as elsewhere in developing countries [1]. The growing popularity of traditional medicine, particularly herbal medicine is based on their observed effectiveness in the treatment and prevention of diseases. This belief is that, one, traditional medicines are 'natural' and therefore safe; in the other hand, lack of success in treating different alignments by modern medicine due to drug resistance and unfavorable side effects. However, these believes has led to indiscriminate use over a long period of time without appropriate dosage monitoring and undermining danger associated with the potential toxicity of medicinal plant therapy. There is a documented incidence of renal and hepatic toxicity resulting from the long-time administration of medicinal plants [2,3]. Therefore, this thought has necessitated us to document scientific information on the safety/toxicic risk potentials of Albizia gummifera.

*A. gummifera* is a member of Leguminosae family and Minosaideae sub family. This plant is a large deciduous tree with flattened canopy, growing up to 35 m high and trunk up to 75 cm in diameter. It is found in east Africa, the Democratic Republic of Congo, Madagascar, and West Africa, ranging from dry or wet lowlands to up land forest edges, and in riverine forest, at an altitude of 2400 m above sea level. It is indigenous in few countries namely; Angola, Cameroon, Democratic Republic of Congo, Ethiopia, Kenya, Madagascar, Nigeria, Tanzania, Uganda, and Zambia. Traditionally stem bark decoction of *A. gummifera* is used to treat malaria and an extract from fresh crushed pods is used to treat stomach pains. The seeds and stem bark of the plants have shown antibacterial activities against both gram positive and gram negative bacteria [4], molluscidal activities against Biomphalaria pfeifferi, Bulinus sp. and physaacuta [5], larvicidal activity against Aedes agypti, Aedes africanus, and Culex quinquefasciatus [6]. Its roots are used to cure skin diseases such as acne, itching and eczema. Moreover, crude hydro-alcoholic (20-80%) extracts of *A. gummifera* was effective against reference strain of N. gonorrhoeae [7].

Although Albizia gummifera has many useful health benefits, to our knowledge no literature exists on its toxicity profile. This study was therefore undertaken to evaluate the acute and sub-chronic toxicities of the ethanolic extract of *A. gummifera* seeds on biochemical, hematological and histopathological indices of albino Wistar rats.

## Materials and Methods

### Plant collection and processing

The seeds of *A. gummifera* were collected from Mettu, Illu Aba-Bora, Ethiopia which is 400 km west of Addis Ababa in the wild at altitudinal range of 900-3900 meter above sealevel. The plants identity was authenticated by taxonomist using standard Flora, and voucher specimens of *A. gummifera* (Voucher Number AG-2006), which were pre-deposited in the Herbarium of the Traditional and Modern Medicine Research, Ethiopian Public Health Institute, Addis Ababa, Ethiopia.

### Plant material extraction

The dried seeds of the plant were crushed to powder using wooden-made pestle and mortar. About 1250 gm of the powdered seeds of *A. gummifera* was macerated with hydroalcohol (70% ethanolic) in 1:4 solutes to solvent ratio and placed in orbital shaker at room temperature for 72 h. The procedure was repeated three times to extract exhaustively until the extract gave faint or no coloration. The extract was then filtered through Whatman filter paper No.1 to remove any residue, and then, it was evaporated by a vacuum rotary evaporator and further concentrated by water bath at 40°C to obtain the crude extract. Then, the gummy residue extract was and kept in air tight brown glass bottles with proper label and kept in a refrigerator at 4°C until used.

### Experimental animals

Swiss albino rats, 4 to 5 weeks of age, weighing between 100 to 120 g, that were bred at Animal Breeding Unit, Ethiopian Public Health Institute (EPHI) was used in this study. The animals were housed in sanitary cages and had access to tap water and food. The room temperature was controlled at 24 to 26°C in a 12 h light/dark cycle. All procedures involving the animals were conducted with strict adherence to standard guidelines and procedures. The male and female rats were kept in separate cages. They were all acclimatized for one week to the laboratory environment prior to drug administration. The leftover food and water were changed daily and the cages were cleaned with the husk changed every three days. All the animals seemed healthy.

### Acute oral toxicity test

The rats were randomly grouped in to twelve experimental groups (Group I to XII) and one control groups of female rats with four rats in each group. The rats were fasted overnight but allowed free access to drinking water prior to experimentation. The animals in the group I-XII received *A. gummifera* seed extract at single oral doses of 50, 100, 150, 250, 500, 1000, 1500, 2000, 2500, 3000, 3500, and 4000 mg/kg body weight, respectively, in attempt to see sign of toxicity and to

determine the $LD_{50}$ of the extracts of the plants. The control group received only distilled water. The animals were kept under observation after post-treatment in order to observe any death or any behavioural and/or clinical manifestations such as CNS effect (excitement, ataxia, and sleep), altered feeding, vomiting and diarrhoea. At the end of two weeks, one animal from each group was randomly sacrificed humanely after anaesthesia (diethyl ether) by cervical dislocation and post-mortem gross observations were carried out on the internal organs.

### Sub-chronic toxicity test

Fifteen male and 15 female Wistar rats were randomly allocated to the treatment and control groups to investigate the effect of sub chronic treatment with *A. gummifera* seed extracts on general body weight and weight of the organs (liver and kidneys); and on blood parameters as well as histopathology of liver and kidney tissues. The rats were randomly assigned to three groups of ten animals, five males and five females. One group was assigned as control group; animals in one group from the treatment group received single daily dose of 125 mg/kg body weight and the second group was administered with a single daily dose of 250 mg/kg body weight of *A. gummifera* seed extract for 90 days. Throughout the experimental period, the female and male rats were housed in separate cages. The control group received only distilled water, daily throughout the period of study. The body weight of each rat in each group was measured before the beginning of drug administration and once a week thereafter throughout the study period. Throughout the study period, animals in all the study group were carefully monitored/ followed/ for any clinical signs of toxicity, body weight changes and mortality and were later sacrificed for haematological and biochemical investigations and organs histological changes.

### Biological specimen collection

At the end of dose administration, blood samples were collected through cardiac puncture using a gauge needle mounted on a 5 ml syringe. Before specimen collection all animals were anesthetized with diethyl ether. Blood from each animal were collected into non-anti-coagulated and Ethylene Diamine Tetra-Acetic Acid (EDTA) anti-coagulated tubes and allowed to clot for 3 h. The collected blood was centrifuged within 30 min of collection at 3,000 rpm for 10 min and the serum was collected for blood chemistry (biochemical assay). After blood collection, each rat in the treated and control groups were quickly humanly sacrificed by cervical dislocation. The animals were placed in the supine position on dissection board. The limbs were stretched and fixed to make the autopsy of the organs of interest easy. At autopsy, liver and kidneys were visually examined for any signs of gross lesions. The organs removed from each rat were blotted on the filter paper. Then each of these organs was weighed on a semi-microbalance. After rinsing in normal saline, sections were taken from each of these organs. These specimens were placed in a pre-labeled sample bottles containing fixative (10% neutral buffered formalin) and used for histopathological studies.

### Hematological and biochemical analyses

Hematological and serum biochemical parameters were analyzed at Core Laboratories, Ethiopian Public Health Institute, Addis Ababa, Ethiopia. Hematological parameters including RBC count, WBC count, HCT, HGB, RDW, PLT count, and differential count of each of the WBCs were measured in an automatic hematology analyzer, cell-DYN-3700 (Abbott Diagnostic Division, USA). In addition, red cell indices such as MCV, MCH and MCHC were also analyzed with the automatic analyzer. Similarly, serum biochemical parameters including ALP, ALT, AST, and urea were determined in clinical chemistry analyzer, Human star 80 (Human GmbH, Germany).

## Histopathological Studies

### Tissue processing

For histopathological studies under light microscopy, tissue samples taken at autopsy were processed in Histology laboratory, Department of Anatomy, College of Health Sciences, Addis Ababa University. Each of the tissue samples harvested from liver and kidneys of all extract treated and non-treated animals were fixed separately in 10% neutral buffered formalin. Following fixation, the tissues were rinsed in running water overnight to remove excess fixative. The wet fixed tissues were dehydrated with progressively increasing concentrations of ethanol. After dehydration, the tissues were passed through xylene solution to clear the ethanol and facilitate molten paraffin wax infiltration (55°C). The tissues were transferred to liquid paraffin wax. The wax impregnated tissues were then embedded in paraffin blocks. All tissue blocks were labelled and allowed to dry at room temperature. These tissue blocks were sectioned with a Leica Rotary Microtome (Leica Rm2125RT, Model Rm2125, China) at 5-6 μm thickness. The ribbons of these sections were collected and gently floated on a tissue flotation water bath at a temperature of 20°C to stretch the paraffin wax impregnated tissue. The stretched floated ribbons were picked up on glass microscopic slides. The slides were placed in a warm oven overnight to help the slice adhere to the slides. The slides were allowed to cool at room temperature and kept ready for routine staining steps.

### Tissue staining

Before carrying out the staining of tissues, the sections were deparaffinised by xylene. Then the tissues were hydrated successively by running through decreasing concentration of alcohols. The slides were then rinsed in distilled water followed by Harris' haematoxylin stain. These slides were washed in tap water and dipped into 1% acid alcohol for differentiation and remove excess stain. The sections were rinsed briefly in running tap water to remove excess acid. The slides were then dipped in bluing solution followed by counter stain in eosin. The H and E stained sections were dehydrated by running through increased grade of ethyl alcohols. Lastly, these slides were mounted using DPX mountant and glass cover slips.

### Microscopy and Photomicrography

Microscopic slides of organs under study were examined carefully under compound light microscope at Histology Laboratory of Anatomy Department, College of Health Sciences, AAU. Slides from the extract treated groups were evaluated for any toxic insult to the organs compared to slides from their respective control groups. Finally, photomicrographs of selected slides were taken using (LEICA ICC50 HD, Germany) automated built-in digital photo camera.

### Statistical Analysis

The numerical data obtained from the experiment were analysed statistically on SPSS version 20, computer software package. The values of body weight changes were analysed and the results were expressed as M ± SEM. Differences between the treated and control groups were compared by using one-way analysis of variance (ANOVA), followed by Dunnett's t-test to determine their level of significance. Differences at $p < 0.05$ were considered statistically significant.

## Results

### Acute toxicity study

The acute toxicity study was a single dose toxicity test conducted to estimate lethal dose of the 70% ethanolic seeds extract of *A. gummifera* in rats' model. The administration of the extract orally at 50, 100, 150, 250, 500, 1000, 1500, 2000 and 2500 mg/kg body weight did not produce mortality of the administered group for seeds extract of *A. gummifera*. While two rats died among the 4000 mg/kg *A. gummifera* seed extract treated group. The LD 50 of *A. gummifera* was therefore found as 4000 mg/kg. These animals have shown some behavioral changes such as altered feeding, low locomotion and pilio-erection before death. Also acute manifestation like diarrhea and loss of appetite were observed. No abnormal gross necropsy of liver and kidneys were observed.

### Sub-chronic toxicity study

**Effect of the extract of both plants on general health and body weight:** During the 90 days of sub-chronic toxicity evaluation, all the male and female rats that were orally administered with the repeated doses of both 125 mg/kg and 250 mg/kg body weight showed no extract related noticeable changes in their general behaviour as compared to the control group for both of the plant extracts. The effect of the seed extracts of *A. gummifera* on the body weight of male and female rats during the 13 weeks of sub-chronic treatment are summarized in (Table1).

Body weight of both the treated and control groups increased with increasing duration. As it can be seen from (Figure 1 and 2), the body weight increase patterns of the male and female rats during the sub-chronic treatment with both of the plants extracts seem to be normal. In the seeds extract of *A. gummifera* administered groups, no significant difference ($p > 0.05$) was observed in the mean values of the body weights of male and female rats treated with 125 mg/kg body weight and males treated with 250 mg/kg body weight as compared with their respective controls. However, significant difference was observed in the mean body weight of female rats treated with 250mg/kg body weight as it decreased at the 9th week by 8.7% and further decreased by 12.8% at the 10th week as compared with the control group.

| Period | Sex | Control | Treatment groups (mg/kg body weight/ day) | |
| --- | --- | --- | --- | --- |
| | | | 125 | 250 |
| WK1 | Male | 166.4 ± 1.75 | 168.2 ± 3.35 (0.24) | 166.8 ± 2.49 (0.51) |
| | Female | 164.8 ± 2.13 | 167.6 ± 3.36 (0.40) | 167.8 ± 3.67 (0.32) |
| WK2 | Male | 175.2 ± 2.15 | 179.6 ± 4.13 (0.24) | 176 ± 5.09 (0.12) |
| | Female | 172.2 ± 3.65 | 179.2 ± 5.12 (0.53) | 178.6 ± 3.44 (0.91) |
| WK3 | Male | 191.8 ± 2.18 | 191.2 ± 4.08 (0.25) | 171.6 ± 5.29 (0.11) |
| | Female | 186.6 ± 2.98 | 189.6 ± 3.97 (0.59) | 187.2 ± 4.25 (0.51) |
| WK4 | Male | 201.6 ± 2.80 | 189.8 ± 3.48 (0.68) | 196.2 ± 5.90 (0.18) |

| | | 197.6 ± 3.28 | 196.2 ± 4.12 (0.67) | 202 ± 4.15 (0.66) |
|---|---|---|---|---|
| | Female | 197.6 ± 3.28 | 196.2 ± 4.12 (0.67) | 202 ± 4.15 (0.66) |
| WK5 | Male | 209.8 ± 2.85 | 205.2 ± 2.08 (0.56) | 216.8 ± 4.91 (0.32) |
| | Female | 205.2 ± 3.06 | 209.4 ± 5.42 (0.29) | 225.2 ± 3.47 (0.81) |
| WK6 | Male | 216.8 ± 2.75 | 209.4 ± 1.29 (0.17) | 218.8 ± 3.65 (0.59) |
| | Female | 213 ± 2.76 | 211.6 ± 4.27 (0.42) | 217.2 ± 2.94 (0.90) |
| WK7 | Male | 223.6 ± 2.50 | 214.4 ± 1.89 (0.59) | 219.8 ± 4.83 (0.23) |
| | Female | 220.4 ± 3.76 | 207.2 ± 4.62 (0.70) | 226.8 ± 2.08 (0.28) |
| WK8 | Male | 231 ± 2.51 | 221.4 ± 1.80 (0.54) | 220.8 ± 3.80 (0.44) |
| | Female | 227 ± 4.89 | 210.6 ± 4.61 (0.91) | 229.8 ± 2.39 (0.19) |
| WK9 | Male | 242.2 ± 2.35 | 226.6 ± 1.99 (0.75) | 222.2 ± 4.59 (0.22) |
| | Female | 235.6 ± 4.53 | 212.2 ± 7.77 (0.32) | 215.2 ± 1.39 (0.23) |
| WK10 | Male | 252.6 ± 2.42 | 233.8 ± 2.15 (0.83) | 234.8 ± 4.53 (0.25) |
| | Female | 247.8 ± 3.65 | 223 ± 6.40 (0.32) | 216 ± 7.07* (0.04) |
| WK11 | Male | 261.6 ± 6.77 | 238.8 ± 2.35 (0.06) | 237.6 ± 3.47 (0.22) |
| | Female | 255.2 ± 3.76 | 219.4 ± 6.52 (0.31) | 220.6 ± 2.06 (0.27) |
| WK12 | Male | 265 ± 4.82 | 249.6 ± 3.43 (0.53) | 240.2 ± 5.11 (0.43) |
| | Female | 265.4 ± 4.53 | 225.6 ± 5.81 (0.64) | 226.4 ± 3.47 (0.62) |
| WK13 | Male | 269.2 ± 4.22 | 258.8 ± 3.53 (0.74) | 248.4 ± 3.33 (0.20) |
| | Female | 274.4 ± 4.00 | 223.8 ± 5.99 (0.45) | 232.6 ± 2.60 (0.42) |

Values are given as Mean ± S.E.M. for each male and female subgroup. The figures under the brackets indicate the calculated p values of the treatment groups as compared to the controls.

*=significant (p<0.05). The mean difference is considered significant at p<0.05. (n=10 (5 male and 5 females in each group)).

**Table 1:** Effect of the sub-chronic administration of *A. gummifera* seeds extract on the body weight of male and female rats.

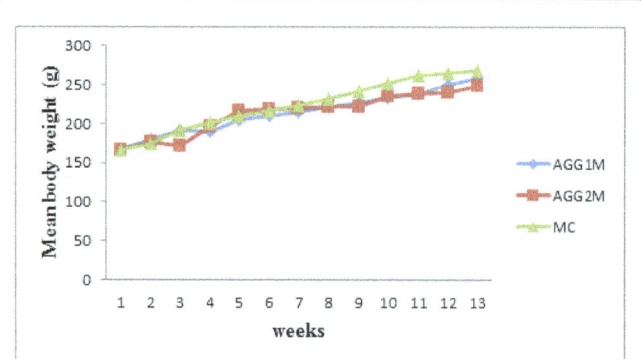

**Figure 1:** Time course and effect of seeds extract of *A. gummifera* on body growth pattern of male rats treated with 125 mg/kg body weight and 250 mg/kg body weight as compared to the controls. Each value point represents mean ± S.E.M. Note: AGG1M=*A. gummifera* administered group I male rat, AGG2M= *A. gummifera* administered group II male rat & MC= male control rat.

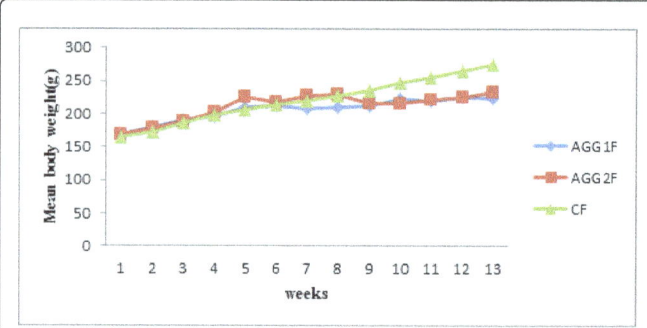

**Figure 2:** Time course and effect of seeds extract of *A. gummifera* on body growth pattern of female rats treated with 125mg/kg body weight and 250mg/kg body weight as compared to the controls. Each value point represents mean ± S.E.M. Note: AGG1F=*A. gummifera* administered group I female rat, AGG2F=*A. gummifera* administered group II female rat & CF= female control rat.

**Effect of *A. gummifera* hydro alcohol seeds extract on hematological parameters:** The effect of sub-chronic treatment of the seed extract of *A. gummifera* on hematological parameters of male rats as compared to the controls is illustrated in (Table 2).

| Hematological Parameters | Control (G3) | 125 mg/kg body weight (G1) | 250 mg/kg body weight (G2) |
|---|---|---|---|
| WBC (× 103/µL) | 7.99 ± 1.08 | 12.24 ± 2.18 (.19) | 10.94 ± 1.49 (.39) |
| RBC (× 106/µL) | 9.94 ± 0.17 | 10.14 ± .14 (.54) | 10.00 ± .11 (.93) |
| HGB (g/dL) | 18.50 ± 0.25 | 18.26 ± .38 (.80) | 17.53 ± .23 (.10) |
| HCT (%) | 54.36 ± 1.12 | 54.30 ± 1.06 (.99) | 52.73 ± .49 (.41) |
| MCV (fL) | 54.66 ± .44 | 53.50 ± .36 (.25) | 52.73 ± .66 (.06) |
| MCH (pg) | 18.63 ± .06 | 18.00 ± .20 (.04)* | 17.53 ± .14 (.004)* |
| MCHC (g/dL) | 34.03 ± .33 | 33.63 ± .18 (.49) | 33.23 ± .23 (.12) |
| PLT (x 103/µL) | 901.66 ± 67.49 | 1101.00 ± 81.22 (.11) | 1079.33 ± 23.53 (.15) |
| RDW-CV (%) | 20.16 ± .06 | 21.63 ± .21 (.00)* | 21.90 ± .15 (.00)* |
| NEUT (%) | 15.36 ± 2.01 | 28.30 ± 4.93 (.05) | 32.70 ± 2.20 (.01)* |
| LYMPH (%) | 77.56 ± 1.73 | 66.50 ± 6.24 (.14) | 64.66 ± 1.46 (.09) |
| MONO (%) | 5.30 ± 1.44 | 4.70 ± 1.20 (.90) | 5.60 ± .70 (.97) |
| EO (%) | 1.40 ± .95 | 0.26 ± .08 (.32) | 0.16 ± .06 (.27) |
| BASO (%) | .36 ± .17 | 0.23 ± .13 (.73) | 0.20 ± .10 (.63) |

**Table 2:** Hematological parameters of male rats administered with 125 and 250mg/kg body weight of seed extract of *A. gummifera*.

The sub-chronic treatment with both 125 mg/kg and 250 mg/kg body weight seed extract did not significantly affect haematological parameters except a few of the parameters seen to be significant (p<0.05). Sub-chronic treatment of male rats with 125 mg/kg and 250 mg/kg of seed extracts produced significant change (p<0.05) in the MCH as it decreased by 3.4% in the 125 mg/kg administered group and further decreased by 5.9% in the 250 mg/kg administered group, and RDW-CV as it increased by 7.3% in the 125 mg/kg administered group and further increased by 8.6% in the 250 mg/kg administered group. Besides, the seed extract induced significant change in the NEUT at 250 mg/kg body weight as it increased from 15.36 ± 2.01 to 32.70 ± 2.20.

Hematological parameters such as RBC, WBC and PLT increased in the male rats at both doses compared to the control although not significant. But, parameters such as HGB, HCT, MCV, MCH, LYMPH, EO and BASO were all found decreased in the male rats even though they were statistically not significant.

| Hematological Parameters | Control (G3) | 125 mg/kg body weight (G1) | 250 mg/kg body weight (G2) |
|---|---|---|---|
| WBC (× 103/µL) | 5.27 ± 2.32 | 9.55 ± 1.71 (.42) | 10.48 ± 3.17 (.30) |
| RBC (× 106/µL) | 8.66 ± .31 | 8.99 ± .18 (.51) | 9.32 ± .14 (.14) |
| HGB (g/dL) | 16.86 ± .67 | 17.16 ± .55 (.88) | 17.13 ± .06 (.90) |
| HCT (%) | 49.13 ± 1.74 | 51.36 ± 1.40 (.42) | 50.93 ± .34 (.55) |
| MCV (fL) | 56.76 ± .66 | 57.10 ± .40 (.88) | 54.63 ± .61 (.06) |
| MCH (pg) | 19.46 ± .23 | 19.06 ± .23 (.42) | 18.36 ± .23 (.02)* |
| MCHC (g/dL) | 34.33 ± .14 | 33.63 ± .12 (.03)* | 33.40 ± .20 (.01) * |
| PLT (x103/µL) | 665.00 ± 218.70 | 1029.00 ± 12.34 (.18) | 1222.33 ± 92.09 (.05) |
| RDW-CV (%) | 17.23 ± .98 | 18.60 ± .20 (.26) | 19.43 ± .27 (.07) |
| NEUT (%) | 12.06 ± 2.14 | 20.90 ± 6.96 (.32) | 35.00 ± 1.80 (.02)* |
| LYMPH (%) | 79.83 ± 3.89 | 73.36 ± 8.51 (.67) | 58.13 ± 4.16 (.07) |
| MONO (%) | 4.40 ± .55 | 5.13 ± 1.88 (.94) | 6.53 ± 2.51 (.64) |
| EO (%) | 3.66 ± 3.12 | .50 ± .05 (.40) | .26 ± .12 (.36) |
| BASO (%) | .03 ± .03 | .10 ± .05 (.48) | .06 ± .03 (.81) |

Values are expressed as Mean ± SEM. The figures in brackets indicate the calculated p values of the treatment groups as compared to the control. * =significant (p<0.05). The mean difference is considered significant at p<0.05.

**Table 3:** Hematological parameters of female rats administered with125 and 250 mg/kg body weight of seed extract of *A. gummifera*.

The effect of 13 weeks of sub-chronic treatment of the seed extract of this plant on hematological parameters of female rats is illustrated in (Table 3).The seed extract induced significant change (p<0.05) at 250 mg/kg body weight in the MCH as it decreased by 5.6% and in the MCHC as it decreased by 2.0% at the lowest dose and further by 2.7% at the highest dose. In addition, the seed extract affected the NEUT at 250 mg/kg body weight as it increased from 12.06 ± 2.14 to 35.00 ± 1.80. The parameters like WBC, RBC and PLT increased in the female rats compared to their controls but this increment was not significant. On the other hand, hematological parameters such as EO and MCV decreased at both doses but still the values were not significant.

| Biochemical Parameters | Control (G3) | 125 mg/kg dose (G1) | 250 mg/kg dose (G2) |
|---|---|---|---|
| Albumin (g/dl) | 4.70 ± 0.22 | 4.79 ± 0.26 (0.94) | 4.45 ± 0.19 (0.65) |

| | | | |
|---|---|---|---|
| ALP (U/L) | 135.75 ± 11.69 | 168 ± 12.79 (0.44) | 160.75 ± 29.26 (0.59) |
| ALT (U/L) | 79.75 ± 2.59 | 94.25 ± 5.15 (0.11) | 79.75 ± 6.21 (1.00) |
| AST (U/L) | 179.75 ± 5.20 | 251.5 ± 43.65 (0.34) | 253.75 ± 47.42 (0.32) |
| Urea (mg/dL) | 28.50 ± 0.96 | 33 ± 0.41 (0.09) | 36.75 ± 2.21 (0.005) * |

Values are expressed as Mean ± SEM. The figures in brackets indicate the calculated p values of the treatment groups as compared to the control. * =significant (p<0.05). The mean difference is considered significant at p<0.05.

**Table 4:** Serum biochemical parameters of male rats administered with 125 and 250 mg/kg body weight of seed extract of *A. gummifera*.

**Effect of *A. gummifera* hydro alcohol seeds extract on serum biochemical parameters:** Effects of sub-chronic treatment with hydro-alcoholic seed extract of *A. gummifera* on serum biochemical parameters of male and female rats are shown in (Tables 4 and 5), respectively. Except urea with male administered at 250 mg/kg body weight as it increased by 28.94%, all the parameters measured were not significantly different between the control and extract administered groups at both doses.

| Biochemical Parameters | Control (G3) | 125 mg/kg dose (G1) | 250 mg/kg dose (G2) |
|---|---|---|---|
| Albumin (g/dl) | 5.16 ± 0.19 | 5.01 ± 0.16 (0.79) | 4.87 ± 0.16 (0.42) |
| ALP (U/L) | 75.75 ± 12.49 | 88.75 ± 8.41 (0.79) | 134.75 ± 22.87 (0.05) |
| ALT (U/L) | 63.75 ± 5.66 | 74.75 ± 4.00 (0.26) | 61.50 ± 5.33 (0.93) |
| AST (U/L) | 194 ± 16.92 | 237.25 ± 62.26 (0.65) | 192.25 ± 13.88 (0.99) |
| Urea (mg/dL) | 34.50 ± 2.33 | 38.75 ± 2.49 (0.29) | 37.00 ± 1.08 (0.62) |

Values are expressed as Mean ± SEM. The figures in brackets indicate the calculated p values of the treatment groups as compared to the control. The mean difference was not significant (p ≥ 0.05).

**Table 5:** Serum biochemical parameters of female rats administered with 125 and 250 mg/kg body weight of seed extract of *A. gummifera*

## Macroscopic observations and organ weights

After the period of 90 days of sub chronic-toxicity study, rats that were orally administered with the repeated doses of the extracts at both 125 and 250 mg/kg body weight of both plants showed no abnormal gross findings in the liver and kidneys in the post-mortem macroscopic examination. The mean organ weight of liver and kidney of the seed extract of *A. gummifera* administered groups and control group are shown in Tables 6 and 7, for the male and female rats, respectively. No significant difference (p>0.05) was seen in the organ weights between extract treated and control rats of both sex.

| Group | Dose (mg/kg) | Liver (g) | Kidney (g) |
|---|---|---|---|
| I | 125 | 9.32 ± .18 (.29) | 1.05 ± .02 (.95) |
| II | 250 | 9.18 ± 0.13 (.09) | 0.99 ± 0.05 (.60) |

| III | Control | 9.60 ± .07 | 1.04 ± .04 |
|-----|---------|------------|-----------|

**Table 6:** Organ weights of male rats administered with 125 & 250 mg/kg body weight doses of the seed extracts of *A. gummifera.*

| Group | Dose (mg/kg) | Liver (g) | Kidney (g) |
|-------|--------------|-----------|------------|
| I | 125 | 9.40 ± 0.19 (.32) | 0.91 ± 0.05 (.91) |
| II | 250 | 9.42 ± .09 (.27) | 1.01 ± .03 (.52) |
| III | Control | 9.16 ± .12 | 0.85 ± 0.19 |

**Table 7:** Organ weights of female rats administered with 125 and 250 mg/kg body weight doses of the seed extracts of *A. gummifera.*

## Microscopic observations

**Effect of hydroalcoholic seed extract of** *A. gummifera* **on histopathology of the liver:** Routine hematoxylin and eosin stained sections of liver were examined to assess the effect of the 90 days sub-chronic oral administration with 70% ethanolic seed extract of *A. gummifera* on this tissue. Light microscopic examination of the liver sections of 125 mg/kg of both male and female rats for seed extract of *A. gummifera* administered group showed inflammation and congestions of blood in the central vein (Figure 3). The 250mg/kg administered group also showed congestions of blood in the central vein and in the sinusoids, focal cellular necrosis and pyknosis (Figure 3).

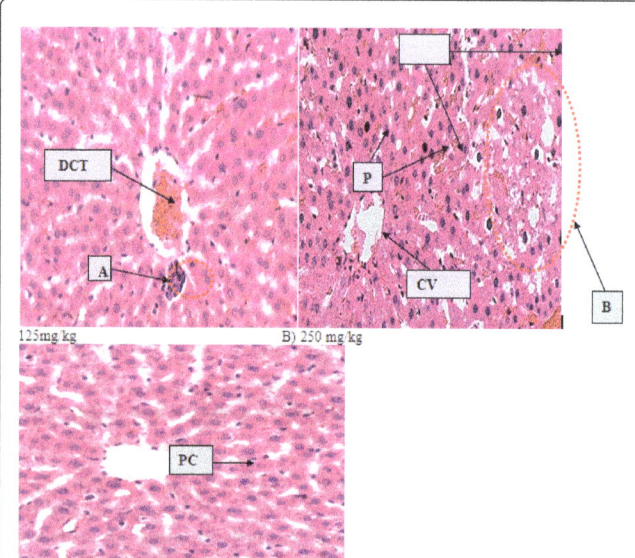

**Figure 3:** Photomicrographof H & E stained liver sections from rats administered with hydroethanolic seeds extracts of *A. gummifera* at 125 mg/kg body weight/day (A), 250 mg/kg body weight/day (B), and control (C) rats.

Different changes were observed in the sections from the hydro ethanolic extract administered rat including: inflammations around central vein (I) and congestion of blood in the central vein (BCCV) in rat administered at 125 mg/kg body weight/day (A); focal cellularnecrosis (N),congestion of blood in the central vein (BCCV),

congestion of blood in the sinusoids (BCS) and pyknosis (P) in rats administered 250 mg/k body weight/day (B); While there was no histopathological changes visible in the sections of the control (C) rats. (Magnifications, all X2000).

**Effect of hydroalcoholic seed extract of** *A. gummifera* **on histopathology of the kidneys:** Histological examinations of sections of the kidney from rats administered with the seeds extract of *A. gummifera* at 125 mg/kg in both male and female rats have shown peritubular blood congestions (Figure 4). Kidney histology of both sex administered with 250 mg/kg body weight have also shown congestions,atrophy of glomeruli and formation of focal protein cast in the renal interstitium (Figure 4).

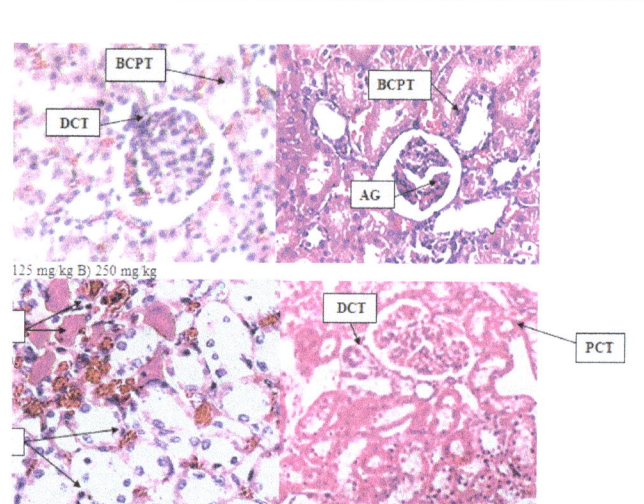

**Figure 4:** Photomicrographof H&E stained kidney sections from rats administered with hydroethanolic seeds extracts of *A. gummifera* at 125mg/kg body weight/day (A), 250 mg/kgbody weight/day (B&C), and control (D) rats.Note: PCT=Proximal convoluted tubule, DCT=Distalconvoluted tubule& CD= Collecting duct.

Various changes were observed in the sections from the hydroethanolic extract administered rats: congestion of blood in the peritubular areas (BCPT) in rat administered at 125 mg/kg body weight/day (A); congestion of blood in the peritubular areas (BCPT),atrophy the glomeruli (AG) and protein cast in the kidney interstitium (PC) in rats administered 250 mg/k body weight/day (B and C); While there were no histopathological changes visible in the sections of the control rat (D). All the changes were observed under 2000 magnifications.

## Discussion

Acute toxicity test is carried out on laboratory animals, in this particular case on albino rats receiving different doses of the substances in question. The oral administration of the aqueous extracts of *A. gummifera* seeds did not show any signs of toxicity nor did they produce lethality in rats up to 3000 mg/Kg. As this dose is minimal it is very unlikely to associate the death of the animal with the extract. 50% of the animals died with 4000 mg/kg for *A. gummifera* seeds extract treated groups. This has, therefore, indicated that the LD50 of these plants were found to be 4000 mg/kg body weight, respectively. The LD

50 of *A. gummifera* is in agreement with an earlier work on the aqueous leaf extract of A. chevalieri by Saidu and associates [8], that the extract has an LD 50 of greater than 3000 mg/kg body weight. In line with this finding, a previous study [6], has indicated that in the mice the LD 50 of *A. gummifera* whose effective dose are 125 mg/kg, through the oral administration, were 2300 body weight. As the effective doses for the plants have been found as 125 mg/kg body weight [9,10], it could be suggested that the lethal dose is more than twenty times greater than the effective dose.

The seeds extract of both plants had no harmful effect on body growth patterns of test groups. Body weight of both the treated and untreated animals of both sexes increased as the duration increased. However, during the 9th week, although statistically not significant, there was a slight decrease in the body weight of female rats treated with *A. gummifera* seeds extract in a dose dependent manner as compared with the controls. But statistically significant difference in body weight was observed in female rats during 10th week at 250 mg/kg body weight. Such changes in the body weight is in line with the results of toxicity studies following administration of aqueous extract of Vernonia amygdalina [11] and administration of aqueous extract of Clerodendrum myricoides [12] which results in suppression of weight gain of the extract treated animals.

As was described by Amacher [13] biological markers are used to recognize, characterize and monitor treatment-related responses following exposure to xenobiotic agents. Biomarkers serve three primary applications in toxicology: to confirm exposure to a deleterious agent, to provide a system for monitoring individual's susceptibility to a toxicant, and to quantitatively assess deleterious effects of a toxicant to an organism or individual. One of such biomarkers is blood profile as manifestation of abnormal changes in metabolism due to underlying disease conditions. In toxicological studies, changes in hematological as well as biochemical parameters are used as indices of toxicities [14].

Measurement of RBC count, HCT also sometimes referred to as a PCV, and HGB can be used to determine anemia which could be due to a decrease in the total number of erythrocytes, MCV, MCH or MCHC [15-17]. More recently RDW-CV, automated parameter providing information on the degree of variation of individual red cell size, has been used in conjunction with the traditional red cell indices in order to narrow down the possible causes of anaemia in an individual patient [17]. The mitotic capacity of different hematopoietic cell lineages predominates in marrow at different times. On direct marrow examination, the great majority of mitoses (74% to 90%) were of erythroid lineage; only a few (0% to 10%) were granulocytic [18]. The alteration in number of RBC count and HGB content may be due to defective haematopoiesis, inhibited erythropoiesis or an increase in destruction of red blood cells [19,20].

In the present study of 125 and 250 mg/kg body weight/ day of *A. gummifera* seeds extract treated group, did not decrease total RBC count, PLT, WBC, LYMPH, MONO, EO, BASO, HCT and HGB in the male rats as compared with the male control group. This observation is in agreement with other findings in which the values of the various RBC and WBC parameters of oral administration of saponins isolated from A. lebbeck bark extract which were found to be comparable with those of the control group [21-27]. The seeds extract of *A. gummifera*, however, significantly increased the NEUT at 250 mg/kg as compared to the control. The seeds extract of this plant did not decrease the levels of two red blood cell indices (MCV and MCHC) but, significantly decreased the level of MCH and increased the RDW-CV at both doses

as compared to the male control. This indicates the seeds extract of *A. gummifera* may slightly induce anemia in male rats.

The seeds extract of this plant did not decrease total RBC count, PLT, WBC, LYMPH, MONO, EO, BASO, HCT, HGB and RDW-CV in the female rats. But have significantly increased the NEUT at 250 mg/kg as compared to the control. The plant seeds extract did not decrease the level of MCH but, decreased MCV at 250 mg/kg administered group and MCHC at both doses (125 and 250 mg/kg body weight) in the female rats as compared to the female control. This also indicates the plant seeds extract may induce anemia. This may happen in both of male and female rats because of the seeds extract of *A. gummifera* may have effect on iron metabolism or/and erythropoiesis.

Another biomarker to toxic effect is serum biochemical profile. This effect can be detected or quantified by measuring the various serum biochemical parameters. ALT is primarily localized in liver tissue, and trace amount is found in skeletal muscle and heart tissue. Its cellular localizations are cytoplasm and mitochondria. This biochemical parameter could leak out from damaged tissues because of histopathological lesion particularly during hepatocellular necrosis [13,21,22]. AST is localized in liver, heart, muscle, brain and kidney tissues. Similarly, its cellular localizations are cytoplasm and mitochondria. This may also leak out from damaged tissues mainly because of hepatocellular necrosis [21-23]. ALP is localized in liver, bile duct, bone, placenta, kidney and intestine. Its cellular localization is the cell membrane. Therecould be over production and release in blood because of hepatobiliary injury and cholestasis [24,25]. Albumin is produced and localized in liver tissue, and is released into blood plasma. Because of hepatic dysfunction it is decreased in synthesis [26].

In the seeds extract of *A. gummifera* administered group, the serum biochemical parameters analyzed for male rats are not found to be significant. Similarly, all the biochemical parameters analyzed for female rats as compared to the control were found insignificant. This result is in agreement with the previous studies by Saidu and associates [8] on aqueous leaf extract of Albizia chevalieri and oral administration of saponins isolated from Albizia lebbeck bark by Gupta and associates [27] which showed no significant effect on serum liver and kidney function and biochemical parameters. Serum urea was increased at 250 mg/kg body weight as compared to the male control. This indicates the seeds extract of *A. gummifera* may induce renal toxicity in male rats at higher doses. This result is supported by other findings in that drug-induced nephrotoxicity may be gender related [28]. The serum levels of creatinine and urea in different drug-induced nephrotoxicity were higher in males than females [28-31]. Usually urea is increased in acute and chronic intrinsic renal diseases, which is characterized by decrement in effective circulating blood volume within the kidney [32]. This explains why urea level increase in blood is one of the good indicators for kidney damage.

Analysis of the organ weight is usually employed to determine whether the size of the organ has changed, as indicator of the adverse effect of the toxicants on that organ. According to [33], the mean kidney weight of the male rats was higher than those of females in both African giant rats and wistar rats, although the difference was not significant. In addition to these, the mean weight of the right kidney was heavier than that of the left kidney in both African giant rats and wistar rats. In this study, both of plant seeds extracts did not produce any detectable and meaningful change in the organ weight of liver and kidneys in both male and female rats at all doses.

Analysis of the toxic potential of a therapeutic agent on target organs is incomplete without gross and histopathological assessments. It is more rationale that all functional studies in toxicology should be coupled with appropriate morphologic pathology studies. Liver and kidney microscopic pathology serve as important tools for identifying and characterizing liver and kidney injuries respectively, whether or not biochemical and macroscopic changes are also identified. Some of the main patterns of liver injury during hepatotoxicity include zonal necrosis and vascular lesions [34]. Similarly, general pathology of renal structures include glomeruli hyper cellularity which may result from increased intrinsic cells or from accumulation of leukocytes in capillary lumina, tubular necrosis is elicited as manifestations of either local metabolic abnormalities or systemic processes (characterized by loss of brush border staining for proximal cells, diffuse flattening of cells with resulting dilatation of lumina, loss of individual lining cells, and sloughing off of cells into lumina [35]. It is worthwhile to note that the kidneys of African giant rats and wistar rats are reddish brown with the African giant rat having a darker red colour *in vivo* [33].

The present study, rats that were orally administered with repeated doses of the extracts at both 125 mg/kg and 250 mg/kg body weight for both of the plants showed no abnormalities of the liver and kidneys in the post mortem macroscopic evaluation. The present study noted the presence of histopathological changes in the liver and kidney tissue of the seeds extract of *A. gummifera* administered rats. Histopathological changes in the liver at the lowest dose were not detected for *A. gummifera* except for sign of congestion and haemorrhage. But, histopathological changes in the liver at 250 mg/kg body weight showed few pyknotic cells and minor focal necrosis. This result is in agreement with herbal plants like Atractylis gummifera and Callilepsi slaureola reported by Larrey [35]. In contrast to the investigation of Larrey [35], rat liver, kidney and heart tissues analysed histopathologically were normal after acute and sub-chronic administration of the aqueous leaf extract of A. chevalieri [8]. Such disagreement between the results may be due to absence of compound responsible for toxic insult in the aqueous leaf extract of A. chevalieri or duration for administration periods as the aqueous leaf extract of Albizia chevalieri has been administered to rats for only about 28 days at a dose between 0-1500 mg/kg body weight.The seeds extract of *A. gummifera* may possess a class of compound that has caused interluminal eosinophilic protein cast, congestion and minor necrosis in the kidney tissue. This is in agreement with previous study on aqueous leaf extract of A. chevalieri that elicited congestion and eosinophilic tubular protein cast [8].

## Conclusion

From the present investigation, the hydro-alcoholic seeds extract of Albizzia gummifera has increased NEUT at 250 mg/kg body weight in both male and female rats. The seeds extract of this plant decreased MCH and increased RDW-CV at both doses in the male rats. Similarly, the extract decreased MCHC at both doses and MCV at higher dose in the female rats. Hence, the hydro alcoholic seeds extract of *A. gummifera* may induce anemia in both male and female rats. All serum chemistry analysed in this study for the seeds extract of the plant were found normal in both male and female rats, except for the elevated serum urea in the male rats at 250 mg/kg body weight. The hydro-alcoholic seeds extract of *A. gummifera* has brought some histopathological alterations in liver such as inflammation at 125 mg/kg body weight and congestions, pyknosis and focal cellular necrosis at the 250 mg/kg body weight. The extract has resulted in some histopathological alterations in the kidney too, such as protein cast and atrophy of glomeruli at 250 mg/kg body weight.

The present study demonstrated sub-chronic toxicity of hydro-ethanolic seeds extract of *A. gummifera* extract in albino wistar rats. However, further studies are needed to identify active ingredients responsible for toxic insult and mechanism of action of the extract for the toxic effects, to examine the toxic effects of these plants on other organs using similar animal model, to assess the toxic effects of these plants on blood parameters and histopathology of internal organs on other animal models and to investigate if changes observed may also be same in humans.

## References

1. WHO, Traditional medicine strategy 2002-2005. Geneva.
2. Tédong L, Dzeufiet PD, Dimo T, Asongalem EA, Sokeng SN, et al. (2007) Acute and Subchronic toxicity of Anacardium occidentale Linn (Anacardiaceae) leaves hexane extract in mice. Afr J Tradit Altern Med 4: 140-147.
3. Ogbonnia S, Adekunle AA, Bosa MK, Enwuru VN (2008) Evaluation of acute and subacute toxicity of Alstonia congensis Engler (Apocynaceae) bark and Xylopia aethiopica (Dunal) A. Rich (Annonaceae) fruits mixtures used in the treatment of diabetes. Afr J Biotechnol 7: 701-705.
4. Geyid A, Abebe D, Debella A, Makonnen Z, Aberra F, et al. (2005) Screening of some medicinal plants of Ethiopia for their anti-microbial properties and chemical profiles. J Ethnopharmacol 97: 421-427.
5. Woldemicheal T (2003) Screening of some medicinal plants of Ethiopia for their molluscidal activities and phytochemical constituents. PhOL 3: 245- 258.
6. Debella A (2007) Screening of some Ethiopian medicinal plants for mosquito larvicidal effects and phytochemical constituents. Pharmacologyonline 3: 231-243.
7. Tefera MA, Geyid A, Debella A (2012) In vitro anti-Neisseria gonorrhoeae activity of Albizia gummifera and Croton macrostachyus. Revista CENIC,Ciencias Biológicas 41: 1-11.
8. Saidu Y (2007) Acute and sub-chronic toxicity studies of crude aqueous extract of Albizzia chevalieri Harms (Leguminosae). Asian J Biochem 2: 224-336.
9. Karunamoorthi K, Bishaw D, Mulat T (2009) Toxic effects of traditional Ethiopian fish poisoning plant Milletia ferruginea (Hochst) seed extract on aquatic macroinvertebrates. Eur Rev Med Pharmacol Sci 13: 179-185.
10. Taye B, Giday M, Animut A, Seid J (2011) Antibacterial activities of selected medicinal plants in traditional treatment of human wounds in Ethiopia. Asian Pac J Trop Biomed 1: 370-375.
11. Amole O (2006) Toxicity studies of the aqueous extract of Vernonia amygdalina. Biomed Res 17: 39-40.
12. Kebede H (2011) The Effect of Clerodendrum Myricoides Aqueous Extract on Blood, Liver and Kidney Tissues of Mice. MEJS : 3.
13. Amacher DE (2002) A toxicologist's guide to biomarkers of hepatic response. Hum Exp Toxicol 21: 253-262.
14. Bin-Jaliah I (2014) Derangement of hemopoiesis and hematological indices in Khat (Cathaedulis)-treated rats. Afr J Biotechnol : 13.
15. Hume R, Dagg JH, Goldberg A (1973) Refractory anemia with dysproteinemia: long-term therapy with low-dose corticosteroids. Blood 41: 27-35.
16. Sagone AL Jr, Lawrence T, Balcerzak SP (1973) Effect of smoking on tissue oxygen supply. Blood 41: 845-851.
17. Ris MM, Deitrich RA, Von Wartburg JP (1975) Inhibition of aldehyde reductase isoenzymes in human and rat brain. Biochem Pharmacol 24: 1865-1869.
18. Sysmex H (2016) Educational enhancement and development. Seed Hematology.

Evaluations of Biochemical, Hematological and Histopathological Parameters of Subchronic Administration of Ethanol...

79

19. Keinänen M, Knuutila S, Bloomfield CD, Elonen E, de la Chapelle A (1986) The proportion of mitoses in different cell lineages changes during short-term culture of normal human bone marrow. Blood 67: 1240-1243.

20. Selmanoglu G, Barlas N, Songür S, Koçkaya EA (2001) Carbendazim-induced haematological, biochemical and histopathological changes to the liver and kidney of male rats. Hum Exp Toxicol 20: 625-630.

21. Choudhari C, Deshmukh P (2007) Acute and subchronic toxicity study of Semecarpus anacardium on Hb% and RBC count of male albino rats. J Herbal Med and Toxicol 1: 43-45.

22. Dufour DR, Lott JA, Nolte FS, Gretch DR, Koff RS, et al. (2000) Diagnosis and monitoring of hepatic injury. I. Performance characteristics of laboratory tests. Clin Chem 46: 2027-2049.

23. Dufour DR, Lott JA, Nolte FS, Gretch DR, Koff RS, et al. (2000) Diagnosis and monitoring of hepatic injury. II. Recommendations for use of laboratory tests in screening, diagnosis, and monitoring. Clin Chem 46: 2050-2068.

24. Ozer J, Ratner M, Shaw M, Bailey W, Schomaker S (2008) The current state of serum biomarkers of hepatotoxicity. Toxicology 245: 194-205.

25. Belansky ES, Cutforth N, Chavez R, Crane LA, Waters E, et al. (2013) Adapted intervention mapping: a strategic planning process for increasing physical activity and healthy eating opportunities in schools via environment and policy change. J Sch Health 83: 194-205.

26. Saukkonen JJ, Cohn DL, Jasmer RM, Schenker S, Jereb JA, et al. (2006) An official ATS statement: hepatotoxicity of antituberculosis therapy. Am J Respir Crit Care Med 174: 935-952.

27. Ramaiah SK (2007) A toxicologist guide to the diagnostic interpretation of hepatic biochemical parameters. Food Chem Toxicol 45: 1551-1557.

28. Thapa BR, Walia A (2007) Liver function tests and their interpretation. Indian J Pediatr 74: 663-671.

29. Gupta RS, Chaudhary R, Yadav RK, Verma SK, Dobhal MP (2005) Effect of Saponins of Albizia lebbeck (L.) Benth bark on the reproductive system of male albino rats. J Ethnopharmacol 96: 31-36.

30. Bennett WM, Parker RA, Elliott WC, Gilbert DN, Houghton DC (1982) Sex-related differences in the susceptibility of rats to gentamicin nephrotoxicity. J Infect Dis 145: 370-373.

31. Goodrich JA, Hottendorf GH (1995) Tobramycin gender-related nephrotoxicity in Fischer but not Sprague-Dawley rats. Toxicol Lett 75: 127-131.

32. Halaris AE, Belendiuk KT, Freedman DX (1975) Antidepressant drugs affect dopamine uptake. Biochem Pharmacol 24: 1896-1897.

33. Laniado-Laborín R, Cabrales-Vargas MN (2009) Amphotericin B: side effects and toxicity. Rev Iberoam Micol 26: 223-227.

# 14

# Nonclinical Safety Evaluation of a Transforming Growth Factor β Receptor I Kinase Inhibitor in Fischer 344 Rats and Beagle Dogs

Anja J Stauber[1*], Kelly M Credille1, Lewis L Truex[1], William J Ehlhardt[1] and Jamie K Young[2]

[1]Lilly Research Laboratories, Toxicology and Pathology, Eli Lilly and Company, Indianapolis, IN, 46285, USA

[2]Covance Laboratories Inc., Greenfield, Indiana, 46140, USA

Corresponding author:Anja J Stauber, Ph.D, D.A.B.T, Lilly Corporate CenterEli Lilly and Company, Indianapolis, Indiana 46285, USA, Email: anja_stauber@lilly.com

## Abstract

**Objective:** The transforming growth factor β (TGF-β) pathway regulates diverse cellular functions and plays a prominent role in diseases such as cancer, autoimmune disorders and cardiovascular disease. LY2157299 monohydrate (LY2157299) is a potent and selective inhibitor of TGF-β receptor I kinase that is under clinical evaluation for the treatment of advanced cancer.

**Methods:** This paper characterizes the toxicity profile of LY2157299 in Fischer 344 rats and beagle dogs for up to six months of daily oral dosing. LY2157299 is well tolerated in the rat and dog for up to one month of daily dosing at doses of 150 and 20 mg/kg, respectively.

**Results:** In the rat, LY2157299 is well tolerated after three months of 2 weeks on/2 weeks off intermittent dosing schedule at 50 mg/kg. Chronic (≥3 months) oral administration results in multiple target organ toxicities involving the cardiovascular, gastrointestinal, immune, bone/cartilage, reproductive, and renal systems.

**Conclusion:** Defining the appropriate dose and schedule led to a better understanding of how to define safety margins and thus enable the clinical investigation of LY2157299 in cancer patients.

**Keywords:** TGF-β Inhibitor; Kinase; Drug-associated cardiovascular toxicity; Rats; Dogs

## Introduction

Transforming growth factor β (TGF-β) signaling leads to pleiotropic activation, including regulation of cell growth, migration, and differentiation [1-3]. TGF-β ligands are differentially expressed across a variety of tissues including hematopoietic, cartilage, bone, cardiac, and neuronal tissues in both endothelial and epithelial cells [4]. The ligands TGF-β1, TGF-β2, and TGF-β3 signal through binding to the TGF-β type I and type II Ser/Thr kinase receptors. Upon ligand binding-mediated activation, phosphorylation of the type II receptor activates the Type I receptor resulting in phosphorylation and activation of downstream Smad proteins, which are the intracellular effectors of TGF-β signaling [5].

Because of its pleiotropic role, genetically altered animals can provide useful insights on the relevance of TGF-β signaling during development and normal physiology. Genetic manipulation of the TGF-β signaling pathway in mice demonstrates its crucial role in embryonic development in controlling vasculogenesis, angiogenesis, and inflammation. The phenotypes of TGF-β1, β2, or β3 knockout models all result in high embryonic lethality or mortality shortly after birth. TGF-β1 and TGF-β2 knockouts have vascular, aortic arch, and cardiac septal defects [6,7]. TGF-β1 knockout mice die shortly after birth due to cardiopulmonary complications with severe tissue inflammation [6]. Ablation of TGF-β receptors I and II results in embryonic lethality with vascular and angiogenesis defects [8,9]. The

Smad proteins are the downstream signal transducers of TGF-β signaling, and genetic knockdown of key regulators such as Smad 2 and 3 are similarly embryonic lethal or affected mice experience a reduced lifespan with abnormalities consisting of mucosal inflammation, skeletal defects, and colon cancer [10]. Based upon the key role that TGFβ signaling plays in embryonic development and survival as well as its central role in certain cancers and other disease states, inhibition of this important signaling pathway may be anticipated to have adverse consequences on animals.

Blocking TGF-β signaling can be achieved via different mechanisms, including neutralizing antibodies and small molecule inhibitors that interrupt the phosphorylation of the TGF-β receptor I kinase (RIK) [11]. Within the last 5 years, a small number of publications have disclosed the effects of TGF-β inhibition in nonclinical toxicology species. Inhibition of TGF-β signaling results in a physeal dysplasia that is observed in rats administered small molecule inhibitors of TGF-β RIK [12,13]. Rats administered repeated doses of small molecule TGF-β RIK inhibitors develop a valvulopathy that is characterized by inflammation, hemorrhage and stromal hyperplasia [12-14]. Valvulopathy in rats is likely a result of direct inhibition of the TGF-β signaling pathway, rather than an "off-target" effect, because multiple structurally diverse small molecule inhibitors have produced similar effects. In contrast, large molecule inhibitors of this pathway appear to have a somewhat different toxicity profile. Monkeys administered GC1008, a human IgG4 pan-neutralizing TGF-β antibody for six months developed a dose- and time-dependent increase in epithelial hyperplasia of the gingiva and bladder [15].

These nonclinical findings from pharmaceutical companies have led to termination of several small molecule drug development programs targeting the TGF-β signaling pathway based on an apparent lack of acceptable safety margins for clinical testing [16].

Here, we disclose the nonclinical toxicology profile of LY2157299, a potent and selective oral TGF-β RIK inhibitor in Fisher 244 rats and Beagle dogs. This inhibitor is being developed for the treatment of patients with advanced cancer. Administration of LY2157299 was associated with several toxicological findings that involved multiple organ systems including cardiovascular, gastrointestinal, immune, bone/cartilage, reproductive, and renal. Toxicities were dose and duration dependent, some evident within days at high doses, whereas others were only evident in studies of 6 months' duration. Despite these serious adverse nonclinical toxicities, careful evaluation of various dosing regimens provided sufficient data to ensure the safety of patients in clinical trials.

## Materials and Methods

### Test compound

LY2157299, (4-[2-(6-methyl-2-pyridyl)-5,6-dihydro-4H-pyrrolo[1,2-b]pyrazol-3-yl]quinoline-6-carboxamide hydrate), a specific and potent inhibitor of TGF-β receptor 1 kinase, was synthesized by Lilly Research Laboratories, a division of Eli Lilly and Company. Dosing suspensions were prepared and stored within established stability parameters in 1% (w/v) carboxymethylcellulose, 0.25% (v/v) Polysorbate 80, and 0.05% (v/v) Dow Corning® Antifoam 1510-US in purified water. LY2157299 monohydrate was prepared in 500mM phosphate buffer (pH 1.8 to 2.2) for administration in dogs.

### Animals and husbandry

Eight oral nonclinical toxicology studies are described in this manuscript: a 2-week pilot study; 1-month, two 3-month studies, and a 6-month study in rats; two 1-month studies and a 6-month study in dogs. With the exception of the 2-week rat pilot study, all studies were conducted to conform to the United States Food and Drug Administration (CFR 21 – Part 58) and Organization for Economic Cooperation and Development (OECD) Good Laboratory Practice standards in place at the time of study initiation.

Male and female Fischer 344 rats (obtained from Taconic, Germantown, NY) were used for nonclinical toxicity studies up to 6 months in duration. All animals were between 6-11 weeks old at the start of treatment with initial body weights ranging from 100 to 300 grams. Clinically acceptable male and female rats were randomly assigned to dose groups to ensure equivalent distribution of body weights. Rats were housed individually in stainless steel cages and offered Certified Rodent Diet and were provided water ad libitum. Animals were fasted overnight prior to euthanasia.

Beagle dogs obtained from Marshall Farms (North Rose, NY) for the three dog studies were approximately 7-10 months of age at the start of treatment. Clinically acceptable male and female dogs were randomly assigned to dose groups to ensure equivalent distribution of body weights. Dogs were individually housed in stainless steel cages with suspended mesh floors and offered Certified Canine Diet and were provided water ad libitum. Animals were fasted overnight prior to euthanasia.

In all studies, animal care and use were done in accordance with federal and local laws, policies, regulations, and standards in effect at the time of their conduct, e.g., Animal Welfare Act and Regulations. Laboratories conducting these studies were accredited by the Association for Assessment and Accreditation of Laboratory Animal Care International and all study protocols were approved by each laboratory's Institutional Animal Care and Use Committee.

### Experimental procedures

Nonclinical toxicology studies were conducted in Fisher 344 rats and Beagle dogs. Table 1 describes the study designs for all studies conducted with LY2157299 reported in this paper. Rats were administered control vehicle or compound orally via gavage, while dogs were administered control vehicle or LY2157299-filled capsules. Plasma for measuring systemic exposure were taken on the first day of dosing and on the last day of dosing in all studies in addition to periodic intervals in studies lasting 3 months or longer. Plasma was analyzed for LY2157299 concentration using the same validated liquid chromatography/mass spectrometry method used for analysis in human plasma [17], except the method was validated over the range of 0.5-500 ng/mL in rat and dog plasma.

| Species | Duration (weeks) | Recovery (weeks) | Dosing Regimen | N (sex/group) | Doses (mg/kg) |
|---|---|---|---|---|---|
| Rat | 2 | None | Daily | 5 | 0, 50, 300, 1200 |
|  | 4 | 4 | Daily | 10 | 0, 15, 50, 150 |
|  | 12 | None | Daily | 10 | 0, 50, 150, 250 |
|  | 12 | None | 2 weeks on 2 weeks off | 10 | 0, 50, 150, 250 |
|  | 8 | 6 | Daily | 10 (control) 35 (treated) | 0, 250 |
|  | 26 | None | Daily | 15 | 0, 50, 150, 250 |
| Dog | 4 | 4 | Daily | 3 | 0, 50, 250, 500 |
|  | 4 | None | Daily | 3 | 0, 2, 8, 20 |
|  | 26 | None | Daily | 4 | 0, 8, 20, 60 |

Table 1: Nonclinical Studies Conducted with LY2157299.

Animals were observed at least once daily for mortality and clinical signs; body weights and food consumption were analyzed weekly. Electrocardiograms (ECGs) were collected at pretest in order to screen for preexisting ECG abnormalities and to provide baseline ECG data for later comparisons. During the live phase, ECGs were collected before dosing and after dosing during the first week of treatment and at 1 month and near the end of the reversibility phase (for 1-month study containing reversibility). For the 6-month study, ECGs were also collected at 3 months and 6 months.

Blood samples for complete blood counts, coagulation, and serum biochemical assays were collected from rats and dogs at the end of the treatment and/or reversibility phases. In the dog, these analyses were evaluated prior to initiation of treatment, around the start of the study and at other time points during the study. Cardiac troponin I was also evaluated in some studies.

Urine samples were collected by cystocentesis at necropsy. Urine was collected from rats overnight using metabolism cages at the end of treatment in the 6-month study and from a subset of rats in the 1-month study. Samples were analyzed for appearance/color, microscopic examination of sediment, bilirubin, blood, glucose, ketones, pH, protein, specific gravity, urobilinogen, and volume.

Rats were anesthetized with isoflurane or carbon dioxide inhalation, euthanized by exsanguination and necropsied. Dogs were administered a barbiturate overdose, exsanguinated and necropsied. Necropsies were conducted in all rats and dogs and any observations were recorded. Tissues collected at necropsy for microscopic evaluation included adrenals, aorta, bone marrow smear, bone with marrow, brain, brown fat (interscapular), cecum, cerebellum with pons or medulla oblongata, cerebrum, epididymides, esophagus, eyes with optic nerves, femur with knee joint, gastrointestinal tract (cecum, colon, duodenum, esophagus, ileum, jejunum, stomach), gross lesions, heart, kidneys, liver, lungs (including bronchi), lymph nodes (mandibular and mesenteric), mammary gland, ovaries with oviducts, pancreas, sciatic nerve, pituitary, prostate, salivary glands, seminal vesicles, skeletal muscle (rectus femoris), skin, spinal cord (cervical), spleen, sternum, testes, thymus, thyroids with parathyroid, tongue, trachea, urinary bladder, uterus with cervix, and vagina. Tissues were preserved in 10% buffered neutral formalin, trimmed, processed routinely, and embedded in paraffin. Paraffin blocks were microtomed and sections stained with hematoxylin and eosin (H&E). The trimming procedure for hearts consisted of longitudinally bisecting these along a plane perpendicular to the plane of the pulmonary artery to expose the right atrioventricular, left atrioventricular, and aortic valves. Each hemisection was embedded in paraffin with the cut surface down. In addition to H&E stained sections, some sections of heart immunostained for alpha-smooth muscle actin (α-SMA) using standard immunohistochemical methods. The tissue sections were examined by light microscopy by board-certified members of the American College of Veterinary Pathologists (ACVP). All studies were peer reviewed by ACVP-certified veterinary pathologists [18].

## Results

LY2157299 was dosed to Fischer 344 rats and Beagle dogs for up to 6 months (Table 1). Daily oral administration was the dose schedule in the rat and the dog except for a study in the rat in which an intermittent dose schedule of 2 weeks on/2 weeks off was investigated. LY2157299 was well tolerated in the rat as a single dose up to 2000 mg/kg (data not shown). In repeat dose studies in the rat, LY2157299 caused mortality at progressively lower doses as the duration of treatment increased. Mortality was observed in rats administered 1200 mg/kg of LY2157299 in a 14-day study. In the 3- and 6-month studies, mortality occurred in animals receiving daily doses of 150 mg/kg (6-month study) and 250 mg/kg (3- and 6-month study) beginning on days 83 and 54, respectively. At a dose of 1200 mg/kg in rats, a gross change of sternal deviation consistent with acquired pectusexcavatum occurred, rarely with concurrent rib deformities, as early as nine days after initiation of dosing.In the longer term (>3 months) rat studies,

most of the deaths that occurred prior to the schedule termination were attributed to compound-related inflammation and rupture of the aorta and/or distributing arteries at or near the base of the heart resulting in hemothorax and/or hemoabdomen.

LY2157299 was evaluated in beagle dogs up to 500 mg/kg. All animals tolerated LY2157299 for the duration of the study with the exception of a single animal administered 500 mg/kg which was euthanized shortly following the end of the treatment period in a 1-month study due to deteriorating condition. This animal was found to have severe necrotizing cholecystitis.

LY2157299 is well absorbed following oral dosing and exposures appear to be dose linear in the rat and dog. In rats, exposures in females are higher than in males and are consistent with the toxicity data in which female rats are more affected than males. No exposure differences are observed between sexes in the beagle dog.

## Cardiovascular toxicology

In both rats and dogs, the heart and great vessels were identified as the major target organs for toxicity. Cardiovascular findings in F344 rats treated with LY2157299 included degenerative and inflammatory valvular lesions (valvulopathy), myocardial degeneration and necrosis, aortitis with rupture, vasculitis/perivasculitis, and increased heart weights. The cardiovascular lesions were dose- and duration-dependent in rats and dogs, respectively (Figures 1 and 2). These cardiovascular lesions were not accompanied by chronic pulmonary or hepatic congestion that would have been suggestive of congestive heart failure, even after 6 months of daily dosing.

## Valvulopathy

The earliest microscopic changes included heart valve lesions and myocardial degeneration at the insertion point of the valves which occurred in less than 2 weeks in the rat at a 1200-mg/kg dose and was also observed in the 3-month and 6-month daily dosing studies at ≥50 mg/kg. No cardiac lesions were observed following 1 month of daily dosing study in the rat at doses of 15 mg/kg, 50 mg/kg, and 150 mg/kg. In the dog, valve lesions were observed following one month of daily dosing at ≥50 mg/kg or at doses as low as 8 mg/kg following 6 months of daily dosing.

In both species, the valvulopathy was characterized by valve thickening, hemorrhage, hemosiderin-laden macrophages, inflammation, stromal and endothelial hyperplasia and increased myxomatous matrix (Figure 3). The inflammation was typically a mixture of lymphocytes and macrophages, but occasionally included neutrophils. The stromal hyperplasia and valve thickening were similar to spontaneous mitral valvulopathy [19], but occurred at a high incidence in the rat and were usually associated with other lesions such as hemorrhage or inflammation. Both atrioventricular and semilunar valves had lesions, and often multiple valves were affected in a given animal. Increased smooth muscle actin (SMA) immunolabeling of the valve consistently occurred when light microscopic lesions were present and indicated valvular interstitial cell activation with transdifferentiation into myofibroblast-like cells. However, because increases in SMA expression were always concurrent with morphologic changes, this finding was not useful as a premonitory marker for the morphologic changes (data not shown).

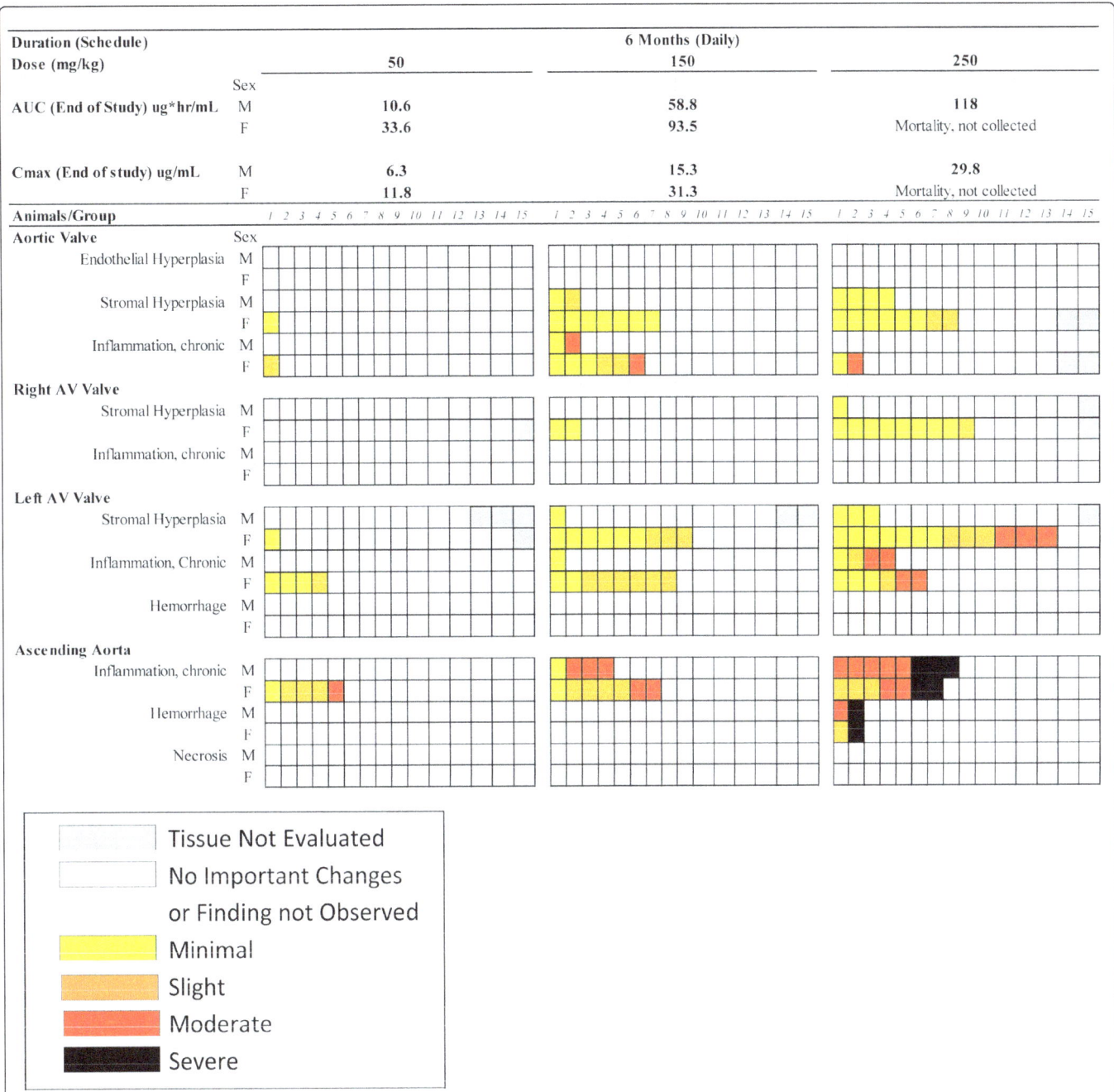

Figure 1: Incidence and severity of cardiac lesions in rats following daily administration of LY2157299 for six months. Exposure was determined at the end of the study in a group of satellite animals receiving compound for six months.

The incidence, severity, and chronicity of valvulopathy were similar in the 3- and 6-month daily dosing studies in rats at all dose levels. In the dog at the end of the 6-month dosing period, most animals in the 20 mg/kg and 60 mg/kg dose groups had at least one valve affected, whereas the 8-mg/kg dose group had fewer affected animals. The valvular lesions were still present in the rat and dog following a treatment-free recovery period. A partial recovery in the rat was observed when rats were dosed with 250 mg/kg LY2157299 daily for 2 months, a dose known to produce virtually 100% incidence of valvular lesions. Rats allowed a 6-week recovery period still had lesions present; however, there was a decrease in severity and incidence, indicating partial reversibility. A chronic end stage lesion characterized by scarring and valvular insufficiency was not recognized microscopically, although valvular function was not assessed in vivo. This could suggest that the onset of the valvular injury occurred at different time points throughout the dosing period.

## Vascular lesions

Vascular lesions occurred when dogs and rats were administered LY2157299 at doses of ≥8 and ≥50 mg/kg in the dog and rat, respectively, for prolonged time periods (≥3 months). In the rat, the earliest lesions were typically periarteritis and intramural hemorrhage that progressed to transmural inflammation, necrotizing vasculitis, and vascular rupture (Figure 4). Vascular lesions were most prominent in the thoracic cavity and involved the aortic arch, coronary arteries, and other distributing arteries originating from the aorta in the thoracic and cranial abdominal cavities. Lesions were often pronounced at the base of the aorta and where distributing arteries branched from the proximal aorta, a site of high pressure and increased turbulence. In a subset of rats, severe degenerative and inflammatory changes were associated with vascular rupture resulting in fatal hemothorax or hemoabdomen. The intramural hemorrhage was compatible with aortic dissection, although vascular dilation and aneurysms were not apparent. There were no lesions in the standard section of thoracic descending aorta.

Changes in the dog aorta did not occur in the 1-month studies but were noted in the 6-month study. While the valvular lesions in the dog were similar to those described in the rat, the aortic vascular change differed. The changes in the base of the ascending aorta of dogs were characterized by focal to multifocal degeneration and disorganization of the mural elastic lamellae, increased prominence of mucopolysaccharide-rich ground substance, but without accompanying inflammation or intramural hemorrhage (Figure 5). In the most affected animals, irregular separation between the elastic layers occurred. There were no findings in the standard section of thoracic descending aorta. Although the microscopic changes likely compromised aortic structural integrity, there were no changes diagnostic of aneurysm.

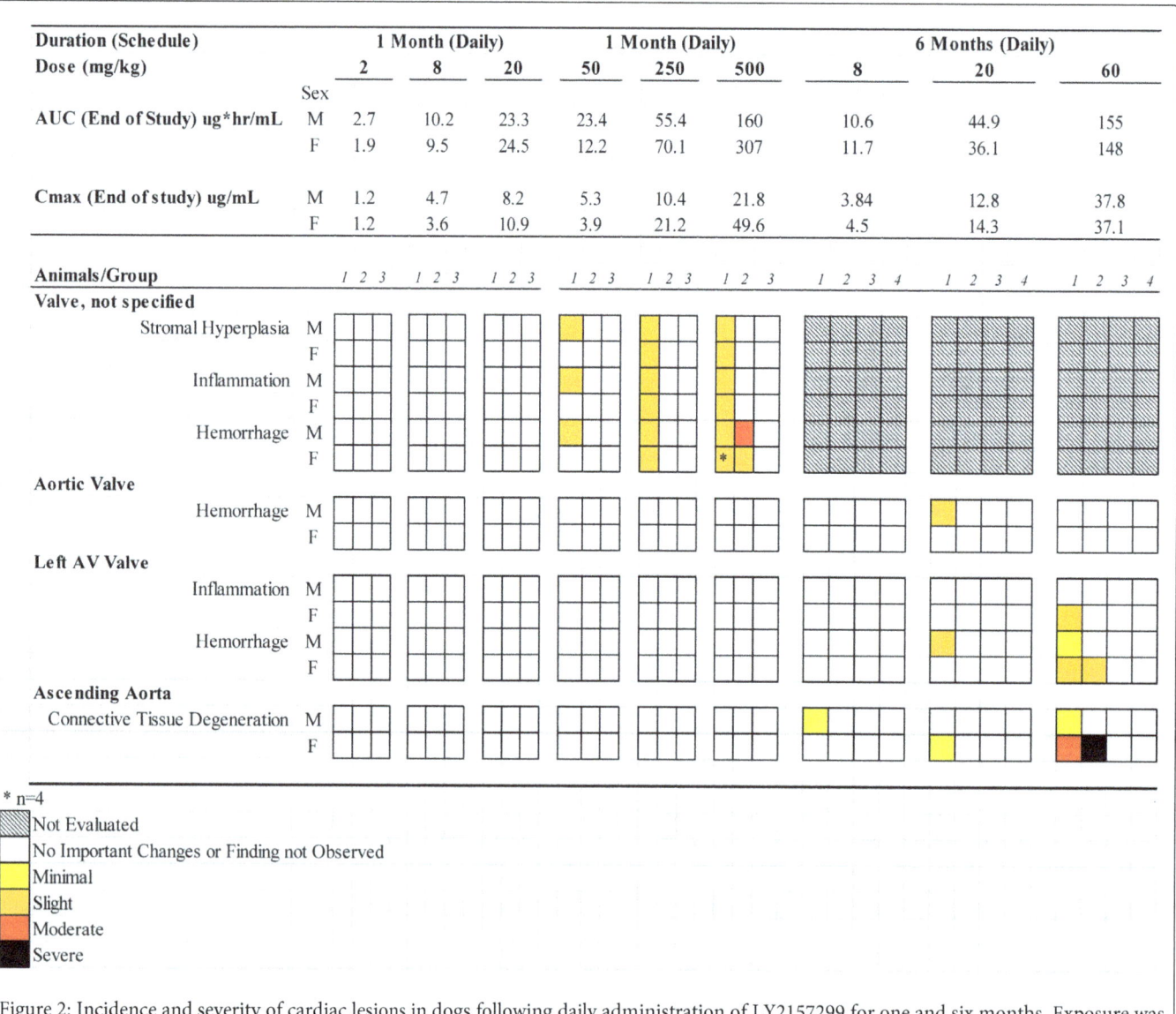

Figure 2: Incidence and severity of cardiac lesions in dogs following daily administration of LY2157299 for one and six months. Exposure was determined at the end of the study.

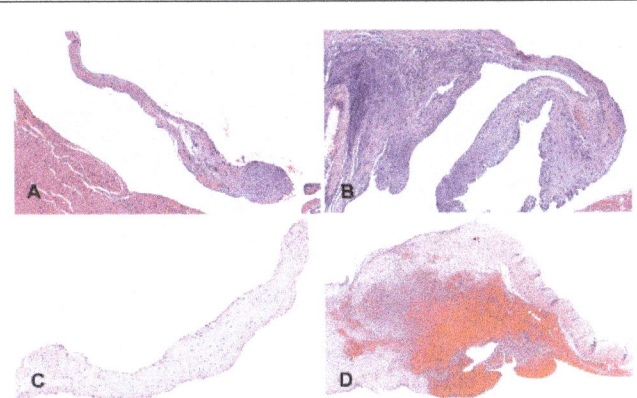

Figure 3: Hematoxylin and eosin stain of atrioventricular heart valves (A) Control rat demonstrating some mild spontaneous myxomatous change at the distal end of the valve. (B) Rat dosed for 3 months with LY2157299. A chronic valvulopathy characterized by expansion of the valve leaflet with increased myxomatous matrix, inflammatory cells, and hemorrhage. (C) Control dog. (D) Valve from a dog dosed for 1 month with LY2157299. An acute valvulopathy characterized by marked expansion due to hemorrhage, edema, and inflammatory cells.

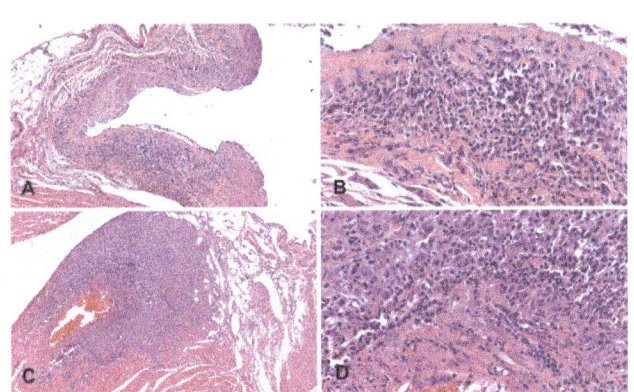

Figure 4: (A and B) Low- and high-magnification images (hematoxylin and eosin stain) of the ascending aorta including the origin of the coronary artery from a rat dosed for 14 weeks with LY2157299. The origin of the coronary artery has disruption of the tunica media with transmural infiltration by mixed inflammatory cells. (C and D) Low- and high-magnification images from a rat dosed for 6 months with LY2157299. The coronary artery has a pronounced perivascular infiltration of mixed inflammatory cells with only limited involvement of the tunica media.

## Additional cardiac findings

Myocardial degeneration and necrosis occurred in rats that had the most pronounced valvular and/or aortic changes, and were interpreted as secondary to the valvular and coronary artery changes rather than a primary test article effect.

Multifocal myocardial degeneration and necrosis typically involved the base of the heart, at the base of the valves, and the ventricles, and

was generally minimal in severity. Microscopic cardiovascular changes were rarely associated with increases in cardiac troponin I concentrations, most likely due to timing of the serum collection and the relatively mild myocardial degenerative changes.

LY2157299 induces slight-to-moderate decreases in blood pressure and increases in heart rate in dogs. These changes were not considered adverse. No biologically relevant change in QT/QTcf, test-article related arrhythmia, or altered waveforms were identified.

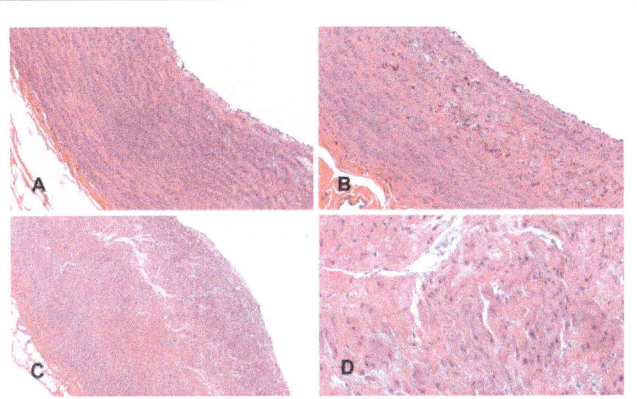

Figure 5: Ascending aorta from dogs dosed for 6 months with LY2157299 (hematoxylin and eosin). (A) Control dog. (B) Focally extensive disruption of the internal elastic laminae within the tunica media. (C and D) Marked disruption of the tunica media resulting in disorganization with loss of the laminar arrangement, increased prominence of mucopolysaccharide-rich ground substance, and cleft formation.

## Characterizing a Non Observed Effect Level for Cardiac Lesions

In order to support the clinical development of LY2157299 with the cardiovascular changes described above, an additional nonclinical toxicology study was conducted in rats to determine if a no observed effect level (NOEL) for cardiovascular changes could be identified using an alternative dosing schedule consisting of 2 weeks on treatment followed by 2 weeks off treatment.

The duration of this study was 3 months and compared daily dosing to the alternative dosing schedule. This duration supports the clinical time interval relevant to patients who are enrolled and then reassessed for disease status 2 months after receiving study drug. Based on the previous 6-month study in rats that identified when early mortality occurred due to cardiac events, a 3-month treatment duration was considered sufficient to induce a high incidence of cardiac lesions with a daily dosing schedule. The doses used for this study were 50 mg/kg, 150 mg/kg, and 250 mg/kg. As expected, mortality due to vascular rupture was observed in rats administered 250 mg/kg daily. In contrast, the rats on the 2-weeks-on/2-weeks-off dosing schedule at all doses survived until the scheduled termination of the study.

Rats administered 150 mg/kg and 250 mg/kg on a 2-weeks-on/2-weeks-off dosing schedule had cardiovascular lesions similar to those in the daily dosing groups, however, the incidence and often severity were lower in rats administered LY2157299 on the intermittent dosing schedule (Figure 6).

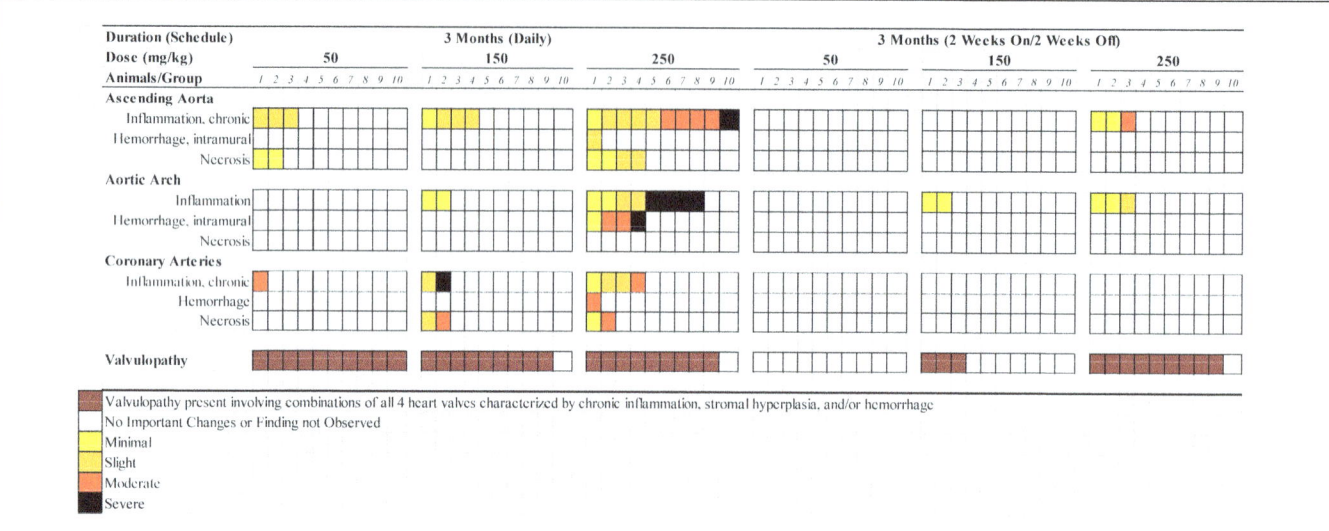

Figure 6: Comparison of incidence and severity of the cardiac lesions in female Fischer 344 rats given LY2157299 in two different dosing schedules for three months.

## Immune system

Numerous changes occurred in multiple organs of the rat and dog that were consistent with altered immune responses, both proinflammatory and also suggestive of immune dysfunction. These patterns occurred most often in organs such as the gastrointestinal tract and skin that are exposed to environmental antigenic stimulation and host commensal bacteria.

Increased mixed inflammatory cell infiltrates within the lamina propria of the large intestines, and less commonly the small intestines and stomach, occurred in studies of at least 1 month in duration. Additionally, increased inflammatory cell infiltrates occurred in the kidneys, lung, gallbladder, and/or prostate gland depending on the species. Rats in the 6-month toxicity study also had multiple subcutaneous abscesses, and acute inflammation involving the preputial and clitoral glands, suggesting immune dysfunction and/or alterations in the innate immune responses.

## Gastrointestinal system

Gastrointestinal changes frequently involved the large intestine, but at higher doses also included the small intestines, stomach, and gallbladder. Findings in the large intestine were most apparent in the 6-month studies and included mucosal inflammation in dogs and rats, and mucosal epithelial hyperplasia and neoplasia in rats. In the cecum of the rat, a continuum was identified with numerous rats showing increased mononuclear inflammatory cell infiltrates within the lamina propria of the mucosa, and fewer animals displaying enterocyte hyperplasia, and adenoma formation. In the colon, fewer rats had increased mucosal inflammation, possibly because of higher background infiltrates; however, some rats had epithelial hyperplasia and adenocarcinoma (Figure 7). Some of the adenocarcinomas were quite large and were the cause of adverse clinical signs, early euthanasia and/or death. Similar inflammatory and hyperplastic changes also involved the rectum.

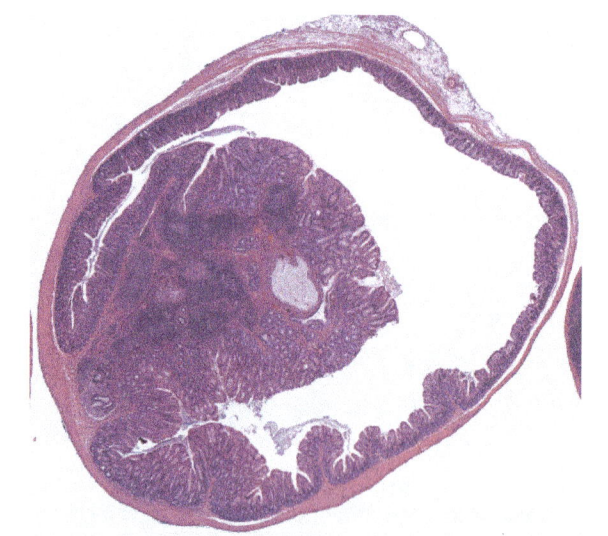

Figure 7: Adenocarcinoma of the colon from a rat that was euthanized after 23 weeks of daily dosing with LY2157299 (hematoxylin and eosin stain).

Dogs in the 1-month toxicity study at high doses (≥50 mg/kg) had acute intestinal changes with more pronounced lesions in the small intestine than the large intestine. These microscopic findings included inflammation and hemorrhage, and increased numbers of mucosal cysts. These dogs also had inflammation of the gallbladder that in one dog included necrotizing cholecystitis with rupture that resulted in bile peritonitis. At the highest dose, some dogs had hepatic inflammation and hepatocellular degeneration, changes that may have been secondary to the intestinal changes. Intestinal lesions in dogs in the 6-month toxicity study were uncommon and limited to mild inflammatory cell infiltrates within the large intestine that ranged from acute to chronic, and sometimes included increased numbers of eosinophils and/or plasma cells. These dogs also had chronic inflammation of the gastric mucosa with glandular atrophy and vasculitis that was most prominent in the cardia.Increased amounts of mucus within the gallbladder occurred in some dogs.

## Skeletal system

Osseous changes included physeal and subphyseal changes in the femur, tibia, and sternum of rats that occurred after just 14 days of dosing and were similar to those previously described with TGF-β inhibition [12,13]. The zones of maturation and hypertrophy were expanded in the physes of the long bones and endplates of the sternabrae, and the primary and secondary spongiosa were denser with increased connectivity (Figure 8). These changes were orderly and appeared to result in relatively normal endochondral ossification. In animals that had a recovery phase, these osseous changes were characterized by a band of metaphyseal hyperostosis (increased trabecular density) that was separated from the physis by a zone of normal endochondral ossification, presumably the result of an earlier alteration in endochondral ossification that had reversed. Microscopic osseous changes were often more pronounced in rats that had the pectus excavatum defect. Similar physeal changes occurred in the sternebrae of the dog after 6 months of dosing. In addition to the physeal lesions, rats dosed for 6 months had additional changes of multifocal cartilaginous degeneration in the joints of the sternebrae and stifle.

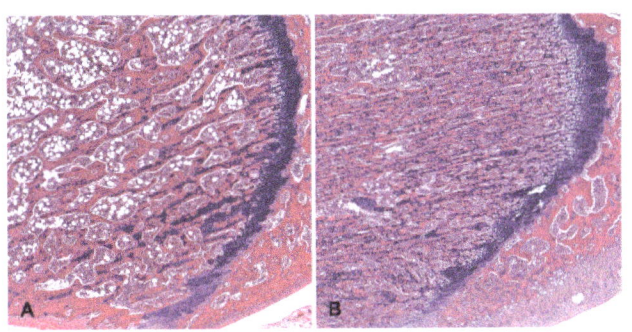

**Figure 8:** Proximal femur including the physis (hematoxylin and eosin stain). (A) Control rat. (B) Rat dosed for 6 months with LY2157299 had expansion of the physeal zones of maturation and hypertrophy, increased density and interconnectivity of the subphyseal primary and secondary spongiosa, and an orderly increase in the trabecular bone density.

## Discussion

TGF-β plays a key role in several disease states, including cancer, cardiovascular disease, and fibrosis, which has made the TGF-β signaling pathway a logical and attractive target of pharmaceutical development. However, TGF-β signaling has posed a challenge with respect to understanding safe therapeutic doses that do not confer toxicities associated with prolonged inhibition of this critical pathway [16]. We characterized the toxicity profile of LY2157299 in nonclinical species for up to 6 months of daily dosing. LY2157299 was well tolerated in the rat and the dog for one month of daily dosing and in the rats for 3 months of intermittent dosing. Long-term daily dosing of ≥3 months caused alterations in the gastrointestinal, immune, musculoskeletal, renal and cardiovascular systems of animals, which is

anticipated based on the integral role for TGF-β signaling for maintaining homeostasis.

Other pharmaceutical companies have published similar valvular toxicities with inhibitors from their development efforts, indicating that the lesions described are likely an on target effect [12,13]. Many explanations have been considered to understand mechanism of this phenomenon; no definitive explanation has been provided at this time [12]. TGF-β is a required mediator for valve structural and functional homeostasis [20]. In response to injury, valvularmyofibroblasts are activated by TGF-β and results in increases in α-SMA expression [21]. This paradoxical inhibition of TGF-β signaling with LY2157299 - treated animals resulting in increased SMA in their heart valves is not understood and awaits further clarification.

We have characterized cardiac effects in nonclinical species that extend beyond the previously reported valvulopathy and, in contrast to the valvulopathy, constituted a pathologic lesion defined as dose limiting within the context of a given study. In both species, the aorta and arteries of the heart are major target organs for toxicity. The vascular lesions in the rat are characterized by inflammation and hemorrhage with associated disruption of the mural organization, sometimes resulting in vessel rupture and hemorrhage into the thoracic cavity. In contrast to the rat, the dog showed changes in the base of the ascending aorta, characterized by degeneration and disorganization of the mural elastic lamellae and often increased prominence of mucopolysaccharide-rich ground substance without accompanying inflammation. The reason for this apparent species difference is unknown.

Our findings support that TGF-β plays a pleiotropic role in cell growth and on the extracellular matrix. It is important in both production of matrix proteins and the degradation of the matrix [22]. Two well-studied genetic diseases Marfan syndrome (MFS) and Loeys-Dietz syndrome (LDS) affect the skeletal, ocular, and cardiovascular systems [23]. Clinically, these syndromes present with overlapping symptoms including aortic aneurysms, dissections and mitral valve prolapse [24]. MFS is caused by mutations in the gene encoding fibrillin-1 that interacts with latent TGF-β binding protein to upregulate TGF-β bioavailability and activity [25]. LDS is an autosomal dominant aortic aneurysm syndrome caused by mutations in the promoter of TGF-β R1 and R2 with increased TGF-β activity [23,26]. In LDS, the microscopic aortic lesion is characterized by fragmentation of elastic fibers, loss of elastin content, and accumulation of amorphous matrix components in the aortic media, changes very similar to those observed in the 6-month dog study with LY2157299 [23]. In cardiac tissue from affected patients and mouse models of MFS, TGF-β signaling is increased, potentially due toaltered receptor processing or alternative pathways responsible for upregulation of TGF-β [27]. Mutations in the TGF-β signaling pathway that should lead to decreased TGF-β signaling resulting in an upregulation of this pathway underscores that in vivo, precise regulation of multiple members is required to maintain homeostasis and that canonical and non-canonical signaling pathways play an important role [28,29].

The findings described in the aorta and cardiac arteries in the toxicology studies in the rat and the dog, based on similarity with genetic syndromes, appear to be more consistent with an upregulation rather than inhibition of the TGF-β pathway. The contributions of the non-canonical TGF-β signaling are not yet understood. Activation of the ERK pathway contributes to progression of aneurysms in *Fbn1*mice. RDEA119, a selective MEK inhibitor, reduced aortic root growth independent of increased *Smad2* activation, suggesting that non-canonical pathway modulation may contribute to progression to aneursyms in *Fbn1*mice [28]. As with MFS and LDS, which are genetic mutations resulting in a clinical phenotype, additional genetic differences may also play a role in susceptibility to cardiac injury observed in nonclinical studies with inhibitors of TGF-β signaling. Behmoaraset al. evaluated seven genetically different strains in rats for their differences in composition of the extracellular matrix and noted a differentiation among strains with respect to matrix composition and occurrence of internal elastic lamina rupture [30].

The changes to the heart following long-term treatment of LY2157299 at toxicologically relevant doses are of largest concern with respect to clinical safety, inhibition of TGF-β signaling resulted in changes to several other organ systems in both the rat and dog. LY2157299 resulted in changes to the bone similar to previous reports [12,13]. Reversibility of bone changes was assessed following the 1-month study in rats revealing a band of increased trabecular density that was separated from the normal physis by a zone of normal endochondral ossification. Following 6 months of treatment in the rat, degeneration in the joints of the sternebrum and stifle was reported. Dominant negative mutant TGF-β receptor II mice are reported to have bifurcated xiphoid process and sternum as well as a progressive osteoarthritis-like disease [31]. Dogs used in the 6-month study were between 6-8 months of age and are expected to still have active longitudinal growth in their bones; therefore, alterations in the endochondral cartilage similar to what was described in the rat may be anticipated [32].

TGF-β also plays a critical role in epithelial biology, acting as a tumor suppressor or promoter [33]. Alteration in TGF-β signaling is common in many cancers [34]. Disruption of TGF-β signaling in either epithelial or stromal cells increases inflammatory responses that promote tumor initiation, progression, and metastasis [35]. *TGFβ1-/-Rag2 -/-* mice develop inflammation-associated adenomas and carcinomas through an inability to maintain epithelial tissue organization [36]. Mice genetically deficient in TGF-β R2 signaling have increased susceptibility to cancer [37]. Similarly, inactivation of downstream proteins *Smad3*and *Smad4* results in carcinomas of the intestine [38,10]. The observations of hyperplasia, adenoma, and carcinoma of the intestine in rats treated with LY2157299 for 6 months are consistent with the well-characterized biology.

The use of intermittent dosing is common practice in oncology: clinicians will reduce the dose or permit a drug holiday to allow the patient to recover from toxicities prior to receiving another dose. Studies have shown that anticancer agents were more tolerable and efficacious when administered in intermittent dosing schedules [39,40]. In contrast to a dosing schedule based on clinical findings, clinical dosing with LY2157299 proactively applied an indirect model to support a clinical dosing regimen that would support a desired pharmacologic effect and avoid unwanted toxicity. Buenoet al. have been able to relate plasma concentrations to pSmad inhibition [41]. Tumor growth inhibition was then linked to pSmad inhibition, providing a tool to titrate the dose required for efficacy. Furthermore, the data support the concept of intermittent dosing in maintaining a similar tumor response. The ability to maintain plasma concentrations required for efficacy lower than those observed to cause adverse toxicities in nonclinical species is important, especially when considering drugs targeting signaling pathways such as TGF-β that have been demonstrated to be critical in maintaining normal function. We demonstrate continuous administration of LY2157299 at high doses or durations ≥3 months in nonclinical species results in adverse toxicities to numerous organ systems including cardiovascular, gastrointestinal, immune, bone/cartilage, reproductive, and renal. The cardiovascular system appears to be most sensitive to abrogation of TGF-β signaling with the small molecule inhibitor LY2157299. Our data have defined a NOEL for cardiovascular lesions of 150 mg/kg and 20 mg/kg, in rat and dog, respectively, after one month of daily dosing and 50 mg/kg for 3 months on a 2-week-on/2-week-off dosing schedule in the rat. An intermittent dosing paradigm demonstrated that the severity and incidence of cardiac lesions could be lessened. The data from the 3-month intermittent dosing study in rats along with the absence of cardiovascular lesions in the 1-month rat and dog study established a nonclinical data package that supports a clinical dosing schedule of 2 weeks on/2 weeks off LY2157299. Successful development of such inhibitors will need to have a thorough characterization of nonclinical toxicity and an understanding of schedule and plasma concentrations needed to demonstrate anti-tumor effect and determine if a sufficient therapeutic window exists to test the clinical efficacy of molecules involved in inhibiting key pathways.

## Funding

This work was supported by Eli Lilly and Company, Indianapolis, IN, USA.

## Acknowledgements

We would like to thank Drs. Michael Lahn, Marcus Andrews, Kyla Carroll, and Armando Irizarry for the critical review of this manuscript. We are thankful to Dr. DurisalaDesaiah for writing assistance of this manuscript.

## References

1. Siegel PM, Massagué J (2003) Cytostatic and apoptotic actions of TGF-beta in homeostasis and cancer. Nat Rev Cancer 3: 807-821.

2. Akhurst RJ, Hata A (2012) Targeting the TGFβ² signalling pathway in disease. Nat Rev Drug Discov 11: 790-811.

3. Massagué J, Blain SW, Lo RS (2000) TGFbeta signaling in growth control, cancer, and heritable disorders. Cell 103: 295-309.

4. Millan FA, Denhez F, Kondaiah P, Akhurst RJ (1991) Embryonic gene expression patterns of TGF beta 1, beta 2 and beta 3 suggest different developmental functions in vivo. Development 111: 131-143.

5. Feng XH, Derynck R (2005) Specificity and versatility in tgf-beta signaling through Smads. Annu Rev Cell Dev Biol 21: 659-693.

6. Kulkarni AB, Ward JM, Yaswen L, Mackall CL, Bauer SR, et al. (1995) Transforming growth factor-beta 1 null mice. An animal model for inflammatory disorders. Am J Pathol 146: 264-275.

7. Sanford LP, Ormsby I, Gittenberger-de Groot AC, Sariola H, Friedman R, et al. (1997) TGFbeta2 knockout mice have multiple developmental defects that are non-overlapping with other TGFbeta knockout phenotypes. Development 124: 2659-2670.

8. Larsson J, Goumans MJ, Sjöstrand LJ, van Rooijen MA, Ward D, et al. (2001) Abnormal angiogenesis but intact hematopoietic potential in TGF-beta type I receptor-deficient mice. EMBO J 20: 1663-1673.

9. ten Dijke P, Arthur HM (2007) Extracellular control of TGFbetasignalling in vascular development and disease. Nat Rev Mol Cell Biol 8: 857-869.

10. Zhu Y, Richardson JA, Parada LF, Graff JM (1998) Smad3 mutant mice develop metastatic colorectal cancer. Cell 94: 703-714.

11. Li HY, McMillen WT, Heap CR, McCann DJ, Yan L, et al. (2008) Optimization of a dihydropyrrolopyrazole series of transforming grow

factor-beta type I receptor kinase domain inhibitors: discovery of an orally bioavailable transforming growth factor-beta receptor type I inhibitor as antitumor agent. J Med Chem 51: 2302-2306.

12. Anderton MJ, Mellor HR, Bell A, Sadler C, Pass M, et al. (2011) Induction of heart valve lesions by small-molecule ALK5 inhibitors. ToxicolPathol 39: 916-924.

13. Frazier K, Thomas R, Scicchitano M, Mirabile R, Boyce R, et al. (2007) Inhibition of ALK5 signaling induces physeal dysplasia in rats. ToxicolPathol 35: 284-295.

14. Stauber AJ, Zimmermann JL, Berridge BR (2006) Pathobiology of a valvulopathy in Fischer 344 rats given a transforming growth factor-ß RI kinase inhibitor. Society of Toxicology, 290.

15. Lonning S, Mannick J, McPherson JM (2011) Antibody targeting of TGF-Î² in cancer patients. Curr Pharm Biotechnol 12: 2176-2189.

16. Garber K (2009) Companies waver in efforts to target transforming growth factor beta in cancer. J Natl Cancer Inst 101: 1664-1667.

17. Gueorguieva I, Cleverly AL, Stauber AJ, Pillay NS, Rodon JA, et al (2013) Defining a therapeutic window for the novel TFG-ß inhibitor LY2157299 monohydrate based on a pharmacokinetic/pharmacodynamic model. Br J ClinPharmacol 77:796-807.

18. Morton D, Sellers RS, Barale-Thomas E, Bolon B, George C, et al. (2010) Recommendations for pathology peer review. ToxicolPathol 38: 1118-1127.

19. Donnelly KB (2008) Cardiac valvular pathology: comparative pathology and animal models of acquired cardiac valvular diseases. ToxicolPathol 36: 204-217.

20. Walker GA, Masters KS, Shah DN, Anseth KS, Leinwand LA (2004) Valvularmyofibroblast activation by transforming growth factor-beta: implications for pathological extracellular matrix remodeling in heart valve disease. Circ Res 95: 253-260.

21. Skalli O, Pelte MF, Peclet MC, Gabbiani G, Gugliotta P, et al. (1989) Alpha-smooth muscle actin, a differentiation marker of smooth muscle cells, is present in microfilamentous bundles of pericytes. J HistochemCytochem 37: 315-321.

22. Jones JA, Spinale FG, Ikonomidis JS (2009) Transforming growth factor-beta signaling in thoracic aortic aneurysm development: a paradox in pathogenesis. J Vasc Res 46: 119-137.

23. Loeys BL, Chen J, Neptune ER, Judge DP, Podowski M, et al (2005) A syndrome of altered cardiovascular, craniofacial, neurocognitive and skeletal development caused by mutations in TGF?R1 or TGF?R2. Nat Genet 37: 275-281.

24. Ramirez F, Dietz HC (2007) Marfan syndrome: from molecular pathogenesis to clinical treatment. CurrOpin Genet Dev 17: 252-258.

25. Horbelt D, Guo G, Robinson PN, Knaus P (2010) Quantitative analysis of TGFBR2 mutations in Marfan-syndrome-related disorders suggests a correlation between phenotypic severity and Smad signaling activity. J Cell Sci 123: 4340-4350.

26. Loeys BL, Schwarze U, Holm T, Callewaert BL, Thomas GH, et al. (2006) Aneurysm syndromes caused by mutations in the TGF-beta receptor. N Engl J Med 355: 788-798.

27. Carta L, Smaldone S, Zilberberg L, Loch D, Dietz HC, et al. (2009) p38 MAPK is an early determinant of promiscuous Smad2/3 signaling in the aortas of fibrillin-1 (Fbn1)-null mice. J Biol Chem 284: 5630-5636.

28. Holm TM, Habashi JP, Doyle JJ, Bedja D, Chen Y, et al. (2011) Noncanonical TGFÎ² signaling contributes to aortic aneurysm progression in Marfan syndrome mice. Science 332: 358-361.

29. Ng CM, Cheng A, Myers LA, Martinez-Murillo F, Jie C, et al. (2004) TGF-beta-dependent pathogenesis of mitral valve prolapse in a mouse model of Marfan syndrome. J Clin Invest 114: 1586-1592.

30. Behmoaras J, Osborne-Pellegrin M, Gauguier D, Jacob MP (2005) Characteristics of the aortic elastic network and related phenotypes in seven inbred rat strains. Am J Physiol Heart CircPhysiol 288: H769-777.

31. Serra R, Johnson M, Filvaroff EH, LaBorde J, Sheehan DM, et al. (1997) Expression of a truncated, kinase-defective TGF-beta type II receptor in mouse skeletal tissue promotes terminal chondrocyte differentiation and osteoarthritis. J Cell Biol 139: 541-552.

32. Yonamine H, Ogi N, Ishikawa T, Ichiki H (1980) Radiographic studies on skeletal growth of the pectoral limb of the beagle. Nihon JuigakuZasshi 42: 417-425.

33. Dumont N, Arteaga CL (2003) Targeting the TGF beta signaling network in human neoplasia. Cancer Cell 3: 531-536.

34. Derynck R, Akhurst RJ, Balmain A (2001) TGF-beta signaling in tumor suppression and cancer progression. Nat Genet 29: 117-129.

35. Achyut BR, Yang L (2011) Transforming growth factor-Î² in the gastrointestinal and hepatic tumor microenvironment. Gastroenterology 141: 1167-1178.

36. Engle SJ, Hoying JB, Boivin GP, Ormsby I, Gartside PS, et al. (1999) Transforming growth factor beta1 suppresses nonmetastatic colon cancer at an early stage of tumorigenesis. Cancer Res 59: 3379-3386.

37. Lu SL, Herrington H, Reh D, Weber S, Bornstein S, et al. (2006) Loss of transforming growth factor-beta type II receptor promotes metastatic head-and-neck squamous cell carcinoma. Genes Dev 20: 1331-1342.

38. Xu X, Brodie SG, Yang X, Im YH, Parks WT, et al. (2000) Haploid loss of the tumor suppressor Smad4/Dpc4 initiates gastric polyposis and cancer in mice. Oncogene 19: 1868-1874.

39. Boss DS, Schwartz GK, Middleton MR, Amakye DD, Swaisland H, et al. (2010) Safety, tolerability, pharmacokinetics and pharmacodynamics of the oral cyclin-dependent kinase inhibitor AZD5438 when administered at intermittent and continuous dosing schedules in patients with advanced solid tumours. Ann Oncol 21: 884-894.

40. Wang X, Zhang L, Goldberg SN, Bhasin M, Brown V, et al. (2011) High dose intermittent sorafenib shows improved efficacy over conventional continuous dose in renal cell carcinoma. J Transl Med 9: 220.

41. Bueno L, de Alwis DP, Pitou C, Yingling J, Lahn M, et al. (2008) Semi-mechanistic modelling of the tumour growth inhibitory effects of LY2157299, a new type I receptor TGF-beta kinase antagonist, in mice. Eur J Cancer 44: 142-150.

# 15

# Individual and Combined Effects of Subchronic Exposure of Three Fusarium Toxins (Fumonisin B, Deoxynivalenol and Zearalenone) in Rabbit Bucks

Judit Szabó-Fodor[1*], Mariam Kachlek[1], Sándor Cseh[3], Bence Somoskői[3], András Szabó[1,2], Zsófia Blochné Bodnár[2], Gábor Tornyos[2], Miklós Mézes[4], Krisztián Balogh[4], Róbert Glávits[5], Dóra Hafner[2] and Melinda Kovács[1,2]

[1]Faculty of Agricultural and Environmental Sciences, MTA-KE Mycotoxins in the Food Chain Research Group, Kaposvár University, Hungary

[2]Faculty of Agricultural and Environmental Sciences, Kaposvár University, Hungary

[3]SZIU Faculty of Veterinary Science, István, Hungary

[4]SZIU Faculty of Agricultural and Environmental Sciences, Hungary

*Corresponding author: Judit Szabó-Fodor, Faculty of Agricultural and Environmental Sciences, MTA-KE Mycotoxins in the Food Chain Research Group, Kaposvár University, Hungary, E-mail: fodor.judit@ke.hu

## Abstract

Objective of the study was to determine reproductive toxicity of Fusarium toxins orally at three subchronic doses on adult Pannon White male rabbits. The four treatments were: control (C, toxin-free diet), F (5 mg/kg FB1), DZ (1 mg/kg DON+0.25 mg/kg ZEA), FDZ (5 mg/kg FB1+1 mg/kg DON+0.25 mg/kg ZEA) for 65 days (n=15/treatment). The doses were pre-determined according the EU limits in finished feed for young pig (in the absence of limits for rabbits' feed; based on the European Commission Recommendation 2006/576/EC and the European Commission Directive 2003/100/EC). The most pronounced effects of the toxins were exerted on the reproductive processes. The ratio of spermatozoa showing progressive forward motility decreased (P<0.05) from 80% to 67% in the FDZ group by day 60. Differences were found between the groups DZ (66.3% ± 23.7) and C (80.2% ± 11.2) in spermatozoa morphology. GnRH treated animals produced less testosterone in FDZ animals, compared to the other three groups (P<0.05). In the comet assay the individual fumonisin treatment resulted in significantly less 0 comets (intact cells), compared to all others. Based on the prevalence of score, lower (P<0.0001) damage was observed in FDZ group, as compared to F and DZ. Among the mycotoxins studied, additive or less than additive effect was found in case of spermatogenesis and sperm cell morphology, synergism in testosterone production, while FB1 acted antagonistically against DON+ZEA in comet assay. All mycotoxins provoked moderate lipid-peroxidation, based on the changes of glutathione concentration, glutathione peroxidase activity and formation of malondialdehyde and conjugated dienes and trienes, and exerted slight genotoxicity based on comet assay, FB1 being antagonistic towards DON+ZEA. In F, DZ and FDZ animals the intensity of spermatogenesis decreased by 43, 31 and 64%, respectively, which was reflected by lack of differentiated spermatozoa, thinning of the germinal epithelium, the appearance of multinuclear giant cells, indicative of the disturbance of meiosis and mitosis of the germinal epithelial cells and in some cases the lack of spermatogonia.

**Keywords:** Fumonisin; Deoxynivalenol; Zearalenon; Spermatogenesis; Testosterone production; Rabbit

## Introduction

The worldwide contamination of foods and feeds with mycotoxins is a significant problem. Studies have shown extensive mycotoxin contamination in both developing and developed countries [1-3], as effect of global climate change [4].

The toxicity of mycotoxins differs depending on the kind of toxin, and in animals it is related to the species, the dose ingested, the duration of the exposure, and their gender and age. The main classes of Fusarium mycotoxins with respect to animal health and production are the non-oestrogenic trichothecenes such as deoxynivalenol (DON) and T-2 toxin (T-2), the myco-oestrogens including zearalenone (ZEA) and its zearalenol metabolites [5] and fumonisins.

Fumonisins (B1 and B2) are cancer-promoting metabolites of *Fusarium proliferatum* and *Fusarium verticillioides* that have a long-chain hydrocarbon unit (similar to that of sphingosine and sphinganine), which plays a role in their toxicity. Fumonisin B1 (FB1)

is the most toxic and has been shown to promote tumour in rats and cause equine leukoencephalomalacia and porcine pulmonary oedema. FB, the most abundant of the numerous fumonisin analogues, was classified by the IARC as a Group 2B carcinogen (possibly carcinogenic in humans) [6].

Although DON is the least toxic type of trichothecene, it can cause significant harmful effects in animals and humans [7]. DON causes a broad variety of toxic effects in animals, and its toxicity is well recognized in mammals. The main effect at the cellular level is the inhibition of protein synthesis via binding to the ribosomal subunit [8]. Chronic oral exposure induces anorexia, decreased weight gain, reduction in feed conversion, gastrointestinal hemorrhaging, inflammation and immune system alterations.

ZEA competes with the naturally produced hormone estradiol-17β for binding sites (estradiol receptors) in various organs in the body of both genders. ZEA can obstruct normal steroid hormone (estradiol, testosterone, progesterone) synthesis in the ovaries and testicles of livestock.

ZEA is found, especially, as a contaminant in corn. ZEA, which is produced mainly by *F. graminearum* and *F. culmorum* and commonly co-occurs with DON and its derivatives. It is among one of the most frequently encountered mycotoxins in grain from FHB (fusarium head blight)-diseased small-grain cereals throughout the Mediterranean countries. It may co-occur with DON in grains such as wheat, barley, oats and corn and fumonisins in corn [9]. Generally, DON is found in higher doses than ZEA when this occurs [10]. Most studies indicate that in artificial environment high moisture favours the production of both classes of mycotoxins, but the optimum temperatures for trichothecene and ZEA production in Fusarium-infected grain appears to be specific to the substrate, species and individual metabolites. The accumulated data revealed definite geographical differences in the level and frequency of DON, NIV and ZEA in wheat and barley. Streit et al. [11] reviewed mycotoxin co-occurrences in animal feed in Europe since 2004. Since Fusarium species are the most frequent fungal pathogens on field crops, it was not surprising that B-trichothecenes (DON), ZEA, and FBs were the major co-contaminants.

Reproductive efficiency is a very important economic factor in animal production. Exposure to several Fusarium mycotoxins have been linked to reproductive disorders as it was reviewed by Cortinovis et al [12]. The effect of these toxins on reproduction has been widely studied in female animals, while knowledge about their effect on reproduction processes in males is limited. As far as it is known they can affect spermatogenesis, and sperm quality, Leydig cell function (testosterone production), gonadotropin secretion, and fertility [13-18].

Humans and animals are generally exposed to multiple mycotoxins in parallel, as some mycotoxins typically co-occur in cereals. However, toxicological data, risk assessments are based on, are provided by studies in which only the individual effects of certain toxins are investigated. The simultaneous exposure of animals to more than one toxin is of concern and requires more study [19]. Synergistic effects may explain why animals sometimes respond negatively to mycotoxin levels much lower than those reported in scientific studies as able to cause mycotoxicoses.

In a survey conducted over a period of 4.5 years in countries of Southern Europe (Portugal, Spain, Italy, Greece and Cyprus) the Fusarium mycotoxins were found to be the major contaminants (fumonisins, type B trichothecenes and ZEA) of feed material and compounded feed samples [20]. There are several studies about mycotoxins' interaction (mainly in vitro), but only a few report the combined effects of three specific Fusarium mycotoxins which are more likely to co-occur; i.e. FB, DON and ZEA. Although there are studies about the three aforementioned mycotoxins very few focus on tertiary mixtures [21-24]. In rabbit bucks, ZEN impairs spermatogenesis and decreases libido, although only at high doses (117.3 mg/kg feed) [25]. Pregnant rabbit does fed on a DON-contaminated diet (0.3 and 0.6 mg/kg) showed marked bodyweight loss, but teratogenic effect was not proven [26]. FB1 was found to be nephron- and hepatotoxic in rabbits [27], and it has also been shown to negatively influence haematopoiesis by impairing bone marrow function [28]. Lung oedema was found only in a small number of rabbits fed a FB1-contaminated diet [29]. The teratogenic effect of FB1 was also described using an oral dose of 300 mg/d for 14 d [18] but a lack of embryotoxicity was found at lower (0.1, 0.5 or 1.00 mg/d) oral doses [30].

Grenier and Oswald [31] performed a meta-analysis of published raw data on mycotoxin interactions in vivo which varies according to the animal species, the dose of toxins, the length of exposure, but also

the parameters measured; and classified the interaction into the following categories: synergistic, additive, less than additive, and antagonistic. The authors also differentiated between three types of synergistic effects and two types of antagonisms. Such characterization of mycotoxin interactions is helpful in experimental designs and interpretations of combined toxicity outcomes and should be included into further investigations on mycotoxin interactions.

The aim of this experiment was to study the dietary, low-dose of FB, DON and ZEA mycotoxins' individual and combined effects on breeding rabbit bucks, in particular with regards to reproductive toxicity.

## Materials and Methods

### Experimental animals, housing and feeding

The experimental animals were Pannon White rabbit breeding bucks (24 weeks of age, $4.0 \pm 0.5$ kg mean bodyweight, n=60). They were individually housed in wire mesh cages ($42 \times 50$ cm) in a closed building, with 16 light h/day. Average temperature ranged from 16°C to 18°C and the farm had overpressure ventilation.

The animals received a commercial diet containing 10.3 MJ digestible energy/kg, 15.5% crude protein, 4.0% crude fat and 14.7% crude fibre for a total of 65 feeding days. The feedstuffs provided were available ad libitum, and the rabbits also had free access to drinking water.

### Toxin production

*Fusarium verticillioides* (for FB1) and *Fusarium graminearum* (for DON and ZEA) (NRRL 20960 [MRC 826] and NRRL 5883, respectively) fungal culture (7 days old) was grown on 0.5 strength potato dextrose agar (PDA; Chemika-Biochemica, Basle, Switzerland). Agar discs (5 mm) were prepared with cork borer (Boekel Scientifica, Pennsylvania, USA), which were then stored at 10°C in darkness in test tubes containing sterile distilled water (10 discs/10 ml).

For toxin production, maize (40 g) was soaked in distilled water (40 ml) at room temperature for 1 hour in Erlenmeyer flasks (500 ml), closed with cotton wool plugs. This was followed by the addition of the inoculated agar discs (10 agar discs per flask) to the two-times autoclaved (20 min.) matrix. The cultures were then stored and incubated at 24°C (FB1), 28°C (DON) and 18°C (ZEA) for 3 weeks, respectively. The flasks were shaken twice every day during the first week of incubation. When the incubation time was complete the fungus-infected cereal was dried at room temperature and ground.

The homogenized fungal cultures contained FB, DON and ZEA at concentrations of 3300, 2010 and 1298 mg/kg, respectively. The European Commission has made recommendations (2006/576/EC) regarding the maximum level of several mycotoxins in complete diets (European Commission, 2006) and introduced regulations (2003/100/EC) regarding aflatoxins (European Commission, 2003). However, these only apply to certain cases, particularly with regard to rabbit feed. Thus in this study doses were pre-determined according the EU limits (based on the European Commission Recommendation 2006/576/EC and the European Commission Directive 2003/100/EC) in finished feed for young pig as the most sensitive animal towards these fusarium mycotoxins among livestock. Fungal cultures were mixed into the feed of experimental animals, based on the presented dose in Table 1.

| Group | Mycotoxin concentration (mg/kg) of the feed | n |
|---|---|---|
| C (control) | 0 | 15 |
| F (FB1) | 5 | 15 |
| DZ (DON+ZEA) | 1+0.25 | 15 |
| FDZ (FB1+DON+ZEA) | 5+1+0.25 | 15 |

Table 1: Experimental groups.

## LC-MS analysis

LC-MS analysis was performed by a Shimadzu Prominence UFLC separation system equipped with a LC-MS-2020 single quadrupole (ultra-fast) liquid chromatograph mass spectrometer (Shimadzu, Kyoto, Japan) comprised a vacuum degasser, a binary pump (20AD), a column oven (CTO 20A) autosampler (SIL 20ACHT), and mass analyser (MS 2020) with both atmospheric-pressure chemical ionization (APCI) and electrospray ionization (ESI) systems. Optimized mass spectra were obtained with an interface voltage of 4.5 kV, a detector voltage of 1.05 kV in negative mode, 1.25 kV in positive mode. Heat block temperature was 200°C and a desolvation gas temperature was 200°C. For nebulizing and drying gas, nitrogen was used (1.5 L/min and 15 L/min flow rate, respectively). Chromatographic separation was performed at 50°C and achieved on an RP-18 (2.1 × 100 mm, 2.6 μm, Kinetex$^{TM}$ Phenomenex USA) stationary phase applying gradient elution 0.3 mL/min eluent total flow rate for mycotoxins and 0.4 mL/min for silymarin flavonoids, with A: 0.1% AcOH and B: 0.1% AcOH in methanol as eluent. With optimum method performance characteristics analytes were quantified using external calibration.

Rabbit-feed samples were milled and extracted using 1% AcOH containing 75:25=MeOH:H$_2$O (V/V) for F-2 CH$_3$CN:water 1:1 (V/V) for FB1 and water for DON and ZEA as extraction solvent. The extracts were shaken at room temperature for an hour then decanted and the supernatant was collected. 1 mL of clean water extract was applied to the immunoaffinity column (IAC; Vicam, DON test) which contains specific antibodies for DON for purification. The IAC was washed with 5 mL water, and DON was slowly eluted in 2 mL methanol. ZEA and FB1 were measured by dilute and shot method. Romer Mix 4 (containing trichotecenes+zearalenon at 10 mg/L) and Romer MIX 3 (containing FB1-2 at 50 mg/L) primary stock solution used as reference. 1 μL of each samples were analysed with a gradient: (0 min) 5% B, (3 min) 60% B, (8 min) 100% B, followed by a holding-time of 3 min at 100% eluent B and 3 min column re-equilibration at eluent A pumped at a flow rate of 0.3 mL/min. DON is detected as [M+AcO]– at m/z=355, ZEA at m/z=317 as [M-H]–, FB1 at m/z=722[M+H]+. The limit of detection (LOD) for FB, ZEA and DON was 3.0, 5.0 and 5.0 μg/kg, while the limit of quantification was (LOQ) 10, 1.0 and 2.0 μg/kg, respectively.

## Experimental design

Bucks were divided into 4 experimental groups. One group of the experimental animals served as control, while into the feed of the other three groups fungal culture was mixed in a pre-defined concentration (Table 1).

The daily feed intake was registered by measuring back the left-over feed amount (in the first 3 weeks daily, and weekly thereafter), while bodyweight was recorded once every week.

The health status of the animals was observed throughout the experiment, morbidity and mortality was logged daily.

On days 30 and 60 blood and sperm was sampled (n=15/group), and a gonadotropin-releasing hormone (GnRH) test was performed (blood samplings related to GnRH test: n=6/group). Blood was sampled from the marginal ear vein, while sperm was collected after a training period into artificial vaginas and seminal plasma was separated with centrifugation.

At the end of the study (on day 65) animals were exsanguinated after stunning. The weight of liver, kidneys, testicles and spleen was measured and macroscopic changes were analyzed and recorded. After dissection (n=15/group) samples were taken for histopathological analysis; the testis, liver and kidney was fixed in 10% neutrally buffered formalin. For the analysis of antioxidant status 2-2 g samples were taken from the liver.

The experimental protocol was authorized by the Food Chain Safety and Animal Health Directorate of the Somogy County Agricultural Office, under allowance number SOI/31/1679-11/2014.

## Clinical chemical parameters

The plasma total protein (TP), albumin (ALB), globulin (GLOB), total cholesterol (tCHOL), triglyceride (TG), glucose (GLU), fructosamine (FA), creatinine (CREA) and bilirubin (BIL) concentrations, and the activity of aspartate aminotransferase (AST), alanine aminotransferase (ALT), gamma-glutamyl transferase (GGT), lactate dehydrogenase (LDH) and alkaline phosphatase (ALKP) were determined in a veterinary laboratory (Vet-med Laboratory, Budapest, Hungary), using Roche Hitachi 912 Chemistry Analyzer (Hitachi, Tokyo, Japan) with commercial diagnostic kits (Diagnosticum LTD., Budapest, Hungary).

## Antioxidant status

For the determination of lipid peroxidation, the samples of blood plasma, red blood cell (1:9) hemolysate (RBCH) and liver were stored at -70°C until analysis. Lipid peroxidation was determined by the quantification of malondialdehyde (MDA) levels with 2-thiobarbituric acid method in blood plasma and RBCH [32] and liver homogenate [33], and determination of conjugated dienes (CD) and trienes (CT) according to the AOAC [34] method in the liver. Among the components of the antioxidant system some parameters of the glutathione redox system was determined in blood plasma, RBCH and liver. The amount of reduced glutathione (GSH) measured by the method of Sedlak and Lindsay [35] and the activity of glutathione peroxidase (GPx) according to Lawrence and Burk [36].

## GnRH test and determination of testosterone concentration

Experimental and control bucks were treated i.m. with 0.2 ml GnRH analogue (Receptal; Intervet, Boxmeer, The Netherlands) for the analysis of the toxin effect on the Leydig cell function. The levels of testosterone hormone were determined from blood samples taken just prior to GnRH analogue injection (0 min) and thereafter in the subsequent 2 hours in every 25 minutes (a total of 6 blood samplings).

The testosterone concentration was determined with a direct $^3$H-radioimmunoassay method [37] adopted and validated for rodents' (chinchilla rabbit and Angora rabbit) plasma as described previously [38].

## Spermatology

Spermatological analyses covered the following parameters: pH, sperm cell concentration (improved Neubauer cell counting chamber), motility, morphology (native and stained) and acrosomal integrity (Spermac$^{TM}$ staining, Beernem, Belgium) of the spermatozoa. Motility was evaluated with a computer assisted sperm analyzer (Medealab$^{TM}$ CASA System, Erlangen, Germany). Moreover, vital test, hyposmotic and peroxidase tests were carried out. A minimum number of 200 spermatozoa were examined for morphology and 500 for motility evaluation [39].

## Comet assay

For comet assay sperm was sampled on day 60 of the experiment (n=15/group). The method was adapted from human spermium examination protocols [40,41], with the following modifications. The semen was washed three times in PBS and re-suspended in PBS to a final of $10^6$ cell/ml number. Onto the microscope slides pre-coated with 1% NMP agarose 10 μl cell suspensions and 75 μl 1% LMP agarose were loaded. The decondensation was performed in two steps, first the slides were soaked for 1 hour at 4°C in a lysis buffer with dithiothreitol, and second the slides were soaked for 1 hour at 37°C in a lysis buffer with proteinase K. After lysis the slides were washed in sterile redistilled water to eliminate the salt adhered to the gel. Electrophoresis was performed at 300 mA and 25 V for 30 minutes at 4°C. After washing and drying the slides were stained with ethidium bromide. All chemicals used in this study were obtained from Sigma-Aldrich Ltd. (Budapest, Hungary). Specialized chemicals used were: Histopaque-1077 and RPMI-1640 medium (Sigma-Aldrich Ltd., Budapest, Hungary).

The fluorescence images were generated using an Alpha-Optika B-600TiFL fluorescence microscope (Optika Microscopes, Bergamo, Italy). Scoring was carried out according to Singh et al. [42] and Collins et al. [43], in which comets are classified into scores of '0', '1', '2', '3' and '4' according to DNA damage and head/tail migration. Each single comet was scored visually and assigned into an arbitrary unit from 0 to 4, depending on the relative intensity of DNA fluorescence in the tail; 800 cells/group were counted.

## Histopathological analysis

After registering the macroscopic pathological signs on the internal and external organs, testicles, liver, kidneys and spleen were stored in 10% neutrally buffered formalin and were embedded into paraffin. For light microscopic analysis microtome slides of 5 micrometer were prepared and stained with hematoxylin-eosin.

The histopathological analysis was performed according to the Act/2011 (03.30) of the Hungarian Ministry of Agriculture and Rural Development and was in accordance with the ethical guidelines of the OECD Good Laboratory Practice for Chemicals [44].

## Statistical analyses

Statistical analyses were performed using IBM SPSS 20.0 [45] software. Data processing and the mathematical-statistical calculations were performed using the compare means (independent-samples-t-test, oneway ANOVA with Tukey post-hoc test), correlate and descriptive statistics modules. In case of comet assay crosstabs options were used for chi-square test.

# Results

## Feed consumption and body weight

The feed intake of the rabbit bucks was not different among the groups. No significant difference in body weight among groups was detected at any of the 12 time points (data not shown), average body weight of the groups was between 4252 and 4442 g by the end of the experiment.

## Clinico-chemical parameters

No inter-group differences (P ≥ 0.05) were found for ALB, TG, GLU, FA, CREA and BIL concentrations, and AST, ALT, GGT, LDH and ALKP activities.

|  |  | Day 30 |  | Day 60 |  |
|---|---|---|---|---|---|
|  |  | mean | SD | mean | SD |
| TP (g/L) | C | 69.85$^b$ | 5.85 | 62.16$^a$ | 3.02 |
|  | F | 68.57$^b$ | 1.72 | 64.73$^{ab}$ | 3.97 |
|  | DZ | 61.33$^a$ | 4.28 | 65.81$^{ab}$ | 7.34 |
|  | FDZ | 69.57$^b$ | 1.92 | 67.74$^b$ | 3.40 |
| GLOB (g/L) | C | 28.65$^b$ | 3.54 | 22.38$^a$ | 2.23 |
|  | F | 27.13$^b$ | 1.61 | 22.96$^a$ | 2.09 |
|  | DZ | 20.23$^a$ | 3.39 | 24.10$^{ab}$ | 5.95 |
|  | FDZ | 27.98$^b$ | 1.63 | 26.67$^b$ | 3.12 |
| tCHOL (mmol/L) | C | 1.45$^{ab}$ | 0.12 | 1.51$^b$ | 0.35 |
|  | F | 1.62$^b$ | 0.19 | 1.21$^a$ | 0.09 |
|  | DZ | 1.33$^a$ | 0.16 | 1.29$^a$ | 0.14 |
|  | FDZ | 1.58$^{ab}$ | 0.17 | 1.44$^{ab}$ | 0.14 |

$^{a,b}$numbers with different superscripts indicate significant differences (P ≤ 0.05) between groups (C, F, DZ and FDZ).

Table 2: Clinico-chemical parameters of rabbits on day 30 and 60.

Differences in TP, GLOB and tCHOL at the two sampling dates (day 30 and 60) are summarized in Table 2. In spite of the slight significant differences between treatments all data were within the reference ranges, which are 54-75 g/L for TP, 15-27 g/L for GLOB and 0.3-3.00 mmol/L for tCHOL [46]. Only GLOB concentration exceeded the upper limit of 27 g/L in the C and FDZ groups on day 30 (29 and 28 g/L, respectively).

## Antioxidant status

On day 30 only MDA concentration in the RBCH showed significant difference between treatments F (35.7 ± 4.5 mmol/l) and DZ (34.2 ± 1.6 mmol/l), as compared to C (43.4 ± 3.5 mmol/l) and

FDZ (43.7 ± 7.6 mmol/l), but other antioxidant parameters did not change significantly (data not shown).

Parameters showing significant treatment effect on day 60 are summarised in Table 3. At day 60, DZ treatment resulted in significantly increased GPx activity in the red blood cells and MDA formation both in RBCH and plasma, while less GSH concentration in the blood plasma. As a result of peroxidation of dienoic and trienoic fatty acids, the concentration of conjugated dienes and trienes increased as a result of the DZ exposure, as compared to the combined effect of three mycotoxins (FDZ).

| Parameter | Groups | | | |
|---|---|---|---|---|
| | C | F | DZ | FDZ |
| GPx-RBCH[1] | 2.7 ± 1.0[a] | 3.5 ± 1.2[a] | 4.9 ± 1.1[b] | 3.1 ± 0.8[a] |
| MDA-RBCH[2] | 30.3 ± 3.0[ab] | 28.3 ± 3.2[a] | 33.9 ± 7.5[b] | 28.8 ± 3.2[a] |
| GSH-plasma[3] | 2.2 ± 0.2[a] | 2.2 ± 0.5[a] | 2.0 ± 0.2[a] | 2.6 ± 0.5[b] |
| MDA-plasma[2] | 18.9 ± 2.8[a] | 18.7 ± 3.0[a] | 24.5 ± 8.0[b] | 16.8 ± 2.9[a] |
| CD liver[4] | 0.51 ± 0.03[ab] | 0.51 ± 0.02[ab] | 0.53 ± 0.05[b] | 0.48 ± 0.05[a] |
| CT liver[4] | 0.19 ± 0.01[a] | 0.20 ± 0.01[ab] | 0.21 ± 0.04[b] | 0.18 ± 0.01[a] |

[1]U/g protein, [2]μmol/ml, [3]μmol/g protein, [4]Abs 232 nm

[a,b]numbers with different superscripts indicate significant differences (P ≤ 0.05) between groups (C, F, DZ and FDZ)

Table 3: Antioxidant parameters measured on day 60.

## Testosterone concentration

The testosterone concentration was significantly different due to mycotoxin exposure only at day 60 at the sampling minutes of 75, 90 and 115 (Figure 1). Figure 1 clearly demonstrates that Leydig cells of the animals intoxicated with the three mycotoxins in combination (FDZ) for a total of 60 days synthesize significantly less testosterone as a response to exogenous GnRH. In the F group blood testosterone level was slightly lowered, while the two toxin combination (DZ) induced a more expressed decline in the concentration, although the differences were not statistically significant.

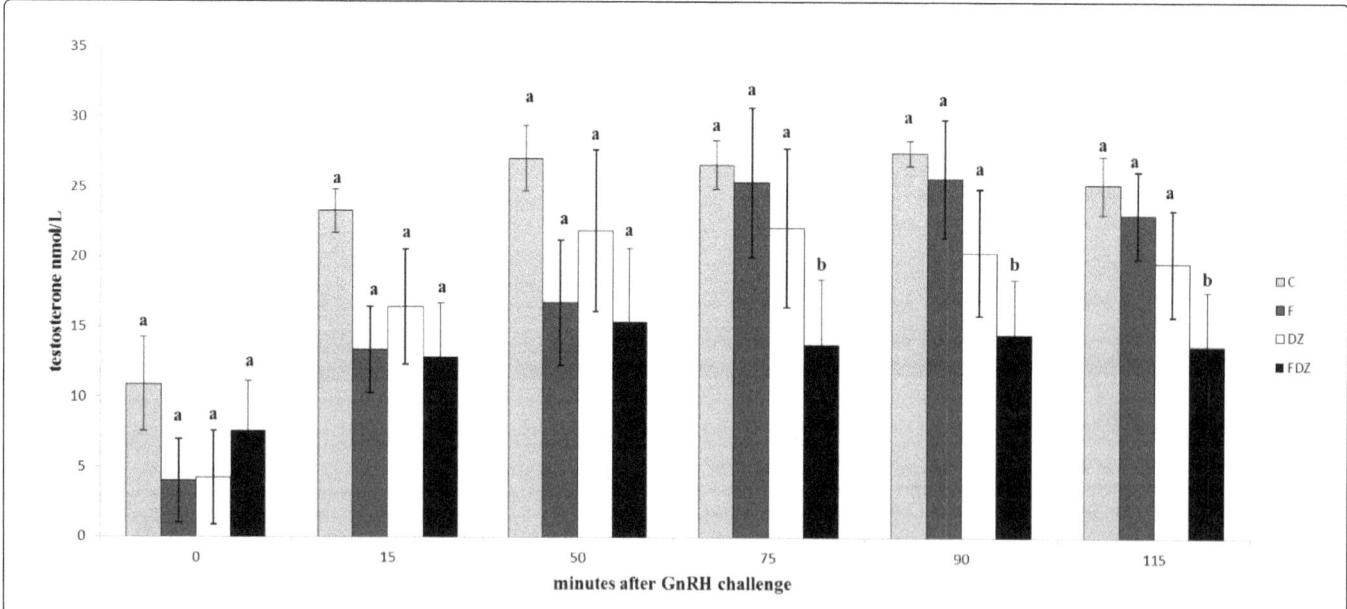

Figure 1: Gonadotropin-releasing hormone (GnRH; mean and standard deviation) induced testosterone production at day 60. [a,b]numbers with different superscripts indicate significant differences (P ≤ 0.05) between groups (C, F, DZ and FDZ).

## Spermatological analysis

No effect of toxin treatment was detected on semen pH (ranging from 6.4 to 8.2 in each group), quantity of the semen (on average 1 ml in each group) and concentration of spermatozoa (ranging from 2.4 to $2.6 \times 10^7$/ml). Comparing the sperm motility between groups, significant effect could also not be proven. The ratio of spermatozoa showing progressive forward motility was around 80% at the beginning of the experiment and decreased from $80 \pm 1.7\%$ to $67 \pm 4\%$ in the semen of FDZ animals showing significant difference when compared to the other three treatment groups. Between the normal morphology of the spermatozoa of the DZ and C animals, statistically significant differences were found (Table 4).

| Group | Spermatozoa with normal morphology |
|---|---|
| C | $80.2 \pm 11.2^b$ |
| F | $76.0 \pm 9.0^{ab}$ |
| DZ | $66.3 \pm 23.7^a$ |
| FDZ | $68.9 \pm 14.1^{ab}$ |
| [a,b]different superscripts in the column indicate significant between-group differences (P ≤0.05) | |

**Table 4:** The ratio of spermatozoa with normal morphology in the semen after 60 days of mycotoxin exposure (%, mean ± SD).

The most frequent morphological abnormalities were: abnormality of the tail, retention of cytoplasmic drop, absence of the acrosome and altered head. A cell was considered altered if at least one defect was present.

## Comet assay

All treatments caused DNA damage and 98.6, 91.6 and 91.8% of the treated cells could be categorized as having 1 to 3 scores in the F, DZ and FDZ group, respectively (Figure 2). Cells with 0 values showed the highest prevalence in group C, while cells with the slightest damage (score 1) were dominant in all toxin treated groups. FB1 resulted significantly less 0 comets (intact cells) compared to the other treatments.

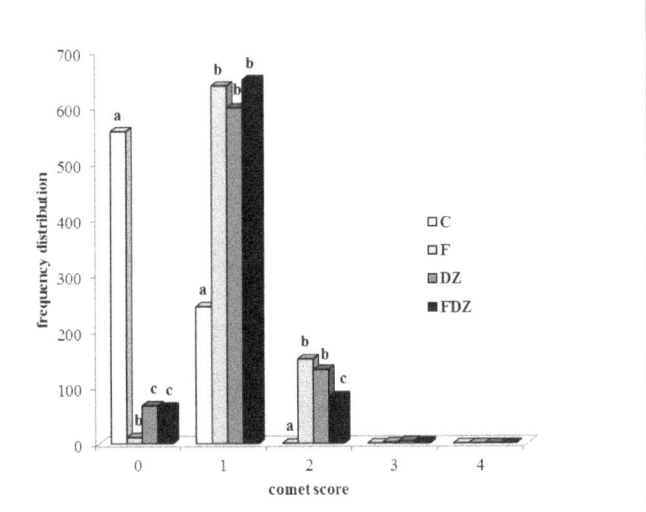

**Figure 2:** Number of cells with the respective comet values (values of comet scores: 0 to 4). [a,b]columns with different superscripts indicate significant differences (P<0.0001).

Cells, with score 1 (Figure 3a) occurred in nearly similar proportions in case of the three toxin treatments. The comet value 2

(Figure 3b) showed the highest prevalence in samples of F and DZ animals, FDZ treatment resulted in significantly less cells of this type. The number of cells with score 3 (Figure 3c) occurred only in 0.6% of the categorized cells. No cells were found with a comet assay score of 4 in the experiment.

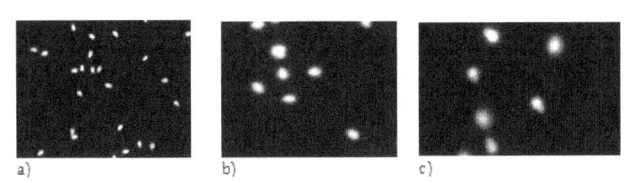

**Figure 3:** Comet assay (DNA damage) scoring: images of comets from bucks' spermatozoa stained with EtBr. Classes 0 (a), 1 (b) and 2 (c) were used for visual scoring.

## Histopathology

No sign of mycotoxicosis was detected. In animals consumed FB1, DZ and FDZ contaminated diet the intensity of spermatogensis decreased by 43, 31 and 64%, respectively (Table 5), which was reflected by the lack of differentiated spermatozoa, thinning of the germinal epithelium, the appearance of multinuclear giant cells indicative of the disturbance of meiosis and mitosis of the germinal epithelial cells and in some cases the lack of spermatogonia.

These histological findings were observed to different severities in the seminiferous tubules. In case of slight alteration (grade 1) disturbance of sperm cell formation was observed in 20-30% of the seminiferous tubules, while in case of grade 2 and 3, 30-70 or 100 % of the tubules, respectively, showed decreased spermatogenesis. Decreased spermatogenesis was manifested in lack of well differentiated sperm cells and less primary, secondary spermatocytes and spermatids, and thinning of the seminiferous epithelium as a consequence (grade 1). In case of intermediate severity (grade 2) these alterations were observed in higher ratio of the tubules, the disturbance of meiosis and mitosis was indicated by the appearance of multinuclear cells. Cases, when all tubules were attacked and moreover, in some tubules even the initial spermiogenetic cells, spermatogonia were also absent, were classified as marked damage (grade 3) (Figures 4 and 5).

| Group | NO | Number of animals showing alteration | | | | |
|---|---|---|---|---|---|---|
| | | 1 | 2 | 3 | All together | % |
| C | 15 | 0 | 0 | 0 | 0 | 0 |
| F | 8 | 6 | 0 | 0 | 6 | 43 |
| DZ | 9 | 4 | 0 | 0 | 4 | 31 |
| FDZ | 5 | 7 | 1 | 1 | 9 | 64 |
| NO=number of animals without alteration, 1=slight/small area/low occurrence frequency, 2=intermediate severity/intermediate area/intermediate occurrence frequency, 3=marked/extensive/high occurrence frequency | | | | | | |

**Table 5:** Decreased intensity of spermatogenesis as revealed by the histopathology of the testicles.

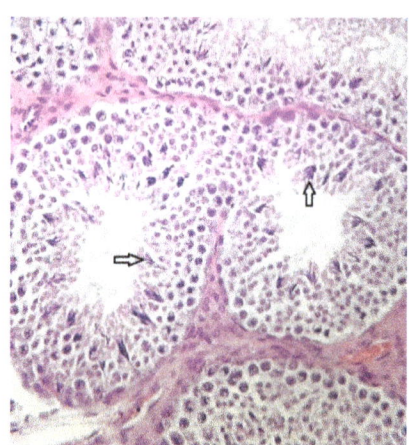

**Figure 4:** Active spermatogenesis in a healthy control animal's seminiferous tubules. The cells at different differentiation levels in the epithelium germinativum (spermatogonia, stage I and II spermatocytes, spermatides and mature spermia (↑) are as well visible. Haematoxylin-eosin staining, 400X.

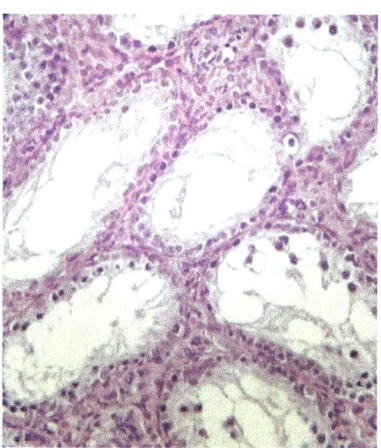

**Figure 5:** A part of the seminiferous tubule after FDZ treatment. The marked lack of germinal epithelialcells is visible. Haematoxylin-eosin staining, 400X.

In the testicles of the toxin treated animals the cytomorphology and the proportion of the Leydig interstitial cells was not significantly different from the controls. In the Malpighian bodies of the spleen of every DZ and FDZ animal, slight lymphocyte depletion (slight thinning of the T and B dependent zones of the Malpighian tubules) was observed. However, the cytomorphology of lymphoblast and lymphocyte cells was not different from the control. In the livers and kidneys no detectable alteration attributable to mycotoxins was found.

**Organ masses**

Among all organs which were measured for weight (testicles, liver, kidneys, spleen) only the weight of the spleen was significantly different between groups. It was the most ($1.84 \pm 0.49^b$) in DZ animals, and least ($1.46 \pm 0.38^a$) in C, while $1.65 \pm 0.30^{ab}$ and $1.65 \pm 0.37^{ab}$ in F

and FDZ, respectively. However the relative organ mass values (data not shown) of the different groups were not significantly different.

**Discussion**

The present study intended to determine the negative effect of a combined, 65-day oral Fusarium mycotoxin administration on the reproductive traits of 24-week old breeding Pannon White rabbit bucks. The low toxin exposure levels were chosen taking the limit values given by the 2006/576/EC recommendation into consideration. The in feed concentrations of FB, DON and ZEA (5, 1 and 0.25 mg/kg feed, respectively) revealed 169-193 µg FB1/kg BW, 33.7-38.7 µg DON/kg BW, and 8.5-9.7 µg ZEA/kg bw exposure. Results indicate that a prolonged low-dose mycotoxin exposure may adversely affect male reproduction as it has been previously demonstrated in case of T-2 toxin. The combined toxin effect indicates highly complex interactions among the mycotoxins, appearing differently in the divergent physiological processes. Among the mycotoxins studied here additive, synergistic, as well as antagonistic effects were detected (Table 6).

| Parameter examined | Type of interaction |
|---|---|
| feed intake | antagonism (not significant) |
| lipid peroxidation (MDA, GPx, CD, CT) | antagonism |
| testosterone production | synergism |
| spermatogenesis by histology | additive |
| sperm cells with normal morphology | less than additive |
| weight of the spleen | antagonism |
| genotoxicity | antagonism |

**Table 6:** Summary of the interactions between FB, ZEA and DON experienced in the experiment (classified according to Grenier and Oswald, 2011).

**Feed consumption and body weight**

The only observation to mention concerning feed consumption and body weight (BW) was that the mean feed intake (FI) of DZ and FDZ animals was somewhat lower, as compared to F and C (significance was not proven). This result may mostly be attributed to DON, since this is the most well-known characteristic effect of trichothecene mycotoxins [47]. In the study of Hewit et al. [48] using naturally contaminated (4.2 mg/kg DON) corn for Fusarium mycotoxin exposure in growing rabbits, no feed refusal was observed and the toxin treated animals had slightly increased BW gain, suggesting that rabbits are less sensitive to this mycotoxin. Deep discussion of a mere tendency is void, but observing data at weeks 4 and 5 again indicate the "likewise positive effect" of low-dose FB, since the lowest FI was found for DZ, but FDZ and F were less suppressed. This is supported by the result on non-human primates of Gelderblom et al. [49], where long-term feeding of FB1 alone had no negative effect on FI and BW, even at higher doses. In that study apparent no-effect threshold in terms of kidney and liver damage was estimated at 8.21 and 13.25 mg total fumonisin/kg diet, being about the double exposure, as compared to the present study. Also no effect on final live weight and weight gain was observed when male rabbits were fed diets containing 12.3 and 24.5 mg/kg FB1 for 5 weeks [50]. Summarized, our study indicates that

DON provides its characteristic feed-intake lowering effect in a slight, but insignificant rate at the dose according to Commission Recommendation (2006/576/EC), while fumonisin shows no determinative effect on BW and FI at these concentrations, in breeding rabbit bucks.

## Clinical chemical parameters and antioxidant status

The health status of the animals can be monitored by regular determination of certain clinical chemical parameters. Despite that the liver and the kidney is considered to be the primary target organs of many mycotoxins (like trichothecenes and FB1) in all species examined, gross hepatic lesions and disorder was not induced by any of the treatments, as underscored by the unaltered ALT, AST, GGT and CREA values, the identical liver and kidney mass values and the lack of histopathological alterations in all groups. These organs were likewise tolerant towards the exposure of low dose of these mycotoxins, without providing degenerative processes. Sprando et al. [14] described an analogous observation, namely few lesions of various tissues in control and treated animals, either incidental or related to experimental techniques (gavage) and unrelated to the test substance. The effects of low (10 mg/kgBW) and high (100 mg/kgBW) oral doses of purified ZEN were studied by Čonková et al [47] in rabbits. Low ZEN doses resulted in a significant increase in ALP activity, while high ZEN doses showed significant increases of AST, ALT, AP, GGT, and LDH activity, indicating possible liver toxicity due to the chronic effects of the toxin.

The alteration found in the TP was attributed to the concentration changes of globulin, since albumin concentration was constant. According to Kim et al. [51], DON stress lowers immunoglobulin expression in mice, but ZEA was found to have no influence on it. This could be the reason of the slight temporary decrease in GLOB and TP of DZ animals at day 30. The results at day 60 are difficult to explain, because difference between groups was rather attributable to the lowered GLOB level in control animals than toxin treatments. However fumonisin treatment decreased GLOB concentration at day 60, compared to day 30. Results of the FDZ group on day 60 are in accordance with those of Tessari et al. [52], describing that FB1 (added to an aflatoxin B1 containing diet) has primary additive effect on the immunological response in birds. It is interesting to highlight that FB1 alone and in higher doses (8 mg/kg feed) had a sex-dependent immunosuppressive effect, male pigs being more prone [53]. The FDZ treatment evokes the question, whether the low dose of FB1 or the interaction between these toxins augmented the immune response. Some kind of anomaly in the immune system was supported by histology, in that in both DZ and FDZ animals, slight lymphocyte depletion (slight thinning of the T and B dependent zones of the Malpighian tubules) was observed in the spleen, without any change in the cytomorphology of lymphoblasts and lymphocytes. In the experiment Sprando et al. [14] similar finding was described when rats orally exposed with 5 mg/kg DON.

The pathophysiological significance of the changes in tCHOL level, which was around 5-20%, is questionable, taking the broad physiological ranges (0.3-3.00 mmol/L) into consideration.

The increased GPx activity in the red blood cells of DZ animals by day 60 reflects more lipid hydroperoxide production, as the role of the enzyme is to reduce lipid hydroperoxides to their corresponding alcohols and this way to reduce free hydrogen peroxide to water. This is supported by the highest MDA concentrations both in the red blood cells and the blood plasma, referring to augmented in vivo lipid

peroxidation [54], and also by the decreased GSH, as co-substrate of GPx, level in plasma. One of the mechanisms by which DON exerts its toxicity is inducing oxidative stress within the cells [55]. ZEA is also known to induce generation of reactive oxygen species (ROS) and consequently lipidperoxidation, while fumonisin was characterised as moderate oxidant mycotoxin [56]. Our results show general agreement with those of Minervini et al. [57], reporting that in vitro FB1 dose at the level of the EC Regulation is not inducing oxidative stress in intestinal cells. On the other hand FB1 has proven to induce ROS production in broiler chicks, but only at extreme high (100 mg/kg feed) dose [58]. Our findings suggest that FB1 in low dose may act antagonistically towards Z and D, which has not been reported yet. Though there is no literature on the mitigating property of FB1 on lipid peroxidation. We thus summarize DZ combination was the most harmful in terms of initial (CD and CT) and terminal (MDA) phases of lipid peroxidation after long-term exposure (60 days); meanwhile FB1 at the EC Regulation level did not cause significant oxidative stress, even more relieved those effects triggered by ZEA and DON.

## Gn-RH induced testosterone production

The testosterone concentration was not significantly influenced by one (F) and two toxins (DZ), but the FDZ treatment dramatically lowered its synthesis and/or release from the Leydig cells by the end of the sampling intervals (minutes 75, 90 and 115), suggesting synergistic effect. As far as the authors are aware, there exists only a single study on male reproduction traits as affected by orally administered DON, which was performed in rats [14]. In this study 0.5, 1, 2.5 and 5 mg/kg DON was applied, and the authors found a dose-dependent down-regulation of testosterone synthesis after 28 days of exposure. Trichothecene toxins may decrease the testosterone production of the Leydig cells by inhibiting early steps of the steroidogenic pathway, i.e. the conversion of pregnenolone to progesterone [25], as it was also observed in our previous study in case of T-2 exposure [38]. These Fusarium toxins may act indirectly as well, on the pituitary gland, or affect Sertoli cell inhibin production, as shown in case of DON [14]. In present study a direct effect of the mycotoxin on Leydig cells was not supported by the histopathological findings.

In fact not DON, but zearalenone is the most potent factor, directly inhibiting testosterone biosynthesis in the Leydig cells, adding that this inhibition is concentration- and time-dependent, happening via changing the nuclear estrogen receptor signaling [59], however the exact molecular mechanism is not known yet. For FB1 direct toxicological studies are lacking, but according to Lu et al. [60], elevated ceramide levels are directly apoptotic towards Leydig cells, which is inhibited by FB, a ceramide-synthase blocking substance. Thus FB1 had no deleterious effect on the rat testicular Leydig cell function in vitro. In summary the main, testosterone synthesis blocking effect in our study was primarily attributed to ZEA. Some kind of synergistic effect occurred between FB1 and DON+ZEA. Taking the common cellular modes of actions of these toxins into consideration, this might be explained with respect to the DNA-synthesis inhibiting effect. FB1 affected the DNA synthesis together with ZEA in a more than additive, rather synergistic way in a DNA inhibition assay, although this effect was not fully confirmed when it was further analysed in a second stage [61].

## Spermatology, histopathology and comet assay

Toxin effect and interaction between the Fusarium toxins applied, manifested in lower sperm motility (FDZ), less spermatozoa with normal morphology (DZ), additive effect in the decreased intensity of spermatogenesis as shown by the histology of the testes, while antagonism concerning genotoxicity measured by comet assay.

Concerning the individual effects of these mycotoxins on sperm motility, only a few data are available. FB1 fed with male rabbits at 7.5 and 10.0 mg/kg dietary levels decreased sperm motility by approximately 18%, the possible explanation was the inhibition of cyclic 3'5'AMP activity and calcium ion transport, or, the decreased formation of the acidic epididymidal glycoprotein synthesis required to maintain motility [50]. Changes, after increasing oral exposure of DON were not consequent, and considered to be random [14], while in an in vitro study no significant effect of DON on motility was found using rabbit spermatozoa (Medvedová et al., 2012). Boeira et al. [62] reported compromised spermatozoa motility after feeding mice with ZEA, while 12 mg daily ZEA exposure for 8 weeks did not alter sperm motility in adult rams [63]. Further data from in vitro studies support no effect of ZEA on boar spermatozoa [64], while on the contrary Rajkovic et al. [65] and Tsakmakidis et al. [66] described impairment of progressive motility. Interestingly in an in vitro study with stallion sperm ZEA caused hyperactivation in motility [67].

As the cellular level effects by which the above described mycotoxins may adversely influence motility are not well described yet, the combined effect is also difficult to explain. Decreased sperm motility caused by the exposure of the three mycotoxins (FDZ) by day 60 might be attributable also to the decreased testosterone concentration as a result of synergistic effect between FB, DON and ZEA observed also by day 60. The male reproductive organs are strongly androgen-dependent in respect of structure, as well as function. Testosterone supports spermatogenesis, sperm maturation, seminal plasma production and sexual functions [68]. So the decreased testosterone secretion may give an explanation also for the more morphologically abnormal cells, and the decreased intensity of spermatogenesis shown by histology. However, direct effect of the particular toxins is also presumable. Interestingly FB1 had only a slight adverse effect on the cell morphology and spermatogenesis. The characteristic toxic effect of FB1 is the inhibition of the sphingolipid synthesis, thus causing cellular ceramide depletion and elevation of shinganine, which is cytotoxic, and has growth inhibitory and pre-apoptotic effects [69]. This results in disturbances of cell growth, differentiation and morphology. In rabbits orally administered FB1 caused similar morphological and structural abnormalities in sperm morphology and spermatogenesis, and 7.5 mg/kg in the diet for FB1 as LOAEL (lowest observed adverse effect level) was suggested [50]. In our study even lower dose, 5 mg/kg had exerted adverse effect; however sensitivity to toxic substance is influenced by several factors. Compared to F group, DZ was similarly compromised. In case F and DZ, disturbance of sperm cell formation was observed only in 20-30% of the seminiferous tubules, however the combined treatment of DON and ZEA resulted in more cells of abnormal morphology. After exposure of the three toxin (FDZ) in 1 animal 30-70, while in another 100% of the seminiferous tubules were concerned, indicating additive effect. The effect of ZEA on spermatogenesis is more thoroughly studied compared to FB1 and DON. In orally exposed mice Zatecka et al. [70] detected decreased sperm concentration, and increased number of morphologically abnormal and also apoptotic spermatozoa. No pathological patterns in the seminiferous tubules were observed and the spermatogenesis was not interrupted, only the number of spermatogonia and spermatocytes were lower (not significantly) in exposed animals (25 μg/kg BW). Kim et al. [71] highlighted that apoptosis is the main effect by which ZEA causes germ cell depletion

and atrophy of the testes. Germ cell apoptosis and thus impaired spermatogenesis was described also by Cho et al [72].

The in vitro exposure to ZEA induced cytotoxicity in boar sperm cells [64]. DON in 2.5 and 5 mg/kg concentration caused germ cell degeneration, decreased sperm cell release and abnormal cell development [14]. As the authors reported, DON may inhibit protein, RNA and DNA synthesis, and be cytotoxic to certain cells, which could cause the harmful effect in the most sensitive pre-leptotene spermatocytes.

Genotoxicity of Fusarium mycotoxins on sperm cells has been reported previously in case of FB1 [17] and ZEA [17,64,66,67], using sperm chromatin structure assay (SCSA), while no data on genotoxicity of DON related to sperm cells are available. A recent study showed that DON decreased cell viability, caused damage to the membrane, the chromosomes and the DNA in human lymphocytes, and potentially induced genotoxicity by the depletion of the antioxidant capacity. On the other hand according to Golli-Bennour and Bacha [56] DON is a non-oxidant mycotoxin, and its genotoxicity is the result of a direct effect on DNA fragmentation and caspade-dependent apoptosis.

In case of FB, Minervini et al. [17] found high degree of individual variability, when chromatin structure stability was checked in vitro, using equine spermatozoa. Interestingly no increase in ROS production was observed even in those cases when genotoxicity was detected, so the damage was attributed to mitochondrial dysfunction related to the altered ceramide metabolism. This mode of action might influence motility as well, knowing that spermatozoa are used as biosensors when testing mitochondrial toxicity, because of the strong influence of mitochondrial function on motility [17].

When we examined the single and combined genotoxic effect of FB1 and DON+ZEA on rabbit sperm cells, an antagonistic effect was observed, highly in accordance with the antioxidant parameters of the same experiment. It is also worth to mention, that none of the toxins had strong genotoxic effect as shown by the total lack of highly damaged cells (score 4). To our knowledge this is the first study analyzing the DNA damage on sperm cells by comet assay in orally mycotoxin exposed animals. There is only one in vitro study using sperm cells for comet assay in mycotoxin genotoxicity studies [73-75], in which human spermatozoa and lymphocytes were assessed for their sensitivity to the genotoxic effect of DON. It was described that spermatozoa are more sensitive towards DON (in terms of DNA damage) as compared to lymphocytes. The reason may be that spermatozoa are a highly specialized cell types with no cytoplasm and extremely condensed chromatin, which seems to be prone towards toxic stimuli. Thus the moderate genotoxic effect of DON has been proven and spermatozoa comet assay as a rapid test for genotoxicity recommended.

## Conclusions

In this study three orally administered fusariotoxins (FB, DON and ZEA) were tested in adult male rabbits, focusing primarily on their reproduction endpoints. The dietary levels were relatively low according to the EU limits in finished feed for young pig, in the absence of limits for rabbits' feed (based on the European Commission Recommendation 2006/576/EC and the European Commission Directive 2003/100/EC). Results indicate that a prolonged low-dose mycotoxin exposure may adversely affect male reproduction. Reproductive processes show higher sensitivity to toxic effects, shown by the different parameters examined. Among the mycotoxins studied additive or less than additive effect was found in case of spermatogenesis and sperm cell morphology, synergism in testosterone production, while FB1 acted antagonistic against DON +ZEA on feed intake, lipid-peroxidation, and genotoxicity. All mycotoxins provoked moderate lipid-peroxidation and exerted slight genotoxicity.

## Acknowledgements

The research was supported by the Hungarian Academy of Sciences (within the frame of the MTA-KE "Mycotoxins in the food chain" Research Group), by the National Scientific Research Fund (OTKA PD 104823) to KB and János Bolyai Research Grants of the Hungarian Academy of Sciences (BO/261/13 and BO/499/13) to KB and JSzF.

## References

1. Jelinek CF, Pohland AE, Wood GE (1989) Worldwide occurrence of mycotoxins in foods and feeds-an update. J Assoc Off Anal Chem 72: 223-230.

2. Placinta CM, D'Mello JF, Macdonald AC (1999) A review of worldwide contamination of cereal grains and animal feed with Fusarium mycotoxins. Animal Feed Science and Technology 78: 21-37.

3. Bennett JW, Klich M (2003) Mycotoxins. Clin Microbiol Rev 16: 497-516.

4. Marroquín-Cardona AG, Johnson NM, Phillips TD, Hayes AW (2014) Mycotoxins in a changing global environment-a review. Food Chem Toxicol 69: 220-230.

5. Glenn AE (2007) Mycotoxigenic Fusarium species in animal feed. Animal Feed Science and Technology 137: 213-24.

6. IARC Working Group on the Evaluation of Carcinogenic Risks to Humans (2002) Some traditional herbal medicines, some mycotoxins, naphthalene and styrene. IARC Monogr Eval Carcinog Risks Hum 82: 1-556.

7. Wegulo SN1 (2012) Factors influencing deoxynivalenol accumulation in small grain cereals. Toxins (Basel) 4: 1157-1180.

8. Pestka JJ, Zhou HR, Moon Y, Chung YJ (2004) Cellular and molecular mechanisms for immune modulation by deoxynivalenol and other trichothecenes: unraveling a paradox. Toxicol Lett 153: 61-73.

9. González HH, Martínez EJ, Pacin AM, Resnik SL, Sydenham EW (1999) Natural co-occurrence of fumonisins, deoxynivalenol, zearalenone and aflatoxins in field trial corn in Argentina. Food Addit Contam 16: 565-569.

10. Osweiler GD (1986) Occurrence and clinical manifestations of trichothecene toxicoses and zearalenone toxicoses. In: Richard JL, Thurston JR (eds.) Diagnosis of mycotoxicoses. National Animal Disease Center, Ames, Iowa, USA.

11. Streit E, Schwab C, Sulyok M, Naehrer K, Krska R, et al. (2013) Multi-mycotoxin screening reveals the occurrence of 139 different secondary metabolites in feed and feed ingredients. Toxins (Basel) 5: 504-523.

12. Cortinovis C, Pizzo F, Spicer LJ, Caloni F (2013) Fusarium mycotoxins: effects on reproductive function in domestic animals-a review. Theriogenology 80: 557-564.

13. Young LG, King GJ (1983) Prolonged feeding of low levels of zearalenone to young boars. Journal of Animal Science 57: 313-314.

14. Sprando RL, Collins TF, Black TN, Olejnik N, Rorie JI, et al. (2005) Characterization of the effect of deoxynivalenol on selected male reproductive endpoints. Food Chem Toxicol 43: 623-635.

15. Gbore FA, Egbunike GN (2008) Testicular and epididymal sperm reserves and sperm production of pubertal boars fed dietary fumonisin B(1). Anim Reprod Sci 105: 392-397.

16. Gbore FA1 (2009) Reproductive organ weights and semen quality of pubertal boars fed dietary fumonisin B1. Animal 3: 1133-1137.

17. Minervini F, Lacalandra GM, Filannino A, Nicassio M, Visconti A, et al. (2010) Effects of in vitro exposure to natural levels of zearalenone and its derivatives on chromatin structure stability in equine spermatozoa. Theriogenology 73: 392-403.

18. Kovács M, Tornyos G, Matics Z, Mézes M, Balogh K, et al. (2013) Effect of chronic T-2 toxin exposure in rabbit bucks, determination of the No Observed Adverse Effect Level (NOAEL). Anim Reprod Sci 137: 245-252.

19. Speijers GJ, Speijers MH (2004) Combined toxic effects of mycotoxins. Toxicol Lett 153: 91-98.

20. Griessler K, Rodrigues I, Handl J, Hofstetter U (2010) Occurrence of mycotoxins in Southern Europe. World Mycotoxin Journal 3: 301-309.

21. Kouadio JH, Dano SD, Moukha S, Mobio TA, Creppy EE (2007) Effects of combinations of Fusarium mycotoxins on the inhibition of macromolecular synthesis, malondialdehyde levels, DNA methylation and fragmentation, and viability in Caco-2 cells. Toxicon 49: 306-317.

22. Lei M, Zhang N, Qi D (2013) In vitro investigation of individual and combined cytotoxic effects of aflatoxin B1 and other selected mycotoxins on the cell line porcine kidney 15. Exp Toxicol Pathol 65: 1149-1157.

23. Wan LY, Turner PC, El-Nezami H (2013) Individual and combined cytotoxic effects of Fusarium toxins (deoxynivalenol, nivalenol, zearalenone and fumonisins B1) on swine jejunal epithelial cells. Food Chem Toxicol 57: 276-283.

24. Wan LY, Woo CS, Turner PC, Wan JM, El-Nezami H (2013) Individual and combined effects of Fusarium toxins on the mRNA expression of pro-inflammatory cytokines in swine jejunal epithelial cells. Toxicol Lett 220: 238-246.

25. Fenske M, Fink-Gremmels J (1990) Effects of fungal metabolites on testosterone secretion in vitro. Arch Toxicol 64: 72-75.

26. Khera KS, Whalen C, Angers G (1986) A teratology study on vomitoxin (4-deoxynivalenol) in rabbits. Food Chem Toxicol 24: 421-424.

27. Gumprecht LA, Marcucci A, Weigel RM, Vesonder RF, Riley RT, et al. (1995) Effects of intravenous fumonisin B1 in rabbits: nephrotoxicity and sphingolipid alterations. Nat Toxins 3: 395-403.

28. Mariscal-Quintanar MG, Garcia-Escamilla RM, Garcia-Escamilla N, Torres-Lopez J, Bautista-Ordonez JA, et al.(1997) Effect of ingesting Aspergillus flavus and Fusarium moniliforme on the cytology of bone marrow and blood and on serum albumin and globulin concentrations. Veterinaria Mexico 28: 75-81.

29. Orova Z (2003) Investigations on the teratogenic effects of fumonisin B1 in swine and rabbit. Thesis, University of Kaposvár, Kaposvár.

30. LaBorde JB, Terry KK, Howard PC, Chen JJ, Collins TF, et al. (1997) Lack of embryotoxicity of fumonisin B1 in New Zealand white rabbits. Fundam Appl Toxicol 40: 120-128.

31. Grenier B, Oswald I (2011) Mycotoxin co-contamination of food and feed: meta-analysis of publications describing toxicological interactions. World Mycotoxin Journal 4: 285-313.

32. Placer ZA, Cushman LL, Johnson BC (1966) Estimation of product of lipid peroxidation (malonyl dialdehyde) in biochemical systems. Anal Biochem 16: 359-364.

33. Botsoglou NA, Fletouris DJ, Papageorgiou GE, Vassilopoulos VN, Mantis AJ, et al. (1994) Rapid, sensitive and specific thiobarbituric acid method for measuring lipid peroxidation in animal tissue, food and feedstuff samples. Journal Agricultural and Food Chemistry 42: 1931-1937.

34. AOAC (1984) Official Methods of Analysis (14thedn.) Association of Official Analytical Chemists, Arlington, VA, USA.

35. Sedlak J, Lindsay RH (1968) Estimation of total, protein-bound, and nonprotein sulfhydryl groups in tissue with Ellman's reagent. Anal Biochem 25: 192-205.

36. Lawrence RA, Burk RF (1978) Species, tissue and subcellular distribution of non Se-dependent glutathione peroxidase activity. J Nutr 108: 211-215.

37. Csernus V (1982) Antibodies of high affinity and specificity for RIA determination of progesterone, testosterone, estradiol-17ß and cortisol. In: Görög S (eds.) Advances in steroid analysis. Academic Press, Budapest, Hungary.

38. Kovács M, Tornyos G, Matics Z, Kametler L, Rajli V, et al. (2011) Subsequent effect of subacute T-2 toxicosis on spermatozoa, seminal plasma and testosterone production in rabbits. Animal 5: 1563-1569.

39. World Health Organisation (1999) WHO laboratory manual for the examination of human semen and sperm-cervical mucus interaction. (4thedn.) Cambridge University Press, UK.

40. Simon L, Carrell DT (2013) Sperm DNA damage measured by comet assay. Methods Mol Biol 927: 137-146.

41. Gopalan RC, Emerce E, Wright CW, Karahalil B, Karakaya AE, et al. (2011) Effects of the anti-malarial compound cryptolepine and its analogues in human lymphocytes and sperm in the Comet assay. Toxicol Lett 207: 322-325.

42. Singh NP, McCoy MT, Tice RR, Schneider EL (1988) A simple technique for quantitation of low levels of DNA damage in individual cells. Exp Cell Res 175: 184-191.

43. Collins A, Dusinská M, Franklin M, Somorovská M, Petrovská H, Duthie S, et al. (1997) Comet assay in human biomonitoring studies: reliability, validation, and applications. Environ Mol Mutagen 30: 139-146.

44. OECD Principles of Good Laboratory Practice (as revised in 1997). OECD Environmental Health and Safety Publications (OECD).

45. IBM SPSS 20 for Windows. SPSS Inc. Chicago, IL. USA.

46. Rotter BA, Prelusky DB, Pestka JJ (1996) Toxicology of deoxynivalenol (vomitoxin). J Toxicol Environ Health 48: 1-34.

47. Harcourt-Brown F (2002) Textbook of rabbit medicine (1stedn.) Elsevier Science. New York, USA.

48. Hewitt MA, Girgis GN, Brash M, Smith TK (2012) Effects of feed-borne Fusarium mycotoxins on performance, serum chemistry, and intestinal histology of New Zealand White fryer rabbits. J Anim Sci 90: 4833-4838.

49. Gelderblom WC, Seier JV, Snijman PW, Van Schalkwyk DJ, Shephard GS, et al. (2001) Toxicity of culture material of Fusarium verticillioides strain MRC 826 to nonhuman primates. Environ Health Perspect 109 Suppl 2: 267-276.

50. Ewuola EO, Egbunike GN (2010) Effects of dietary fumonisin B1 on the onset of puberty, semen quality, fertility rates and testicular morphology in male rabbits. Reproduction 139: 439-445.

51. Kim EJ, Jeong SH, Cho JH, Ku HO, Pyo HM, et al. (2008) Plasma haptoglobin and immunoglobulins as diagnostic indicators of deoxynivalenol intoxication. J Vet Sci 9: 257-266.

52. Tessari EN, Oliveira CA, Cardoso AL, Ledoux DR, Rottinghaus GE (2006) Effects of aflatoxin B1 and fumonisin B1 on body weight, antibody titres and histology of broiler chicks. Br Poult Sci 47: 357-364.

53. Marin DE, Taranu I, Pascale F, Lionide A, Burlacu R, et al. (2006) Sex-related differences in the immune response of weanling piglets exposed to low doses of fumonisin extract. Br J Nutr 95: 1185-1192.

54. Mead JF, Alfin-Slater RB, Howton DR, Popják G (1986) Lipids: Chemistry, biochemistry and nutrition. Plenum Press, NY, USA.

55. Mishra S, Tripathi A, Chaudhari BP, Dwivedi PD, Pandey HP, et al. (2014) Deoxynivalenol induced mouse skin cell proliferation and inflammation via MAPK pathway. Toxicol Appl Pharmacol 279: 186-197.

56. El Golli-Bennour E, Bacha H (2011) Hsp70 expression as biomarkers of oxidative stress: mycotoxins' exploration. Toxicology 287: 1-7.

57. Minervini F, Garbetta A, D'Antuono I, Cardinali A, Martino NA, et al. (2014) Toxic mechanisms induced by fumonisin b1 mycotoxin on human intestinal cell line. Arch Environ Contam Toxicol 67: 115-123.

58. Poersch AB, Trombetta F, Braga AC, Boeira SP, Oliveira MS, et al. (2014) Involvement of oxidative stress in subacute toxicity induced by fumonisin B1 in broiler chicks. Vet Microbiol 174: 180-185.

59. Liu Q, Wang Y, Gu J, Yuan Y, Liu X, et al. (2014) Zearalenone inhibits testosterone biosynthesis in mouse Leydig cells via the crosstalk of estrogen receptor signaling and orphan nuclear receptor Nur77 expression. Toxicol In Vitro 28: 647-656.

60. Lu ZH, Mu YM, Wang BA, Li XL, Lu JM, et al. (2003) Saturated free fatty acids, palmitic acid and stearic acid, induce apoptosis by stimulation of ceramide generation in rat testicular Leydig cell. Biochem Biophys Res Commun 303: 1002-1007.

61. Tajima O, Schoen ED, Feron VJ, Groten JP (2002) Statistically designed experiments in a tiered approach to screen mixtures of Fusarium mycotoxins for possible interactions. Food Chem Toxicol 40: 685-695.

62. Boeira SP, Funck VR, Borges Filho C, Del'Fabbro L, de Gomes MG, et al . (2015) Lycopene protects against acute zearalenone-induced oxidative, endocrine, inflammatory and reproductive damages in male mice. Chem Biol Interact 25: 50-57.

63. Milano GD, Odriozola E, Lopez TA (1991) Lack of effect of a diet containing zearalenone on spermatogenesis in rams. Vet Rec 129: 33-35.

64. Benzoni E, Minervini F, Giannoccaro A, Fornelli F, Vigo D, et al. (2008) Influence of in vitro exposure to mycotoxin zearalenone and its derivatives on swine sperm quality. Reprod Toxicol 25: 461-467.

65. Rajkovic A, Uyttendaele M, Debevere J (2007) Computer aided boar semen motility analysis for cereulide detection in different food matrices. Int J Food Microbiol 114: 92-99.

66. Tsakmakidis IA, Lymberopoulos AG, Alexopoulos C, Boscos CM, Kyriakis SC (2006) In vitro effect of zearalenone and alpha-zearalenol on boar sperm characteristics and acrosome reaction. Reprod Domest Anim 41: 394-401.

67. Filannino A, Stout TA, Gadella BM, Sostaric E, Pizzi F, et al. (2011) Dose-response effects of estrogenic mycotoxins (zearalenone, alpha- and beta-zearalenol) on motility, hyperactivation and the acrosome reaction of stallion sperm. Reprod Biol Endocrinol 9: 134.

68. de Kretser DM, Kerr JB (1994) The cytology of testis. In: Knobil E, Neill JD (eds.) The physiology of reproduction. Raven Press Ltd, New York, USA.

69. Müller S, Dekant W, Mally A (2012) Fumonisin B1 and the kidney: modes of action for renal tumor formation by fumonisin B1 in rodents. Food Chem Toxicol 50: 3833-3846.

70. Zatecka E, Ded L, Elzeinova F, Kubatova A, Dorosh A, et al. (2014) Effect of zearalenone on reproductive parameters and expression of selected testicular genes in mice. Reprod Toxicol 45: 20-30.

71. Kim IH, Son HY, Cho SW, Ha CS, Kang BH (2003) Zearalenone induces male germ cell apoptosis in rats. Toxicol Lett 138: 185-192.

72. Cho ES, Ryu SY, Jung JY, Park BK, Son HY (2011) Effects of red ginseng extract on zearalenone induced spermatogenesis impairment in rat. J Ginseng Res 35: 294-300.

73. Baumgartner A, Kurzawa-Zegota M, Laubenthal J, Cemeli E, Anderson D (2012) Comet-assay parameters as rapid biomarkers of exposure to dietary/environmental compounds - an in vitro feasibility study on spermatozoa and lymphocytes. Mutat Res 743: 25-35.

74. Conková E, Laciaková A, Pástorová B, Seidel H, Kovác G (2001) The effect of zearalenone on some enzymatic parameters in rabbits. Toxicol Lett 121: 145-149.

75. Marína MA, Kalafová M, Schneidgenová N, Maruniaková N (2012) The effect of deoxynivalenol on rabbit spermatozoa motility in vitro. Journal of Microbiology, Biotechnology and Food Sciences 2: 368-377.

# 16

# Assessment of Hematological, Biochemical and Histopathological Effects of Acute and Sub-Chronic Administration of the Aqueous Leaves Extract of *Thymus schimperi* in Rats

**Nigatu Debelo**[1], **Mekbib Afework**[2], **Asfaw Debella**[3], **Eyasu Makonnen**[4], **Wondwossen Ergete**[5] **and Bekesho Geleta**[3*]

[1]*Department of Anatomy, College of Medicine and Health Sciences, Ambo University, Ambo, Ethiopia*

[2]*Department of Anatomy, School of Medicine, College of Health Sciences, Addis Ababa University, Addis Ababa, Ethiopia*

[3]*Directorate of Traditional and Modern Medicine Research, Ethiopian Public Health Institute, Addis Ababa, Ethiopia*

[4]*Department of Pharmacology, School of Medicine, College of Health Sciences, Addis Ababa University, Addis Ababa, Ethiopia*

[5]*Department of Pathology, School of Medicine, College of Health Sciences, Addis Ababa University, Addis Ababa, Ethiopia*

\***Corresponding author:** Bekesho Geleta, Ethiopian Public Health Institute, P.O Box 1242, Addis Ababa, Ethiopia, E-mail: bekeshog@gmail.com

## Abstract

**Background:** *Thymus* species are widely used herbal medicinal plants for various ailments throughout the developing world *Thymus schimperi*. *T. schimperi* is one of the species that is used as spices and traditional medicine for various ailments in Ethiopia.

**Objective:** This study was designed to assess the acute and subchronic toxic effects of the aqueous leaves extract of *T. schimperi* on blood parameters, histopathology and biochemicals of liver and kidney of rats.

**Methods:** The aqueous leaves extract of *T. schimperi* was tested for toxicity study. Wistar rats were randomly divided into control and treatment groups. The doses for acute toxicity study were single doses of 300, 2000, 5000 and 10,000 mg/kg body weight of animal. Whereas, subchronic toxicity study daily administration of doses of 200 and 600 mg/kg of the aqueous extract were used for 90 consecutive days. Biomarkers and hematological parameters, microscopic examination of liver and kidney tissue and body weight of rats were evaluated following the test period besides recording the signs of toxicity.

**Results:** Acute toxicity study did not reveal any signs of toxicity; hence the $LD_{50}$ was higher than 10,000 mg/kg. There was no significant change ($p > 0.05$) in general body weight and most of evaluated hematological and biochemical parameters after 90 days of sub-chronic treatment. The kidneys and liver of treatment group appear normal in their texture, shape, size or color compared to the control in gross and histopathological examination. However, the light microscopic examination reveals that there was localized mononuclear lymphocytic infiltration and mild blood congestion within the hepatic portal and central veins in liver at higher dose (600 mg/kg).

**Conclusion:** The findings revealed that the aqueous leaves extract of *T. schimperi* relatively nontoxic in rats.

**Keywords:** *Thymus schimperi*; Aqueous extract; Acute toxicity; Subchronic toxicity; Biochemicals; Hematology; Histopathology

## Introduction

Herbal remedies and alternative medicines are used throughout the world and in the past herbs often represented the original sources of most drugs [1]. Herbal-derived substances remain the basis for a large proportion of the commercial medications used today for the treatment of heart disease, high blood pressure, pain, asthma and other illnesses [2]. Today a great number of modern drugs are still derived from natural sources, and 25% of all prescriptions contain one or more active ingredients from plants [2].

Because herbs are plants, they are often perceived as "natural" and therefore safe [3]. However, as recent reports have shown, in addition to the many benefits there are also risks associated with the different types of Traditional Medicine/Complementary and Alternative Medicine. Although consumers today have widespread access to various TM/CAM treatments and therapies, they often do not have enough information on what to check when using them in order to avoid unnecessary harm [4].

Traditional herbal products are heterogeneous in nature. Side effects are caused from biologically active constituents from herbs, contaminants, and herb-drug interactions. A common toxicity to herbal medicines involves pyrrolizidine alkaloids, which are complex molecules found in certain plants that may be used or inadvertently added to herbal medicines (including comfrey, which is still available in the United States). These alkaloids produce hepatotoxicity through a characteristic veno-occlusive disease that may be rapidly progressive and fatal [5].

Thymus species are among the medicinal plants commonly used in Ethiopia. The genius Thymus includes about 350 species worldwide and is distributed widely in temperate zones [6]. Many species of Thymus yield the commercially important thyme oil, which exhibits highly antimicrobial effect [7]. Among the various species *T. schimperi* and *T. serrulatus*, are indigenous to Ethiopia locally known as 'Tosign'. The leaves of Thymus are used in Ethiopia as spices to flavor a wide range of food products as well as medicines [8].

Thymus species are one of the widely used herbal medicinal plants for treatment of renal diseases, hypertension, inflammation, infections, pain, to wash skin and used as mouth wash in Ethiopia [9-12]. The volatile oil from thyme was found to contain p-cymene, γ-terpine, carvacrol, rosmarinic acid, eugenol and thymol [8,10]. The volatile oil not only has carminative action, but also antiseptic, antimicrobial and antifungal activities [13]. Thyme is prepared as infusion to treat spasmodic cough, laryngitis, bronchitis urinary infections, renal diseases, hypertension, and Tinea capitis [9]. It is also used as a decongestant, to reduce flatulence and to fight parasites. External uses of thyme include preparations to wash skin wounds or infections [12]. In the Ethiopian traditional medicine the plant has many medicinal applications. Some of the reported applications are for the treatment of gonorrhea, cough, inflammation, spasm, thrombosis, mental illness, eye disease, toothache, urinary retention, stomach problems, leprosy, lung TB, acne and ascariasis [13].

The fresh or dried leaves of both species are used locally as condiments in the preparation of stew, bread and tea. Thyme is often used to flavor meats, soups and stews. It is often used as a primary flavor with lamb, tomatoes and eggs. Even though it's flavorful, but it does not overpower and blends well with other herbs and spices. Thymus contains about 2.5% but not less than 1.0% of volatile oil. The composition of the volatile oil fluctuates depending on the chemotype under consideration. The principal components of Thymus are thymol and carvacrol (up to 64% of oil), along with linalool, p-cymol, cymene, hymene, α- pinene, apigenin, luteolin, and 6-hydroxyluteolin glycosides, as well as di-, tri- and tetra-methoxylated flavones [11].

The rationale of conducting this study is that some herbs that we are using for any purposes may contain harmful chemicals that may cause serious side effects to the host system [14]. *T. schimperi*, have been used by the community for many years for a dietary and medicinal purpose without investigation of the safety of the plant. Therefore, it is necessary to investigate the toxicity of local medicinal plants which are employed by herbalists or communities for therapeutic or diagnosis purposes by gross observation and histopathological examination of liver and kidney. The liver and kidney are major organs of early screening efforts in the preclinical research and a major target organ in the repeated-dose non-clinical safety studies used to support clinical trials [15]. Therefore, the aim of conducting this study was to investigate the toxic effects of using *T. Schimperi* that is used as spices and traditional medicine for various ailments.

## Material and Methods

### Plant material collection and extraction

The fresh leaves of *Thymus schimperi* were collected from south eastern Ethiopia around Dinsho, about 400 km far from Addis Ababa on March 2014. The plant material was authenticated by a botanist in the Ethiopian Public Health Institute and a voucher number HH-001 was deposited in the herbarium for future reference.

About 520 g of the powdered leaves of *T. schimperi* were macerated with distilled water for 2 hours with intermittent agitation by orbital shaker. Then, the supernatant part of agitated materials were decanted and filtered with 0.1 mm$^2$ mesh gauze from the undissolved portion of

the plants. The filtrates of the plants were freeze-dried at lower temperature and reduced pressure, and then lyophilized to form crude extract. A yield of 60.2 g (11.57% w/w) of *T. schimperi* was obtained. Then it was kept in a desiccator at room temperature until used.

### Preparation of experimental animals

For this study male and female healthy Wistar rats of 9 to 10 weeks of age obtained from the animal breeding unit of Ethiopian Public Health Institute were employed. Females were nulliparous and non-pregnant.

Animals of the same sex were grouped into experimental and control groups in a standard cages with six animals per group (n=6) and were kept under standard conditions (at a temperature of 20°C (± 2°C), with natural 12 hrs light/12 hrs dark cycle). For feeding, conventional rodent laboratory diets was used with an unlimited supply of drinking water. The animals were acclimatized to laboratory conditions for one week prior to the experiment to alleviate any non-specific stress [16].

### Method of extract administration

Each group of animal was given different doses of aqueous leaf extracts of *T. schimperi* orally using intra-gastric catheter. For acute toxicity study, the extracts were given once after the animals were fasted of food for 18 hours with a free access for water. After the period of fasting, the animals were weighed and the dose was calculated according to the body weight, then the test substance was administered accordingly [17]. For the sub-chronic toxicity study, the animals were given the aqueous leaves extract of *T. schimperi* for 90 consecutive days. Whereas, animals in the control group were given distilled water. All equipment used were cleaned and placed in an oven after each administration to prevent any contamination.

### Acute toxicity study

The lethal dose for fifty percent (LD$_{50}$) for aqueous leaf extracts of *T. schimperi* was determined using female Wistar rats according OECD protocol [16]. Total of five animals (n=5) per group were used for each dose level investigated. Four test and one control groups were used for the study. The time interval between dosing of each animal at each level was determined by the onset, duration, and severity of toxic signs. A period of 24 hours was allowed between the dosing of each animal. All animals of each level were observed for 14 days. All experimental animals were observed closely for any acute toxicity responses. Treatment of animals at the next dose was given after the previously dosed animals survive. A period of 3 days was allowed between dosing at each dose. According to fixed dose test, the selected starting test dose was 300 mg/kg, because of no available evidences of the toxicity of the plant. The following doses, 300 mg/kg for group-1, 2000 mg/kg for group-2, 5000 mg/kg for group-3, and 10,000 mg/kg for group-4 were given for the experimental animals. The animals in the control group were received distilled water.

### Sub-chronic toxicity study

The study was carried out by using 30 Wistar rats (15 male and 15 female). The rats were randomly grouped in to two experimental and one control groups, containing 10 rats per group (5 male and 5 female in separate cage). Animals of different sexes were placed in the separate cages.

The animals in the experimental group were treated with the aqueous leaves extract of *T. schimperi* at doses of 200 mg/Kg and 600 mg/kg with the intervals of 24 hours for 90 days. All animals have a free access to determined standard pellet and tap water. All groups were closely observed for any physical, food intake, behavioral alterations and signs of abnormalities throughout the study.

## Body weight measurement

Body weight of all experimental animals was taken by using digital electronic balance before commencing the first oral administration and then weekly till last day of oral administration of the extract.

## Cage side observations

For the acute toxicity study animals were observed individually at least once during the first 30 minutes after dosing and periodically during the first 24 hours (with special attention given during the first 4 hours [16]. Whereas, for sub-chronic toxic study, animals were observed daily in group immediately before and after administration of extract.

## Blood collection

At the end of the experiment, all experimental animals were fasted overnight, cervically dislocated, and blood samples were collected by cardiac puncture into tube with anticoagulant ethylene di-amine tetra acetic acid (EDTA) for hematology and into a tube without anticoagulant for blood chemistry. Blood samples in test tubes containing EDTA were immediately processed for hematological parameters using Automated Hematological Analyzer, SYSMEX XT-1800i (SYSMEX CORPORATION, Japan). White blood cell count (WBC), red blood cell count (RBC), the hemoglobin concentration (HGB), hematocrit (HCT), mean corpuscular volume (MCV), mean corpuscular hemoglobin (MCH), mean corpuscular hemoglobin concentration (MCHC), and platelet count (PLC) were determined. For biochemical analysis, the blood samples in the plain test tubes were allowed to stand for 3 hours for complete clotting and then centrifuged at 5000 rpm for 15 minutes using a bench top centrifuge (HUMAX-K, HUMAN-GmbH, Germany). The plasma was withdrawn and transferred into other clean vials. The sera were kept at -20°C until analysis for clinical biochemistry measurements. The concentrations of alanine aminotransferase (ALT), aspartate aminotransferase (AST), urea, albumin and creatinine were automatically determined using COBAS INTEGRA-400 plus Analyzer (ROCHE DIAGNOSTICS, Japan).

## Organs weight measurements and tissue sample

All experimental animals were sacrificed at the end of 90 days treatment after body weight had been measured. Then the animals were dissected and the target organs in the study were removed. After the organs has been removed from the body they were kept in 1% normal saline for a few minutes to clean off any extraneous tissues, further the organs were weighted with the precision balance; and tissue samples were taken from liver and kidney. Sample tissues were placed in a test tube containing 10% buffered formalin for 24 hours and thoroughly rinsed over running tap water overnight. Then the fixed tissues were dehydrated and cleared in a graded series of ethanol and xylene respectively. Then the tissues were infiltrated with molten paraffin wax and embedded in paraffin blocks. The blocks were sectioned at thickness of 5-6 μm using Leica rotary microtome (LEICA

RM 2125 RT, China, checked in Germany). Ribbons of the tissue sections were gently collected using a forceps and laid onto the surface of a water bath heated at 30-40°C. After the sections were thoroughly spread on the water bath, they were placed over tissue glass slides. The slides were then arranged in slide racks and placed in an oven at a temperature of 20-40°C overnight to facilitate the fixation of the specimens onto the glass slides. The thin sections then were undergoes through different stages of xylene and alcohol, being stained with heamatoxylin and eosin [18].

## Light microscopy and photomicrography

Stained tissue sections of the liver and kidney were carefully examined under binocular compound light microscope (OLYMPUS CX41, Japan). Tissue sections from the treated groups were examined for any evidence of histopathologic changes with respect to those of the controls. After examination, photomicrograph of selected slides from both the treated and control groups were taken under a magnification of x40 and x20 objective by using (EVOS XI, China) automated built-in digital photo camera.

## Data processing and analysis

All data which are represented by numbers were packed and analyzed by SPSS statistical software. All values of parameters were expressed in mean ± SEM (standard error of mean). Treatment over time were compared between control and treated groups by using one-way analysis of variance (ANOVA), followed by Dunnett's t-test to determine their level of significance. Differences at $p < 0.05$ were considered statistically significant.

## Ethical consideration

The study was conducted after the ethical and clearance letter was obtained from Ethiopian Public Health Institute. Animals those were used in this study were kept from any unnecessary painful and terrifying situations and handled humanely throughout the study period [16].

## Results

### Acute toxicity

Intragastric administration of extract at different doses of 300, 2000, 5000, and 10,000 mg/kg did not produce any sign of morbidity and mortality in female animals during the period of experiment for acute toxicity. This result indicates that the $LD_{50}$ was above 10,000 mg/kg for the aqueous leaf extract of *T. schimperi*.

### Sub-chronic toxicity

Effects of extract on the body weight: The changes in the mean values of the initial and final body weights of male rats treated with 200 mg/kg and 600 mg/kg of aqueous extract of *T. schimperi* is displayed in Table 1.

The progressive body weight gains were recorded in nearly all groups of rat with time over the period of the experiment. In respect to male rats exposed to *T. schimperi* at the dose of 200 mg/kg compared to control caused a significant increase ($p < 0.05$) in change in mean body weight on the 7th to 10th week and 13th week (Table 1, Graph 1, Graph 2).

| Groups | Body weight of male rats (g) | | | Body weight of female rats (g) | | |
|---|---|---|---|---|---|---|
| | Initial | Final | Change | Initial | Final | Change |
| TS-200 M | 130 ± 11.7 | 255.6 ± 11.01 | 125.6 | 158.4 ± 21.3 | 229.0 ± 9.28 | 70.6 |
| TS-600 M | 117 ± 18.8 | 239.0 ± 14.3 | 122 | 106.4 ± 16.4 | 200.6 ± 4.41 | 94.2 |
| TS-conM | 111 ± 29.08 | 235.2 ± 12.63 | 124.2 | 129.6 ± 12.5 | 204.4 ± 14.01 | 74.8 |

**Table 1:** The mean body weight of rats treated with *T. schimperi* at different weeks and different doses. Values are expressed as mean ± SEM; *=p<0.05. TSc-200M: rats that received extract at dose of 200 mg/kg; TSc-600M: rats that received extract at dose of 600 mg/kg; TSc-conM: rats that received distilled water (control group).

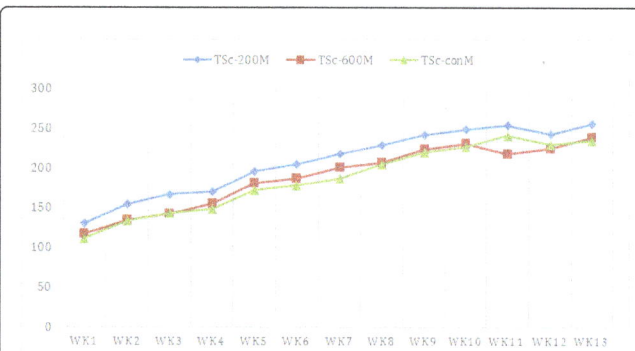

**Graph 1:** Effect of aqueous leaves extract of *T. schimperi* on mean body weight of male rat. The changes in the mean values of the initial and final body weights of female rat treated with 200 and 600 mg/kg of aqueous extract of *T. schimperi* is displayed in Table 1. Concerning female rats, compared to control, *T. schimperi* at the dose of 200 mg/kg caused significant increase (p<0.05, 0.03) in change in body weight on weeks 10th and 11th. At the dose of 600 mg/kg, the herbal remedy does not elicit any significant effect.

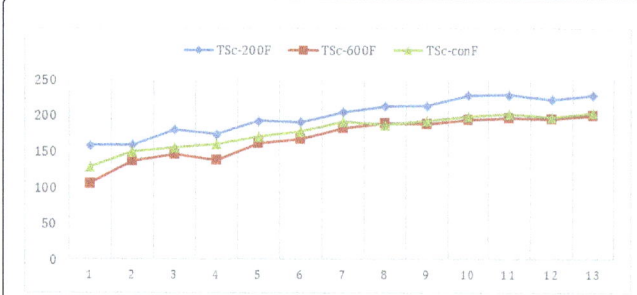

**Graph 2:** Effect of aqueous leaves extract of *T. schimperi* on mean body weight of female rat of different groups.

### Effects of extract on hematological and biochemical parameters

Effect of *T. schimperi* on hematological parameters of female and male rats was listed in Table 2. The aqueous extract of the *T. schimperi* did not produce any significant effect on hematological parameters

after the 90 days administration except in respect of basophils count in which there was a significant decrease (p<0.05) in the female group treated at the dose of 200 mg/kg (0.003 ± 0.003 × $10^{3}$/μl) when compared with the group treated with distilled water (0.016 ± 0.002 × $10^{3}$/μl) (Table 2). There was also a significant decrease (p<0.05) in the proportion of basophils in the male groups treated with *T. schimperi* at doses of 200 mg/kg (0.01 ± 0.004 × $10^{3}$/μl) and 600 mg/kg (0.01 ± 0.002) compared to control group (0.02 ± 0.01 × $10^{3}$/μl) (Table 2).

| Hematological Parameters | Female rats group | | | Male rats group | | |
|---|---|---|---|---|---|---|
| | TS-200 | TS-600 | TS-conF | TS-200 | TS-600 | TS-conF |
| WBC (x10³/μL) | 3.85 ± 1.29 | 3.15 ± 0.17 | 3.648 ± 0.58 | 4.07 ± 0.65 | 5.56 ± 1.14 | 5.66 ± 0.32 |
| RBC (x10⁶/μL) | 8.9 ± 0.075 | 8.79 ± 0.18 | 8.67 ± 0.13 | 9.32 ± 0.06 | 9.7 ± 0.20 | 9.64 ± 0.33 |
| HGB (g/dL) | 17.4 ± 0.49 | 16.8 ± 0.37 | 16.72 ± 0.25 | 17.4 ± 0.22 | 18.2± 0.35 | 18.05 ± 0.95 |
| HCT (%) | 51.4 ± 0.78 | 50 ± 1.12 | 49.42 ± 0.78 | 52 ± 0.64 | 54.6 ± 1.04 | 53.55 ± 2.05 |
| MCV (fL) | 57.8 ± 0.61 | 56.8 ± 0.12 | 57.02 ± 0.32 | 55.7 ± 0.35 | 56.3 ± 0.16 | 55.55 ± 0.25 |
| MCH (pg) | 19.5 ± 0.45 | 19.1 ± 0.05 | 19.26 ± 0.08 | 18.6 ± 0.12 | 18.8 ± 0.14 | 18.75 ± 0.35 |
| MCHC (g/dL) | 33.8 ± 0.44 | 33.6 ± 0.05 | 33.84 ± 0.13 | 33.4 ± 0.05 | 33.4 ± 0.25 | 33.7 ± 0.5 |
| PLT (x10³/μL) | 856 ± 61.86 | 831± 0.00 | 772 ± 45.9 | 804 ± 45.21 | 716 ± 43.81 | 839.5 ± 7.5 |

**Table 2:** The subchronic effect of aqueous leaves extract of *T. schimperi* on hematological parameters in rats; Values are expressed as mean ± SEM; *=p<0.05.

Effect of *T. schimperi* on serum biochemical parameters of female rat after the 90 days administration is displayed in Table 5. There was a significant decrease (p<0.05) in the concentration of albumin in the female group treated with the extract at the dose of 200 mg/kg (5.02 ± 0.27707 g/dl) compared to the group treated with distilled water (5.75 ± 0.559) (Table 3). On the other side there was also a significant increase (p<0.05) in the concentration of creatinine level in the female groups treated with *T. schimperi* at doses of 200 mg/kg (0.86 ± 0.14) compared to the group treated with distilled water (0.635 ± 0.081).

The concentration of urea were significantly increased (p<0.001) in the female groups that received *T. schimperi* at a dose of 600 mg/kg (44.2 ± 2.28) compared to the group treated with distilled water (32 ± 5.83). Moreover the concentration of other parameters such as ALP, ALT and AST did not show a significant change in the female groups that received *T. schimperi* at a dose of 200 mg/kg and 600 mg/kg compared with the group treated with distilled water (Table 3).

Regarding the male groups that receive the same dose as the female groups the extract did not cause significant effect at all doses compared to control, except for AST level which significantly decrease in the male groups that received *T. schimperi* at doses of 200 mg/kg (216.8 ± 3.85) and 600 mg/kg (227.2 ± 8.51) compared to a group treated with distilled water (520.4 ± 2.55) (Table 4).

| | Parameters | | | | | |
|---|---|---|---|---|---|---|
| **Groups** | **Creatinine (mg/dl)** | **Albumin (g/dl)** | **ALP (U/ L)** | **ALT (U/ L)** | **AST (U/L)** | **Urea (mg/dl)** |
| TSc-200 F | 0.86 ± 0.14[*] | 5.02 ± 0.27[*] | 93.4 ± 22.27 | 84.8 ± 14.86 | 190 ± 2.98 | 37.8 ± 2.48 |
| TSc-600 F | 0.694 ± 0.083 | 5.19 ± 0.47 | 75.6 ±19.14 | 87.2 ± 7.563 | 232.6 ± 5.35 | 44.2 ± 2.28[*] |
| TSc-conF | 0.635 ± 0.081 | 5.75 ± 0.56 | 89.2 ± 9.99 | 141.4 ± 10.26 | 335.2 ± 2.14 | 32 ± 5.831 |

**Table 3:** The sub-chronic effect of aqueous leaves extract of *T. schimperi* on serum biochemical parameters of female rats. Values are expressed as mean ± SEM; [*]=p<0.05.

| | Parameters | | | | | |
|---|---|---|---|---|---|---|
| **Groups** | **Creatinine (mg/dl)** | **Albumin (g/dl)** | **ALP (U/ L)** | **ALT (U/ L)** | **AST (U/L)** | **Urea (mg/dl)** |
| TSc-200 M | 0.75 ± 0.03 | 4.76 ± 0.88 | 155.2 ± 34.71 | 99.8 ± 10.26 | 216.8 ± 3.85[*] | 44.4 ± 15.04 |
| TSc-600 M | 0.694 ± 0.11 | 5.02 ±.55 | 187 ± 101.80 | 95.6 ± 11.72 | 227.2 ± 8.51[*] | 35.6 ±1.14 |
| Tsc-conM | 0.76 ± 0.14 | 4.64 ± 0.21 | 104.4 ± 44.53 | 161.2 ± 71.26 | 520.4 ± 2.55 | 35.2 ± 2.77 |

**Table 4:** The sub-chronic effect of aqueous leaves extract of *T. schimperi* on some serum biochemical parameters of male rats. Values are expressed as mean ± SEM; [*]=p<0.05.

### Effects of extract on the weights of liver and kidney

Effect of aqueous leaf extract of *T. schimperi* did not produce any significant effect on weights of liver and kidneys of rats after the 90 days administration in the group treated with the preparation at the doses of 200 mg/kg and 600 mg/kg compared with the group treated with distilled water. The values are indicated in Table 5.

| | Male organ weight (g) | | Female organ weight (g) | |
|---|---|---|---|---|
| **Groups** | **Liver** | **Kidney** | **Liver** | **Kidney** |
| TS-200 | 6.78 ± 0.32 | 0.65 ± 0.07 | 7.14 ± 0.85 | 0.66 ± 0.06 |
| TS-600 | 7.04 ± 0.67 | 0.612 ± 0.04 | 6.52 ± 0.37 | 0.60 ± 0.07 |
| TS-con | 6.52 ± 0.76 | 0.624 ± 0.04 | 6.52 ± 0.76 | 0.64 ± 0.04 |

**Table 5:** The sub-chronic effect of aqueous leaves extract of *T. schimperi* on the weight of liver and kidneys of male and female rats. Values are expressed as mean ± SEM; [*]p<0.05.

### Gross Pathologic Observations

On the examination of the gross appearance of internal organs of treated rat (Figures 1A-1F), such as liver and kidney did not show any abnormal changes in texture, shape, size or color compared to the control. There was no sign of necrosis or lesion was appreciated on the organs of all treated groups.

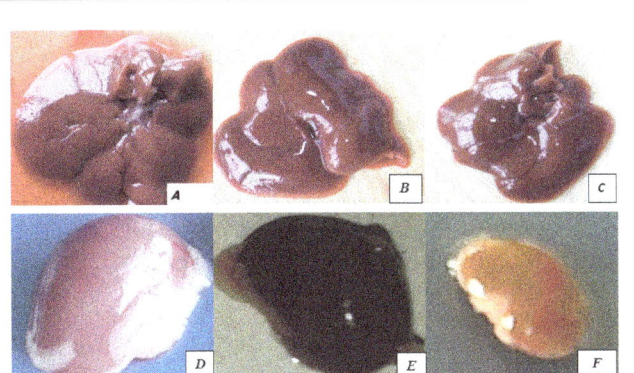

**Figure 1:** The gross appearance of liver (control rat (A), rat treated with 200 mg/kg (B), and rat treated with 600 mg/kg (C) and of kidney (control rat (D), rat treated with 200mg/kg (E), and rat treated with 600 mg/kg (F).

### Light microscopy of liver

The microscopic examination of liver sections of control group rat (Figures 2A and 2B) showed the normal architecture of structural units of the liver, the hepatic lobules, formed by cords of hepatocytes separated by hepatic sinusoids.

There were no significant histopathological presentations observed in the groups treated with distilled water and treatment groups. The liver appeared normal with preserved hepatic architecture, hepatocytes arranged as radial plates, and having eosinophilic cytoplasm and basophilic central nuclei. No cytoplasmic inclusions were seen and no portal inflammation (Figures 2A-2F). Mild blood congestion was observed in the rat liver at dose of 600 mg/kg within the hepatic portal and central veins (Figures 2E and 2F).

### Light Microscopy of Kidney

On the microscopic examination of kidney sections of rats there were no adverse histopathological presentations observed in all the treatment groups. Normocellular glomerular tufts were displayed on a background containing tubules. Examination of kidney sections of rat treated with the aqueous extract of *T. schimperi* (Figures 3C-3F) at doses of 200 mg/kg and 600 mg/kg doses indicated no structural difference compared to the control groups (Figures 3A and 3B) rat. The microscopic architecture of sections of kidney in treated groups had a similar appearance to that of the controls in which renal corpuscles maintaining their normal size of urinary space and normal tubular structures are examined. No necrosis was observed.

### Discussion

Worldwide, various medicinal plants and botanical drugs have been widely adapted as primary therapeutic agents or supplements for treating various human illnesses [19]. The safety study is accomplished by the implementation of general pre-clinical toxicity experiments to uncover potential poisonous effects of any drug majorly in liver and kidney of animals [20]. If there is mild inflammation and tissue damage to these organs, the permeability of the cell membrane will increase and release cytoplasmic enzymes such as LD, ALP, and AST, while necrosis will release mitochondrial ALT as well as AST leaking into the blood and increase in levels [21,22]. Toxicity screening models provide important preliminary data to help select natural remedies with potential health beneficial properties for future work [23]. The first toxicity test performed on the formulation was the evaluation of acute toxicity determined from the administration of a single exposure. It was conducted to determine the safety margin of the formulation [19]. Accordingly, the aqueous leaf extracts from the *T. schimperi* did not induce lethality in rats when administered orally up to doses of 10,000 mg/kg. Therefore, this result suggests the LD50 of aqueous extract of *T. schimperi* was estimated to be greater than 10,000 mg/kg because of no morbidity and mortality were recorded up on oral administration of this dose. Hence, the herbal preparation can be said to be safe when orally administered substance does not produce lethality up to 10, 000 mg/kg [24]. Visible signs of acute or delayed toxicity were not observed in acute toxicity study. This result goes in line with the previous study [25,26]. Observations by the naked eye on organs like the liver and kidneys of the treated animals after 2 weeks did not show any gross pathological change such as in color, organ swelling, texture and atrophy or hypertrophy after single administration of the formulation when compared with the control group.

toxicity related information which is not only detected by direct examination of organs and body weight analysis. Studies on hematological parameters can easily reveal abnormalities in body metabolic processes, and the blood profile usually provides important information on the response of the body to injury or lesion, deprivation and stress [27]. Therefore, the extent of toxic effect of drugs and/or plant extracts can be determined by assessment of hematological parameters [28].

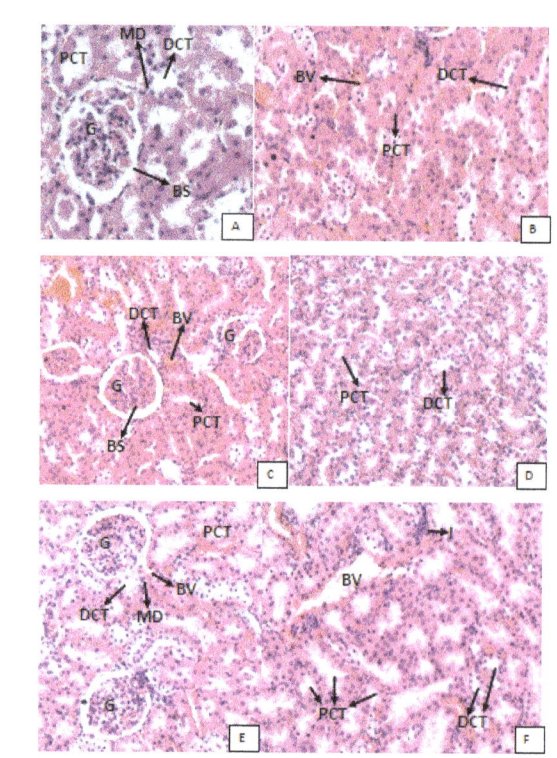

**Figure 3:** Photomicrographs of kidney sections of control group rats (A & B), rats treated with 200 mg/kg (C & D), Rats treated with 600 mg/kg body weight/day (E&F) of the aqueous leaves extract of *T. schimperi*. G=Glomeruli, BS=Bowman's space, DCT=Distal convoluted tubule, PCT=proximal convoluted tubule, I=Infiltration, MD=Macula densa, BV=Blood vessel. (Sections were stained with H & E).

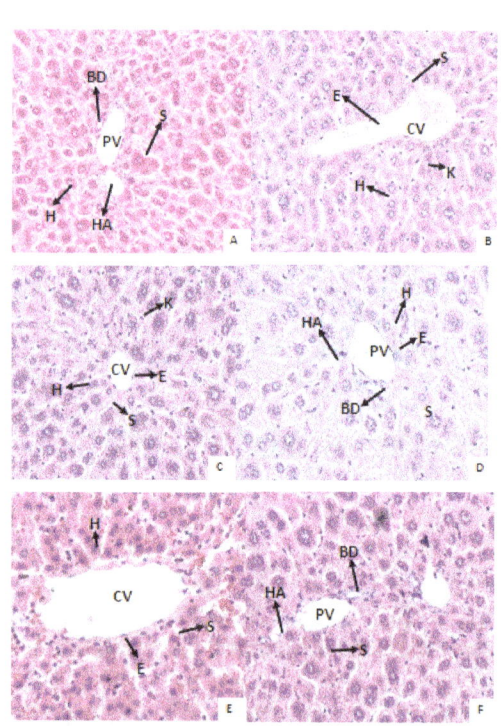

**Figure 2:** Photomicrographs of liver sections of control group rats (A & B), rats treated with 200 mg/kg (C & D), rats treated with 600 mg/kg body weight/day (E & F) of the aqueous extracts of *T. schimperi*. (CV=Central vein, E=Endothelial cells, PV=Portal vein, BD=Bile duct, H = Hepatocytes, S=Sinusoids, HA=Hepatic artery, K=Kupffer cells, I=Infiltration. (Sections were stained with H and E).

Daily treatment with both doses of the aqueous leaf extracts of *T. schimperi* to male and female Wistar rats for a period of 12 weeks did not show any toxicity related morbidities and mortalities. Hematological parameters were also evaluated to obtain further

Red blood indices such as the mean corpuscular volume (MCV), mean corpuscular hemoglobin (MCH) and mean corpuscular hemoglobin concentration (MCHC) are the most useful indicators in the diagnosis of anemia in most animals [29]. As indicated on (Table 2) the effect of the aqueous leaf extract of *T. schimperi* on MCV, MCH, and MCHC were insignificant in treated group compared to the control. These observations demonstrate that the aqueous extract of the leaves in this study did not cause significant toxic effect on the levels of calculated red blood cell (RBC) indices at both doses. Hence, subchronic treatment with the aqueous leaf extract of *T. schimperi* has shown no effect on the size of RBCs and in hemoglobin weight per RBC in rats. This effect clearly suggested that the aqueous leaf extracts did not cause macrocytic and microcytic anemia [30]. This finding is in agreement with other findings in which the values of the various RBC parameters of extract treated rabbits were found to be comparable with those of the control group [31]. The changes in RBC count, average hemoglobin (Hgb) and hematocrit (HCT) levels of treated group animals were also insignificant (p>0.05) compared with that of vehicle received rats.

In the hematological analysis the white blood cell (WBC) count also was performed. In herbal toxicity studies, increase in WBC may indicate the impact of plant extracts in inducing the immune response of treated animals [32]. On the other hand, significant decrease in the WBC of the blood indicates a decline in the production of leukocytes called leukopenia, means that the body is less able to fight off infections. However, the hematological analysis in this study demonstrated that the estimated total WBC count after sub-chronic administration of the formulation was not significantly changed in response to the administered aqueous leaf extract of T. schimperi at doses of 200 mg/kg and 600 mg/kg compared to the control. This result may indicate that the aqueous leaf extract in this study does not possess chemicals capable of inducing leukocytosis, which is an abnormally high number of WBC in the blood circulation or in suppression of normal production of WBC [29]. Also, similar results were obtained by previous study that found no changes in the WBC count with different groups compared with control groups [31].

In platelet count, thrombocytopenia is a condition of abnormally low number of platelets in the circulation, may result from decreased production or increased destruction of platelets [32]. Some drugs provoke platelet antibodies and platelet destruction, resulting in thrombocytopenia [29]. On the other hand, thrombocytosis is an abnormal increase in the number of circulating platelets [33]. However, in this study the change in the platelets count as compared to the control group is insignificant in both treated group of rats. This result suggests that the aqueous leaf extract at both doses used in this study has no effect in inducing neither thrombocytopenia nor thrombocytosis.

Elevated serum levels of enzymes produced by the liver or nitrogenous wastes to be excreted by the kidney might be indications to their spillage into the blood stream as a result of necrosis of the tissues [34]. Because of the liver's strategic location between intestinal tract and rest of body it's the first organ to encounter ingested nutrients, vitamins, metals, drugs, and environmental toxicants as well as waste products of bacteria that enter portal blood [19]. So the liver is a primary destination for any toxic substance entered to the body, especially through gastrointestinal route, the liver suffers first. Because of its wide range of functions, any abnormal change in liver will definitely affect complete metabolism of an animal [35]. Liver chemistry tests include several serum chemistries that reflect liver function. The most commonly used serum liver chemistry tests include serum transaminases (alanine aminotransferase (ALT), aspartate aminotransferase (AST)), serum alkaline phosphatase (ALP), Gamma-glutamyl transpeptidase (GGT), bilirubin and albumin. The major intracellular enzymes of the liver are alanine aminotransferase (ALT) and aspartate aminotransferase (AST). However, injuries of liver cells (hepatocytes) allowing for escape of these enzymes into the bloodstream raises their levels in the blood [36]. The levels of ALP and GGT in the serum are important parameters for evaluation of hepatobiliary route. For hepatocellular evaluation, measurement of a minimum of two scientifically appropriate blood tests is recommended, e.g ALT, AST, sorbitol dehydrogenase, glutamate dehydrogenase, or total bile acids [28].

AST is not specific for liver. AST is also present in red blood cells, cardiac muscle, skeletal muscle, kidney and brain tissue, and may be elevated due to damage to these sources as well. AST is defined as a biochemical marker for the diagnosis of acute myocardial infarction [37]. Therefore, it is an absolute prerequisite not to take in consideration of extra-hepatic tissue damage as a possible source of serum AST when evaluating the enzyme in relation to the liver. Beside this, only about 20% of AST is cytosolic and the rest is found in mitochondria of hepatocytes and other cells [38]. Unlike AST, ALT is fairly specific being found largely in the liver and it is commonly used as a biomarker for liver problems [39]. ALT is purely cytosolic and is more specific for hepatocytes. Elevation of serum levels of both AST and ALT can occur with states of altered hepatocellular membrane permeability. Because ALT is located only in the cytosol, serum levels tend to be relatively higher than AST. Since majority of AST is found within mitochondrial of cells, it is released slowly in comparison to ALT [37]. Hence, serum transaminases, especially ALT, are the most important markers of hepatic injury [39].

In the present study, the toxicological effects of 200 mg/kg and 600 mg/kg body weight doses of the aqueous leaf extracts of T. schimperi on liver biochemical parameters were investigated in rats. In liver function test, there were no significant changes in the serum level of ALT and AST in most animal groups treated with both doses of the aqueous leaf extracts of T. schimperi in comparison to the control group. The non-significant change of these enzymes between the control and treated group animals after 12 weeks administration indicates that the aqueous leaf extract did not cause adverse toxic effect or hepatic damage on the liver. There was also significant decrement in the level AST was observed in male rats treated at both doses compared with the control group. The result signifies that Thymus species had no liver damage effect on AST. AST levels are usually not as high in chronic liver injury, often less than 4 times the highest normal level [38]. This result was supported by previous study conducted on rats states that administration of 500 mg/kg of the extract of T. vulgaris could significantly improve altered enzyme levels as well as the histological architecture of liver [40].

Kidney is a sensitive organ, whose function is known to be aected by a number of factors such as drugs including phytochemicals of plant origin that ultimately lead to renal failure. Kidney function test is a collective term for a variety of individual tests and procedures that can be done to evaluate how well the kidneys are functioning [41]. Accordingly, renal function can be assessed by measuring the levels of plasma creatinine, urea and uric acid concentrations [41]. Assessment of possible renal damage due to aqueous leaf extract of plants in this study was made by assaying plasma urea and creatinine levels [42]. Results show in most of the groups of animals no significant alteration in the blood urea nitrogen (BUN) and creatinine levels due to T. schimperi treatment. The female rat treated at 200 mg/kg had shown significant increased creatinine values compared with control group. Even if the values has shown significant increment but still all values are under the normal range (i.e 0.2-0.8 mg/dl) [43].

Histopathological examinations provide information to strengthen the findings on biochemical and heamatological parameters [44]. The present histological examination indicated that liver sections of rats treated with aqueous leaf extract of T. schimperi at both 200 mg/kg and 600 mg/kg doses did not show focal necrosis and pyknosis. In addition, the general histological architecture and its functions were not affected in any of the treatment group rats compared to the control. This was strengthened by study done in rats over 8 weeks indicated that the altered renal tissue could be assisted by the aqueous extract of Thyme [45].

Moreover, there were no eect on the levels of AST and ALT, which is considered to be sensitive indicators of hepatocellular damage and within limits, can provide a quantitative evaluation of the degree of damage to the liver [37]. It is reasonable to deduce, therefore, that *T. schimperi* did not induce any damage to the liver or kidneys. This is further confirmed by the histological assessment of these organs [46]. No dierence was observed in the weight and structure of the liver and kidney between the control and the treated groups. In agreement with these results, the findings of another study demonstrated no changes of liver weight were reported in broiler chickens fed 1 g/kg thyme powder [47]. Altogether, the sub-chronic study indicates that *T. schimperi* ingestion did not induce detrimental changes and morphological alterations in these organs.

## Conclusion

The acute toxicity test suggests that oral single dose (10,000 mg/kg) administration of *T. schimperi* is practically non-toxic to Wistar rats. The sub-chronic toxicity study suggests that *T. schimperi* are do not caused a significant effect in liver, kidney and blood parameters when administered orally at doses of 200 mg/kg and 600 mg/kg in Wistar rats. Therefore, with respect to results from liver and kidney, the aqueous leaf extract of *T. schimperi* can be considered as relatively nontoxic in rats.

## Acknowledgements

The authors are grateful for financial support of this study which was provided by Ministry of Finance and Economic Development (project number OBN6.34/2006) through Ethiopian Public Health Institute and the School of Graduate Studies of Addis Ababa University. Staffs of the Traditional and Modern Medicine Research Directorate, and Finance, plan & monitoring sincerely appreciated for their direct and indirect contribution during the work.

## References

1.  Cooper EL (2004) Drug Discovery, CAM and Natural Products. Evid Based Complement Alternat Med 1: 215-217.

2.  Saad B, Azaizeh H, Said O (2005) Tradition and perspectives of arab herbal medicine: a review. Evid Based Complement Alternat Med 2: 475-479.

3.  Ernst E (1998) Harmless herbs? A review of the recent literature. Am J Med 104: 170-178.

4.  Barrett B, Kiefer D, Rabago D (1999) Assessing the risks and benefits of herbal medicine: an overview of scientific evidence. Altern Ther Health Med 5: 40-49.

5.  Stickel F, Patsenker E, Schuppan D (2005) Herbal hepatotoxicity. J Hepatol 43: 901-910.

6.  Ramon MV (1997) Synopsis of the genus thymus in the mediterranean area. CSIC - Real Jardín Botánico p 249-262.

7.  Nzeako BC, Al-Kharousi ZS, Al-Mahrooqui Z (2006) Antimicrobial activities of clove and thyme extracts. Sultan Qaboos Univ Med J 6: 33-39.

8.  Dagne E, Hailu S, Bisrat D, Worku T (1998) Constituents of the essential oil of Thymus schimperi. Bull Chem Soc Ethiop 12: 79-82.

9.  Parvev N, Yadav S (2010) Ethnopharmacology of single herbal preparations of medicinal plants in Asendabo district, Jimma, Ethiopia. Indian Journal of Traditional Knowledge 9: 727-728.

10. Anthony, Mescher L (2012) Junquiria's Basic Histology; text and atlas, 12th edition p16.

11. Panizzi L, Flamini G, Cioni PL, Morelli I (1993) Composition and antimicrobial properties of essential oils of four Mediterranean Lamiaceae. J Ethnopharmacol 39: 167-170.

12. Debella A, Debebe D, Urga K (2003) Medicinal plants and other useful plants of Ethiopia, Ethiopian Health and Nutritional Institute, Berhanena Selam Printing Press, Addis Ababa, Ethiopia p9-17.

13. WHO (2002) Traditional medicine strategy, Geneva.

14. Effendi W, Siti-Nurtahirah J, Hussin Z (2006) The side effects of Kacip fatimah Extract on Liver and kidney of white rats. Journal of Sustainability Science and Management 1: 40-46.

15. Coolborn AF, Bolatito B, Clement AF (2012) Study of acute and subchronic toxicity of Spathodea campanulata P Beav leaf. Int Proc Chem Biol Environ Eng 41: 76-80.

16. OECD (2008) Guidelines for the testing of new chemicals revised draft guideline 425; acute oral toxicity.

17. Dapar L, Maxwell P, Aguiyi, John C, Wannang, et al. (2007) The histopathologic effects of Securidaca longepedunculata on heart, liver, kidney and lungs of rats. African Journal of Biotechnology 6: 591-595.

18. Forysth A (2005) Tissue processing: from the cut-up to the H&E slide.

19. Curtis DK (2007) Casarett and Doull's Toxicology: The basic science of poisons, 7th edition, The McGraw-Hill Companies p18-40.

20. Farzamfar B, Abdollahi M, Ka'abinejadian S, Heshmat R, Shahhosseiny MH, et al. (2008) Sub chronic toxicity study of a novel herbal-based formulation (Semelil) on dogs. DARU J Pharmaceutical Sciences 16: 15-19.

21. Arneson W, Brickell J (2007) Clinical chemistry-laboratory perspective. F.A Davis company, Philadelphia.

22. Hall AP, Elcombe CR, Foster JR, Harada T, Kaufmann W, et al. (2012) Liver hypertrophy: a review of adaptive (adverse and non-adverse) changes--conclusions from the 3rd International ESTP Expert Workshop. Toxicol Pathol 40: 971-994.

23. Rosenthal N, Brown S (2007) The mouse ascending: perspectives for human-disease models. Nat Cell Biol 9: 993-999.

24. Pour BM, Latha LY, Sasidharan S (2011) Cytotoxicity and oral acute toxicity studies of Lantana camara leaf extract. Molecules 16: 3663-3674.

25. Clarke EG, Clarke ML (1977) Veterinary Toxicology. London: Cassel and Collier Macmillian Publishers p268-277.

26. Fachini-Queiroz FC, Kummer R, Estevão-Silva CF, Carvalho MD, Cunha JM, et al. (2012) Effects of Thymol and Carvacrol, Constituents of Thymus vulgaris L. Essential Oil, on the Inflammatory Response. Evid Based Complement Alternat Med 2012: 657026.

27. Bosco AD, Gerencser Z, Szendro Z, Ugnai C, Cullere M, et al. (2014) Dietary supplementation of spirulina (Arthrospira platensis) and Thyme (Thymus vulgaris) on rabbit meat appearance, oxidative stability and fatty acid profile during retail display. Meat Sci 96: 114-119.

28. Raza M, Al-Shabanah OA, El-Hadiyah TM, Al-Majed AA (2002) Effect of prolonged vigabatrin treatment on haematological and biochemical parameters in plasma, liver and kidney of Swiss albino mice. Pharmace Scien 70: 135-145.

29. Weingand K, Brown G, Hall R, Davies D, Gossett K, et al. (1996) Harmonization of animal clinical pathology testing in toxicity and safety studies. The Joint Scientific Committee for International Harmonization of Clinical Pathology Testing. Fundam Appl Toxicol 29: 198-201.

30. Rogers K (2011) Blood: Physiology and Circulation (The Human Body), 1st edition. Encyclopædia Britannica 42: 121-225.

31. Mbaka GO, Adeyemi OO (2010) Toxicity study of ethanol root extract of Sphenocentrum Jollyanum (Menispermaceae) Pierre. Asian J Experi Biolo Scien 14: 869-874.

32. Tousson E, El-Moghazy M, El-Atrsh E (2011) The possible effect of diets containing Nigella sativa and Thymus vulgaris on blood parameters and some organs structure in rabbit. Toxicol Ind Health 27: 107-116.

33. Aajibade TO, Olayemia FO, Arowolo ROA (2012) The haematological and biochemical effects of methanol extract of the seeds of Moringa oleifera in rats. J Medic Plants Res 6: 615-621.

34. Mikhael M, Orr R, Amsen F, Greene D, Singh MA (2010) Effect of standing posture during whole body vibration training on muscle morphology and function in older adults: a randomised controlled trial. BMC Geriatr 10: 74.

35. Paliwal A, Gurjar RK, Sharma HN (2009) Analysis of liver enzymes in albino rat under stress of ?-cyhalothrin and nuvan toxicity. Biol and Medic 2: 70-73.

36. Thapa BR, Walia A (2007) Liver function test and their interpretation. Indian J Pediatr 74: 663-671.

37. Gaze DC (2007) The role of existing and novel cardiac biomarkers for cardioprotection. Curr Opin Investig Drugs 8: 711-717.

38. Thierry A, Acha AE, Paulin N, Aphrodite C, Pierre K, et al. (2011) Sub-acute toxicity study of the aqueous extract from Acanthus montanus Djami Tchatchou. Electronic J Biol 7: 11-15.

39. Giboney PT (2005) Mildly elevated liver transaminase levels in the asymptomatic patient. Am Fam Physician 71: 1105-1110.

40. Amacher DE (1998) Serum transaminase elevations as indicators of hepatic injury following the administration of drugs. Regul Toxicol Pharmacol 27: 119-130.

41. Abdel-kader MA, Mohamod NZ (2012) Evaluation of protective and antioxidant activity of thyme (Thymus vulgaris) extract on paracetamol-induced toxicity in rats. Australian Journal of Basic and Applied Sciences 6: 467-474.

42. Stark JL (1980) BUN/creatinine: your keys to kidney function. Nursing 10: 33-38.

43. Paula AF, Mark AB (2011) Kidney function test p35-43.

44. Harrison L, Johnson-Delaney CA (1996) Exotic Animal Companion Medicine Handbook for Veterinarians. Zoological Education Network p1-3.

45. El Hilaly J, Israili ZH, Lyoussi B (2004) Acute and chronic toxicological studies of Ajuga iva in experimental animals. J Ethnopharmacol 91: 43-50.

46. Kensara OA, Elsawy NA, Nutr PJ (2012) Aqueous extract of Thymus Vulgaris-induced prevention of kidney damage in hypertensive adult male albino rat: Biochemical and ultrastructural study. Pakistan Journal of Nutrition 11: 367-374.

47. Demir E, Kilinc K, Yildirim Y, Dincer F, Eseceli (2008) Comparaitive effect of mint, sage, thyme and flavomycin in wheat-based broiler diets. Arch Zootec 11: 54-63.

# 17

# Neurotoxic Manifestation of Snake Bite in Bangladesh

**Mohammad Robed Amin**[1*], **SM Hasan Mamun**[2], **Nazmul Hasan Chowdhury**[3], **M Rahman**[4], **Mohammad Ali**[5], **Abdullah Al Hasan**[1], **MR Rahman**[6] and **M A Faiz**[7]

[1]*Dhaka Medical College, Bangladesh*

[2]*Chittagong Medical College, Bangladesh*

[3]*Comilla Medical College, Bangladesh*

[4]*Shahabuddin Medical College, Dhaka, Bangladesh*

[5]*Bogura Medical College, Bangladesh*

[6]*Begum Khaleda Zia Medical College, Dhaka, Bangladesh*

[7]*Sir Salimullah Medical Medical College, Dhaka, Bangladesh*

[*]**Corresponding author:** Dr. Md. Robed Amin, Assistant Professor of Medicine, Department of Medicine, Dhaka Medical College, Dhaka, Bangladesh. E-mail: robedamin@yahoo.com

## Abstract

**Introduction:** Snake bite is a potentially life threatening emergency situation physician has to encounter in rural areas of tropical countries in South-East Asia including Bangladesh. Among the venomous snakes in Bangladesh, Neurotoxic snakes like Cobra and Krait are the commonest. In this study neurotoxic manifestation of venomous snakes are clinically observed.

**Methods:** In this series a total 35 snakebite patients with neurological features from May 1999 to June 2001 were included and preexisting neurological cases were excluded.

**Results:** Among the 537 total snake bite cases, the neurotoxic snake bite was 10% with 51 cobra bite and 12 kraits bite. The victims age are in the range of 3.5 years to 85 years with 70% cases are under 30 years of old. There is slight male preponderence with almost same number of bite at home and outside. The common clinical neurotoxic features are ptosis, (100%) external ophthalmoplegia, dysphagia, dysphonia and broken neck sign. The chest movements were reduced in 20 % cases. All 35 cases (100%) were treated with Haffkine polyvalent anti snake venom with 8.6% cases needed 2nd dose. All 35 cases with neurotoxic features were also treated with anti cholinesterses (100%) and among them 14.2% needed ventilatory support. Anti-snake venom reaction was very common in the with pyrogenic reaction (80.64%) and anaphylactic reaction (64.51%). The outcome of snake bite was excellent with 97% recovery with one residual neurological deficit and no fatality.

**Conclusion:** The neurotoxic snake bite has definite characteristics neurological sign and symptoms which could lead to fatality with respiratory paralysis.

**Keywords:** Neurotoxic; Venomous; Snake

## Introduction

Snake bite is a potentially life threatening and important emergency situation a physician has to encounter in rural areas of tropical countries in South-East Asia including Bangladesh (Warrell, 1995). The importance of snake bite has been emphasized by the WHO [1]. In a recent study conducted in 1995-1996 it has been shown that incidence of snake bite is 4.3 per 100,000 populations with mortality of 20%.Epidemiological aspects of snake bite and clinical presentation following bite has been described from different countries. Several measures were taken to characterize the venoms and standardize the antivenoms [2-4].

There are about 82 species of snakes in Bangladesh amongst which 28 species are venomous and others are non-venomous. The venomous snakes of medical importance in our country is *Cobra, Naja, Gokhra ; Krait, Bangarus , Shakhini, Kewtey; Russells Viper, Doboia russelii, Chandrabora; Green snakes, Trimeresurus, Gal tawa;*

*King cobra, Ophiophagus, Shankachur or Khalandar,* and all species of sea snakes. Medically important snake species are the ones that fill into one of the three categories: a) commonly cause death or serious disability, b) uncommonly cause bites but are recorded to cause serious effects, c) commonly because bites but serious effects are very uncommon [1].

Effects of snake bite involve different systems depending upon species of snakes causing bite [5]. Cobra and Krait bites are associated with prominent neurotoxicity. Local envenoming with soft tissue necrosis has also been described in some countries including Bangladesh following Cobra bite [6,7] but the krait bite is not associated with any local envenomation. Russell's viper bite is associated with coagulation abnormalities and renal failure with occasional reports of neurotoxicity, pituitary necrosis and increased vascular permeability [8]. Green snake bite is associated with swelling of the bitten part and coagulation abnormality. The sea snake bite is associated with neurotoxicity, myotoxicity and renal failure. The common serious envenoming is neurotoxicity which is characterized by ptosis, external ophtalmoplegia, dysphagia, dysphonia, weakness of facial muscles, broken neck sign (weakness of neck muscles leading to unable to flex the neck), loss of tendon jerks and respiratory paralysis [9]. Considerable geographical variation in clinical presentation has been described following bite by some species of snakes including Cobra and Russell's viper [10]. Diagnosis of species of snake responsible for bite is essential for management of patients. Estimation of venom antigen from swab from wound site, serum or urine by Enzyme Linked Immunosorbent Assay (ELISA) technique has been found to be useful in some countries [11]. In absence of such facilities, good epidemiological study by identification of brought dead snake may be helpful in correlating clinical features with type of snakes. Careful documentation of clinical features following bite by different snakes is needed in Bangladesh. Most often people seek treatment from traditional healers called 'ozha'. As a result doctors in the community are not appropriately aware of various aspects of snake bite and its management. Venomous snake bite with neurotoxic features consist the major venomous bite in our country. Unfortunately many of the published cases of neurotoxic snake bite are poor to describe due to lack of detailed examination and observation. An attempt has been made in this study to describe clinical presentation of patients of snake bite presented with neurological features. Species identification of the offending snake was also attempted to define the snake in our country which causes neurotoxicities after venomous bite.

## Materials and Methods

In this series a total 35 snakebite patients with pure neurological features were included. All patients having one or other neurological manifestation with or without local envenomation after snake bite were admitted and treated in snake bite study clinic (SBSC) under medicine unit-III in Chittagong Medical College Hospital. (Only unit where all the patients of snake bite is admitted in C.M.C.H.). This study was carried out over the period of 2 years ranging from May 1999 to June, 2001.

Any patient, who presented with one or more of the recognized neurotoxic features developed after snakebite of all ages and both sexes, was included in this study. However, patients having history of pre-existing neurological disease were excluded from the study. Venomous snake bite leading to cardiotoxicity, renal failure or coagulopathy was also excluded from the study. The patients who received antihistamine, sedative or steroids in pre hospital or primary care management were also not included in this study.

A detailed history was taken from each of the patient and/or attendant and relevant points for example: time and place of bite, sequence of occurrence of symptoms with progression, pre-hospital treatment history etc. was specially sought. Simultaneously thorough physical examination especially detailed neurological examination was done. Local examination was also done minutely to note fang marks, swelling, tenderness, blistering, enlarged and tender lymph nodes etc.

Special inquiry was done to identify the offending snake by asking the party to bring the snake (if it had been killed) for direct identification. The identification of snakes that were not brought to hospital was done by showing photographs or preserved samples.

Some investigations were done to search probable complications like excessive muscle breakdown, cardiotoxicity, coagulation abnormality etc. Investigations carried out routinely include Haemoglobin level, TC and DC of WBC, serum CPK, ECG and 20 min whole blood clotting test (20 min WBCT). Bed side peak expiratory flow rate (PEFR) was done in every patients except those presented with ventilatory failure or unconscious. All patients were observed for 5 days in hospital to see recovery, anti-snake venom reaction and any early residual neurological deficit present or not. If the patients developed neurological deficit or local envenomation, further observation by neurologist and surgical specialist was done.

All enrolled patients with features of neurotoxicity (one or more) were treated with polyvalent anti-venom and in Neostigmine. In some cases artificial ventilation were given for variable durations. The outcome of treatment was noted in all cases. The collected data is preserved and analysis done with EP Info 6 manual and expressing results in percentage and number.

## Results

During the study period (May 1999 to June 2001) a total 537 snake bite patients were admitted. 365 patients were non venomous and 172 patients were venomous bite patients. Green pit bites (102 pt) were highest among the venomous patient. 63 patients (cobra-51 and krait-12) presented with neurotoxicity with or without local envenoming. The other venomous bite patients were sea snake (05) and Russell's viper bite (02). Among the venomous bites, 35 patients presented with neurological manifestations with or without local necrosis were included in the study. The other 28 neurotoxic patients were excluded due to presence of prior neurological disease, prior treatment with antihistamine, sedative or steroids in prehospital or primary health care.

**Age:** The age of the studied patients ranged from 3.5 to 85 years. Most of the victims were between 5 to 30 years that comprised 70% of total patients (Table 1).

| Age (years) | Number of patient | Percentage |
|---|---|---|
| 1-5 | 1 | 2.85 |
| 6-10 | 6 | 17.14 |
| 11-20 | 11 | 31.42 |
| 21-30 | 8 | 22.85 |
| 31-40 | 4 | 11.42 |
| 41-50 | 2 | 5.71 |
| >50 | 3 | 8.57 |

**Table 1:** Age distribution (n=35) of neurotoxic snake bite.

**Sex:** Among the patients, males were a bit predominant (54.2%).

**Pre-hospital treatment:** All patients received some types of treatment before coming to the hospital. Most of those treatments were traditional and harmful. All patients received multiple tight tourniquets over the bitten limb, some of which were tight enough to cause arterial occlusion. Others include suction of bitten site, application of stone/seeds, multiple incisions over bite vicinity, attempt of induced vomiting, recitation by 'ozha' (Table 2).

| Example | Number of patient | percentage |
|---|---|---|
| Application of multiple ligature | 35 | 100 |
| Immobilization | 0 | 0 |
| Suction of bitten limb | 7 | 20 |
| Application of stone/seed | 6 | 17.14 |
| Incision at bite vicinity | 10 | 28.57 |
| Attempt of induced vomiting | 6 | 17.14 |
| Recitation by Ozha | 17 | 48.57 |

**Table 2:** Pre-hospital treatment (n =35).

## Clinical features

### Neurological manifestations

Most common neurological manifestation observed was ptosis of varying degrees, which was present in all patients (Table 3).

| Features | Number of patient | Percentage |
|---|---|---|
| Ptosis | 35 | 100 |
| External ophthalmoplegia | 33 | 94.2 |
| Broken neck sign | 28 | 80 |
| Dysphagia | 27 | 77.1 |
| Dysphonia/nasal voice | 24 | 68.5 |
| Weakness of grip | 23 | 65.7 |
| Depressed reflexes | 9 | 25.7 |

**Table 3:** Neurological features (n=35).

The next common was external ophthalmoplegia. Others were broken neck sign (weakness of neck muscles), dysphonia particularly nasal Voice, dysphagia, weakness of grip, inability to open mouth, depressed reflexes, generalized weakness. Patients presented in primary care hospital with sign and symptoms of neurotoxicity and referred with documentation were also entered in the data process. Three patients presented with unconsciousness in SBSC were seen in primary health care with ptosis, opthalmoplegia, dysphonia, dysphagia etc and were referred early for management. All patients had some amount of weakness of limb muscles.

### Chest movement

Chest movement was diminished in 7 patients of whom five patients developed complete respiratory paralysis and needed artificial ventilator support.

### Features of local bite area

On local examination, typical double fang marks were found in 20 patients and single fang mark in the 13 patients. The affected area was tender in all cases, hot in 23 cases (65.71%) and the limb was swollen in 26 (74.28%). In 18 cases enlarge and tender local lymph nodes were palpable (Figure 1).

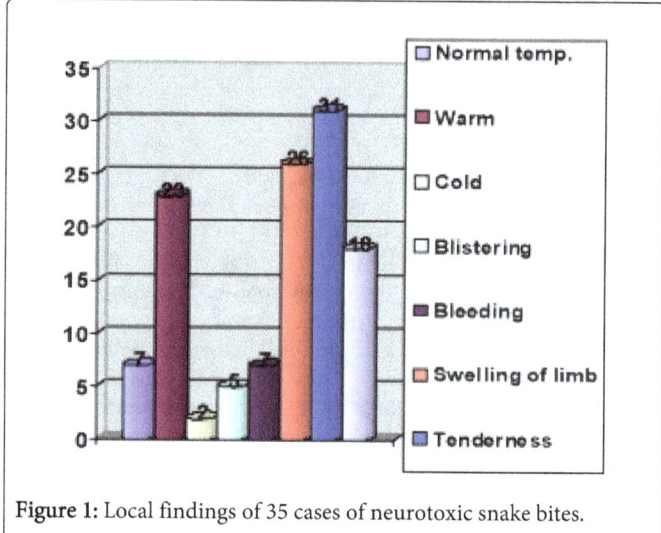

**Figure 1:** Local findings of 35 cases of neurotoxic snake bites.

## Investigations

Regarding investigations 23 patients had neutrophil leukocytosis (Table 4).

| Investigation | Number of patient | Percentage |
|---|---|---|
| Polymorph leukocytosis | 23 | 65.7 |
| Urinary albumin | 19 | 54.2 |
| Abnormal ECG | 2 | 5.7 |
| 20 min. WBCT abnormal | 35 | 0 |

**Table 4:** Investigations findings (n=35) of Neurotoxic snakebite cases.

Urinary albumin was found in 54% cases. Bedside 20-min. whole blood clotting test was normal in all cases indicating no coagulation abnormality. ECG was abnormal only in two patients.

## Identification of snakes

The offending snakes were identified in 15 cases; the snake was Monocellate Cobra (*Naja kaouthia*) in all those cases. Nine patients could bring the snake and six patients could identify the offending snake by seeing the photograph of Cobra. The identification process of brought snake, photograph or preserved specimen did not identify the other 20 snakes. The victims saw snakes in brief period in those cases and it could be either cobra or krait.

## Treatment

All enrolled patients were treated with polyvalent antivenom. The criteria for antivenom administration were one or more neurological manifestations. Single doses (10 vials) in saline solution were given initially to all patients and 3 patients needed 2nd dose of antivenom due to lack of response.

## Auxiliary treatment

Along with anti-snake venom the anticholinesterase Neostigmine was given to all patients. Five patients required artificial ventilation for variable duration.

## Anti-venom reaction (Type)

31 cases developed one or many anaphylactic reactions. Among them 20 patient developed early anaphylactic reactions, 25 patient developed pyrogenic reaction and 14 patient developed both anaphylactic and pyrogenic reaction.

## Anaphylactic reaction

In these series 20 patients out of 35 developed anaphylactic reaction in different ways. Most cases (16 patients) presented with urticaria with itching. The next common presentation was nausea and vomiting (8 patient). The same number of patient (8) was also have vigorous presentation with bronchospasm which was clinically presented with wheeze, rhonchi, crepitation etc. Only 2 patient developed angioedema in this series. The other uncommon presentation was with cough (3 pt), headache (2 pt), fever (3pt), tachycardia and palpitation (2 pt).

## Time of recovery

After anti-venom therapy, time required to recover from neurological manifestations ranged from 0.5 hour to 48 hours with a median of 4 hours (Figure 2).

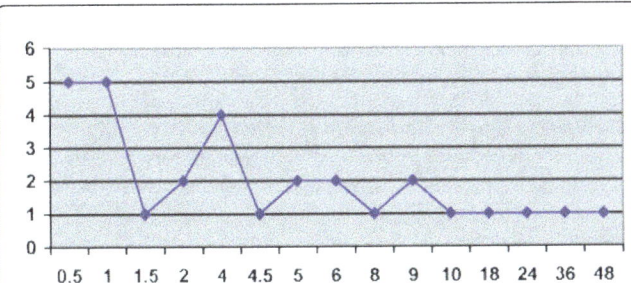

**Figure 2:** Time of recovery (in hours) from neurological features after A/V therapy.

## Outcome of treatment

In this series 34 cases of neurological manifestation were completely recovered. There was a single case with persistent neurological sequelae. There was no death in this study group of patient.

## Discussion

The age of the patients range from 3.5 years to 85 years. Most of the victims were between 5-30 years of age comprised (70%). It indicates that, growing and active parts of the society are bitten by the snakes [12,13]. Males are higher than the females as they are in special risk of out-side activity especially during cultivating and harvesting seasons. Thus this is an occupational hazard of young and active males especially those who work in hilly area and forest [12,13].

All the patients bitten by snakes with neurotoxic envenomation in our study showed a similar pattern of neurological manifestations. Two outstanding and severe clinical effects were noted in the present series. First was neuromuscular curare like effects, esp. the effect on respiratory muscles which frequently led to breathing failure and second was its necrotic effect on skin and subcutaneous tissue around the bite site, which in many cases resulted in wide slough lesions.

When the time of onset of the paralysis (Blurring vision, double vision, difficulty in swallowing or opening mouth etc all indicate commencement of muscle paralysis) could be reasonably determined (35 patients) the average time between the bite and the development of symptoms attributable to the paralysis was 4 ½ hours, with a range 1 to 10 hours. The overt neuroparalysis with many features developed 45 min to 10 hours after the first symptom of envenomation, indicating that there was a significant latent period between the first evidence of the absorption of venom and the development of paralysis. This study is consistent with the study of study in Thailand [14] where the interval was 8 hours and Campbell, C. H in which the interval was 5 ½ hours [15]. So it can be said that the envenoming process takes time to develop (hours) and there is a latent period between interaction with snake and gross neuroparalysis.

The first sign of neurotoxicity is ptosis (incomplete or complete) with external ophthalmoplegia in most cases in this study (100% for ptosis and 94.2% for ophthalmoplegia) showed that the paralysis always appears first in the muscles supplied by the cranial nerves, usually in the external ocular muscles or the muscles which elevate the upper eye lids. This observation is also consistent with the study in Thailand by Mitrakul C. where ptosis predominantly presented in 63% of cases [14] and study in Papua by Campbell CH [15]. The next common sign observed in this series was dysphagia 27 patients (77.1%) and dysphonia 24 patients (68.5%), which indicate the relatively early involvement of muscles of tongue, palate, pharynx and jaw rather than limbs or chest muscles [16]. The pooling of secretion and inability to open or close the mouth is frequently observed in this series, which also dictates the statement to be a correct one. 28 patients in this series showed broken neck sign (80%), which was associated with weak neck flexion in most of the patients. Weakness of grip was seen in 23 of the cases (65.7%) and loss or depressed of deep reflex was seen in only 9 cases (25.7%). The huge involvement of neck muscle explained the traditional belief of sequential muscle paralysis is not true rather several muscles group are frequently involved together [15,17]. In the clinico-epidemiological study done by Faiz et al. in 1999 in CMCH, the neurological manifestations among the venomous bites were similar to this study. Diminished chest movement were present in 7 cases out of whom 5 patients (14.2%) developed severe respiratory paralysis requiring artificial ventilatory support for variable duration (Ranged from 1hour to 48 hours with a median of 15 hours). In this group, two patients (both female of middle age) presented with apnoea as well as imperceptible pulse and blood pressure. Sensory function was intact in all cases except three, who were unconscious at presentation as well. Consciousness level was all right in rest of the cases even when they were under ventilator. It suggests that the neurotoxic venom acts mainly on peripheral nervous system [17].

In this study, commonest (70%) abnormal laboratory result during first few days after bite was mild to moderate leukocytosis with neutrophilia. Raised serum CPK was found in 50% cases with most of them had tight tourniquet for long duration suggesting muscle damage by pressure effect. ECG was abnormal in 5 cases. One female middle-aged patient had fast atrial fibrillation, which persisted later. This AF might have present from beforehand. Another female patient of 50 years had some ECG features of hypokalaemia. It was confirmed by doing serum electrolyte levels where serum potassium was 3.3

mmol/L. This may be due to imbalance in I/V fluid infusion. In other 3 cases there were features of partial Right Bundle Branch Block. The normal 20 min. whole blood clotting test in all cases confirmed that there was no clotting disturbance, which is consistent with Elapid bites of our country.

Identification of an offending snake is not very easy, because the incident is very sudden and mostly accidental and in most cases happens in dark bushy areas or at night. In spite of above facts, in this study offending snake was identified in 15 cases (42%), all were Mono-cellate Cobra (*Naja kauthia*). In nine cases the party brought the snake along with them-7 dead and 2 alive. Other 6 patients described the snake specifically and identified the snakes by seeing photographs. All these 15 cases of definitive cobra bite also had features of local envenoming (pain, swelling, and necrosis) along with neurotoxicity. Among the unidentified cases, twelve patients had exactly similar features; thus they would be cobra bite as well. Remaining 8 cases had no/minimal features of local envenomation and possibly they could be due to krait bite. Thus it can be simply said that most common venomous snake with neurological manifestations in this region is monocellate cobra, *Naja kauthia*.

All patients of this study were treated with Haffkine's polyvalent anti-venom. This anti-venom is effective against envenomation by Cobra, Krait, Russell's viper and Saw-scaled viper. A single dose of A/V consists of 10 vials (each-10 mg). Most of the patients respond to single dosage of A/V. In 3 cases, second dose was needed as they did not show any improvement (even deterioration occurred) after 2-3 hours of first dose. Definitive improvement was observed after 2nd dose. Only one patient who required two doses of A/V that were given at 3-4 hours interval had neurological sequelae. The number of doses required was not proportionate to the time between bite and hospitalization. Two patients required two doses even they were admitted within 2-3 hours of bite. On the other hand, one patient, who was admitted 23 hours after the bite, responded very well to single dose. May be the amount of injected during bites and reversibility of binding of venom with neuromuscular junction play the main role. All patients of this study also received anticholinesterase-Neostigmine for variable duration depending upon the severity of neurotoxicity. This was proved to be very much effective [18,19] especially when there was impending respiratory failure as evident by diminished chest movement.

Respiratory failure, the most ominous sign (present in 5 pts) in this study was consistently heralded by other milder neuromuscular changes. Nonetheless, in many cases apnea had quite an early onset, as early as 2.5 hours after the bite. This was also observed by Mitrakul et al. [14]. Victims of cobra bite or suspected victims should therefore be observed closely for neurological signs immediately after the bite and for at least 24 hours, regardless of the severity of the early local changes. Mechanical ventilation was required in 5 patients; the duration ranged from 1 hour to 48 hours. All these patients could die of snakebite without the facility of artificial ventilation. Therefore, facilities for endotracheal intubation and artificial ventilation are mandatory for total and comprehensive management of neurotoxic snake bite.

As the anti-venom that was used was horse serum, A/V reaction was very common. But all reactions could be managed easily with recommended regimen as requires [19]. It indicates that, frequent A/V reactions should not be taken as frightening thing and A/V therapy must be given in all cases where indicated.

All patients survived after effective management. Complete recovery was observed in 34 cases, the recovery time (from neurotoxicity) ranging from 0.5 hour to 48 hour with a median of 4 hours. Only one patient recovered after getting 2 doses of A/V with some distinctive neurological sequel in the form of generalized tonic-clonic seizure, myoclonus, cerebellar and extrapyramidal features. These features persisted months after his discharge (till last follow-up). CT scan and MRI of brain were done but no definitive lesion could be detected. Consultation was done with expertise and it was inferred that these sequel are due to hypoxic brain damage, which occurred during the brief period of apnea before starting mechanical ventilation.

## Conclusion

Although most of the snake bite is nonvenomous, it is important to differentiate it from venomous snake bite that needs immediate attention and specific management. The venomous snake bite may present with local or systemic envenoming in the form of neurotoxicity, vasculotoxicity, myotoxicity, cardiotoxicity etc. The neurotoxic snake bite with respiratory paralysis is the prime cause of death in venomous bite in Bangladesh.

The Elapidae group of snakes are (especially cobra and krait) the neurotoxic with or without local envenoming in our country. The neurotoxic features are ptosis, external ophthalmoplegia, broken neck sign, dysphagia, dysphonia, weakness, depressed reflex which can lead to fatal respiratory paralysis. Although the identification of snake is sometimes troublesome there is 'Syndromic Approach' to ameliorating the problem. Handling the snake is dangerous but it is wise and helpful for management if the dead specimen is brought to the health facility.

The diagnosis is straightforward if there is gross neurotoxicity and the specimen is brought in front. Although laboratory investigation is nonspecific, ELISA method to detect and analysis the venom components is matter of huge interest to medical scientist. Venom antigenimia, electrophysiology, histopathology, genetics etc all are currently involved in diagnosis and management of snake bite.

## Acknowledgements

The authors gratefully acknowledge the kind support of all members of the health professionals of the study hospitals for management of the cases.

## References

1. WHO (1981) progress in the characterization of venoms and standardization of antivenoms Geneva: World Health Organization.

2. Harvey AL, Banfaraz A, Thomas E, Faiz MA, Preston S, et al. (1994) Screening of snake venoms for neurotoxic and myotoxic effects using simple in vitro preparations from rodents and chicks. Toxicon 32: 257-266.

3. Barfaraz A, Harvey AL (1994) The use of the chick biventer cervicis preparation to assess the protective activity of six international reference antivenoms on the neuromuscular effects of snake venoms in vitro. Toxicon 32: 267-272.

4. Theakston RDG, Reid HA (1983) Development of simple standard assay procedures for the characterization of snake venoms. Bull World Health Organ 61: 949-956.

5. Khan MAR, Sareesrip Prani (1987) Bangladesher Bannya Prani Dhaka. Bangla Academy 42:168.

6. Wüster W, Thorpe RS (1991) Asiatic cobras: systematics and snakebite. Experientia 47: 205-209.

7. Faiz MA, Raman MR, Das JC (1994) Neurotoxicity and tissue necrosis following bite by cobra (Naja). Dhaka Congress.

8. Warrell DA (1989) Snake venoms in science and clinical medicine. 1. Russell's viper: biology, venom and treatment of bites. Trans R Soc Trop Med Hyg 83: 732-740.

9. Minton SA (1990) Neurotoxic snake envenoming. Semin Neurol 10: 52-61.

10. Chippaux JP, Williams V, White J (1991) Snake venom variability: methods of study, results and interpretation. Toxicon 29: 1279-1303.

11. Silamut K, Ho M, Looareesuwan S, Viravan C, Wuthiekanun V, et al. (1987) Detection of venom by enzyme linked immunosorbent assay (ELISA) in patients bitten by snakes in Thailand. Br Med J (Clin Res Ed) 294: 402-404.

12. Devkota UN, Steinmann JP, Shah LN (2000) Snake bite in Nepal- A study from Sihara district. Journal of Nepal Medical Association 39: 203-209.

13. Islam QT, Azhar MA, Ekram ARMS (1999) Snake bite in the northern Bangladesh: a hospital based study of 68 cases. Taj 12: 135-138.

14. Mitrakul C, Dhamkrong-At A, Futrakul P, Thisyakorn C, Vongsrisart K, et al. (1984) Clinical features of neurotoxic snake bite and response to antivenom in 47 children. Am J Trop Med Hyg 33: 1258-1266.

15. Campbell CH (1969) A clinical study of venomous snake bite in Papua.

16. Sethi PK, Rastogi JK (1981) Neurological aspects of ophitoxemia (Indian krait)- A clinico-electromyographic study. Indian J Med Res 73: 269-276.

17. CAMPBELL CH (1964) Venomous Snake Bite in Papua and its Treatment with Tracheotomy, Artificial Respiration and Antivenene. Trans R Soc Trop Med Hyg 58: 263-273.

18. Theakston RD, Phillips RE, Warrell DA, Galagedera Y, Abeysekera DT, et al. (1990) Envenoming by the common krait (Bungarus caeruleus) and Sri Lankan cobra (Naja naja naja): efficacy and complications of therapy with Haffkine antivenom. Trans R Soc Trop Med Hyg 84: 301-308.

19. Sutherland SK (1992) Antivenom use in Australia. Premedication, adverse reactions and the use of venom detection kits. Med J Aust 157: 734-739.

18

# Oral Glycine and Sodium Thiosulfate for Lethal Cyanide Ingestion

Matthew Brenner[1,2], Sarah M Azer[1], Kyung-Jin Oh[3], Chang Hoon Han[4], Jangwoen Lee[1], Sari B Mahon[1], Xiaohua Du[5], David Mukai[1], Tanya Burney[1], Mayer Saidian[1,6*], Adriano Chan[7], Derek I Straker[7], Vikhyat S Bebarta[8] and Gerry R Boss[7]

[1]Beckman Laser Institute, University of California, Irvine, California, USA

[2]Division of Pulmonary and Critical Care Medicine, Department of Medicine, University of California, Irvine, California, USA

[3]Department of Urology, Chonnam National University Medical School, South Korea

[4]Department of Internal Medicine, National Health Insurance Service Ilsan Hospital, Goyang-si, Geonggi-do, South Korea

[5]Pulmonary Department, The First Affiliated Hospital of Kunming Medical University, Kunming, Yunnan, China

[6]The Institute for Drug Research, School of Pharmacy, Hebrew University of Jerusalem, Jerusalem Israel

[7]Department of Medicine, University of California, San Diego, La Jolla, CA, USA

[8]Department of Emergency Medicine, University of Colorado School of Medicine, Aurora, CO, USA

*Corresponding author: Mayer Saidian, Beckman Laser Institute, University of California, Irvine, California, USA, E-mail: msaidian@uci.edu

## Abstract

**Objective:** Accidental or intentional cyanide ingestion is an-ever present danger. Rapidly acting, safe, inexpensive oral cyanide antidotes are needed that can neutralize large gastrointestinal cyanide reservoirs. Since humans cannot be exposed to cyanide experimentally, we studied oral cyanide poisoning in rabbits, testing oral sodium thiosulfate with and without gastric alkalization.

**Setting:** University research laboratory.

**Subjects:** New Zealand white rabbits.

**Interventions:** Seven animal groups studied; Groups 1-5 received high dose oral NaCN (50 mg, >LD100) and were treated immediately with oral (*via* nasogastric tube): 1) saline, 2) glycine, 3) sodium thiosulfate or 4) sodium thiosulfate and glycine, or 5) after 2 min with intramuscular injection of sodium nitrite and sodium thiosulfate plus oral sodium thiosulfate and glycine. Groups 6-7 received moderate dose oral NaCN (25 mg, LD70) and delayed intramuscular 6) saline or 7) sodium nitrite-sodium thiosulfate.

**Measurements and Main Results:** All animals in the high dose NaCN group receiving oral saline or glycine died very rapidly, with a trend towards delayed death in glycine-treated animals; saline *versus* glycine-treated animals died at 10.3+3.9 and 14.6+5.9 min, respectively (p=0.13). In contrast, all sodium thiosulfate-treated high dose cyanide animals survived (p<0.01), with more rapid recovery in animals receiving both thiosulfate and glycine, compared to thiosulfate alone (p<0.03). Delayed intramuscular treatment alone in the moderate cyanide dose animals increased survival over control animals from 30% to 71%. Delayed treatment in high dose cyanide animals was not as effective as immediate treatment, but did increase survival time and rescued 29% of animals (p<0.01 *versus* cyanide alone).

**Conclusions:** Oral sodium thiosulfate with gastric alkalization rescued animals from lethal doses of ingested cyanide. The combination of oral glycine and sodium thiosulfate may have potential for treating high dose acute cyanide ingestion and merits further investigation. The combination of systemic and oral therapy may provide further options.

**Keywords:** Oral cyanide poisoning; Sodium thiosulfate; Gastric alkalization; Continuous wave near infrared spectroscopy; Glycine

**Abbreviations:** CWNIRS: Continuous Wave Near Infrared Spectroscopy; OxyHb: Oxyhemoglobin; DeoxyHb: Deoxyhemoglobin.

## Introduction

Cyanide is highly toxic, and exposures can result from accidental or intentional causes, including inhalation or ingestion from industrial processes, chemical weapons, terrorism, or suicidal acts [1-5]. Acute and chronic dietary cyanide ingestion occurs in third-world countries where consumption of unprocessed crops, including cassava, leads to significant oral cyanide exposure [6].

Regardless of exposure method, death from acute cyanide poisoning is usually rapid, within minutes from inhalation, and within minutes to hours following oral ingestion [7]. A major mechanism of cyanide toxicity is inhibition of cytochrome c oxidase, a key component of complex IV of the mitochondrial electron transport system. This induces cellular hypoxia, leading to seizures, respiratory depression, cardiac arrhythmias, and cardiovascular collapse, with characteristic elevation of plasma lactate and venous oxygen concentrations [4].

Acute toxicity from oral cyanide ingestion is dose dependent, but other factors such as solubility of the ingested cyanide or cyanogenic compound and presence of food in the gastrointestinal tract can affect clinical severity and time until death [4]. The current recommendation for treating acute oral cyanide poisoning is to neutralize absorbed cyanide by intravenously administered drugs such as hydroxocobalamin, nitrites, and sodium thiosulfate, in addition to supportive care. No treatment exists for preventing absorption of the large gastrointestinal reservoir of cyanide that may be present following ingestion. Historical treatments for acutely ingested poisons included induction of vomiting and/or gastrointestinal lavage, with limited effectiveness. Inefficiency of gastric emptying, rapid onset of seizures, loss of consciousness, and aspiration risks has led to abandoning these approaches for oral cyanide poising. Thus, treatments that directly neutralize ingested cyanide within the gastrointestinal (GI) tract are needed.

Sodium thiosulfate acts as a sulfur donor for the enzyme rhodanese, which transfers the sulfur to cyanide generating thiocyanate, a relatively non-toxic product [5,8-10]. At high concentrations, thiosulfate is absorbed from the GI tract [11,12], and, under certain conditions, thiosulfate can react non-enzymatically with cyanide to generate thiocyanate [13,14]. Thus, oral/enteral thiosulfate could potentially neutralize cyanide in the GI tract, as well as metabolize systemically absorbed cyanide. Since sodium thiosulfate is inexpensive, and has minimal toxicity [15], large quantities could be administered enterally.

On exposure to acidic gastric conditions, ingested cyanide ion is rapidly converted to hydrogen cyanide gas due to its pKa of 9.3 and boiling point of 26.3°C. Thus, cyanide is likely absorbed as hydrogen cyanide gas, rather than as cyanide ion [16], and cyanide gas in gastric or intestinal bubbles (as opposed to dissolved gas) may be less accessible to neutralizing antidotes within the GI tract. We hypothesized that raising gastric pH with an orally administered buffer should maintain cyanide primarily as cyanide ion, thus delaying systemic absorption. At a pH above 10.3, >90% of ingested cyanide would be in the ionized form. We recently showed we could rescue rabbits from a lethal dose of oral cyanide using the combination of oral cobinamide and sodium carbonate [17]. However, cobinamide is relatively expensive, is absorbed from the GI tract and has some toxicity when administered parenterally at high doses, and is not FDA approved. Furthermore, while sodium carbonate is an effective and safe buffer, large volumes of $CO_2$ gas form when added to the acidic stomach. This creates a large gas "headspace" where hydrogen cyanide gas may not be as accessible for neutralization. Glycine is also an effective buffer at high pH, but does not generate gas on exposure to acid. Human ingestion of up to 31 g of glycine per day is without serious side effects [18,19]. Thus, we proposed that glycine would be an ideal agent to raise gastric pH to delay cyanide absorption.

Our primary aim is to develop safe and inexpensive methods for treating oral cyanide poisoning. For developing cyanide antidotes, animal studies are equivalent to human clinical trials, since efficacy cannot be tested in humans, and FDA approval is based solely on animal experiments. Some victims of oral cyanide ingestion may be asymptomatic shortly following ingestion, or it may be unknown if ingestion actually occurred, particularly in mass exposure situations. For asymptomatic patients or unexposed persons who think they were exposed, treatment must be safe and inexpensive and preferably by the oral route. Patients who are unconscious or severely symptomatic may require combined systemic and enteral antidote treatment. To investigate this range of possible exposure and severity scenarios, we used lethal rabbit models of moderate and high dose oral cyanide ingestion, assessing survival, physiologic parameters, and metabolic effects of cyanide; the latter were monitored using continuous wave near infrared spectroscopy [20-25]. We found that high dose oral thiosulfate is effective in lethal oral cyanide poisoning.

## Materials and Methods

### Animal preparation

Pathogen free New Zealand White rabbits from 3.5 to 4.5 g were used. All procedures were reviewed and approved by the Institutional Animal Care Committee of the University of California, Irvine. Each rabbit was deprived of food for at least 16 h and water for 3 h prior to the experiment. An Elizabethan collar was placed to prevent coprophagy during the 16 h pre-treatment period.

Animals were anesthetized with a 2: 1 Ketamine HCl (100 mg/ml, Ketaject, Phoenix Pharmaceutical Inc., St. Joseph, MI): Xylazine (20 mg/ml, Anased, Lloyd Laboratories, Shenandoah, IA) intramuscular injection. A 23 gauge 1-inch catheter was then inserted in the marginal ear vein for intravenous access. The animals were intubated using a 3.5 mm cuffed endotracheal tube, which was connected to a Bickford non-rebreathing circuit. Animals continuously inhaled a mixture of 1.5-2.5% isoflurane and room air through an Ohmeda V.M.C anesthesia machine. A 14 French naso-tracheal suctioning catheter connected to a three-way stopcock was introduced through the mouth into the stomach. Position was confirmed by auscultation of injected air and withdrawal of gastric fluid contents. Heart rate and oxygen saturation ($SpO_2$) were monitored through a pulse oximeter (Biox 3700 Pulse Oximeter, Ohmeda, Boulder, CO) ear probe (Datex-Ohmeda TS-E4-H) placed on the animal's cheek. Respiratory rate, end tidal $CO_2$, and end tidal $O_2$ were monitored through a Datex Ohmeda, General Electric, S/5 Patient Monitor connected to the endotracheal tube. The femoral artery and vein in the left groin were isolated by blunt dissection, and catheterized with 12 inch, 18 g catheters (C-PMA-400-FA, Cook Inc, Bloomington, IN), with three-way stopcocks connected to each catheter. Blood pressure was measured by a calibrated pressure transducer (TSD104A Transducer and MP100 WSW System Biopac Systems, Inc., Santa Barbara, CA) connected to the arterial line.

### Gastric fluid sampling

Gastric fluid was sampled at baseline, after sodium thiosulfate and glycine administration, and at 2.5, 7.5, 15, 30, 45, and 60 min post sodium cyanide installation.

### Blood sampling and data Collection

Cyanide analysis, blood gasses, $SpO_2$, and metabolic data were obtained from blood samples collected at baseline, at the time of cyanide administration, and at 2.5, 5, 10, 15, 30, 45, and 60 min post cyanide administration. Blood pressure was monitored continuously and recorded every minute for the first 10 min after cyanide installation, then every 15 min thereafter.

Animals that survived until 60 min post cyanide administration were considered to have survived and were euthanized with 1 cc of

Euthasol (390 mg Pentobarbital Sodium/50 mg Phenytoin Sodium) (Euthasol, Virbac AH, Inc., Fort Worth, Texas) administered through the marginal ear vein. Animals that died before 60 min were considered "non-survivors."

## Antidotes and reagents

For use in moderate and high dose cyanide experiments, 25 or 50 mg NaCN (Sigma-Aldrich), respectively, was dissolved in 10 ml of 0.9% saline (Revival Animal Health). Glycine (2 M, Sigma-Aldrich) was adjusted to pH 11 with 10 N NaOH, and 5 to 12 cc were given through the gastric tube in 2.5 cc increments to adjust stomach pH to >9. Averages of 7.5 cc of glycine were needed to reach the target stomach pH. Sodium thiosulfate pentahydrate (2.5 M, Sigma-Aldrich) was given orally (4 cc in 2 doses given 5 min apart) or by intramuscular injection (0.62 cc). Sodium nitrite (Sigma-Aldrich) was given intramuscularly as 0.32 cc of an 800 mM solution.

## Study design and treatment groups

Rabbits were divided into seven groups of seven animals per group, except the moderate cyanide dose group treated with saline (Group 6), where 10 animals were used. Thus, a total of 52 animals were studied.

Glycine was administered as a 2 M solution adjusted to pH 11 with NaOH; 5-12 cc (average: 7.5cc) were administered to achieve a gastric pH >9. Sodium thiosulfate was administered as two equal instillations of 4 cc of a 2.5 M solution, given five minutes apart after gastric alkalization, in groups 3 and 4. In the high dose delayed treatment Group 5, 30 cc of oral thiosulfate with 7.5 cc 2 M glycine plus simultaneous IM injections of 0.64 cc 2.5 M thiosulfate and 800 mM NaNO were administered after apnea onset or at 2 min post-cyanide exposure, whichever came first. In the moderate dose Group 7, simultaneous IM injections of 0.64 cc 2.5 M thiosulfate and 800 mM NaNO were administered immediately post-cyanide exposure.

The seven groups are as follows:

High Dose Cyanide (50 mg NaCN) with Simultaneous Oral Therapy

Group 1: Saline (control group),

Group 2: Glycine,

Group 3: Sodium thiosulfate,

Group 4: Glycine and sodium thiosulfate,

High Dose Cyanide (50 mg NaCN) with Delayed Oral and Intramuscular Therapy,

Group 5: Oral glycine and thiosulfate plus intramuscular nitrite-thiosulfate given at apnea or 2 minutes post ingestion, whichever came first,

Moderate Dose Cyanide (25 mg NaCN) with Delayed Intramuscular Therapy,

Group 6: Saline (control group),

Group 7: Intramuscular nitrite-thiosulfate given at apnea or 2 min post ingestion, whichever came first

Six of the 10 animals in Group 6 were previously used as controls and reported in a prior study of oral cobinamide treatment [17].

## CWNIRS measurements

The CWNIRS system was designed to optimize detection of a metabolic poison such as cyanide [26]. It consists of a light source (HL 2000, Ocean Optics, FL), a CCD spectrometer (BTC111E, B&WTek, DE), and customized optical fiber guides. It acquires a full spectrum of transmitted light (600~1000 nm) every second and collects light intensity values at five wavelengths (732, 758, 805, 840, 880 nm) to calculate changes in tissue oxyhemoglobin (OHb) and deoxyhemoglobin (RHb) using a modified Beer-Lamberts' law. The two wavelengths below 805 nm, an isosbestic point, have good sensitivity for detecting deoxyhemoglobin and the two wavelengths above the isosbestic point have good sensitivity for detecting oxyhemoglobin.

CWNIRS recovery times were compared to midpoint return of oxyhemoglobin toward baseline. Rate of return was analyzed by slope analysis from 25 to 75% of recovery from peak to baseline. Maximal change was determined from baseline to peak values.

## Measurement of Red Blood Cell (RBC) cyanide concentration

Cyanide in blood is bound almost exclusively to ferric (met) hemoglobin in RBCs; thus, the blood cyanide concentration can be measured by measuring cyanide in RBCs [27]. Whole blood collected from animals was immediately cooled to 4°C, centrifuged, and the plasma and RBC fractions separated. Samples were kept at 4°C and analyzed within 48 h. The RBCs were lysed in ice-cold water, and the lysates were placed into the outer compartment of a Conway micro-diffusion cell. A volume of 10% trichloroacetic acid equal to the lysate volume was also added to the outer compartment, and an alkalized cobinamide solution was added to the center compartment. The cell was capped, and the lysate was mixed with the tricholoracetic acid by gently tilting the chamber. The trichloroacetic acid denatures the hemoglobin and releases hydrogen cyanide gas, which was trapped in the cobinamide solution. The resulting dicyanocobinamide is measured spectrophotometrically as described previously [28]. Cyanide concentrations were determined from standard curves using freshly prepared KCN dissolved in 1 mM NaOH. Sample duplicates showed <15% variation.

## Measurement of plasma and gastric fluid thiocyanate concentration

Thiocyanate in the plasma was reduced to cyanide using potassium permanganate as described previously [29]. The resulting cyanide was measured as described above.

Samples of gastric fluid were withdrawn from the stomach *via* the nasogastric tube at baseline, after alkalization, and at 2.5, 7.5, 30, and 45 min post cyanide administration. Thiocyanate in the fluid was measured by adding samples to acidic ferric nitrate, which yields a yellow-orange product that can be quantified spectrophotometrically at 460 nm. The thiocyanate concentration was determined from standard curves, with sample duplicates showing < 15% variation.

## Measurement of cyanide reaction with sodium thiosulfate

We assessed reaction rates of sodium thiosulfate with sodium cyanide under conditions simulating the intragastric milieu, both under native conditions and after adding glycine buffer. Thus, we incubated 750 mM sodium thiosulfate with 40 mM NaCN at 37°C. We conducted the experiment at low and high pH (pH 2.0 and 10.0, respectively), and measured thiocyanate production over varying periods of time from 5 to 60 min using the acidic ferric nitrate reagent described above. We compared results to a standard curve of sodium thiocyanate.

## Statistical analysis

Survival time curves were compared by Kaplan Meier survival analysis (Systat Software, San Jose, CA) with significance calculated by log-rank (Mantel-Cox) tests (Prism 6 Software, Graphpad, Inc., La Jolla, CA), and overall survival assessed by a Chi-square analysis between individual groups with adjustment for multiple comparisons. Gastric pH, concentrations of cyanide and metabolites, and recovery rates across groups were compared by ANOVA with repeated measures (Systat Software, San Jose, CA).

## Power analysis

For the primary outcome variable of survival, power analysis yielded 6 animals per group in animals treated with high dose cyanide, if mortality is 100% in control animals and survival is >70% in treated animals, with two tailed $p < 0.05$ and beta error avoidance at >80%. CWNIRS recovery times were compared by time to midpoint return of oxyhemoglobin curves to baseline, and rate of return was analyzed by slope analysis comparison by ANOVA.

## Results

### Measurement of cyanide reaction with sodium thiosulfate

Cyanide can react directly with thiosulfate, generating thiocyanate, but relatively high concentrations of both reactants are needed and the reaction is favored under alkaline conditions [14,30]. We investigated whether the reaction could occur under conditions that simulated those of our *in vivo* experiments. We found that at pH 2, with 750 mM sodium thiosulfate and 40 mM NaCN, the rate of thiocyanate production was 20 nmol/min, whereas at pH 10, thiocyanate production was about eight-fold faster or 155 nmol/min.

### Gastric pH measurements

Gastric pH measurements were performed in the high dose cyanide animals at intervals pre- and post-cyanide exposure (Figure 1). All animals had baseline gastric pH <2. Group 1 animals (cyanide alone) died before serial gastric pH measurements could be made and are not shown in Figure 1.

Group 2 animals that received cyanide and glycine had sustained gastric pH values above 8 until death (mean pH range 9.6-10, following glycine and cyanide). Group 3 animals that received cyanide and sodium thiosulfate had low pH values initially (pH~1) that rose slowly to 3.8+0.3 at 60 min.

Group 4 animals administered glycine plus sodium thiosulfate and cyanide continued to have more alkaline pH in the stomach than group 3 animals, 9.7+0.3 after administration, but did have a gradual decrease in pH to 6.4+1.5 at 60 min (p<0.01 by ANOVA across groups).

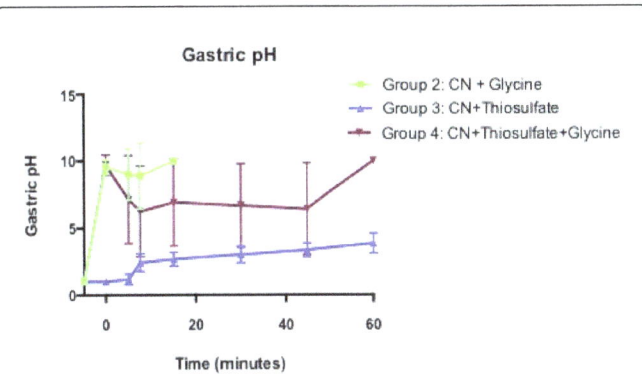

**Figure 1:** Gastric pH in the high dose cyanide treatment groups. Baseline pH was measured prior to instillation of drugs or cyanide. Time 0 is immediately following instillation of drugs and cyanide. Results are shown for Groups 2, 3, and 4. Group 1 animals (cyanide alone) did not survive long enough for multiple measurements. The increase in pH following glycine administration is significantly different from non-glycine-treated animals p<0.01 by ANOVA.

### Survival with high dose cyanide exposures

**Effect of High Dose Oral Cyanide (Group 1):** Animals in Group 1, receiving saline with high dose cyanide, survived an average of 10.3 ± 3.9 min (range 3 to 14 min, 95% CI 6.7 to 13.9) (Figure 2). All animals in Group 1 became apneic between 2 and 3.5 min post cyanide ingestion (mean 2.6+0.7 min, 95% CI 2.0-3.3 min). Thus, the model is rapidly and uniformly lethal (Figure 2).

**Effect of Glycine (Group 2):** Animals in Group 2, receiving glycine buffer with high dose cyanide, survived an average 14.6 ± 5.9 min (range 7.5-24, 95% CI 9.2 to 20.1 min) (Figure 2). Thus gastric alkalization prolonged time to death by ~40% (p=0.13 compared to Group 1 animals), but did not prevent death.

**Effect of Sodium Thiosulfate (Group 3):** Animals in Group 3, receiving oral sodium thiosulfate, recovered slowly as demonstrated by CWNIRS monitoring of oxy- and deoxyhemoglobin (see below), but all survived the 60 min experimental period (Figure 2; p<0.01 for survival compared to Groups 1 and 2).

**Effect of Glycine and Sodium Thiosulfate (Group 4):** Animals in Group 4, receiving glycine buffer and sodium thiosulfate, recovered quickly and survived the full 60 min (Figure 2); p<0.01 for survival compared to Groups 1 and 2.

**Delayed Combined Oral and Intramuscular Antidote Treatment (Group 5):** Group 5 animals were not treated until onset of apnea or at 2 min post-cyanide, when they were severely compromised clinically. Two of seven animals (29%) survived (Figure 2), and the median survival time increased from 10 to 32 min (Figure 2; p<0.01 for survival compared to Groups 1 and 2).

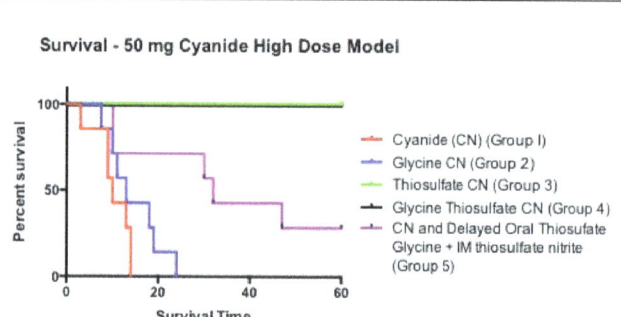

**Figure 2:** Survival Curves of High Dose Cyanide Groups. Group 1, cyanide alone and Group 2, cyanide plus glycine, animals all died. Group 3 animals receiving oral thiosulfate survived the full 60 min, as did Group 4 animals receiving glycine and sodium thiosulfate (compared to Group 1 and 2 animals, p<0.01 by Log-rank analysis). Of Group 5 animals receiving high dose cyanide followed by delayed intramuscular thiosulfate nitrite and oral thiosulfate plus glycine, 29% survived (p<0.01 compared to Group 1 and 2 animals).

## Blood cyanide and thiocyanate analysis

All animals had similar, low baseline blood cyanide concentrations (mean 2.9 μM, range 2.6 to 3.1 μM) (Figure 3 top), and plasma thiocyanate concentrations (mean 52.1 μM, range 49.3 to 53.6 μM) (Figure 3 middle).

Group 1 cyanide alone animals demonstrated a rapid increase in the blood cyanide concentration, which peaked at 72+15 μM at 5 min post cyanide instillation (Figure 3 top). In contrast to the large rise in cyanide concentrations, Group 1 animals exhibited only a small rise in plasma thiocyanate concentrations, peaking at 57.2+4.7 μM at 10 min post exposure (Figure 3 middle), consistent with minimal conversion of cyanide to thiocyanate in this group.

Group 2 animals, receiving glycine and cyanide, exhibited a slower rise in blood cyanide concentrations compared to Group 1 animals, yielding 31.5+6 μM at 5 min, but the cyanide concentration continued to rise until expiration, with a mean concentration of 52.2+15 at 15 min (Figure 3 top). Similar to Group 1 animals, Group 2 animals showed no significant change in thiocyanate concentrations, yielding 53.6+4.8 μM at 10 min (Figure 3 middle) (p=NS compared to CN controls), again consistent with limited conversion of cyanide to thiocyanate.

Group 3 animals, receiving sodium thiosulfate, and group Group 4 animals, receiving both glycine and sodium thiosulfate, exhibited a similar initial rise in the blood cyanide concentration. In both these groups, the blood cyanide concentration peaked by 15 min and began to fall subsequently. The blood cyanide concentration was statistically lower in Group 3 and 4 animals compared to Group 1 animals (p<0.01).

The thiocyanate concentration in Group 3 and 4 animals increased at a rate significantly greater than that of Group 1 and 2 animals, consistent with increased conversion of cyanide to thiocyanate in these groups. During the first 10 min following cyanide ingestion (corresponding to when rapid clinical deterioration occurs in control animals), the plasma thiocyanate concentration rose significantly faster in Group 4 than Group 3 animals, pointing to a beneficial effect of the

glycine: at baseline, Group 3 and 4 animals had equivalent plasma thiocyanate concentrations [50.1+3.1 (95% CI 42 to 58) and 53.6+4.2 μM (95% CI 48 to 59), respectively], but at 5 min, corresponding concentrations were 95.6+8.0 (95% CI 76 to 116) and 130.0+11.1 μM (95% CI 116 to 144), and at 10 min, they were 119+7 (95% CI 101 to 138) and 129+10 μM (95% CI 116 to 141) (p<0.02 ANOVA with repeated measures).

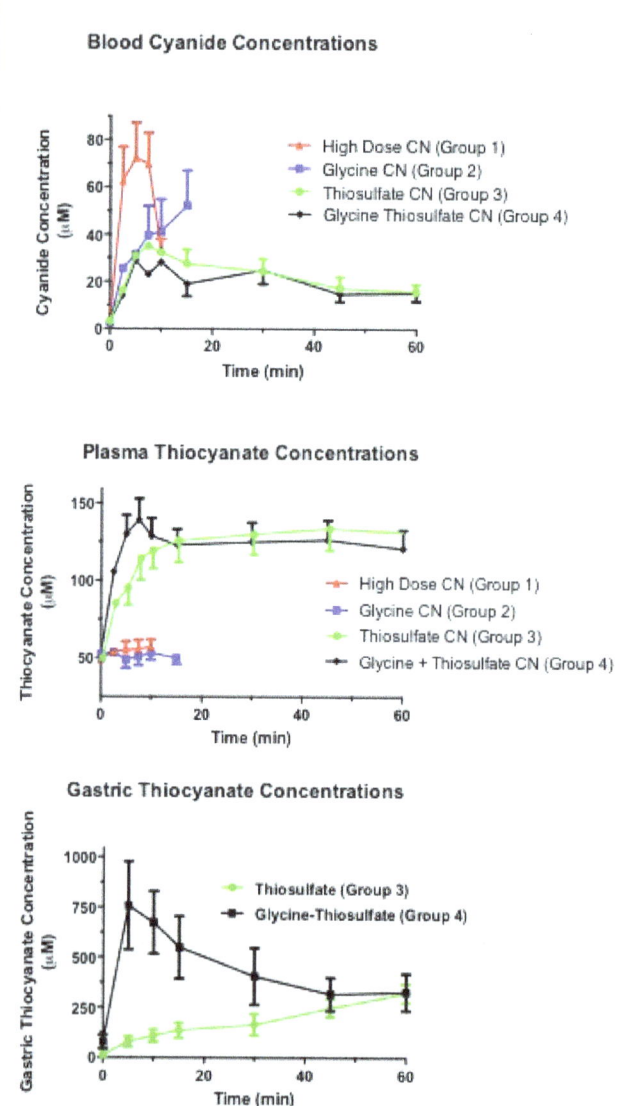

**Figure 3:** Blood, plasma and gastric cyanide and thiocyanate concentrations: The blood cyanide concentration rose rapidly in control animals (Group 1 cyanide alone), and all expired by 15 min. In Group 2 animals (cyanide plus glycine), the rate of cyanide absorption was significantly lower, but continued to climb until death. In Group 3 and 4 animals receiving sodium thiosulfate or sodium thiosulfate plus glycine, the cyanide concentration rose at the same rate as glycine alone (Group 2 animals), but leveled off and began to decrease by 10 min post ingestion.

## Gastric thiocyanate

We measured the gastric fluid thiocyanate concentration in Group 3 and 4 animals, and found it rose very rapidly in the Group 4 animals from 78+59 at baseline to 758+219 µM by 5 min post ingestion (Figure 3 bottom). This is in contrast to a smaller increase in the Group 3 animals, from 13+7µM at baseline to 80+53 µM at 5 min (p<0.05 ANOVA with repeated measures comparing Group 4 to Group 3), demonstrating greater gastric conversion of cyanide to thiocyanate in alkaline conditions *in-vivo*.

## Rate of recovery in surviving animal groups - CWNIRS analysis

We continuously monitored oxygenated hemoglobin (OxyHb) and deoxygenated hemoglobin (DeoxyHb) by CWNIRS over the brain region. In Group 1 and 2 animals, the oxy hemoglobin concentration rose initially for a brief period, then decreased rapidly as the animals expired from cyanide poisoning. The deoxy hemoglobin concentration also rose briefly, but then fell in the terminal phases and tissue blood voume decreased (serial data not shown due to rapid death).

Base excess graph showing changes beginning immediately following ingestion of cyanide in four rabbit groups. Group 1 rabbits administered cyanide alone died rapidly, before 15 min blood gas measurements could be obtained. In Group 2 animals receiving glycine and cyanide, rapid decrease in base excess developed prior to death. Group 3 animals administered sodium thiosulfate with cyanide, showed a rapid sustained decrease in base excess. Group 4 animals that received both sodium thiosulfate and glycine had a gradual mild decrease in base excess following cyanide ingestion (p<0.03 compared to Group 3, ANOVA with repeated measures).

In Group 3 and 4 animals, the OxyHb concentration rose initially as cyanide was absorbed and animals became progressively unable to extract oxygen from the tissues, but it returned relatively quickly to baseline values in the Group 4 animals. The time to recovery was significantly faster in Group 4 animals averaging 2.4+5.4 min, compared to group 3 animals 17.1+1.9 min (p<0.05) (Figure 4, top).

## Base excess

Base excess is reduced quickly in this model due to cyanide-induced lactic acid production. Base excess was equivalent in all groups at baseline (mean 2.6+3.0 mmol/L, 95% CI 1.4 to 3.1 mmol/L; p>0.7 across groups; Figure 4, bottom). Base excess rapidly decreased in Group 2 animals to (-)5+0.9 mmol/l (95% CI: (-)3.6 to (-)6.4 mmol/L) at 15 min (p<0.01 compared to baseline). Group 3 animals also showed a significant decrease in base excess to (-) 4.9+3.2 mmol/L (95% CI (-)1 to (-9) mmol/L) by 15 min, with a further progressive decrease over the 60 min study period to (-)9.6+2.9 mmol/L (95% CI (-)5 to (-)11) (p<001 compared to baseline). In contrast, in Group 4 animals, base excess decreased at a more gradual rate to 0.9+2.6 mmol/L (95% CI: 1.9 to (-)3.6 mmol/L) at 45 min, and (-)2.7+3.0 mmol/L (95% CI: 07 to (-)4.9 mmol/L) at 60 min (Figure 4 ) (p=0.01 compared to group 3 animals ANOVA with repeated measures).

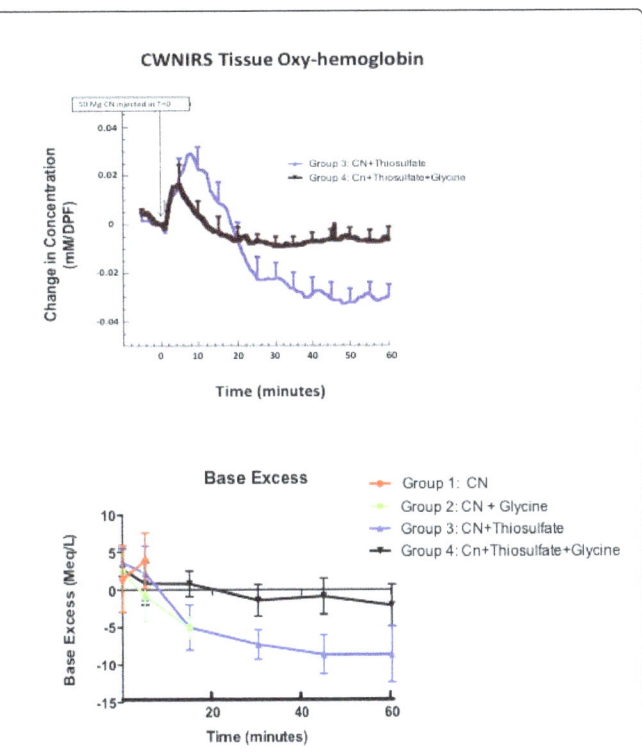

**Figure 4:** Rate of recovery–CWNIRS and Base Excess, CWNIRS composite curves show changes in brain oxyhemoglobin concentration immediately following ingestion of cyanide in the rabbit groups that recovered. Group 3 animals that received sodium thiosulfate with cyanide had a slower recovery time to baseline than Group 4 animals that received both sodium thiosulfate and glycine (p<0.05).

## Blood pressure

Baseline blood pressures were similar in all groups, with a mean arterial pressure (MAP) of 45+10 mmHg (95% CI 41-48). The MAP did not differ significantly between Group 3 and Group 4 animals at any time point, gradually decreasing to 31+8 mmHg (95% CI 30-58 mmHg) and 36+10 mmHg (95% CI 26-45 mmHg) at 60 min in Group 3 and 4 animals, respectively (p>0.5).

## Delayed treatment in moderate cyanide dose poisoning

In order to investigate delayed antidote administration and intramuscular administration, the efficacy of intramuscular administration alone was studied in animals using lower dose oral cyanide ingestions (since intramuscular injection alone was previously found not to rescue animals receiving 50 mg of cyanide).

Thirty percent of Group 6 animals that received 25 mg of cyanide and were treated with intramuscular saline placebo survived, with a median survival time of 21 min (compared to 10 min for Group 1 animals that received 50 mg cyanide) (Figure 5, p<0.001, Log-rank for difference between the Group 6 and Group 1). Of Group 7 animals that received delayed intramuscular injection of sodium nitrite and sodium thiosulfate after CN ingestion, 71% survived (p<0.05 compared to Group 6 animals; Figure 5).

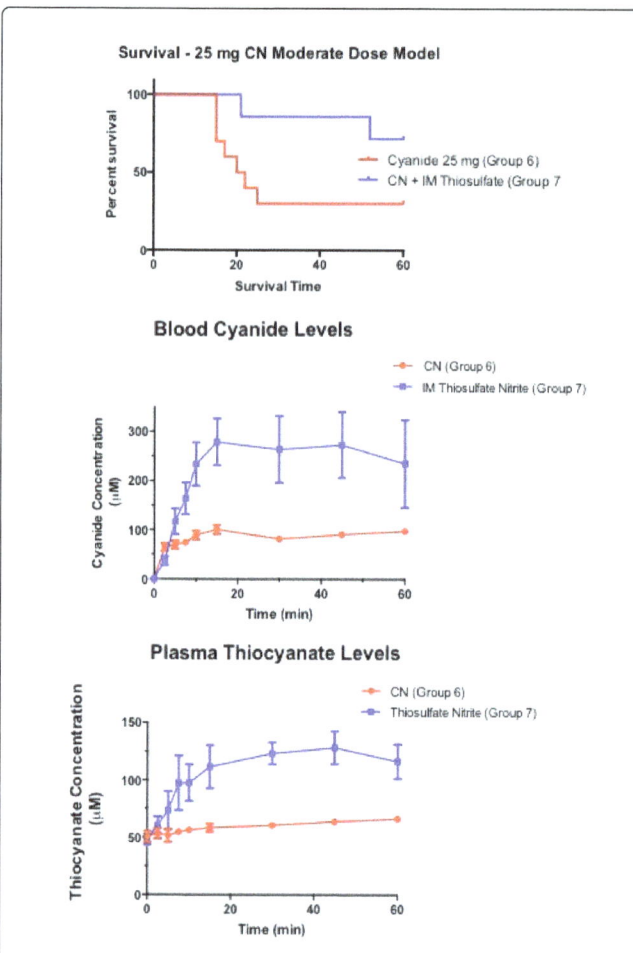

**Figure 5:** 25 mg intramuscular treatment model. Survival: Survival time curves following moderate dose ingested cyanide. Cyanide 25 mg alone (group 6) had 30% survival. Group 7 animals administered ingested cyanide plus intramuscular thiosulfate nitrite had 72% overall survival (p<0.05).

Blood CN Concentration: easured blood CN levels rose higher in animals receiving intramuscular thiosulfate thiosulfate/sodium nitrate than in animals receiving cyanide alone in this model despite significantly greater survival (p<0.01). The measured levels in these animals are also higher than levels in animals given high dose oral thiosulfate antidote (Groups 3 and 4). This is likely due to conversion of some blood hemoglobin to met-hemoglobin with greater carrying capacity for cyanide from the sodium nitrite administered with the intramuscular injection.

Plasma Thiocyanate Concentration: Plasma thiocyanate levels were higher in the sodium thiosulfate/sodium nitrite intramuscular treated animals as well (p<0.01), due to increased conversion of CN to thiocyanate, and similar to the oral thiosulfate treated animals (Groups 3 and 4).

## Discussion

This investigation was designed to study treatment for various scenarios of oral cyanide poisoning, including moderate and high dose ingestions. We focused on approaches that could be safely applied to

individual or mass casualty settings, as well as to cases of suspected but unconfirmed exposures. All of the drugs we used are inexpensive and stable, have minimal side effects, and are FDA approved in some form (though not for this route, mode, dose or indication).

The 50 mg cyanide dose we used was very high, resulting in death in less than 15 min in Group 1 animals. Gastric alkalization by glycine could not be expected to prevent death, since all cyanide would eventually be absorbed, but we hypothesized that it could increase survival time. Thus, Group 2 animals that received glycine alone showed a trend toward longer survival, at 14 min compared to 10 min in Group 1 animals, but this difference was not statistically significant. Further studies would be required to determine whether higher glycine doses would further increase survival time, but this seems unlikely, since we confirmed that the gastric pH remained 9 in the animals that received glycine.

Group 3 animals that received sodium thiosulfate alone showed more signs of cyanide poisoning than Group 4 animals treated with sodium thiosulfate plus glycine, and although Group 3 animals slowly recovered, their base excess (reflecting lactate concentrations), and CWNIRS tissue hemoglobin oxygenation did not return to baseline. The gastric fluid of these animals developed a cloudy appearance, that we suspect is precipitated sulfur from acid instability of sodium thiosulfate [31]. This may be another contributing factor to the greater effectiveness of sodium thiosulfate when administered in alkaline conditions.

In contrast, Group 4 animals that received glycine and sodium thiosulfate showed rapid recovery and 100% survival. We hypothesize that gastric alkalization by glycine maintained the administered NaCN as CN- ion, rather than shifting to HCN gas as would occur in the acid milieu of the stomach. The hypothesis that gastric alkalization likely delayed systemic cyanide absorption, allowing sodium thiosulfate more time to neutralize cyanide, is supported by data in Figure 3 showing that blood cyanide concentrations increased at a slower rate in animals given glycine than in the control group.

Other possible mechanisms for the effectiveness of glycine and sodium thiosulfate include non-enzymatic conversion of cyanide to thiocyanate in the stomach at an elevated pH, or more systemic absorption of thiosulfate with enzymatic conversion of cyanide to thiocyanate. These possibilities were suggested by the more rapid and sustained rise in the plasma thiocyanate concentration in the glycine plus sodium thiosulfate-treated animals (Figure 3). To evaluate these two possible mechanisms, we measured thiocyanate in gastric fluid. Gastric samples obtained at baseline showed no significant thiocyanate. In Group 3 animals that received sodium thiosulfate and cyanide, a modest gradual increase in gastric thiocyanate was found. In contrast, in Group 4 animals that received glycine, cyanide, and sodium thiosulfate, the thiocyanate concentration increased rapidly. Thiocyanate is easily absorbed, and hence intra-gastric conversion of cyanide to thiocyanate likely occurred. However, some component of the oral thiosulfate effect appears to be due to systemic absorption and enzymatic conversion of cyanide to thiocyanate. This is evidenced by the relatively rapid rise in plasma thiocyanate in Group 3 animals (oral thiosulfate alone), despite low gastric thiocyanate concentrations at 10-20 min post ingestion and treatment (Figure 3 bottom and middle graphs).

Some of the administered glycine was likely absorbed, but it is unlikely that glycine absorption contributed to maintaining higher base excess concentrations in Group 4 animals since: 1) CWNIRS concurrently showed improved tissue hemoglobin oxygen curves, 2) the gastric thiocyanate concentrations were higher in Group 4 animals receiving glycine plus thiosulfate, and 3) Group 2 animals receiving glycine with cyanide showed rapid drop in base excess. Together, these findings support that stomach alkalization by glycine increased thiosulfate reaction with cyanide to generate thiocyanate in the stomach.

We used previously published methods [21,26,32-37] for applying near infrared technology to optically monitor the rate of cyanide poisoning and reversal by tracking tissue hemoglobin oxygenation. The CWNIRS data support the effectiveness of glycine and sodium thiosulfate for reversing metabolic parameters of cyanide poisoning in parallel with improvement in survival. In animals given glycine alone, tissue oxyhemoglobin concentrations quickly deteriorated as the animals began to succumb to cyanide toxicity. In contrast, animals given both sodium thiosulfate and glycine exhibited an initial rise in oxyhemoglobin and fall in deoxyhemoglobin due to inability of cyanide-poisoned cells to extract oxygen from hemoglobin. Subsequently, these animals recovered, and optical metabolic parameters returned toward baseline, due to effective neutralization of cyanide by sodium thiosulfate. Animals given cyanide alone or glycine plus cyanide demonstrated only a very brief rise in oxyhemoglobin, followed by precipitously decreased oxyhemoglobin associated with the rapid onset of terminal cardiovascular collapse.

Thus, the data show that gastric alkalization by glycine in conjunction with sodium thiosulfate appears to be effective in rescuing animals receiving supra-lethal doses of oral cyanide. Our *in-vitro* data showed that at high concentrations, non-enzymatic reaction between sodium thiosulfate and cyanide does occur, and is more rapid at alkaline pH. Chemical analysis of reaction rates between cyanide and sodium thiosulfate suggest the reaction can occur when the concentrations of cyanide and sodium thiosulfate are as high as those used in the current study (~40 mM cyanide and 0.75 M sodium thiosulfate) [14,30]. Reaction rates are expected to be faster at alkaline pH, than at acid pH [14,30], as we observed *in-vitro* and *in-vivo*.

Several important limitations of this study will need to be addressed in subsequent animal studies before considering oral glycine and sodium thiosulfate as antidotes for oral cyanide poisoning. Most importantly, rabbits have a very rapid metabolic rate compared to humans and we administered an extremely high dose of cyanide (50 mg), which is close to a lethal dose for a full grown adult human. Thus, the therapeutic time-window for antidote administration was extremely short, and we administered the glycine and sodium thiosulfate concurrently with the oral cyanide in the 50 mg dose animal groups. A combination of initial systemic (intravenous or intramuscular) antidote followed by oral antidote may be preferable for acute oral cyanide ingestion, particularly in high dose symptomatic cases. In the lower dose, 25 mg oral cyanide exposed animals, improved overall survival (71%) was achieved with delayed intramuscular antidote injection alone group animals, but 29% still expired. In the severely poisoned (50 mg cyanide ingestion group where apnea occurs between 1 and 3.5 min without treatment), delayed treatment animals receiving combined intramuscular and oral antidote had increased survival time compared to controls, and 29% of the animals were able to survive. The systemic (intramuscular) antidote is available very rapidly neutralize absorbed cyanide, while the oral antidote is used neutralize the gastrointestinal reservoir. Such combination therapy approaches appear feasible based on our studies.. Large animal models, with metabolic rates more analogous to adult humans and consequently, a longer potential therapeutic time window, will need to be studied using longer delays in antidote administration that more closely parallel treatable human exposures. Second, the effects of food in the stomach and GI tract on the response to treatment need to be investigated. Food delays cyanide absorption [38, 39], but could affect the ability of glycine to raise pH, and could possibly interfere with the ability of sodium thiosulfate to neutralize cyanide. Additionally, in apneic patients, oral antidote alone would not likely be a clinical consideration, because it would not be effective quickly enough and cannot be administered until the airway has been secured and a nasogastric tube placed.

Therefore, we speculate that oral antidote administration in mass casualty situations may be limited to known or possible ingestion victims who are alert enough to swallow safely, while in severe symptomatic ingestion cases, enteral administration (*via* nasogastric tube) will likely only be administrable once airway protection has been secured.

In the future, other reactive sulfur containing compounds with higher reported cyanide reaction rate constants with cyanide [14,30] could be considered for further investigation. An important question of whether chronic cyanide toxicity associated with cyanogenic foods could be mitigated by repeated glycine and sodium thiosulfate ingestion is complex and will require careful study. It is conceivable that gastric alkalization could paradoxically lead to exacerbation of the ingestion from greater conversion of cyanide through the intestine due if increased passage of cyanogenic compounds through stomach occurs under alkaline conditions.

The FDA recognizes that antidotes for cyanide poisoning cannot be tested in humans and requires that efficacy be determined in at least two different animal species (preferably non-rodent), under GLP conditions. This study only observed short-term survival, and long-term effects will also require further investigation.

## Conclusions

In conclusion, these studies indicate that the combination of oral glycine and sodium thiosulfate appears to have potential for treating high dose acute cyanide ingestion and merits further investigation. The combination of systemic and oral therapy may provide additional options. The antidote candidates used in this study are safe, inexpensive, and have been FDA approved for other indications.

## Acknowledgement

The authors thank Dr. Kathy Osann, bio-statistician for her consultation, statistical analysis recommendations, and review of the manuscript.

## Funding

This work was supported, in part, by the CounterACT Program, National Institutes of Health Office of the Director (NIH OD), and the National Institute of Neurological Disorders and Stroke (NINDS) grant numbers U54 NS0792, U01 NS058030, and U54 NS063718, and by the Air Force Office of Scientific Research award numbers FA9550-17-1-0193 and FA9550-14-1-0193. Any opinions, findings, conclusions, or recommendations expressed in this material are those of the author(s) and do not necessarily reflect the views of the United States Air Force.

# References

1.  Hall AH, Rumack BH (1986) Clinical toxicology of cyanide. Ann Emerg Med 15: 1067-1074.

2.  Khan AS, Swerdlow DL, Juranek DD (2001) Precautions against biological and chemical terrorism directed at food and water supplies. Public Health Rep 116: 3-14.

3.  Cummings TF (2004) The treatment of cyanide poisoning. Occup Med (Lond) 54: 82-85.

4.  Borron SW, Stonerook M, Reid F (2006) Efficacy of hydroxocobalamin for the treatment of acute cyanide poisoning in adult beagle dogs. Clin Toxicol (Phila) 44 Suppl 1: 5-15.

5.  Coentrão L, Moura D (2011) Acute cyanide poisoning among jewelry and textile industry workers. Am J Emerg Med 29: 78-81.

6.  Tshala-Katumbay D, Mumba N, Okitundu L, Kazadi K, Banea M, et al. (2013) Cassava food toxins, konzo disease, and neurodegeneration in sub-Sahara Africans. Neurology 80: 949-951.

7.  Bhattacharya R (2000) Antidotes to cyanide poisoning: present status, vol. 32.

8.  Sylvester DM, Hayton WL, Morgan RL, Way JL (1983) Effects of thiosulfate on cyanide pharmacokinetics in dogs. Toxicol Appl Pharmacol 69: 265-271.

9.  Meillier A, Heller C (2015) Acute Cyanide Poisoning: Hydroxocobalamin and Sodium Thiosulfate Treatments with Two Outcomes following One Exposure Event. Case Rep Med 2015: 4.

10. Baskin SI, Porter DW, Rockwood GA, Romano JA, Patel HC, et al. (1999) In vitro and in vivo comparison of sulfur donors as antidotes to acute cyanide intoxication. J Appl Toxicol 19: 173-183.

11. Farese S, Stauffer E, Kalicki R, Hildebrandt T, Frey BM, et al. (2011) Sodium thiosulfate pharmacokinetics in hemodialysis patients and healthy volunteers. Clin J Am Soc Nephrol 6: 1447-1455.

12. Schulz V (1984) Clinical Pharmacokinetics of Nitroprusside, Cyanide, Thiosulphate and Thiocyanate. Clinical Pharmacokinetics 9: 239-251.

13. Isom GE, Borowitz JL, Hall AH (2015) Cyanide metabolism and physiological disposition. In: Toxicology of Cyanides and Cyanogens. John Wiley & Sons 54-69.

14. Luthy RG, Bruce SG (1979) Kinetics of reaction of cyanide and reduced sulfur species in aqueous solution. Environmental Science & Technology 13: 1481-1487.

15. Baskin S, Horowitz AM, Nealley EW (1992) The antidotal action of sodium nitrite and sodium thiosulfate against cyanide poisoning. J Clin Pharmacol 32: 368-375.

16. Newhouse K, Chiu N (2010) Toxicological review of hydrogen cyanide and cyanide salts. In. Edited by Agency USEP. Washington, DC: EPA

17. Lee J, Mahon SB, Mukai D, Burney T, Katebian BS, et al. (2016) The Vitamin B12 Analog Cobinamide Is an Effective Antidote for Oral Cyanide Poisoning. J Med Toxicol 1-10.

18. Garlick PJ (2004) The Nature of Human Hazards Associated with Excessive Intake of Amino Acids. J Nutrion 134: 1633S-1639S.

19. Rose WC, Wixom RL, Lockhart HB, Lambert GF (1955) THE AMINO ACID REQUIREMENTS OF MAN: XV. THE VALINE REQUIREMENT; SUMMARY AND FINAL OBSERVATIONS. J Biolo Chem 217: 987-996.

20. Brenner M, Benavides S, Mahon SB, Lee J, Yoon D, et al. (2014) The vitamin B12 analog cobinamide is an effective hydrogen sulfide antidote in a lethal rabbit model. Clin Toxicol 52: 490-497.

21. Lee J, Kim JG, Mahon SB, Mukai D, Yoon D, et al. (2014) Noninvasive optical cytochrome c oxidase redox state measurements using diffuse optical spectroscopy. J biomed optics 19: 055001.

22. Brenner M, Kim JG, Mahon SB, Lee J, Kreuter KA, et al. (2010) Intramuscular cobinamide sulfite in a rabbit model of sublethal cyanide toxicity. Ann Emerg Med 55: 352-363.

23. Lee J, Kim JG, Mahon S, Tromberg BJ, Ryan KL, et al. (2008) Tissue hemoglobin monitoring of progressive central hypovolemia in humans using broadband diffuse optical spectroscopy. J Biomed Opt 13: 064027.

24. Lee J, Kim JG, Mahon S, Tromberg BJ, Mukai D, et al. (2009) Broadband diffuse optical spectroscopy assessment of hemorrhage- and hemoglobin-based blood substitute resuscitation. J Biomed Opt 14: 044027.

25. Brenner M, Kim JG, Lee J, Mahon SB, Lemor D, et al. (2010) Sulfanegen sodium treatment in a rabbit model of sub-lethal cyanide toxicity. Toxicol Appl Pharmacol 248: 269-276.

26. Kim JG, Lee J, Mahon SB, Mukai D, Patterson SE, et al. (2012) Noninvasive monitoring of treatment response in a rabbit cyanide toxicity model reveals differences in brain and muscle metabolism. J biomed optics 17: 105005.

27. Lundquist P, Rosling H, Sörbo B (1985) Determination of cyanide in whole blood, erythrocytes, and plasma. Clin Chem 31: 591-595.

28. Blackledge WC, Blackledge CW, Griesel A, Mahon SB, Brenner M, et al. (2010) New facile method to measure cyanide in blood. Anal Chem 82: 4216-4221.

29. Chan A, Balasubramanian M, Blackledge W, Mohammad OM, Alvarez L, et al. (2010) Cobinamide is superior to other treatments in a mouse model of cyanide poisoning. Clin Toxicol 48: 709-717.

30. Bartlett PD, Davis RE (1958) Reactions of Elemental Sulfur. II. The Reaction of Alkali Cyanides with Sulfur, and Some Single-Sulfur Transfer Reactions. J Am Chemi Socty 80: 2513-2516.

31. LaMer VK, Kenyon AS (1947) Kinetics of the formation of monodispersed sulfur sols from thiosulfate and acid. J Colloid Science 2: 257-264.

32. Bevilacqua F, Berger AJ, Cerussi AE, Jakubowski D, Tromberg BJ (2000) Broadband absorption spectroscopy in turbid media by combined frequency-domain and steady-state methods. Applied Optics 39: 6498-6507.

33. Lee J, Armstrong J, Kreuter K, Tromberg BJ, Brenner M (2007) Non-invasive in vivo diffuse optical spectroscopy monitoring of cyanide poisoning in a rabbit model. Physiol Meas 28: 1057-1066.

34. Lee J, El-Abaddi N, Duke A, Cerussi AE, Brenner M, et al. (2006) Noninvasive in vivo monitoring of methemoglobin formation and reduction with broadband diffuse optical spectroscopy. J Appl Physiol 100: 615-622.

35. Lee J, Keuter KA, Kim J, Tran A, Uppal A, et al. (2009) Noninvasive in vivo monitoring of cyanide toxicity and treatment using diffuse optical spectroscopy in a rabbit model. Mil Med 174: 615-621.

36. Merritt S, Gulsen G, Chiou G, Chu Y, Deng C, et al. (2003) Comparison of water and lipid content measurements using diffuse optical spectroscopy and MRI in emulsion phantoms. Technol Cancer Res Treat 2: 563-569.

37. Pham TH, Coquoz O, Fishikin JB, Anderson E, Tromberg BJ (2000) Broad bandwidth frequency domain instrument for quantitative tissue optical spectroscopy. Rev Sci Instrum 71: 2500-2513.

38. Hayes Jr W (1969) The 90-Dose LD50 and a Chronicity Factor as Measures of Toxicity. Journal of Occupational and Environmental Medicine 11: 53-54.

39. Abraham K, Buhrke T, Lampen A (2016) Bioavailability of cyanide after consumption of a single meal of foods containing high levels of cyanogenic glycosides: a crossover study in humans. Arch Toxicol 90: 559-574.

# 19

# Accidental Substance Abuse Poisoning in Children: Experience of the Dammam Poison Control Center

**Ahmed R. Ragab[1]*, Maha K. Al-Mazroua[2], and Naglaa F. Mahmoud[3]**

[1]Department of Forensic Medicine and Clinical Toxicology, Faculty of Medicine, Mansoura University, Mansoura, Egypt

[2]Dammam Poison Control Center, Dammam, Eastern Region, Ministry of Health, Saudi Arabia

[3]Department of Forensic Medicine and Clinical Toxicology, Faculty of Medicine, Cairo University, Cairo, Egypt

*Corresponding author: Ahmed R. Ragab, Department of Forensic Medicine and Clinical Toxicology, Faculty of Medicine, Mansoura University, Mansoura, Egypt,
E-mail: ahmedrefat1973@yahoo.com

### Abstract

**Introduction:** Cannabis and amphetamines are the most commonly used illegal drugs in adults in Saudi Arabia. Accidental Substance Abuse poisoning is an uncommon form of poisoning in children, but potentially serious.

**Objective:** To describe the clinical presentation, diagnosis and treatment of children with accidental poisoning from various forms of substances of abuse in a pediatric secondary hospital.

**Material and Methods:** We report on14 patients with accidental intoxication by amphetamines, cannabis and opiates.

**Results:** The clinical presentation was variable deterioration in level of consciousness, somnolence, ataxia, tremor, apnea, hypotonia and seizure. The investigation of toxic urine detected benzphetamine, tetrahydrocannabinol (THC) and morphine in all cases of amphetamine, cannabis and heroine intoxication respectively. In all patients with amphetamine and cannabis intoxication supportive measures were established. In only one case of acute heroine intoxication was naloxone therapy given. All cases recovered well and were discharged within 24-48 hours of admission.

**Conclusion:** A high index with early priority of suspicion should be maintained for substances of abuse involving "amphetamines, cannabis or morphine" intoxication in previously healthy children with acute onset of neurological symptoms of unknown etiology. Accidental poisoning by various substances of abuse is, in itself, an alarm signal on the attitude of parents in caring for their children. These families deserve special monitoring by social services, since such accidents may be covering up child abuse.

**Keywords:** Substances of abuse; Amphetamines; Morphine; Coma; Accidental poisoning; Drowsiness; Children

## Introduction

Substance abuse is a common problem in families involved with the child welfare system. There is increasing awareness that the abuse of drugs by parents and other caregivers can have a negative impact on the safety, permanence, and well-being of children [1].

Clinical signs of amphetamines toxicity especially in pediatric population include hyperthermia, tachycardia, tachypnea, mydriasis, tremors, and seizures. In addition, amphetamine intoxication has been reported to cause hyperthermia, hypoglycemia and mild thrombocytopenia [2,3]. Diagnosis can be confirmed by detecting amphetamine in stomach contents or vomitus, or mainly by positive results obtained in urine tests for illicit drugs [4].

Regarding cannabis intoxication; the main psychoactive metabolite is delta-9-tetrahydrocannabinol (THC) [5]. It is the most widely consumed psychoactive drug in Spain, especially among adolescents. Despite stabilization in the prevalence of consumption, it was reported that 11.2% of the population aged 15-64 had ever spent in the last year [6]. In parallel to this high prevalence of consumption there has been an increase in the number of cases of accidental poisoning by this substance in the pediatric population [7].

Opiate poisoning can occur at any time from birth to terminal care. The outcome can range from discomfort such as constipation, to death from respiratory depression. Regarding the epidemiology of acute opiate intoxication in children, it is difficult to get reliable incidence figures [8]. The pediatrics is less liable to poisoning from opiates and less likely to be exposed to them, especially illicit forms of medication. Acute opiate toxicity presents with drowsiness. There may be nausea or vomiting. Respiratory depression may be apparent. Hypotension and tachycardia are possible. There are usually pinpoint pupils but this sign may be absent if other drugs are involved [9].

Because there are so many child cases involving substance abuse, child welfare agencies should begin to use a range of strategies to prevent and treat substance abuse in families, and to improve outcomes for children and families [1].

## Objective

The purpose of this study was to shed light on the problem of accidental substance abuse poisoning among children, to determine the factors related to accidental substance of abuse poisoning by the most common abused agents in poisoned patients who were visited a pediatric ER department.

## Material and Methods

### Study setting

This work was conducted as a cross sectional prospective, (Electronic Medical Review) EMR database review study at Damamm Regional Poison Control Center–Eastern Region, KSA.

### Inclusion criteria

Pediatric patients suspected for substances abuse toxicity in two hospitals (Dammam Medical Complex and Qatif Central Hospital) that were participating in two year-long period from the beginning of January, 2011 until the end of December, 2013.

### Study population parameters

Investigators noted down important and detailed information of all the patients, like their age, and sex as well as their patient code, in-patient or out-patient admission status and medical service type.

At present, the status of electrolytes, renal and liver function values were evaluated at the same time of screening the substance abuse profile kit. Important laboratory activities and investigations such as blood urea nitrogen, serum Creatinine concentration, both serum ALT and AST levels were also conducted.

### Electronic medical records review process

Three reviewers conducted the entire review process – 'physcians. Taking the help of individual patient records, the individual patient records were accessed by way of medical record number access into the EMR. Predefined data points fed into a standard type Excel worksheet was set up on a share drive that was password protected which was to be used by every single reviewer in order to get the abstraction data information. Then every patient was reviewed on an independent basis to be reviewed for agreement purpose followed by checks carried out by the third reviewer to see if there were still any other discrepancies identified. Data extractors had to have total agreement amongst them. The study was approved by the Medical Ethics Committee of the Dammam Regional Poison Control Center/ Ref No 11/2010.

## Results

The description of the clinical case series: Present eight pediatric cases with accidental intoxication by amphetamines. All of them were boys between 14 months and five years old. The clinical presentation was variable (Table 1).

| No | Age | | | Sex | Route of Poisoning | Clinical Presentation | Glasgow Coma Scale | Urine Drug of Abuse Results | Duration of Recovery |
|---|---|---|---|---|---|---|---|---|---|
| | Ys | Ms | Ds | | | | | | |
| 1 | 1 | 11 | 1 | Male | By ingestion | Abnormal behavior, Irritability, Tachycardia | 14 | Amphetamines metabolites, Benzodiazepines | 26 hours |
| 2 | 2 | 3 | 7 | Male | By ingestion | Drowsy, Hallucination, Tachyaponea. | 14 | Amphetamines metabolites | 16 hours |
| 3 | 1 | 2 | 5 | Male | By ingestion | Abnormal Behavior, Hypertonia, Hyperactivity, Hyperreflexia | 13 | Amphetamines metabolites | 22 hours |
| 4 | 2 | 3 | 19 | Male | By ingestion | Abnormal movement in the mouth, Tremors in the tongue | 12 | Amphetamines metabolites and caffeine. | 18 hours |
| 5 | 3 | 9 | 23 | Male | By ingestion | Convulsion, Hypertension | 14 | Amphetamines metabolites | 12 hours |
| 6 | 4 | 2 | 4 | Male | By ingestion | Seizures, Hyperthermia, Tachycardia, Mydriasis | 10 | Amphetamines metabolites Caffeine, Benzodiazepines. | 18 hours |
| 7 | 3 | 1 | 25 | Male | By ingestion | Drowsy, Hallucination, Tachyaponea. | 14 | Amphetamines metabolites | 16 hours |
| 8 | 1 | 4 | 3 | Male | By ingestion | Abnormal Behavior, | 14 | Amphetamines metabolites | 24 hours |

| | | | | | | Abnormal movement, Irritability. | | | |
|---|---|---|---|---|---|---|---|---|---|
| 9 | 5 | 1 | 3 | Male | By ingestion | Drowsy, Convulsions, and Vomiting | 15 | Cannabinoids | 36 hours |
| 10 | 1 | 4 | 2 | Male | By inhalation | Comatose, Convulsion, Tachyaponea, Mydriasis | 10 | Cannabinoids | 22 hours |
| 11 | 3 | 2 | 5 | Male | By ingestion | Comatose, Tachycardia, Tremors, Flushing | 10 | Cannabinoids | 11 hours |
| 12 | 2 | 7 | 14 | Male | By ingestion | Aponea, Drowsy, Irritability, Somnolence, Hallucinations. | 10 | Cannabinoids | 19 hours |
| 13 | 11 | 1 | 1 | Male | By sniffing | Vomiting, Drowsy, Depression | 13 | Morphine and Codeine and 6 MAM | 19 hours |
| 14 | 0 | 0 | 1 | Male | Transplacental | Meiosis, Irritability, Diarrhea, Hypoglycaemia | 9 | Morphine and Codeine | 37 hours |

Table 1: Clinical, diagnostic and resolution time frame table.

Case [1] had a characteristic sudden development of abnormal behavior, irritability and sinus tachycardia. In case [2] we observed a condition characterized by drowsiness, moderate malaise, visual hallucination, and tachyaponea. In patient [3] there was the presence of generalized hyperactivity, hypertonia and hyperreflexia. As regards the fourth case, abnormal movement in the mouth and fine tremors in the tongue were characteristic signs. In patient [5] convulsion and hypertension were the main pathognomonic signs. The sixth patient had characteristic serial attacks of seizures, hyperthermia, tachycardia and mydriasis. In patient [7], hallucination was markedly represented, with drowsiness and tachyaponea. Finally, child number [8] presented at admission a picture characterized by abnormal movement, abnormal behavior and pallor followed by acute episodes of generalized irritability, a few seconds long. Physical examination revealed a significant malaise, mydriasis and peripheral coldness.

Regarding cannabis intoxication we detected four pediatric patients with acute accidental toxicity of cannabis. All of them were males and their ages ranged from 16 months to five years. Patient [9] had a single attack of convulsions, two episodes of vomiting, and presented with marked drowsiness status. In patient [10] we detected a marked disturbed consciousness level with seizures, tachyaponea and mydriasis. Patient [11] presented to the ER department with marked tachycardia, tremors, flushing and coma. The last case of acute accidental toxicity in pediatric patient [12] presented with aponea, irritability, somnolence and hallucinations.

Accidental opiate toxicity in pediatric patient represent in two cases one had 1 day male newborn with transplacental exposure of morphine from an addicted opiate mother and represented with meiosis, irritability diarrhea and hypoglycemia as a result of withdrawal effects. The second case was an eleven-year-old male boy who visited the ER department following recurrent attacks of vomiting and drowsiness with depressive mode after a first episode of exposure to heroin.

While follow up the observed interrogation; how all families, except in the cases of patients 8, 10, and 13 omitted information about the possibility of ingesting toxic abuse substance. The parent of patient 8 reported early the accidental ingestion of a "Capatgone tablet" suspected of street medication of his father. The mother of child [10] suspected cannabis poisoning had occurred during his sleep from inhaling cannabis smoke that released from father smoking set. The last case was a child who had sniffed heroin powder, copying one of his friends, and once his condition had deteriorated he told his mother about his toxic exposure.

In all cases, blood count, and biochemical and acid-base status is assessed on admission. Except for the finding of metabolic acidosis in patient 14, the results of these tests were normal. In all patients, consistent support measures were established in regard to ensure the airway, providing oxygen by face mask, administration of activated charcoal, and gastric lavage. In case 11, for the unknown potential toxicity, naloxone and flumazenil were administered intravenously as coma cocktail. After the maneuvers are implemented and necessary for the stabilization treatment of the patients were investigated urine toxicology by semi-quantitative (Bio Rad ® TOX / See Drug Screen Test). All patients showed THC above 25 ng/dl values, which was confirmed by GC/MS. In patients [1] and [6] we also identified caffeine and benzodiazepines (diazepam dose received for irritability and seizure control). The outcome was satisfactory in all cases, with resolution of symptoms within 24 h , allowing discharge 24-48 hours after admission.

## Discussion

Substance Abuse intoxication in children is a rare form of acute poisoning, but recently an increasing number of cases have been reported to the register.

The primary psychoactive constituents in variable Substance Abuse are THC in cases of cannabis, morphine-3-glucoronide and normorphine in morphine, and benzphetamine in amphetamine. In cases of cannabis the proportion of active constituents varies by consumption in the form of marijuana (3-5%) , hashish (5-20%) or hashish oil ( 16-43%) [8].

The route of intake varies according to the type of Substance Abuse (in cases of amphetamine it is ingestion, in cases of cannabis it is inhalation and in cases of morphine it is injection). In children, poisoning is usually due to accidental ingestion of cannabis material, their effects by ingestion route are slower, durable and variables. Begin to be apparent after 1 h, with a maximum effect at 2-3 h and its action lasts about 5 H [9]. In the present study; only one case by inhalation and the remaining by the ingestion route.

The toxic effects of amphetamine vary widely by age. They include abdominal pain, acne, blurred vision, excessive grinding of the teeth, profuse sweating, dry mouth, loss of appetite, nausea, reduced seizure threshold, tics, and weight loss. The effects of amphetamine on the gastrointestinal tract are unpredictable. Amphetamine may reduce gastrointestinal motility if intestinal activity is high, or increase motility if the smooth muscle of the tract is relaxed [10]. In the current study, abnormal behavior, irritability, tachycardia were the main presented symptoms and signs.

In the present series study the chief characteristic symptom of the studied cases regarding, acute cannabis intoxication was disturbed consciousness level. The symptoms of cannabis intoxication include nausea, vomiting, dry mouth, thirst, hyperorexia, pale skin and conjunctival hyperemia. From a neurological point of view, as regards consciousness disorders, abrupt onset hypotonia, ataxia, mydriasis or miosis, decreased reflexes, mood modification, perceptual disturbances, seizures and even coma may be observed. The most common cardiovascular effect is tachycardia, although high doses may cause bradycardia [11].

Typically, families report information about the possibility of accidental ingestion of a toxin from the maternal side. In our series, ten cases omitted accidental ingestion. Sometimes the version offered is not credible, as in patient 11, whose parents reported that the cannabis intoxication had occurred outdoors, through eating "something on the ground".

Clinical suspicion and prompt detection of the drug are the pillars of substance abuse diagnosis. Differential diagnosis should be made with central nervous system infections, head injuries and metabolic disorders. Thinking of Substance Abuse intoxication as a cause of a sudden decreased level of consciousness in previously healthy and afebrile patients, may allow testing save as CT and lumbar puncture , not without complications [12].

Diagnosis is made through urine toxicology research by semi-quantitative (Bio Rad * TOX/See Drug Screen Test) whose detection threshold is (500 ng/dl in amphetamines, 25 ng/dl in cannabis, 200 ng/dl in morphine). The diagnosis is confirmed by gas chromatography/mass spectrometry, the detection threshold (100 ng/dl in amphetamines, 5 ng/dl in cannabis, and morphine 100 ng/dl).

Treatment in Substance Abuse situations consists of supportive measures which vary according to the severity of symptoms. Performing gastric lavage and administration of activated charcoal is recommended. Care must be taken when performing these procedures, given the risk of aspiration in patients with depressed sensorium. This will isolate the airway in cases where Glasgow is less than 8 and no control coal tape nasogastric tube. Isolated cases have been reported in which intravenous naloxone and flumazenil have been used successfully, aiming to reverse depression neurológica. In cases of severe agitation and irritability, as in amphetamine toxicity diazepam, has been given intravenously.

In cases of cannabis intoxication, unlike in adults, the evolution of the poisoning in children is variable. The most satisfactory evolution sees the disappearance of symptoms within hours after the establishment of supportive measures. However, there are cases that have presented with seizures, respiratory obstruction or coma, that have required intensive pediatric care [13-15].

## Conclusion

The high number of substance abuse users in the current research may be attributed to easy access of pediatric patients to this substance, which explores the increasing number of cases of accidental poisoning by these substances. We cannot rule out this type of poisoning in any home environment, regardless of the inhabitants' socioeconomic status. Monitoring of children is an important responsibility of parents and is the main form of prevention of childhood accidents. Accidental poisoning by various substances of abuse is, in itself, an alarm signal on the attitude of parents in caring for their children. These families deserve special monitoring by social services, since such accidents may be covering up child abuse.

## Acknowledgments

No funding or sponsorship was received for this study. Dr. Ahmed Refat Ragab is the guarantor for this article, and takes responsibility for the integrity of the work as a whole.

## References

1. Office on Child Abuse and Neglect (2009) Protecting Children in Families Affected by Substance Use Disorders Children's Bureau, ICF International.

2. Lemke TL, Williams DA, Roche VF, Zito W (2013) Foye's Principles of Medicinal Chemistry (7th edn). Wolters Kluwer Health/Lippincott Williams & Wilkins, Philadelphia.

3. Berman SM, Kuczenski R, McCracken JT, London ED (2009) Potential adverse effects of amphetamine treatment on brain and behavior: a review. Mol Psychiatry 14: 123-142.

4. Bütefisch CM, Davis BC, Sawaki L, Waldvogel D, Classen J, et al. (2002) Modulation of use-dependent plasticity by d-amphetamine. Ann Neurol 51: 59-68.

5. Schwartz RH (2002) Marijuana: a decade and a half later, still a crude drug with underappreciated toxicity. Pediatrics 109: 284-289.

6. García-Algar O, Gómez A (2010) [Cannabis in paediatric emergencies]. An Pediatr (Barc) 72: 375-376.

7. Spadari M, Glaizal M, Tichadou L, Blanc I, Drouet G, et al. (2009) [Accidental cannabis poisoning in children: experience of the Marseille poison center]. Presse Med 38: 1563-1567.

8. Drug Misuse and Dependence-Guidelines on Clinical Management (1999) Drug Misuse and Dependence – Guidelines on Clinical Management, Department of Health, University of Cambridge.

9.   Macnab A, Anderson E, Susak L (1989) Ingestion of cannabis: a cause of coma in children. Pediatr Emerg Care 5: 238-239.

10.  Fantegrossi WE, Godlewski T, Karabenick RL, Stephens JM, Ullrich T, et al. (2003) Pharmacological characterization of the effects of 3,4-methylenedioxymethamphetamine ("ecstasy") and its enantiomers on lethality, core temperature, and locomotor activity in singly housed and crowded mice. Psychopharmacology (Berl) 166: 202-211.

11.  Heyman RB, Anglin TM, Copperman SM, Joffe A, McDonald CA, et al. (1999) American Academy of Pediatrics. Committee on Substance Abuse. Marijuana: A continuing concern for pediatricians. Pediatrics 104: 982-985.

12.  Appelboam A, Oades PJ (2006) Coma due to cannabis toxicity in an infant. Eur J Emerg Med 13: 177-179.

13.  Borrego Domínguez R, Arjona Villanueva D, Fernández Barrio B, Huidobro Labarga B, Alonso Martín JA (2007) [Comatose state after cannabis intake]. An Pediatr (Barc) 67: 276-278.

14.  Boros CA, Parsons DW, Zoanetti GD, Ketteridge D, Kennedy D (1996) Cannabis cookies: a cause of coma. J Paediatr Child Health 32: 194-195.

15.  Bonkowsky JL, Sarco D, Pomeroy SL (2005) Ataxia and shaking in a 2-year-old girl: acute marijuana intoxication presenting as seizure. Pediatr Emerg Care 21: 527-528.

# 20

# Protective Effect of Vitamins C and E against Nitrocellulose Thinner Induced Nephrotoxicity in Albino Wistar Rats

**Friday E. Uboh**[*], **Saviour U. Ufot, Uduak O. Luke, Godwin O. Igile and Chinelo M. Ozojie**

*Biochemistry Department, Faculty of Basic Medical Sciences, College of Medical Sciences, University of Calabar, P.M.B. 1115, Calabar, Nigeria*

[*]**Corresponding author:** Friday E. Uboh, Biochemistry Department, Faculty of Basic Medical Sciences, College of Medical Sciences, University of Calabar, P.M.B. 1115, Calabar, Nigeria, E-mail: fridayuboh@yahoo.com

## Abstract

Effect of vitamins C (vitamin C) and E (vitamin E) on nitrocellulose thinner (NCT)-induced nephrotoxicity in male rats was assessed. Six groups of six rats each, were orally administered 0.5 ml distilled water, 0.5 ml soybean oil, 40.0 mg NCT/kg bwt, 40.0 mg NCT/kg bwt+200 mg vitamin C/kg bwt, 40.0 mg NCT/kg bwt+200 IU vitamin E/kg bwt, and 40.0 mg NCT/kg bwt+200 IU vitamin E+200 mg vitamin C/kg bwt, respectively, for 30 days. The animals were sacrificed, 24 hours after last experimental treatments, blood and kidney tissues were collected for analyses of indicators of nephrotoxicity using standard methods. The results showed a significant ($p<0.05$) increase in serum creatinine (sCr), urea, uric acid, $K^+$, $HCO_3^-$ and $Cl^-$ and decrease in serum $Na^+$ levels, as well as severe renal histological changes in rats exposed to NCT only, compared to the values obtained for the control groups receiving only distilled water and soybeans oil, respectively. No significant ($p>0.05$) difference was recorded for these parameters in rats receiving soybean oil, compared with control rats receiving distilled water. These results indicated that exposure to NCT induced nephrotoxicity in rats. It was also observed that administration of vitamin C and vitamin E, in combination and singly, to rats exposed to NCT produced relatively normal renal histological status, and levels of the assayed serum nephrotoxicity indicators within the control range; suggesting vitamin C and vitamin E to be potent in preventing NCT-induced nephrotoxicity in rats. However, comparative percentage decreases (CPD) in sCr, uric acid, $K^+$ and $HCO_3^-$ indicated that combined vitamin C and vitamin E administration produced a higher protective potency than single administration; and that vitamin C produced a higher potency than vitamin E against NCT-induced nephrotoxicity.

**Keywords:** Nitrocellulose-thinner; Nephrotoxicity; Vitamins C and E; Nephroprotection

## Introduction

The kidneys are known to play a vital role in the excretion of most hydrophilic metabolic wastes from the body. The renal tissues are therefore the major tissue responsible for the clearance of wastes products of metabolic activities from the body. The functional state of the renal tissues may therefore be assessed by the rate at which the tissues clear or sequester these metabolic wastes from the blood. Abnormality or dysfunction of the renal tissues usually results in the accumulation of these metabolic wastes in the blood, due to the failure of the renal tissues to effectively clear the metabolic wastes from circulation. Hence, the concentrations of most of these wastes substances tend to build or increase in the blood, to the levels that are above the normal range. In routine clinical and research investigations, the plasma or serum concentrations of some wastes metabolites and electrolytes are commonly determined to assess the functional integrity of the renal tissues. Among the waste metabolites that are commonly considered in renal function assessment include creatinine, urea, blood urea nitrogen and uric acid, while sodium, potassium, chloride, bicarbonate, magnesium, and sometimes calcium ions are among the electrolytes that are often used to assess the renal functions [1-3].

The functional state of the renal tissues may be adversely affected by several factors, including chemical insults. Chemical insults to the renal tissues may arise from the exposure to toxic chemical agents, or their metabolites. These toxic substances can interact with the macromolecular constituents of the renal tissues, and produce a compromise in the renal functions. Our previous studies revealed that nitrocellulose thinner is one of the chemical agents that can cause an adverse effect on the functional state of the renal tissues [4,5]. Nitrocellulose thinner (NCT) is an industrial solvents commonly used in furniture, paints and automobile spray-painting industries. It contains such organic chemical agents, as ethylbenzene or toluene and butyl acetate. These chemical substances are known to constitute chemical pollutants in different environments. WHO [6] reported that these chemical pollutants are detectable in household and workplace air. Hence, exposure to chemical pollutants from NCT in indoor and outdoor environments may be common. Individuals may be exposed to this solvent by direct inhalation of the volatile constituents, or ingestion of foods and drinks contaminated by the solvents during use. Particularly, occupational exposures to mixtures of toluene, ethylbenzene and butyl acetate have been reported in painting or lacquering workplaces [7-9].

Exposure to NCT, and related organic solvents has been reported to induce haematotoxicity, hepatotoxicity and nephrotoxicity in humans and experimental animals [4,8-13]. The presence of chemical constituents of nitrocellulose thinner, like other xenobiotics, may activate some drug metabolizing enzymes to transform these chemical substances into various metabolites in the body [14]. These metabolites, which may be very reactive, in the course of their renal excretion are likely to interact with the renal tissues to express some toxic effects [15,16]. These interactions may produce cellular injury, resulting in tissue damage. Damage to the renal tissues is likely to result in the overall compromise of the functional status of the kidneys.

Exposures to certain reactive or toxic metabolites have been reported to produce varying degrees of renal dysfunction in humans and experimental animals [3,17,18].

Most toxicity effect(s) associated with exposure to chemical agents and their metabolites are known to be indication of tissue, or tissue components-reactive metabolite species interactions in the body. The presence of antioxidants has been reported to provide protective mechanism against different toxicity effects associated with the reactive species generated by chemical substances into the body tissues [19]. While some antioxidants are endogenously generated within the body, others (including antioxidant vitamins) may be provided as micronutrients in the diets. According to the report, such antioxidants vitamins as ascorbate (vitamin C) and α-tocopherol (vitamin E) have been demonstrated to provide protection against chemicals induced oxidative stress in different tissues via several mechanisms [20-22].

According to Carr et al. [19], the effectiveness of ascorbate in mitigating the pathophysiological processes of oxidative stress tends to be higher than that of α-tocopherol. The reported increased protective effectiveness of ascorbate against oxidative stress may likely be attributed to its effectiveness in scavenging a wide range of reactive oxygen and nitrogen species, as well as its ability to regenerate α-tocopherol, and possibly tetrahydrobiopterin, from its radical species. Also, ascorbate is known to act as a co-antioxidant and possibly prevent the pro-oxidant activity of α-tocopherol [19,23-26]. However, our earlier study showed that vitamin E is relatively more effective than vitamin C in providing protective measures against gasoline vapour-induced hepatotoxicity in rats [27]. It is therefore possible that co-administration of vitamin C and E may be more effective in protecting the tissues against chemicals induced oxidative stress processes, than singular administration. On the basis of the reported contradicting protective effectiveness of vitamins C and E against chemicals-induced toxicities, this study assessed the protective effectiveness of co-administration and singular administration of vitamins C and E against nitrocellulose thinner induced nephrotoxicity in rats.

## Materials and Methods

### Animal handling and treatment

Thirty six apparently normal matured male albino Wistar rats (180 to 200 g), obtained from Biochemistry Department Experimental Research Animal House of the University of Calabar, Calabar, Nigeria, were used in this study. They were fed with standard laboratory diet and allowed free access to tap water ad libitum. The work was carried out under 12 hours light/dark cycle illumination and prevailing tropical room temperature.

Preliminary acute toxicity studies in mice, gave LD 50 of 16.0 ml/kg (i.e., 160.2 mg/kg, by weight) body weight of nitrocellulose thinner (solubilized in Grand pure soya beans oil). Hence, 4.0 ml/kg (i.e., 40 mg/kg, by weight) body weight concentrations (25% of LD50) were used in this study.

The animals were distributed into six groups, with six rats each, as highlighted below:

Group 1: Comprised of six rats receiving 0.5 ml of distilled water only for thirty (30) days

Group 2: Comprised of six rats receiving 0.5 ml soya beans oil only for thirty (30) days

Group 3: Comprised of six rats receiving 40.0 mg/kg body weight of nitrocellulose thinner (NCT) for thirty (30) days.

Group 4: Comprised of six rats receiving 40.0 mg/kg body weight of NCT + 200 mg/kg body weight of vitamin C for thirty (30) days

Group 5: Comprised of six rats receiving 40.0 mg/kg body weight of NCT + 200 IU/kg body weight of vitamin E for thirty (30) days

Group 6: Comprised of six rats receiving 40.0 mg/kg body weight of NCT + 200 IU and 200mg/kg body weight of vitamins E and C, respectively, for thirty (30) days

The choice of the dosage of the vitamins was based on our previous report that daily administration of vitamins C (200 mg/kg body weight) C and E (200IU/kg body weight) produced protective effect against gasoline-induced hepatoprototoxicity in rats [27]. The vitamins were administered to the rats, one hour after NCT administration, and all the administrations were carried out once daily, six days per week, throughout the experimental period. The animals were sacrificed, 24 hours after the 30th day of experimental period. All animal experiments were carried out according to the Guidelines of Institution's (University of Calabar, Nigeria) Animal Research Ethics Committee, with reference to the Guide for the Care and Use of Laboratory Animals [28].

### Collection and preparation of tissues for analyses

Blood and kidneys were collected for analyses. Blood samples were collected by cardiac puncture, under chloroform vapor anaesthesia, 24 hours after termination of experimental treatments, into sterile plain sample bottles. The blood samples were allowed to clot and centrifuged with Table-top centrifuge (MSE model, England) at 3000 rpm for 10 minutes to obtain the serum, which was used for the biochemical assays. The kidneys collected were dissected out carefully, blotted free of blood, sliced and immersed in 10% phosphate buffer formalin and in 2.5% phosphate buffer glutaraldehyde (pH 7.4) for histological analysis.

### Biochemical analyses

The concentrations of creatinine, urea, uric acid and electrolytes (including $Na^+$, $K^+$, $HCO3^-$ and $Cl^-$) in the serum were determined using referenced standard methods [29-32]. Reagent kits obtained from Biosystems Laboratories (S. A. Costa Brava, Barcelonia, Spain) and Randox Laboratories (United Kingdom) were used in the study. All the reagent kits were of analytical grade.

### Histological analysis

The slices of kidney tissues were fixed in 10% formosaline for 24 hr, after which they were dehydrated with 100% ethanol solution and then embedded in paraffin. They were thereafter sectioned at 7 μm thickness, and stained with haematoxylin and eosin (HE) for histological examination. Images of kidney sections processed by HE were examined under light microscope for morphological changes.

### Statistical analysis

Results were presented as mean ± S.E.M. The data generated from the study were statistically analysed using one-way analysis of variance (ANOVA) with SPSS (version 17.0) and Microsoft Excel programmes. Student "t" test was also used for pair-wise comparison, and differences were considered significant at $p<0.05$.

# Results

The results of this study are presented in figures 1-4 and slides 1a-f. The results showed that serum creatinine, urea, uric acid, K+, HCO3- and Cl- levels were significantly ($p < 0.05$) increased, while the serum Na+ level decreased significantly in rat model, following exposure to NCT, when compared with the control (Figure 1-3). However, there was no significant ($p < 0.05$) difference in the serum creatinine (1.5 ± 0.5 mmol/l), urea (36.3 ± 4.1 mmol/l), uric acid (2.3 ± 0.8 mmol/l), Na+ (142.8 ± 7.1 mEq/l), K+ (1.5 ± 0.6 mEq/l), HCO3- (13.0 ± 2.1 mEq/l) and Cl- 81.1 ± 3.8 mEq/l) levels of rats receiving soybeans oil only, compared, respectively, to the levels (1.5 ± 0.5 mmol/l, 36.9 ± 3.8 mmol/l, 2.4 ± 0.6 mmol/l, 143.6 ± 6.2 mEq/l, 1.6 ± 0.3 mEq/l, 12.8 ± 2.6 mEq/l and 80.7 ± 4.6 mEq/l, respectively) recorded for the control rats receiving distilled water only. Also, administration of vitamins C and E, either singularly or in combination, to rats exposed to NCT produced a significant ($p < 0.05$) decrease in serum creatinine, urea, uric acid, K+, HCO3- and Cl- levels, and increase in serum Na+ level to levels within the control range, compared respectively to the levels obtained for rats exposed to NCT only (Figure 1-3). The levels of these serum indices recorded for rats exposed to NCT and treated with vitamins C and E were not significantly ($p < 0.05$) different from the levels recorded for rats in the control. This observation implies that administration of vitamins C and E to rats exposed to NCT maintained serum creatinine, urea, uric acid, Na+, K+, HCO3- and Cl- levels within the control range.

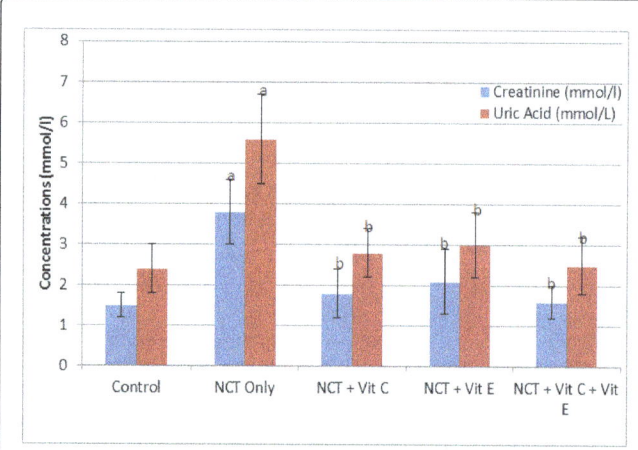

**Figure 1:** Effect of vitamins C (Vitamin C) and E (Vitamin E) on serum creatinine and uric acid concentrations of rats exposed to Nitrocellulose thinner (NCT). a=p<0.05 compared with control; b=p<0.05 compared with NCT only.

Moreover, it was observed from the results of this study that administration of vitamin C only to rats exposed to NCT produced a significant ($p < 0.05$) increase in comparative percentage decrease in serum creatinine and K+ concentrations, compared respectively to the comparative percentage decrease recorded for rats exposed to NCT and administered vitamin E only (Figure 4). However, the comparative percentage decrease in serum creatinine, uric acid, K+ and HCO3- concentration recorded for rats exposed to NCT and treated with vitamins C and E, in combination, was significantly ($p < 0.05$) higher, compared respectively to the comparative percentage decrease in serum creatinine, uric acid, K+ and HCO3- concentration recorded for rats exposed to NCT and treated singularly with vitamins C and E

(Figure 4). The results obtained from this study therefore suggested that vitamin C is more potent than vitamin E in protecting the renal tissues against NCT induced toxicity on one hand, and that on the other hand, combined administration of vitamins C and E produced a higher protective potency against NCT induced renal tissues toxicity than administration of vitamins C and E singly in rats.

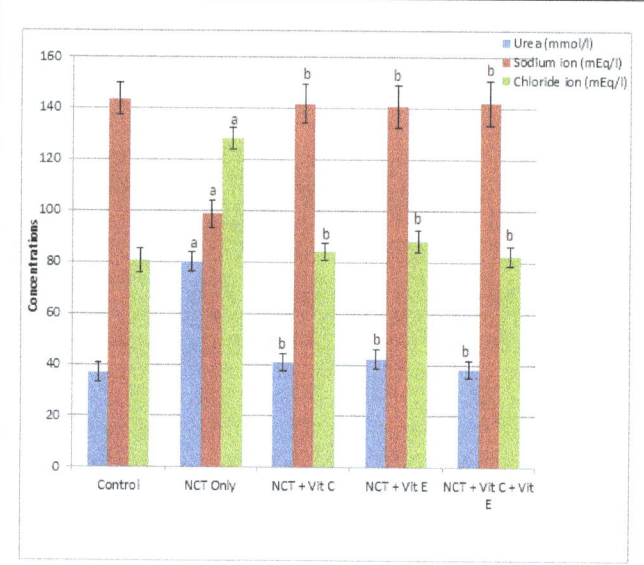

**Figure 2:** Effect of vitamins C (Vitamin C) and E (Vitamin E) on serum urea, sodium and chloride ions concentrations of rats exposed to Nitrocellulose thinner (NCT). a=p<0.05 compared with control; b=p<0.05 compared with NCT only.

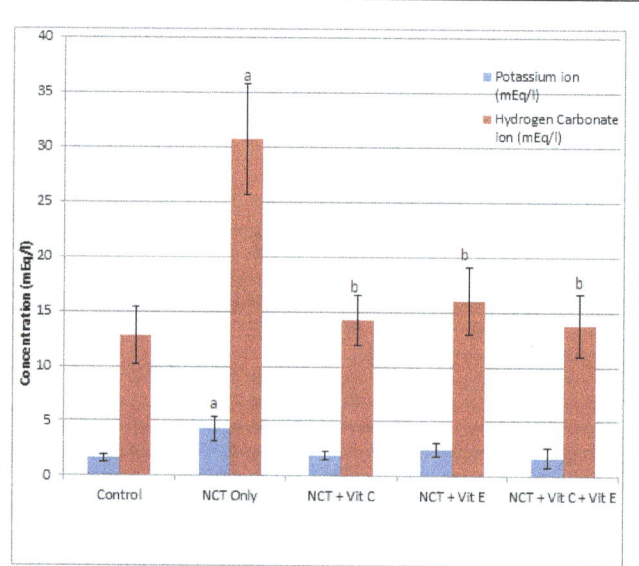

**Figure 3:** Effect of vitamins C (Vitamin C) and E (Vitamin E) on serum potassium and hydrogen carbonate ions level of rats exposed to Nitrocellulose thinner (NCT). a=p<0.05 compared with control; b=p<0.05 compared with NCT only.

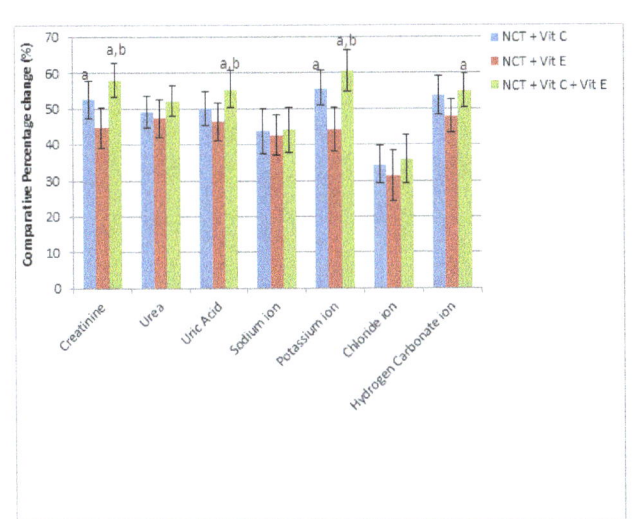

**Figure 4:** Comparative percentage effect of vitamins C (Vitamin C) and E (Vitamin E) on some serum metabolites and electrolytes of renal function assessments in rats exposed to Nitrocellulose thinner (NCT). a=p<0.05 compared with NCT+Vitamin E; b=p<0.05 compared.

Slide 1c shows the various negative changes in renal histological structure following exposure to nitrocellulose thinner, compared to the relatively normal histological structures observed for the control groups (Slides 1b and c), and the groups exposed to nitrocellulose thinner and treated with vitamins C and E (Slides 1 d-f). These results show that exposure to nitrocellulose thinner caused adverse changes in renal tissues histological pattern, such as necrosis of glomeruli and tubules, atrophic glomeruli, glomerular capsule and tubules dilatation. And that administration of vitamins C and E to rats exposed to nitrocellulose thinner-prevented the occurrence of these nitrocellulose thinner induced adverse changes in renal tissues histological integrity in male rats (Slides 1 d-f).

## Discussion

It is generally known that exposure to some chemical solvents, including nitrocellulose thinner, may cause severe organ tissue toxicities. Particularly, previous studies reported that exposure to nitrocellulose thinner is capable of exerting deleterious effects on the renal tissues, hence nephrotoxicity [4,5,33]. In our earlier studies, exposure to nitrocellulose thinner was observed to cause elevation of serum creatinine, urea, BUN, uric acid, $K^+$, and renal tissue malondialdehyde (MDA), as well as decreased serum protein, $Na^+$, $Ca_2^+$, $HCO_3^-$, $Cl^-$ levels and renal tissue superoxide dismutase (SOD) activity in rats [4,5]. Also, a significant distortion in the architectural integrity of the ultrastructural profile of the renal tissues was also observed to be associated with exposure to nitrocellulose thinner in these previous studies. Similar increase in serum creatinine, urea, uric acid, $Na^+$, $K^+$, $HCO_3^-$ and $Cl^-$ levels was observed to be associated with exposure to nitrocellulose thinner in this present study. Also, marked distortions in the architectural integrity of the ultrastructural status of the renal tissues following exposure to nitrocellulose thinner were also recorded in this study. Elevation in serum creatinine, uric acid, urea and blood urea nitrogen has been reported to be strongly associated

with the development of renal disease, hence renal dysfunction or failure [10,34,35]. The observations made from this present study in correlation with our earlier reports [5,27] therefore indicated that exposure to nitrocellulose thinner is among the risk factors for nephrotoxicity, with the possibility of producing renal failure.

Literature reports that some of these chemical substances produce renal toxicity via the generation of **free radicals** and other reactive species in the course of their metabolism [36-38]. The results of this study therefore suggest that nitrocellulose thinner contain some chemical substances with nephrotoxic potentials. It is generally known that when the level of the reactive species, or pro-oxidants, generated in the course of chemical agents' metabolism in the tissues overwhelms the endogenous protective antioxidants, they tend to interact with the tissues' macromolecular components. The interaction of these reactive species, generated from chemical agents' metabolism, with the renal tissues is likely to result in the nephrotic damage and necrosis [39]. It may therefore be assumed that the reactive metabolites of the nitrocellulose thinner's constituents might have interacted with the renal tissues to induce the nephrotoxicity reported in this present work and our previous studies [4,5,13]. The observation made from the results of this study therefore supports of our earlier reports that NCT induced nephrotoxicity in experimental animals [4,5,13]. However, administration of antioxidants supplements have been reported to provide some degree of protection against the chemical agents generated reactive species tissue challenges. Vitamins C and E have been reported to be among the vitamin supplements with effective antioxidant properties in the various biological systems [20-22].

Vitamin C has been reported to mediate its antioxidant effect by scavenging free reactive oxygen specie [40-44]. This indicates that Vitamin C may inhibit the chain reactions of chemical agents-generated free radicals or scavenged the reactive free radicals before reaching their tissue targets; while Vitamin E is reported to act by breaking the antioxidant chain that prevents reactive oxygen species from interacting with membrane macromolecules to produce cell membrane damage [45]. Also, Factor et al. [46], demonstrated that vitamin E can directly reduce ROS production by interfering in the union between the membrane and the NADPH oxidase complex. Also administration of vitamin E, have been reported to play a vital role in the prevention of lipid peroxidation, to protect the tissues against chemical injury [47,48]. In this study, the levels of metabolites and electrolytes assayed were observed to fall within the control range following administration of vitamins C and E to rats exposed to nitrocellulose thinner. Also, relatively normal histological integrity of the renal tissues was observed in rats exposed to nitrocellulose thinner and treated with vitamins C and E. The results of this present study therefore showed that vitamins C and E supplements are capable of providing protection against nitrocellulose induced nephrotoxicity in rats.

In agreement with the report of Car et al. [19], the results of this present study showed that vitamin C is relatively more potent than vitamin E in protecting the renal tissues against NCT induced renal toxicity in rats. However, it was observed that the protective effectiveness of combined administration of vitamins C and E, as a combined therapy, was higher than that of single therapy administration; and that the protection potency of vitamin E was more than that of vitamin C. The specific mechanism(s) of the higher protective potency of the combined, than single, administration of vitamins C and E against nitrocellulose thinner induced nephrotoxicity is a subject for further investigation.

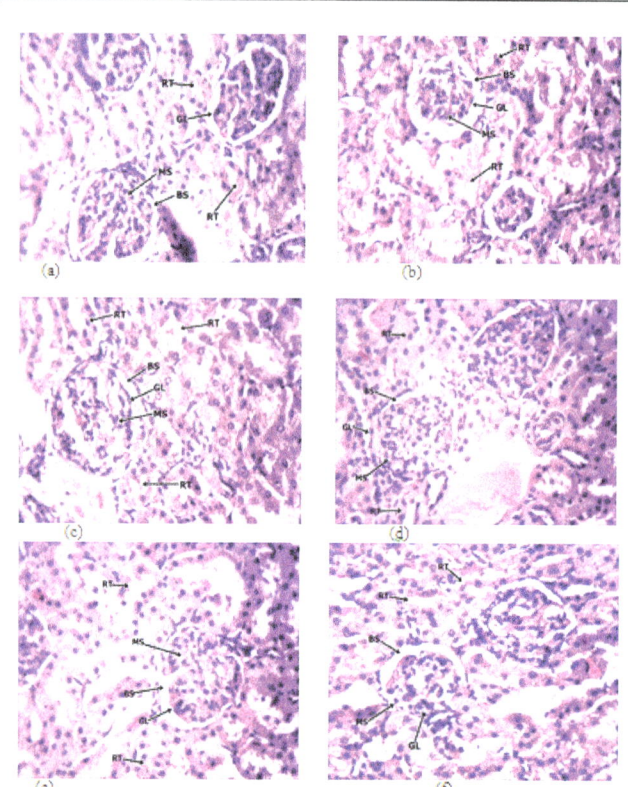

**Slide 1:** Sections of renal tissues of, (a) control rats receiving distilled water only, (b) rats receiving soya beans oil only, (c) rats receiving 40.0mg NCT/kg bwt, (d) rats receiving 40.0 mg NCT/kg bwt+200 mg Vitamin C/kg bwt, (e) rats receiving 40.0mg NCT/kg bwt+200IU Vitamin E/kg bwt and (f) rats receiving 40.0mg NCT/kg bwt+200IU Vitamin E/kg bwt+200mg Vitamin C/kg bwt. Slides 1a and b show normal kidney tissues showing prominent glomeruli (GL) and renal tubules (RT). The glomeruli are surrounded by clear bowman's space (BS) and a cellular mesangium (MS) consisting of deeply stained basophilic oval to round mesangial cells. The renal tubules are closely packed with empty lumen, lined by cuboidal epithelial cells with regular cellular outline. Also, the intervening interstitium is scanty and contains normal blood vessels. Slide 1c shows atrophic glomeruli and some swollen glomeruli with loss of bowman space. Their mesangial cells are scanty with areas of fibrosis. The renal tubules are closely packed and lined by swollen epithelial cells with some tubules showing detachment of epithelial cells from their basement membrane. Also, the intervening interstitium is scanty and contains congested blood vessels and thick wall arterioles. Slide 1d, e and f show prominent glomeruli and renal tubules. The glomeruli are surrounded by clear bowman's space and a cellular mesangium. The renal tubules are closely packed with empty lumen, lined by cuboidal epithelial cells having regular cellular outline and moderate eosinophilic cytoplasm and prominent nuclei with nucleoli. Also, the intervening interstitium is scanty and contains blood vessels.

Based on the results obtained from this study, it may be concluded that coadministration of vitamins C and E is more potent than single administration, in providing protection against nitrocellulose thinner-induced nephrotoxicity in male albino Wistar rat model. Also, it is very likely that the results obtained from this study may be applicable to humans since most biochemical and physiological activities in rats correlate those in human. However, more investigations are needed to verify this assertion.

## References

1. Nwankwo EA, Nwankwo B, Mubi B (2006) Prevalence of impaired kidney in hospitalized hypertensive patients in Maiduguri, Nigeria. Internet. J Inter Med 6 (1).

2. Atangwho JI, Ebong PE, Eteng MU, Eyong EU, Obi AU (2007) Effect of Vernonia amygdalina Del Leaf on kidney function of diabetic rats. Int J Pharmacol 3: 143-148.

3. Crook MA (2007) The kidneys, In: Clinical chemistry and metabolic medicine, 7th edition. Bookpower, Britain pp 36-57.

4. Uboh FE, Akpanabiatu MI, Aquaisua AN Bassey EI (2012) Oral exposure to Nitrocellulose thinner solvent induces Nephrotoxicity in male albino Wistar rats. J Pharmacol Toxicol 7: 78-86.

5. Uboh FE, Ufot S, Mboso S, Eyong EU (2014) Effect of Costus afer Leaves' Juice on Nitrocellulose Thinner Induced Nephrotoxicity in Rats. Res J Environ Toxicol 8: 37-45.

6. World Health Organization (WHO) (2005) Concise International Chemical Assessment Document 64. Butyl Acetates. World Health Organization: Geneva.

7. Seeber A, Sietmann B, Zupanic M (1996) In search of dose-response relationships of solvent mixtures to neurobehavioural effects in paint manufacturing and painters. Food Chem Toxicol 34: 1113-1120.

8. JovanoviÄ JM, JovanoviÄ MM, SpasiÄ MJ, LukiÄ SR (2004) Peripheral nerve conduction study in workers exposed to a mixture of organic solvents in paint and lacquer industry. Croat Med J 45: 769-774.

9. Faber WD, Roberts LSG, Stump DG, Tardif R, Krishnan K, et al. (2006) Two-generation reproduction study of ethylbenzene by inhalation in Crl-CD rats. Birth Defects Res B Dev Reprod Toxicol 77: 10-21.

10. Patil AJ, Bhagwat VR, Patil JA, Dongre NN, Ambekar JG et al. (2007) Occupational lead exposure in battery manufacturing workers, silver jewelry workers, and spray painters in Western Maharashtra (India): effect on liver and kidney function. J Basic Clin Physiol Pharmacol 18: 87-100.

11. Uboh FE, Usoh IF, Nwankpa P, Obochi GO (2012) Effect of oral exposure to Nitrocellulose thinner on Haematological profiles of male albino Wistar rats. AJBMB, 2: 227-234.

12. Uboh FE, Ufot S (2013a) Withdrawal from exposure reverses hematotoxicity and hepatotoxicity caused by oral exposure to Nitrocellulose thinner in male rats. J Clin Toxicol 3: 173.

13. Uboh FE, Ufot SU, Eyong EU (2013b) Comparative effect of withdrawal from exposure on gasoline and diesel induced nephrotoxicity in male albino Wistar rats. J Clin Toxicol 3:170.

14. Hu Z, Wells PG (1994) Modulation of benzo (a) pyrene bioactivation by glucuronidation in lymphocytes and hepatic microsomes from rats with a hereditary deficiency in bilirubin UDP-glucuronosyl-transferase. Toxicol Appl Pharmacol 127: 306-313.

15. Page NP, Mehlman M (1989) Health effects of gasoline refueling vapors and measured exposures at service stations. Toxicol Ind Health 5: 869-890.

16. Nygren J, Cedewal B, Erickson S, Dusinska M, Kolman A (1994) Induction of DNA strand breaks by ethylene oxide in human diploid fibroblasts. Environ Mol Mutagen 24: 161-167.

17. Chatterjea MN, Shinde R (2002) Renal function Tests. In: Textbook of Medical Biochemistry, 5th Edition. JAYPEE Brothers medical publishers Ltd., New Delhi; 564-570.

18. Jimoh FO, Odutuga AA (2004) Histological changes of selected rat tissues following ingestion of thermally oxidized groundnut oil. Biokemistri 16: 1-10.

19. Carr AC, Zhu BZ, Frei B (2000) Potential antiatherogenic mechanisms of ascorbate (vitamin C) and alpha-tocopherol (vitamin E). Circ Res 87: 349-354.

20. Whitehead CC, Keller T (2003) An update on ascorbic acid in poultry. World's Poultry Sc J 59: 161-184.

21. Ayo JO, Minka NS, Mamman M (2006) Excitability scores of goats administered ascorbic acid and transported during hot-dry conditions. J Vet Sci 7: 127-131.

22. Sutcu R, Altuntas I, Buyukvanli B, Akturka O, Ozturka O, et al. (2007) The effects of diazinon on lipid peroxidation and antioxidant enzymes in rat erythrocytes: role of vitamins E and C. Toxicol Ind Health 23: 13-17.

23. Jialal I, Grundy SM (1993) Effect of combined supplementation with alpha-tocopherol, ascorbate, and beta carotene on low-density lipoprotein oxidation. Circulation 88: 2780-2786.

24. Schwarzacher SP, Hutchison S, Chou TM, Sun YP, Zhu BQ, et al. (1998) Antioxidant diet preserves endothelium-dependent vasodilatation in resistance arteries of hypercholesterolemic rabbits exposed to environmental tobacco smoke. J Cardiovasc Pharmacol 31: 649-653.

25. Heitzer T, Ylä Herttuala S, Wild E, Luoma J, Drexler H (1999) Effect of vitamin E on endothelial vasodilator function in patients with hypercholesterolemia, chronic smoking or both. J Am Coll Cardiol 33: 499-505.

26. Huang A, Vita JA, Venema RC, Keaney JF (2000) Ascorbic acid enhances endothelial nitric oxide synthase activity by increasing intracellular tetrahydrobiopterin. J Biol Chem 275: 17399-17406.

27. Uboh FE, Ebong PE, Akpan HD, Usoh IF (2012c) Hepatoprotective effect of vitamins C and E against gasoline vapor-induced liver injury in male rats. Turk J Biol 36: 217-223.

28. NRC (1995) National Research council: Nutrient requirements of laboratory animals. fourth revised edition, National Academy Press. Washington, DC 29-30.

29. Newman DJ, Price CP (1999) Renal function and Nitrogen Metabolites. CA. Burtis, ER Ashwood (Eds.) Tietz Textbook of Clinical Chemistry. (3rd Edn.) Philadelphia. WB Saunders Co Pp: 1204.

30. Tietz NW (1976) Fundamentals of Clinical Chemistry. Saunders WB company, Philadelphia, PA. Pp: 874-880.

31. Trinder P (1957) Analyst, 76: 596-600.

32. Searcy RL, Reardon JE, Foreman JA (1967) A new photometric method for serum urea nitrogen determination. Am J Med Technol 33: 15-20.

33. Patrick-Iwuanyanwu KC, Okon EA, Areh NW, Wegwu MO (2013) Toxicological effect of inhalation exposure to nitrocellulose paint thinner fumes. Arch Appl Sci Res 5: 264-269

34. Mazzali M, Hughes J, Kim YG, Jefferson JA, Kang DH, et al. (2001) Elevated uric acid increases blood pressure in the rat by a novel crystal-independent mechanism. Hypertension 38: 1101-1106.

35. Serrato HMI, Fortoul TI, Martinez RR, Alvarado MLR, Trevino CL et al. (2006) Lead blood concentrations and renal function evaluation: Study in an exposed Mexican population. Environ Res 100: 227-233.

36. Arise RO, Malomo SO (2009) Effects of ivermectin and albendazole on some liver and kidney function indices in rats. Afr J Biochem Res 3: 190-197.

37. Padmini MP, Kumar JV (2012) A histopathological study on gentamycin induced nephrotoxicity in experimental Albino rats. J Dental Med Sci 1: 14-17.

38. Varghese HS, Kotagiri S, Swamy BMV, Swamy PA, Raj GG (2013) Nephroprotective activity of Benincasa hispida (Thunb.) Cogn. Fruit extract against paracetamol induced nephrotoxicity in rats. Res J Pharm Biol Chem Sci 4: 322-332.

39. McGinness JE, Proctor PH, Demopoulos HB, Hokanson JA, Kirkpatrick DS (1978) Amelioration of cis-platinum nephrotoxicity by orgotein (superoxide dismutase). Physiol Chem Phys 10: 267-277.

40. Odigie IP, Okpoko FB, Ojobo PD (2007) Antioxidant Effects of Vitamins C and E on Phenylhydrazine-Induced Haemolysis in Sprague Dawley Rats: Evidence for A better Protection by Vitamin E. Niger Postgrad Med J 14: 1-7.

41. Dogun ES, Ajala MO (2005) Ascorbic Acid and Alpha Tocopherol Antioxidant Status of Type 2 Diabetes Mellitus Patients seen in Lagos. Niger Postgrad Med J 12: 155-157.

42. Chen K, Suh J, Carr AC, Morrow JD, Zeind J, et al. (2000) Vitamin C suppresses oxidative lipid damage in vivo, even in the presence of iron overload. Am J Physiol Endocrinol Metab 279: E1406-1412.

43. Frei B (2004) Efficacy of dietary antioxidants to prevent oxidative damage and inhibit chronic disease. J Nutr 134: 3196S-3198S.

44. Ambali S, Akanbi D, Igbokwe N, Shittu M, Kawu M, et al. (2007) Evaluation of subchronic chlorpyrifos poisoning on hematological and serum biochemical changes in mice and protective effect of vitamin C. J Toxicol Sci 32: 111-120.

45. Brigelius-Flohé R, Traber MG (1999) Vitamin E: function and metabolism. FASEB J 13: 1145-1155.

46. Factor VM, Laskowska D, Jensen MR, Woitach JT, Popescu NC, et al. (2000) Vitamin E reduces chromosomal damage and inhibits hepatic tumor formation in a transgenic mouse model. Proc Natl Acad Sci U S A 97: 2196-2201.

47. Farías RC, Santillán ME, Salinas GJ, Sánchez RN, Cruz M, et al. (2009) Protective effect of some vitamins against the toxic action of ethanol on liver regeration induced by partial hepatectomy in rats. World J Gastroenterol 14: 899-907.

48. Bradford A, Atkinson J, Fuller N, Rand R (2003) The effect of vitamin E on the structure of membrane lipid assemblies. J Lipid Res 44: 1940-1945.

# 21

# Randomized Controlled Trial of Treatment of Chronic Kidney Disease of Uncertain Aetiology with Enalapril

**Mathu Selvarajah**[1], **Shanthi Mendis**[2*], **Saroj Jayasinghe**[3], **Rezvi Sheriff**[4], **Tilak Abeysekera**[5] and **Firdosi Mehta**[6]

[1]*Department of Nephrology, Teaching Hospital Anuradhapura, Sri Lanka*

[2]*Department of Management of Noncommunicable Diseases, World Health Organization, Geneva, Switzerland*

[3]*Department of Clinical Medicine, Faculty of Medicine, University of Colombo, Sri Lanka*

[4]*Faculty of Medicine, University of Colombo, Sri Lanka*

[5]*Nephrology Unit, General Hospital (Teaching), Kandy, Sri Lanka*

[6]*World Health Organization, Colombo, Sri Lanka*

[*]**Corresponding Author:** Dr. Shanthi Mendis, Department of Management of Noncommunicable Diseases, World Health Organization, Geneva, Switzerland, E-mail: prof.shanthi.mendis@gmail.com

## Abstract

**Introduction:** A double blind placebo controlled randomized trial was conducted to investigate the effect of angiotensin-converting-enzyme (ACE) inhibitor enalapril on the progression of Chronic Kidney Disease (CKD) caused by chronic exposure to nephrotoxins.

**Methods:** 263 people aged 18-70 years diagnosed with CKD stages I, II or III who were not taking ACE inhibitors, who had no other chronic disease or contraindication for treatment with ACE inhibitors, were randomly assigned to enalapril or placebo. The main outcomes were albumin to creatinine ratio (ACR) and estimated glomerular filtration rate (eGFR).

**Results:** The mean systolic and diastolic blood pressure levels declined significantly in both enalapril and placebo groups with no significant difference in the two groups. There was a significant improvement in the albumin to creatinine ratio in the enalapril group compared to the placebo group (p<0.005). In the enalapril group, the mean albumin to creatinine ratio declined from 162.0 mg/g (SD 321.7) at baseline, to 55.4 mg/g (SD 122.4) at one year follow up; while in the placebo group, the mean albumin to creatinine ratio increased from 197.9 mg/g (SD 461.6) at baseline to 253.2 mg/g (SD 558.7), at one year follow up. In both groups, the eGFR declined significantly, during the 12 month follow-up, lower in the enalapril group, although with no significant difference. In the enalapril group the mean (eGFR) declined from 71.7 ml/min (SD 22.2) to 57.1 ml/min (SD16.1), while in the placebo group the mean eGFR declined from 73.8 ml/min (SD 24.2) to 54.7 ml/min (SD 20.3).

**Conclusion:** Enalapril is beneficial in reducing albuminuria in patients with chronic kidney disease of uncertain aetiology.

**Keywords:** Enalapril; Nephrotoxins; Chronic kidney disease of uncertain aetiology; Randomized control trial; Proteinuria

## Introduction

Chronic Kidney Disease of uncertain aetiology, which cannot be attributed to diabetes mellitus, hypertension, glomerulonephritis, chronic pyelonephritis or other known etiologies, emerged in the North Central Region of Sri Lanka about two decades ago. Research upto date suggest that the most probable aetiology of this condition is long term exposure to nephrotoxic heavy metals and pesticides, together with deficiency of selenium and genetic susceptibility [1-3]. Chronic Kidney Disease due to longterm exspoure to environmental Nephrotoxins (CKDn) is slowly progressive, probably starting in the second decade of life, and asymptomatic until very advanced. Interstitial fibrosis and tubular atrophy with or without nonspecific interstitial mononuclear cell infiltrate is the dominant histopathological observation [2,4,5]. It has become a major public

health problem causing serious economic and health consequences particularly in the lower socioeconomic communities in the North Central Region region in Sri Lanka. The health care costs for the management of these patients are considerable as those in end stage kidney disease require haemodialysis or transplantation. Further, these high technology interventions are not readily accessible to the majority with CKDn due to economic constraints. This highlights the need to find prevention strategies and treatment modalities for slowing and reversing the progression of CKDn in those with early stages of the disease [6,7].

Main treatment modalities to slow down the progression to chronic renal disease are likely to be through control of blood pressure and proteinuria. The importance of proteinuria as a significant risk factor for end stage kidney disease is well recognized [8]. Proteinuria reduction is considered as a surrogate marker of renoprotection in proteinuric renal disease [9]. Angiotensin II mediates hemodynamic effects as well as inflammation and fibrosis in the kidney, heart, and vasculature [10]. ACE inhibitors can boost renal repair by promoting survival and repair of podocytes, preventing mesangial cell hyperplasia, and inducing glomerular endothelial cell remodeling. Other mechanisms include reduction of the expression of plasminogen activator inhibitor 1, an inhibitor of matrix degradation, decreased expression of collagen I and IV and TGF-b, and increased metalloproteinase activity [11]. Treatment that is targeted at reducing proteinuria has been shown to reduce progression of diabetic and non-diabetic kidney disease [12-18]. In most forms of proteinuric chronic renal disease, glomerular filtration rate continues to decline even when the initial insult has been removed [12]. Angiotensin converting enzyme inhibitors have been shown to be effective in retarding the progress of some forms of proteinuric kidney disease [12-34].

Currently there are no known treatment modalities to retard the progression of tubule-interstitial damage caused by nephrotoxins. If ACE inhibitors are found to be effective in retarding the progress of CKDn it will be a cost effective intervention for controlling this major public health problem in Sri Lanka.

The objective of this prospective double blind controlled study was to investigate the efficacy of enalapril, on the progression of CKDn by comparing and evaluating the effect of enalapril to a placebo on estimated glomerular filtration rate and albuminuria. We hypothesised that treatment with enalapril for 12 months in subjects with CKDn, would blunt decline in glomerular filtration rate and albuminuria compared with placebo.

## Methods

Subjects living in two districts (Anuradhapura and Polonnaruwa) in the North Central Region of Sri Lanka, diagnosed as having CKDn in a population prevalence study (1), who satisfied inclusion criteria of the trial were invited to participate. The trial was registered in the Sri Lanka Clinical Trials Registry. Ethical clearance for the study was obtained from the Ethical Review Committee, Medical Research Institute, Ministry of Health, Sri Lanka. All participants gave written informed consent. Patients were potentially eligible if they were between 18 and 70 years and had albumin to creatinine ratio > 30mg/g and estimated glomerular filtration rate >15 ml/min. The response rate was 70.87% (n=427). Patients who were already on treatment with either an ACE inhibitor or an angiotensin receptor blocker were excluded (n=41). Another 54 patients were excluded based on other exclusion criteria (pregnancy-4, breast feeding-16, renal calculus with urinary tract dilatation-4, diabetes mellitus-7, malignancy-2, eGFR <15 ml/min-8, recent history of acute kidney injury following snake bite-2, rheumatoid arthritis-2, glomerulonephritis-2, not willing to take western medicine-7). Repeat urine albumin to creatinine ratio was <30 mg/g in 69 patients. They were excluded from the study.

The patients with CKDn were graded as follows: (using the Chronic Kidney Disease Epidemiology collaboration (CKD- EPI) equation) (1)

Stage 1: persistent albuminuria (i.e. ACR ≥ 30 mg/g in initial and repeat urine sample) and eGFR >90 ml/min/1.73 m2

Stage 2: persistent albuminuria and eGFR 60-89 ml/ min/1.73 m2

Stage 3: persistent albuminuria and eGFR 30-59 ml/ min/1.73 m2

Stage 4: persistent albuminuria and eGFR 15-30 ml/ min/1.73 m2.

Patients who had no exclusion criteria (n=263) were randomized to treatment and placebo groups (Figure 1), and followed up at the Teaching Hospital Anuradhapura and Base Hospitals Padaviya and Medirigriya.

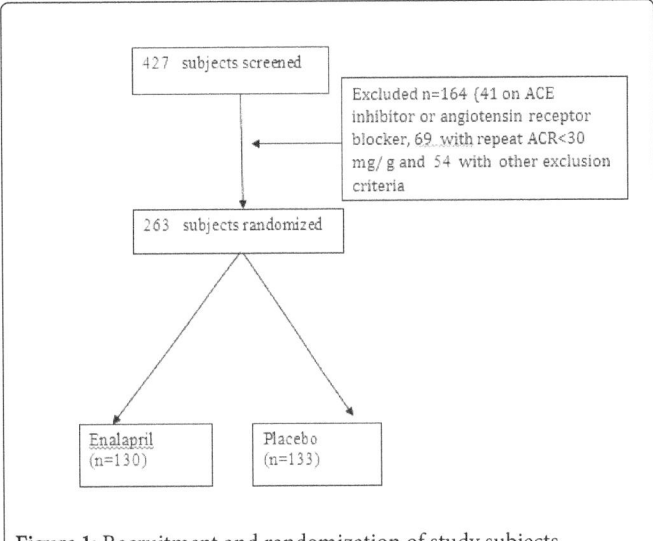

**Figure 1:** Recruitment and randomization of study subjects.

Following informed consent and completion of the baseline assessments, participants were randomized into the trial in a 11 ratio to placebo and enalapril arms. Randomization was provided by the World Health Organization using a computer-generated programme. Patients, investigators, monitoring members and outcome assessors were blinded to group assignment and intervention. The randomization list and blinding codes remained confidential, and only the study statistician had access to the randomization list.

At the baseline visit, laboratory tests were done for urine sediment analysis, urine albumin creatinine ratio, hemoglobin, white cell count and differential count, glucose, urea, HbA1C, uric acid, cholesterol, triglycerides, liver enzymes, bilirubin and 24 hour urine analysis. All analyses were performed according to standard procedures using automatic analyzers. Allocation concealment was extended to the laboratory personnel.

Participants were seen at two pre-randomization visits, and every month after randomization for 12 months. Those who were randomized were commenced on enalapril or placebo. Enalapril or placebo were started at low dose and titrated up based on blood pressure, proteinuria and serum potassium level. All treatments other than enalapril were continued at the discretion of the responsible physician. Blood pressure was measured as the mean of two measurements made in the seated position using a mercury sphygmomanometer. Measurement of urinary albumin creatinine ratio was performed on spot urine samples. During each visit and at the end of follow-up, it was assessed: compliance, symptoms, blood pressure, serum creatinine, and serum potassium and urine albumin to creatinine levels. The abbreviated Modification of Diet in Renal Disease (MDRD) equation was used to estimate eGFR.

Nine patients underwent renal biopsy on clinician direction (not as part of study protocol).

During the course of the study, 5 cases in the enalapril group and one case in the placebo group were switched over to losartan due to persistent dry cough. Five cases were withdrawn due to other reasons (Figure 1). Loss of appetite and hyperkalaemia necessitated the discontinuation of treatment in 2 patients in the enalapril group. One patient in the placebo group was withdrawn from the study due to pregnancy. In the enalapril group, one patient (68 years) suffered a myocardial infarction and one patient (64 years) suffered a stroke.

Confidentiality of participants' data was protected by identifying patients on all study forms by a unique patient identification number. No study forms or other documents collected for the purpose of this study revealed the participant's name. No subject identifiers were presented on any files transmitted to any committee or any institution.

## Statistical Analysis

In order to calculate the sample size and the power estimates two indices of improvement were selected; Estimated Glomerular Filtration rate (eGFR) and urine Albumin Creatinine Ratio (ACR). To ensure a power of at least 80%, at α=5% and to detect up to 14.04 ml/min discrepancies in eGFR rate and up to 20.77 mg/gr discrepancies in ACR rate, 51 cases and 51 controls were required. Assuming that eGRF rate and ACR rate follow a normal distribution with standard deviations of σ=30.84 ml/min and σ=50.52 mg/gr respectively, a sample size of 100 in each arm was required to ensure a statistical power of the test at least 80% at α=5% and account for 25% loss of cases and controls during follow up.

Data collected during the baseline visit and the 12 follow up visits were analyzed to test the change in albuminuria and estimated glomerular filtration rate in participants receiving enalapril and compared to participants receiving the placebo. Intention to treat analysis was used where the baseline allocation to active treatment or control treatment was used over all of the study period. Due to non-symmetric distributions the Wilcoxon rank-sum (Mann-Whitney) test was used for continuous data. Proportions were tested using Fischer's exact test.

## Results

As shown in table 1, there was no significant difference in the baseline characteristics (age, sex distribution, systolic and diastolic blood pressure, albumin to creatinine ratio and eGFR) in the enalapril and placebo groups.

| Characteristics | Enalapril group | Placebo group | P value |
|---|---|---|---|
| | (n=130) | (n=133) | |
| Age (years) | 47.7 (13.3) | 48.3 (13.6) | 0.18 |
| (mean, SD*) | | | |
| Male sex (number, %) | 61 (46.92) | 51 (38.35) | 0.17 |
| Blood pressure (mmHg) | 124.5 (17.9) | 125.2 (18.9) | 0.76 |
| Systolic mean, (SD) | | | |
| Diastolic mean, (SD) | 78.3 (10.6) | 80.4 (11-6) | 0.14 |
| Albumin creatinine ratio (ACR) | 162.0 (321.7) | 197.9 (461.6) | 0.47 |

**Table 1:** Baseline characteristics of patients in enalapril group and placebo group. *SD: Standard deviation.

The mean systolic and diastolic blood pressure levels declined significantly in both enalapril and placebo groups. The mean reduction in systolic blood pressure was 11.6 and 9.9 mm Hg (p=0.005, 0.031), respectively. The mean reduction in diastolic blood pressure was 9.7

and 8.3 mmHg (p ≤ 0.001), respectively. There was no significant difference between the enalapril and placebo groups in the reduction in systolic blood pressure and diastolic blood pressure.

There was a significant improvement in the albumin to creatinine ratio (ACR) in the enalapril group compared to the placebo group (p<0.005). In the enalapril group, the mean albumin to creatinine ratio declined from 162.0 mg/g (SD 321.7) at baseline, to 55.4 mg/g (SD 122.4) at one year follow up; while in the placebo group, the mean albumin to creatinine ratio increased from 197.9 mg/g (SD 461.6) at baseline to 253.2 mg/g (SD 558.7), at one year follow up (Table 2). The trend of ACR by month until the end of study in the placebo group and enalapril group is shown in figure 2 and 3 respectively, enalapril group demonstrating a decline throughout the study period.

| Variable | Enalapril group | Placebo group | P |
|---|---|---|---|
| | (n=56) | (n=48) | |
| Systolic blood pressure (mmHg) | | | |
| mean, (SD*) | 112.9 (15.5) | 115.3 (12.2) | 0.58 |
| Diastolic blood pressure (mmHg) | | | |
| mean, (SD) | 68.6 (12.4) | 72.1 (7.1) | 0.14 |
| Albumin creatinine ratio (mg/g) | | | |
| mean, (SD) | 55.4 (122.4) | 253.2 (558.7) | 0.005 |
| Estimated glomerular filtration rate (eGFR) mean, (SD) | 57.1 (16.1) | 54.7 (20.3) | 0.63 |

**Table 2:** Outcomes of enalapril group and placebo group. * SD: Standard deviation.

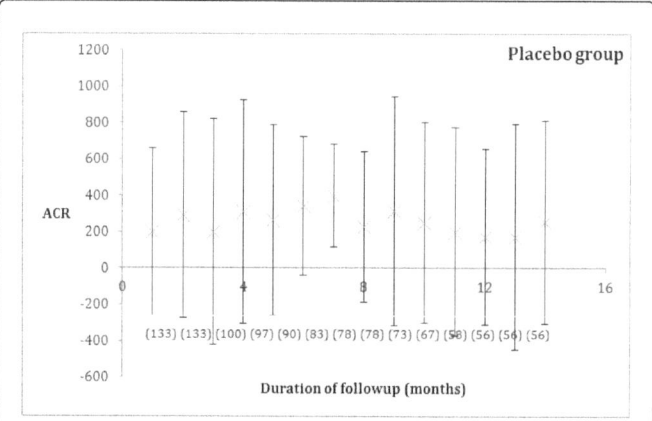

**Figure 2:** Effect of placebo on albumin to creatinine ratio (ACR) during follow up. Number of subjects at each follow up visit is shown in parentheses.

In both groups, the eGFR declined significantly (p<0.001) during the 12 month follow up. In the enalapril group the mean eGFR declined from 71.7 ml/min (SD 22.2) to 57.1 ml/min (SD16.1). In the placebo group the mean eGFR declined from 73.8 ml/min (SD 24.2) to 54.7 ml/min (SD 20.3). The decline in eGFR was less marked in the enalapril group, although there was no significant difference in the rate of decline between the two groups (Table 2). The trend of eGFR in the placebo group and enalapril group during the 12 months is shown in figures 4 and 5 respectively.

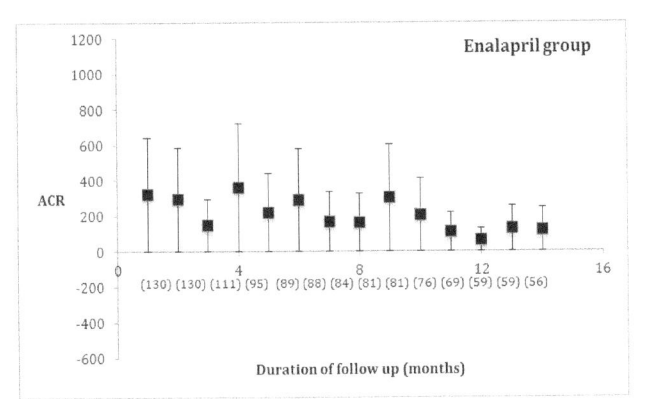

**Figure 3:** Effect of enalapril on albumin to creatinine ratio (ACR) during follow up. Number of subjects at each follow up visit is shown in parentheses. (Difference in ACR between placebo and enalapril groups was significant at all follow up visits after the first 3 months)

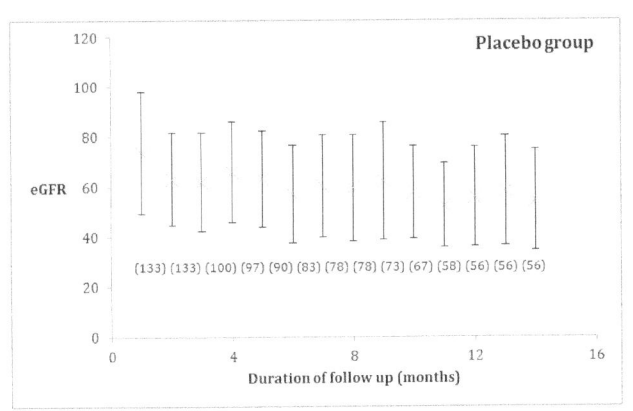

**Figure 4:** Effect of placebo on the estimated glomerular filtration rate (eGFR) during follow up. Number of subjects at each follow up visit is shown in parentheses.

All nine biopsy reports were reported as interstitial fibrosis and tubular atrophy with or without nonspecific interstitial mononuclear cell infiltrate as the dominant histopathological lesion.

## Discussion

This is the first study which has investigated the efficacy of enalapril in the treatment of chronic kidney disease due to nephrotoxins. Our results demonstrate the beneficial effect of enalapril in decreasing ACR, with a significant reduction at the end and throughout the study period. We interpret these results as demonstrating that enalapril was effective in reducing albuminuria in these patients with nephropathy due to longterm exposure to environmental toxins (CKDn).

ACE inhibitors are proven to have beneficial effect on proteinuric chronic kidney disease [12-34]. Proteinuria plays an important role in the progression of both non diabetic and diabetic kidney disease and

the pathological process implicated in this regard [16,35,36]. Ramipril efficacy in Nephrology Study showed that in proteinuric nephropathy of various aetiologies higher proteinuria at inclusion was associated with faster GFR decline. Ramipril therapy slowed glomerular filtration rate decline and end stage kidney disease development effectively [12,34]. The benefit of enalapril on slowing progression of renal disease has also been demonstrated in children with chronic disease [37] and patients on automated peritoneal dialysis [38].

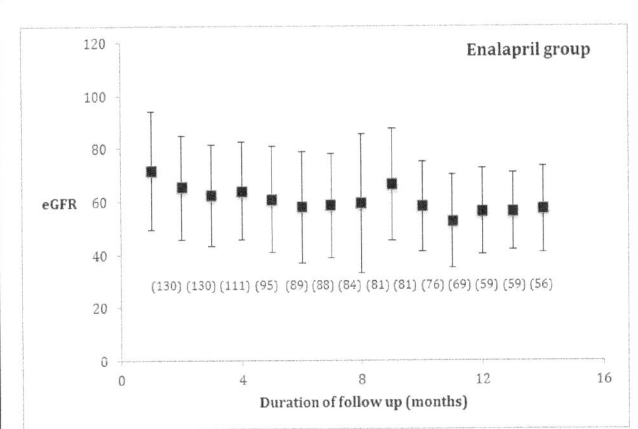

**Figure 5:** Effect of Enalapril on the estimated glomerular filtration rate (eGFR) during follow up. Number of subjects at each follow up visit is shown in parentheses.

In diabetic nephropathy, a 50% reduction in albuminuria was associated with a relative risk reduction for end stage renal disease of approximately 50% (8). Other studies have also shown a renoprotective effect of ACE inhibitors on progression of nondiabetic kidney disease [18,19,25,27,29]. A Cochrane review of 49 studies containing 12 067 diabetic patients at all stages of CKD found that ACEi and angiotensin receptor blockers improved end-stage renal disease and other outcomes (39).

In our study, there was no slowing of the rate of progression of nephropathy in the enalapril group or the placebo group, as reflected in the eGFR during the 12 month follow up. However, eGFR declined less in the enalapril group, although statistically the difference was not significant. A longer follow up period might demonstrate a beneficial effect, as reported in other studies with ACE inhibitors [12].

Blood pressure reduction itself lowers urinary protein reduction rate and retards the rate of GFR deterioration in chronic kidney disease [21,23,30,40]. Blood pressure reduction throughout the study was similar in both enalapril group and the control group. Hence, the beneficial effect of enalapril on proteinuria reduction appear to be independent of the antihypertensive effect and may be attributed to other pleiotropic effects [9,12].

No subjects in the trial were prematurely withdrawn due to acute deterioration of renal function. In the enalapril group 5 patients were switched over to losartan due to persistent dry cough. A meta-analysis of 17 randomized control trials has reported that there is a higher risk of dry cough in patients taking enalapril compared to losartan although the effects of enalapril and losartan on blood pressure and renal function are comparable [41]. Almost 30% of patients in the ACE inhibitor arm developed hyperkalemia higher than 5 mmol/l. However, hyperkalaemia necessitated the discontinuation of treatment only in 2 patients in the enalapril group. ACE inhibitors as well as angiotensin II receptor blockers are known to increase serum potassium concentrations in patients with chronic kidney disease. In a randomized, double-blind study treating stage 3 CKD with olmesartan and enalapril, 37% on olmesartan and 40% on enalapril developed hyperkalemia higher than 5 mmol/L [42].

Despite current available treatments, most patients with chronic kidney disease still continue to have residual proteinuria and progression of disease [13,15,16,18]. For example, in controlled trials, about one fifth of patients with severe diabetic nephropathy who have been intensively treated still progress to end stage renal disease in about 3 years [13,15].

CKDn has a major negative impact on a range of clinical outcomes including quality of life and often result in catastrophic spending due to the high cost of longterm care including renal dialysis. There is therefore a need for the development of new strategies to reduce exposure to nephrotoxins and to arrest the rate of loss of renal function to lessen the need for dialysis. Presence of varying degrees of mononuclear inflammatory cells in different stages of CKDn suggests activation of immune competent cells by the primary nephrotoxic injury. Use of immunosuppression to control the immune activation in selected cases will be a hypothesis to test [43,44].

**Limitations:** Attrition of subjects at different stages was the main limitation of the study. However the effect of enalapril on reduction of proteinuria could be demonstrated at all stages of follow up and was significant after the first 3 months (Figure 3).

At present chronic kidney disease attributed to environmental toxins has been reported from many parts of the world [3]. This study is limited to a sample of individuals from Sri Lanka, diagnosed as having chronic kidney disease attributed to environmental nephrotoxins. However, these results may have implications for treatment of people living in other parts of the world, who have chronic kidney disease due to longterm exposure to environmental toxins such as heavy metals and pesticides. Further studies are needed in different settings to investigate the efficacy of ACE inhibitors in delaying the progress of CKDn.

# Conclusions

Enalapril reduces the mean albumin to creatinine ratio at the end and throughout the study period. The blood pressure reduction was similar in groups, the enalapril and the placebo group; the beneficial effect of enalapril on proteinuria reduction is independent of its antihypertensive effects. Further longterm studies are needed to investigate the beneficial effect of ACE inhibitors on CKDn.

# Funding

The study was funded by the World Health Organization and the National Science Foundation of Sri Lanka.

# Acknowledgement

Dr. Lanka Dissanayake and Mr Sumudu Hewawasam are thanked for providing administrative support for the study.

# References

1. Jayatilake N, Mendis S, Maheepala P, Mehta FR (2013); CKDu National Research Project Team. Chronic kidney disease of uncertain aetiology; prevalence and causative factors in a developing country. BMC Nephrol 14: 180.

2. Nanayakkara S, Senevirathna S, Karunaratne U. Chandrajith R, Harada K, et al. (2012) Evidence of tubular damage in the very early stage of chronic kidney disease of uncertain etiology in the North Central Province of Sri Lanka: a cross-sectional study. Environ Health Prev Med 17:109-17.

3. Shanthi M (2015) Law and Society Trust Review. Chronic kidney disease of uncertain aetiology; policy perspectives 25: 3-12.

4. Nanayakkara S, Komiya T, Ratnatunga N, Senevirathna S, Harada K, et al. (2012) Tubulointerstitial damage as the major pathological lesion in endemic chronic kidney disease among farmers in North Central Province of Sri Lanka. Environ Health Prev Med 17: 213-221.

5. Athuraliya NT, Abeysekera TD, Amerasinghe PH, Kumarasiri R, Bandara P, et al. (2011) Uncertain etiologies of proteinuric-chronic kidney disease in rural Sri Lanka. Kidney Int 80: 1212-1221.

6. Honeycutt AA, Segel JE, Zhuo X, Hoerger TJ, Imai K, et al. (2013) Medical costs of CKD in the Medicare population. J Am Soc Nephrol 24: 1478-1483.

7. Essue BM, Wong G, Chapman J, Li Q, Jan S (2013) How are patients managing with the costs of care for chronic kidney disease in Australia? A cross-sectional study. BMC Nephrology 14: 5.

8. Wilmer WA, Rovin BH, Hebert CJ, Rao SV, Kumor K, et al. (2003) Management of glomerular proteinuria: a commentary. J Am Soc Nephrol 14: 3217-3232.

9. Ruggenenti P, Cravedi P, Remuzzi G (2012) Mechanisms and treatment of CKD. J Am Soc Nephrol 23: 1917-1928.

10. Dzau VJ, Antman EM, Black HR, Hayes DL, Manson J, et al. (2006) The cardiovascular disease continuum validated:Clinical evidence of improved outcomes. Part I: Pathophysiologyand clinical trial evidence (risk factors through stable coronaryartery disease). Circulation 114: 2850-2870.

11. Van der Meer IM, Cravedi P, Remuzzi G (2010) The role of renin angiotensin system inhibition in kidney repair. Fibrogenesis Tissue Repair 3: 7.

12. The GISEN Study Group (1997) Randomized placebo-controlled trial of the effect of ramipril on decline on GFR and risk of terminal renal failure in proteinuric, non-diabetic nephropathy. The GISEN Group. Lancet 349: 1857-1863.

13. Lewis EJ, Hunsicker LG, Clarke WR, Berl T, Pohl MA, et al. (2001) The Collaborative Study Group: Renoprotective effect of the angiotensin-receptor antagonist irbesartan in patients with nephropathy due to type 2 diabetes. N Engl J Med 345: 851-60.

14. Atkins RC, Briganti EM, Lewis JB, Hunsicker LG, Braden G, et al. (2005) Proteinuria reduction and progression to renal failure in patients with type 2 diabetes mellitus and overt nephropathy. Am J Kidney Dis 45: 281-87.

15. Brenner BM, Cooper ME, deZeeuw D, Keane WF, Mitch WE, et al. (2001) RENAAL Study Investigators: Effects of losartan on renal and cardiovascular outcomes in patients with type 2 diabetes and nephropathy. N Engl J Med 345: 861-869.

16. Remuzzi G, Benigni A, Remuzzi A (2006) Mechanisms of progression and regression of renal lesions of chronic nephropathies and diabetes. J Clin Invest 116: 288-296.

17. De Zeeuw D, Remuzzi G, Parving HH, Keane WF, Zhang Z, et al. (2004) Proteinuria, a target for renoprotection in patients with type 2 diabetic nephropathy: Lessons from RENAAL. Kidney Int 65: 2309-20.

18. Jafar TH, Schmid CH, Landa M, Giatras I, Toto R, et al. (2001) Angiotensin-converting enzyme inhibitors and progression of nondiabetic renal disease: A meta-analysis of patient-level data. Ann Intern Med 135: 73-87.

19. Praga M, Gutiérrez E, González E, Morales E, Hernández E (2003) Treatment of IgA nephropathy with ACE inhibitors: a randomized and controlled trial. J Am Soc Nephrol 14: 1578-1583.

20. Parving HH, Hommel E, Nielsen MD, Giese J (1989) Effect of captopril on blood pressure and kidney function in normotensive insulin dependent diabetics with nephropathy. BMJ 299: 533-536.

21. Palmer SC, Mavridis D, Navarese E, Craig JC, Tonelli M, et al. (2015) Comparative efficacy and safety of blood pressure-lowering agents in adults with diabetes and kidney disease: a network meta-analysis. Lancet 385: 2047-2056.

22. Wu HY, Huang JW, Lin HJ, Liao WC, Peng YS, et al. (2013) Comparative effectiveness of renin-angiotensin system blockers and other antihypertensive drugs in patients with diabetes: systematic review and bayesian network meta-analysis. BMJ 347: f6008.

23. Blood Pressure Lowering Treatment Trialists' Collaboration, Ninomiya T, Perkovic V, Turnbull F, Neal B, Barzi F, et al. (2013) Blood pressure lowering and major cardiovascular events in people with and without chronic kidney disease: meta-analysis of randomised controlled trials. BMJ 347: f5680.

24. Lv J, Perkovic V, Foote CV, Craig ME, Craig JC, et al. (2012) Antihypertensive agents for preventing diabetic kidney disease. Cochrane Database Syst Rev 12: CD004136.

25. Cheng J, Zhang X, Tian J, Li Q, Chen J (2012) Combination therapy an ACE inhibitor and an angiotensin receptor blocker for IgA nephropathy: a meta-analysis. Int J Clin Pract 66: 917-923.

26. Vejakama P, Thakkinstian A, Lertrattananon D, Ingsathit A, Ngarmukos C, et al. (2012) Reno-protective effects of renin-angiotensin system blockade in type 2 diabetic patients: a systematic review and network meta-analysis. Diabetologia 55: 566-78.

27. Sharma P, Blackburn RC, Parke CL, McCullough K, Marks A, et al. (2011) Angiotensin-converting enzyme inhibitors and angiotensin receptor blockers for adults with early (stage 1 to 3) non-diabetic chronic kidney disease. Cochrane Database Syst Rev 10: CD007751.

28. Schjoedt KJ, Hansen HP, Tarnow L, Rossing P, Parving HH (2008) Long-term prevention of diabetic nephropathy: an audit. Diabetologia 51: 956-961.

29. Bonne JF, Fournier A, Massy Z, Choukroun G, Fournier A (2006) Overview of randomised trials of ACE inhibitors. Lancet 368: 1152-1153.

30. Strippoli GF, Craig M, Craig JC (2012) Antihypertensive agents for preventing diabetic kidney disease. Cochrane Database Syst Rev 12: CD004136.

31. Barnett AH (2005) Preventing renal complications in diabetic patients: the Diabetics Exposed to Telmisartan And enaprIL (DETAIL) study. Acta Diabetol 42 Suppl 1: S42-49.

32. Mauer M, Zinman B, Gardiner R, Drummond KN, Suissa S, et al. (2002) ACE-I and ARBs in early diabetic nephropathy. J Renin Angiotensin Aldosterone Syst 3: 262-269.

33. Lovell HG (2001) Angiotensin converting enzyme inhibitors in normotensive diabetic patients with microalbuminuria. Cochrane Database Syst Rev 1: CD002183.

34. Ruggenenti P, Perna A, Gherardi G, Gaspari F, Benini R, et al. (1998). Renal function and requirement for dialysis in chronic nephropathy patients on long-term ramipril: REIN follow-up trial. Gruppo Italiano di Studi Epidemiologici in Nefrologia (GISEN). Ramipril Efficacy in Nephropathy. Lancet 352: 1252-6.

35. Remuzzi G, Bertani T (1998) Pathophysiology of progressive nephropathies. N Engl J Med 339: 1448-1456.

36. Schmieder RE, Ruilope LM, Barnett AH (2011) Renal protection with angiotensin receptor blockers: where do we stand. J Nephrol 24: 569-580.

37. Hari P, Sahu J, Sinha A, Pandey RM, Bal CS, et al. (2013) Effect of enalapril on glomerular filtration rate and proteinuria in children with chronic kidney disease: a randomized controlled trial. Indian Pediatr 50: 923-928.

38. Reyes-Marín FA, Calzada C, Ballesteros A, Amato D (2012) Comparative study of enalapril vs. losartan on residual renal function preservation in automated peritoneal dialysis. A randomized controlled study. Rev Invest Clin 64: 315-321.

39. Strippoli GF, Bonifati C, Craig M, Navaneethan SD, Craig JC (2006) Angiotensin converting enzyme inhibitors and angiotensin II receptor antagonists for preventing the progression of diabetic kidney disease. Cochrane Database Syst Rev 4: Cd006257.

40. Peterson JC, Adler S, Burkart JM, Greene T, Hebert LA, et al. (1995) Blood pressure control, proteinuria, and the progression of renal disease. The Modification of Diet in Renal Disease Study. Ann Intern Med 123: 754-762.

41. He YM, Feng L, Huo DM, Yang ZH, Liao YH (2013) Enalapril versus losartan for adults with chronic kidney disease: a systematic review and meta-analysis. Nephrology (Carlton) 18: 605-14.

42. Espinel E, Joven J, Gil I, Suñé P, Renedo B, et al. (2013) Risk of hyperkalemia in patients with moderate chronic kidney disease initiating angiotensin converting enzyme inhibitors or angiotensin receptor blockers: a randomized study. BMC Res Notes 6: 306.

43. Wang YM, Zhou JJ, Wang Y, Watson D, Zhang GY, et al. (2013) Daedalic DNA vaccination against self antigens as a treatment for chronic kidney disease. Int J Clin Exp Pathol 6: 326-333.

44. Zheng G, Wang Y, Xiang SH, Tay YC, Wu H, et al. (2006) DNA vaccination with CCL2 DNA modified by the addition of an adjuvant epitope protects against "nonimmune" toxic renal injury. J Am Soc Nephrol 17: 465-474.

# 22

# Renal and Hepato-Protective Effects of *Irvingia gabonensis* Juice on Sodium Fluoride-Induced Toxicity in Wistar Rats

**Adamma A Emejulu\*, Chinwe S Alisi, Emeka S Asiwe, Chidi U Igwe, Linus A Nwogu and Viola A Onwuliri**

*Department of Biochemistry, Federal University of Technology, PMB 1526, Owerri, Imo State, Nigeria*

\***Corresponding author:** Adamma A Emejulu, Department of Biochemistry, School of Biological Sciences, Federal University of Technology, P.M.B. 1526, Owerri, Imo State, Nigeria, E-mail: adajulu@yahoo.com

## Abstract

**Objective:** Renal and hepato-protective effects of *Irvingia gabonensis* juice on sodium fluoride-induced toxicity was assessed in twenty-four male Wistar albino rats.

**Methodology:** The rats were divided into 4 groups of 6 animals each. All except normal control (NC), were intoxicated with 20 mg.Kg$^{-1}$ body weight of sodium fluoride (NaF) daily by gavage for 35 days. Sodium fluoride control group (NaFC) received only the toxicant. Test group (IG) received *I. gabonensis* juice concurrently with the toxicant, while the standard control (Q+Vit. E) received concurrently, 15 mg.Kg$^{-1}$ body weight of Quercetin+100 mg.Kg$^{-1}$ body weight of α-tocopherol throughout the 35 days. Normal control (NC) group received only standard pelletized diet and water. Serum aspartate aminotransferase (AST), alanine aminotransferase (ALT), total protein, albumin, total cholesterol, serum creatinine and electrolyte levels were assessed among test, standard and control animals.

**Result:** *Irvingia gabonensis* significantly ($p<0.05$) reduced AST activity in the IG group (137.68 ± 12.66 U/L) compared to NaFC group (175.12 ± 10.63 U/L). This compares to the reduction in the AST activity in standard (Q +Vit. E) group (135.69 ± 10.66 U/L). ALT activity was also reduced in the IG group. Effects of *I. gabonensis* on albumin and cholesterol levels were similar to that of the standard group. Administration of *I. gabonensis* also significantly ($p<0.002$) reduced elevated creatinine and Cl$^-$ concentrations, while significantly ($p<0.05$) elevating serum Ca$^{2+}$ and Mg$^{2+}$ ion levels.

**Conclusion:** *Irvingia gabonensis* fruit juice has some renal and hepato-protective potential which may be due to the presence of secondary plant metabolites like flavonoids, tannins and alkaloids found in the plant. The fruit is also rich in Ca$^{2+}$ and Mg$^{2+}$. Increased domestication is encouraged.

## Key words:

Medicinal plant; Chemical toxicity; *Irvingia gabonensis*; Organ functions

## Introduction

African rain forest is filled with varieties of plants. *Irvingia* is a genus of African and Southeast Asian trees in the family Irvingiaceae. *Irvingia gabonensis* (Aubry-Lecomte ex O'Rorke) Baill is commonly known as "wild mango", "bush mango" or 'African mango' and is a commercially indigenous fruit tree of the West and Central Africa. They bear edible mango-like fruits called 'Ugiri' in Igbo land (Nigeria) and 'Dika' in Cameroon, but are especially valued for their fat- and protein-rich nuts called 'ogbono' or 'dika' nuts. The fruits are broadly ellipsoid, about 4-7 cm long, green when unripe and yellow when ripe with a fleshy mesocarp. The fruit pulp is juicy, although the taste varies between sweet and bitter, it has great commercial potentials ranging from the preparation of juices, jams and jellies to wine and soap making [1,2].

In Nigeria, *Irvingia gabonensis* is a widely domesticated and grown perennial fruit tree, enjoyed both for its succulent pulp and its malleable kernels which are domestically used as a substitute for making popular "draw soups". *Irvingia gabonensis* has been shown to possess nutritional or medicinal values [3,4].

The *I. gabonensis* trees grow to about 15-40 m in height and 1m in diameter; they may occur in gregarious clusters. Different parts of the plant are used in traditional and modern medicine for the treatment of several illnesses and in industrial processes [5]. The seeds of *I. gabonensis* have a wide variety of application including its use as a thickener in soup and stews and a source of edible oil. The bark has been widely applied in the treatment of diarrhea [6], dysentery [7], scabby skin [6] and a potent anti-inflammatory agent [7]. Leaf decoction of *I. gabonensis* and the seed extract have been reported to possess hypoglycaemic and hypolipidemic effects [8-10]. Antidiabetic effects of its bark and leaves on streptozocin-induced diabetic rats have also been reported [11].

Although its fruit is widely eaten, it has remained largely understudied. Much that is known on *I. gabonensis* is mostly on the seeds and stem bark. This lack of information on the fruit juice has contributed to its underutilization and under-exploitation. Use of some of this wild fruits can do much to combat malnutrition and sustain life. It has been established that *I. gabonensis* contains elemental micronutrients and we had observed a hypolipidemic effect of the fruit juice on sodium fluoride induced dyslipidemia in rats [12].

Toxicity of sodium fluoride has been well established. It is hepatotoxic, causing among others degenerative and inflammatory changes [13,14]. It is neurotoxic [15,16] and increases oxygen free radicals and its resultant oxidative stress [17]. More recently, low glucose utilization [18], cognitive deficits and anxiety-depression-like behaviors have been described in mice treated with NaF [19].

Increased use of sodium fluoride is witnessed worldwide, with a lot of debate going-on on its continuous usage or non-use especially in fluoridation of water. Children are most vulnerable especially through excessive consumption of toothpastes. Increased risk of fluorosis due to high water-borne fluoride concentrations is threatening many parts of the world [20] and black children are disproportionately affected [16,21] due probably to biologic susceptibility or mere greater fluoride intake [21]. With increasing rate of consumption of fluorides worldwide and particularly in our locality, the present study was therefore designed to investigate the protective effect of *Irvingia gabonensis* fruit juice on the liver and kidney of male wistar rats exposed to sodium fluoride toxicity.

## Materials and Methods

### Chemicals/Reagents

Sodium fluoride (Fluka-Chemie, Switzerland), Quercetin dihydrate (Sigma-Aldrich Mo USA), α-Tocopherol (Fluka-Chemie, Switzerland). ALT test kit (Randox), AST test kit (Randox), Alkaline phosphatase test kit (Randox), Serum Bilirubin, Urea, Creatinine and Cholesterol test kits (Biosystem), Sodium, Potassium, Calcium, Magnesium and Chloride test kits (Teco, USA). All chemicals and reagents used were of analytical grades.

### Plant materials

Apparently healthy fresh, ripe and edible fruits of *I. gabonensis* were collected from a local plantation in Ugiri-Ike, Ikeduru Local Government Area of Imo State, Nigeria.

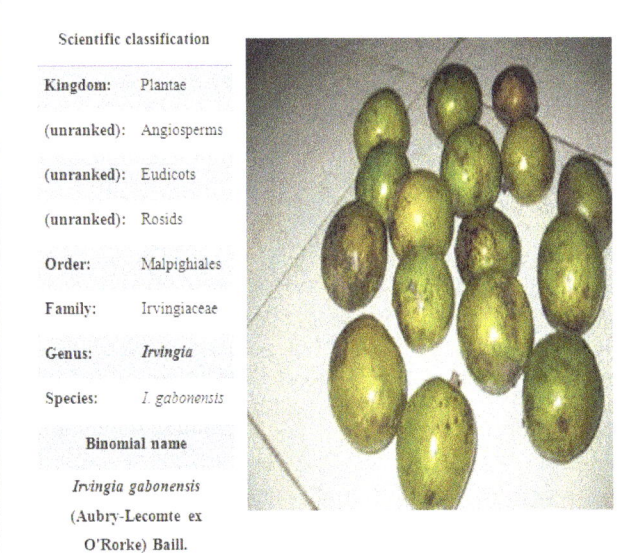

| Scientific classification | |
|---|---|
| Kingdom: | Plantae |
| (unranked): | Angiosperms |
| (unranked): | Eudicots |
| (unranked): | Rosids |
| Order: | Malpighiales |
| Family: | Irvingiaceae |
| Genus: | *Irvingia* |
| Species: | *I. gabonensis* |

**Binomial name**

*Irvingia gabonensis*
(Aubry-Lecomte ex O'Rorke) Baill.

Figure 1: Overview on *Irvingia gabonensis*.

The plant material was authenticated by Dr. F. N. Mbagwu, a plant taxonomist at the Department of Plant Science and Biotechnology, Imo State University, Owerri, Imo State. Plant specimens were deposited in the institution's herbarium with voucher no. IMSUH 0198. These fruits were obtained fresh as at when needed (Figure 1).

### Fruit juice preparation

The ripe and edible fruits of *I. gabonensis* were washed with clean tap water and peeled, seeds removed and the succulent pulp cut into sizeable bits. These were weighed and 250 g portion of the fleshy part of the fruits was extracted with 250 ml of distilled water in a juice extractor (Sinbo SJ3138, China) to obtain the fruit juice. The resultant juice was then stored in a freezer (≤ -4.0°C) until needed. Fresh juice of the fruit was prepared each day of administration.

### Qualitative phytochemical screening

The methods described by [22] were used to evaluate the qualitative phytochemical content of the fruit juice.

### Animals

Twenty four healthy, male albino Wistar rats (*Rattus norvegicus*) weighing 120-150 g were used for the study. The animals were purchased from the animal house of the Department of Veterinary Medicine, University of Nigeria, Nsukka. They were housed in stainless steel cages under standard laboratory conditions of light, temperature (21 ± 2°C) and relative humidity (55 ± 5%). The animals were fed standard rat pellets (Vital finisher, Nigeria) and tap water ad libitum and allowed for a period of two weeks to acclimatize before commencement of the study. The Ethical committee of the University approved the study protocol prior to commencement of study and treatment of the animals was in accordance with the Principles of Laboratory Animal Care (NIH Publication, 1985 to 1993; revised, 1985).

### Grouping of animals

The rats were randomly divided into four (4) experimental groups of six (6) animals each and treatments administered for 35 days as follows:

Group I served as normal control (NC), which received standard pelletized diet and water only throughout the treatment period.

Group II served as intoxicated control (NaFC), which received standard diet and water ad libitum and sodium fluoride toxicant (20 mg/kg b wt) by gavage daily.

Groups III served as intoxicated test group (I.G), which received standard diet and water ad libitum, in addition to *I. gabonensis* fruit juice (IG) and sodium fluoride toxicant (20 mg/kg b wt) daily.

Group IV served as intoxicated standard group (Q +Vit E), which received standard diet and water ad libitum, in addition to Quercetin (15 mg/kg b wt) plus α-tocopherol (100 mg/kg b wt) and the toxicant sodium fluoride (20 mg/kg b wt) daily.

### Blood collection

At the end of thirty five days of daily intoxication and treatment with *I. gabonensis* juice and standard for amelioration, animals were fasted overnight. They were then lightly anaesthetized with dichloromethane, sacrificed by cervical dislocation and blood collected by cardiac puncture. The blood sample (5 ml) of each animal was taken and allowed to clot for 45 min at room temperature. Serum was separated by centrifugation at 600 × g for 15 min and analyzed for various biochemical parameters.

## Biochemical analyses

Serum alanine aminotransferase (ALT) and aspartate aminotransferase (AST) activities [23], ALP activities [24], protein [25] and albumin concentrations [26] were assayed using commercial kits (Randox, UK). Serum total bilirubin [27], total cholesterol [28], urea [29] and creatinine [30] concentrations were determined using commercial kit (Biosysytem). Sodium was determined by the modified method described by [31] and [32], potassium by the method described by [33], chloride by modified method described by [34], magnesium as described by [35] and calcium as described by [36] using commercially available test kits (Teco, USA).

## Statistical analyses

Statistical software "Analyze-it" for Microsoft excel was used for the analysis. Differences between the various groups and the control group were tested at p ≤ 0.05 using one-way analysis of variance (ANOVA) statistic followed by Tukey post-Hoc test.

## Results and Discussion

Phytochemical screening revealed the presence of phenolics, alkaloids, flavonoids, phytosterols, phenols, phlobatanin, tannins and saponins in *I. gabonensis* fruit juice.

Results shown on Figure 2 indicated that serum ALT and AST activities were significantly (p<0.05) elevated by 82% and 88% respectively in NaF-exposed rats compared to controls. Treatment of exposed rats with *I. gabonensis* fruit juice and reference standard resulted in a reduction in serum ALT and AST activities by 35.8% & 21.4% and 48.23% and 22.5% respectively. For AST activity, there was a significant reduction from 175.12 ± 10.63 U/L in the NaF control group to 137.68 ± 12.66 U/L in the *I. gabonensis* group and 135.69 ± 10.66 U/L in the standard group (Q+Vit. E). For ALT activity, it was 50.52 ± 2.42 U/L in the NaFC group, 32.43 ± 3.66 U/L in the *I. gabonensis* group, 26.15 ± 0.45 U/L in the standard and 27.74 ± 4.55 U/L in the normal control.

Similarly, bilirubin concentration was reduced from 11.54 ± 0.21 g/L in the NaFC to 8.76 ± 0.10 g/L in I.G group and 8.96 ± 0.21 g/L in standard group. However, serum total protein and albumin concentrations remained relatively unchanged (Figure 2). Figure 2 also showed that total cholesterol was significantly (p<0.05) increased in the NaF control rats, and in exposed rats treated with the reference standard and *I. gabonensis* fruit juice compared to the normal control.

From these results, it was observed that oral administration of NaF for 35 days to adult male rats resulted in a significant alteration of liver function. The liver is a primary site for xenobiotics detoxification, its metabolism is readily altered by toxicity. Xenobiotic hepatotoxic action is usually expressed by cell respiration disorders that interfere with oxidation and reduction mechanisms; either through impairment in protein, carbohydrate and lipid metabolism or by disturbances in intra- and extracellular transport. Consequently, whole cell or its cytoplasmic organelles can be damaged.

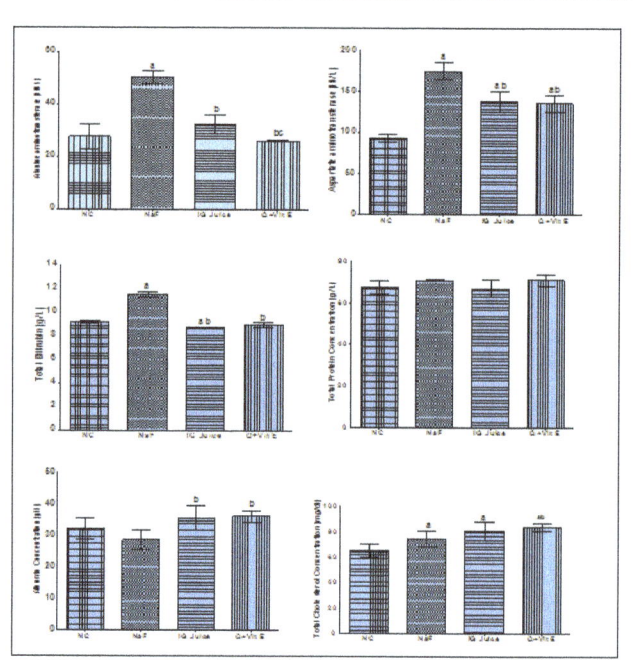

**Figure 2:** Effect of *I. gabonensis* juice administration on liver function of male Wistar albino rats administered 20 mg/kg b wt NaF for 35 days. Values are mean ± standard deviation of 6 determinations. *a* Significantly (p<0.05) different from Normal control (NC); *b* Significantly (p<0.05) different from sodium fluoride (NaF) control; *c* Significantly (p<0.05) different from *I. gabonensis* (IG) juice.

Most frequently the damage occurs as parenchymal vacuolar degeneration, necrosis of hepatocytes or disorders in the activity of metabolic enzymes [37-39] as seen from our study. Adverse effects of NaF on liver function have been reported with marked elevation of ALT and AST in mice [40].

These results are consistent with earlier reports on the hepatotoxicity of NaF. One study [41] reported that NaF induced morphological changes in rat hepatocytes and promoted cells vacuolar degeneration. Pale, granular hepatocytes, compatible with parenchymal degeneration, were observed in mice administered 0.95 mg fluoride/kg/day in drinking water for 7-28 days [42]. Also, liver congestion was observed in sheep given a single intragastric dose of fluoride as low as 9.5 mg fluoride/kg. Mild serum increases of liver enzymes glutamate dehydrogenase (GDH) and gamma-glutamyl transferase (γ-GT) also occurred in sheep administered 38 mg fluoride/kg body weight [43]. However, these alterations in liver enzymes were normalized by *I. gabonensis* fruit juice. Furthermore, the corresponding increase in total bilirubin in our study revealed a deleterious effect of NaF on liver metabolism in line with the elevation of serum transaminases. Hyperbilirubinaemia is characteristic of impaired bilirubin metabolism involving metabolic disturbances in the liver. This could be as a result of defective conjugation, transport and/or excretion of bilirubin, or overproduction of bilirubin caused by an excessive breakdown of red blood cells due to the toxins from the administered chemical. Breakdown of red blood cells frequently occur in humans, as a result of severe falciparum malaria, sickle cell disease, haemolysis associated with glucose-6-phosphate dehydrogenase deficiency and toxins from bacteria or snake venoms etc. Administration of *I. gabonensis* fruit juice resulted in amelioration of liver damage as ALT, AST and total bilirubin levels were significantly reduced in these animals.

Our result showed no significant changes in serum protein and albumin metabolism by *I. gabonensis* juice and our reference standard administration to NaF exposed animals. Albumin is a key metabolite in liver detoxification function. Depletion of albumin concentration usually occurs in correspondence with reduction in total protein as this form the bulk of available serum and liver protein. On the other hand, a decreased albumin concentration could be explained by inflammatory reactions. These inflammatory reactions have been confirmed by histological sections realized on liver of NaF-treated mice in the works of [40]. They observed infiltration of leucocytes in hepatocytes of mothers and their pups, which however was more pronounced in the mothers [40].

Also, result obtained demonstrated a significant increase in total cholesterol of animals exposed to NaF. The *I. gabonensis* juice and reference standard also produced mild increases in cholesterol level. These increases may be an indirect pointer to the ability of these amelioratives to promote cholesterol synthesis. *I. gabonensis* fruit has been widely reported to exert lipid lowering effect by induction of HDL-cholesterol synthesis [8-10]. Hence the increase in total cholesterol observed in our study is believed to be as a result of increased HDL-cholesterol synthesis. Lipid profile studies were not carried out in this study to ascertain the exact cholesterol lipoprotein that was increased, but we had earlier observed a hypolipidemic effect of the fruit juice on sodium fluoride induced dyslipidemia in rats, as a result of increased HDL-C synthesis [12].

Our result in Figure 3 revealed a significant (p<0.05) increase in urea concentration in NaF-treated rats compared to normal control. Administration of the reference standard resulted in a significant (p<0.05) reduction of urea in exposed rats, but this reduction was non-significant in *I. gabonensis* treated rats. Similarly, serum creatinine was significantly (P<0.05) elevated in NaF control rats compared to normal control. This was significantly reduced by both *I. gabonensis* juice and reference standard administration showing a protective effect on the kidney. The effect of *I. gabonensis* on serum urea and creatinine levels were very much similar to that of the standard (Q+Vit E) group, but were not reduced to the level of the normal control. It is well known that ureamia paralleled by elevated serum creatinine is characteristic of intrinsic renal failure [44].

The electrolyte profile results (Figure 3) showed that potassium concentration was not altered by NaF administration. On the other hand, NaF exposure resulted in a significant (P<0.001) elevation of sodium concentration in NaF control rats and among *I. gabonensis* juices and reference standard treated groups compared to control.

The observed increase in sodium concentration may be attributed to an increased retention of sodium ion or may be contributed by Na$^+$ ion resulting from the administered NaF. Also, our result demonstrated a significant (p<0.05) increase in chloride ion concentration across all groups exposed to NaF compared to control. The elevated serum concentration of Na$^+$ and Cl$^-$ ions indicate reduced ability of the kidney to eliminate the toxic metabolic substances and reabsorb the metal and non-metal ions. Increase in chloride concentration may be attributed to retention or a decreased clearance of chloride ion which may be due to a preferential excretion of F$^-$ anion instead of Cl$^-$ anion.

The observed increase in chloride ion concentration is consistent with observed increase in sodium ion concentration.

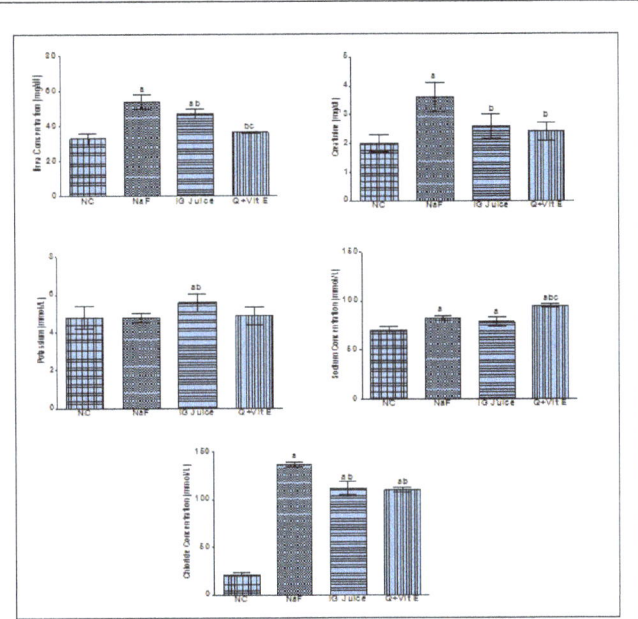

**Figure 3:** Effect of *I. gabonensis* juice administration on kidney function of male Wistar albino rats administered 20 mg/kg b wt NaF for 35 days. Values are mean ± standard deviation of 6 determinations. *a* Significantly (p<0.05) different from Normal control (NC); *b* Significantly (p<0.05) different from sodium fluoride (NaF) control; *c* Significantly (p<0.05) different from *I. gabonensis* (IG) juice.

Potassium ion concentration was not altered by sodium fluoride administration in the NaF control group. However, *I. gabonensis* juice administration resulted in a significant (p<0.05) increase in potassium ion concentration. The observed increase in K$^+$ ion may be as a result of *I. gabonensis* juice serving as a source of this cation. Changes in serum urea, creatinine, Na$^+$, and Cl$^-$ are associated with impairment of renal function [45] and the major route of excretion of fluoride is by the kidneys. The result of our study showed that NaF administration may have caused kidney damage resulting in altered kidney metabolism, dyshomeostasis of electrolyte profile and impairment in kidney clearance of urea and elevated creatinine. Our observed alteration in kidney function by NaF administration is consistent with previous reports [46-49].

NaF exposure had no effect on calcium concentration as can be seen in NaF control group when compared to normal control. However, administration of *I. gabonensis* juice resulted in a 30% increase in serum calcium concentration. We suggest that the ameliorative effect of our juice may be via mechanisms involving calcium retention, or may be as a result of the juice serving as a source of calcium. Similarly, *I. gabonensis* juice and our reference standard resulted in a significant (P<0.05) increase in magnesium concentration compared to both normal and NaF control. These showed that the fruit juice of *I. gabonensis* could serve as a potential source of these important minerals (Figure 4). *I. gabonensis* has been reported to be a rich source of these minerals [50].

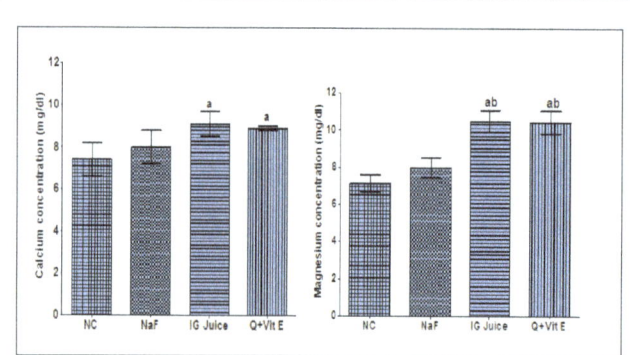

**Figure 4:** Effect of *I. gabonensis* juice administration on serum calcium and magnesium concentrations of male Wistar albino rats administered 20 mg/kg b wt NaF for 35 days. Values are mean ± standard deviation of 6 determinations. *a* Significantly (p<0.05) different from Normal control (NC); *b* Significantly (p<0.05) different from sodium fluoride (NaF) control; *c* Significantly (p<0.05) different from *I. gabonensis* (IG) juice.

Magnesium ion concentration in the NaF exposed rats was low, but was significantly elevated by administration of *I. gabonensis* and our reference standard. Fluoride is known to reduce absorption of calcium and magnesium from the gut [51,52]. These cations are needed by metalloenzymes in transcription, translation and enzymatic cascade mechanisms, acting as secondary messengers [53]. Hypocalcaemia may lead to muscle spasms and weakness, convulsions and cardiac dysrhythmias, coma and respiratory failure may also occur. Hence it is a great advantage that Mg$^{2+}$ concentration was restored in the *I. gabonensis* treated group.

## Conclusion

It can be deduced from our study that *I. gabonensis* fruit juice has some hepatoprotective potential which may be as a result of the presence of some secondary plant metabolites. The fruit is also a good source of Ca$^{2+}$ and Mg$^{2+}$ ions. Further studies are thus required in this area of research as the use of *I. gabonensis* is sustainable and environmentally friendly. Increased domestication of the plant is also encouraged.

## References

1. Leakey R, Schrecheriberg K, Tchoundjev Z (2003) The participatory domestication of West African indigenous fruits. Int For Rev 5: 338-347.

2. Shiembo PN, Newton AC, Leakey RB (1996) Vegetative propagation of Irvingia gabonensis, a West African fruit tree. For Ecol Manage 87: 185-192.

3. Duguma B, Tonye T, Depommier D (1990) Diagnostic survey on local multipurposes trees/shrubs, fallow systems and livestock in Southern Cameroon. CRAF Working pp 34.

4. Ndoye O, Perez MR, Eyebe A (1997) The markets of non-timber forest products in the humid zone of Cameroon. Rural Development Forest Network, Overseas Development Institute, London.

5. Anegbeh PO, Usoro C, Ukafor V, Tchoundjeu Z, Leakey RR, et al. (2003) Domestication of Irvingia gabonensis 3: Phenotypic variation of fruits and Kernels in a Nigeria village. Agroforestry Systems 58: 213-218.

6. Ndoye O, Tchamou N (1994) Utilization and marketing trends for Irvingia gabonensis products in Cameroon. ICRAF-IITA Conference on Irvingia gabonensis, Ibadan, Nigeria.

7. Okolo CO, Johnson PB, Abdurahman EM, Abdu-Aguye I, Hussaini IM (1995) Analgesic effect of Irvingia gabonensis stem bark extract. J Ethnopharmacol 45: 125-129.

8. Ngondi JL, Mbouobda HD, Etame S, Oben J (2005) Effect of irvingia gabonensis Kernel Oil on blood and liver lipids on leam and overweight rats. Journal of food technology 3: 592-594.

9. Ngondi JL, Oben JE, Minka SR (2005) The effect of Irvingia gabonensis seeds on body weight and blood lipids of obese subjects in Cameroon. Lipids Health Dis 4: 12.

10. Dzeufiet DP, Ngeutse DF, Dimo TT, Ngueguim TF, Tchamadeu M, et al. (2009) Hypoglycemic and hypolipidemic effects of Irvingia gabonensis (irvingiaceae) in diabetic rats. Pharmacol online 2: 957-962.

11. Ngondi JL, Djiotsa EJ, Fossouo Z, Oben J (2006) Hypoglycaemic effect of the methanol extract of Irvingia gabonensis seeds on streptozotocin diabetic rats. Afr J Trad Cam 3: 74-77.

12. Emejulu AA, Alisi CS, Asiwe SE, Iheanacho KM, Onwuliri VA (2014) Hypolipidemic effect of Irvinga.gabonensis fruits juice on sodium fluoride induced dyslipidemia in rats. Afr J Biochem Res 8: 151-157.

13. Chinoy NJ, Sharma M, Michael M (1993) Beneficial effects of ascorbic acid on reversal of Fluoride toxicity in male rats, Fluor 26: 45-56.

14. Parihar S, Choudhary A, Gaur S (2013) Toxicity of fluoride in liver of Albino rat and Mitigation after adopting artificial (Vitamin C and D) and natural (Aloe vera) food supplementations. International Journal of Advancements in Research & Technology 2: 1-11.

15. Mullenix PJ, Denbesten PK, Schunior A, Kernan WJ (1995) Neurotoxicity of sodium fluoride in rats. Neurotoxicol Teratol 17: 169-177.

16. Connett P (2012) 50 Reasons to Oppose Fluoridation. Fluoride Action Network.

17. Essiz D, Eraslan G, Altintas L (2008) Antioxidant and Therapeutic Efficacy of Proanthocyanidin in Sodium Fluoride-Intoxicated Mice. Fluor 41: 308-313.

18. Jiang C, Zhang S, Liu H, Guan Z, Zeng Q, et al. (2014) Low glucose utilization and neurodegenerative changes caused by sodium fluoride exposure in rat's Developmental Brain. Neuromolecular Med 16: 94-105.

19. Liu F, Ma J, Zhang H, Liu P, Liu YP, et al. (2014) Fluoride exposure during development affects both cognition and emotion in mice. Physiol Behav 124: 1-7.

20. Vasant RA, Narasimhacharya AV (2012) Amla as an antihyperglycemic and hepato-renal protective agent in fluoride induced toxicity. J Pharm Bioallied Sci 4: 250-254.

21. Center for Disease Control and Prevention (CDC) (2005) Surveillance for dental caries, dental sealants, tooth retention, edentulism, and enamel fluorosis-United States, 1988-1994 and 1999-2002. MMWR Surveill Summ 54: 1-43.

22. Trease GE, Evans WC (1996) Pharmacognosy (13th eds) Bailere Traiadal, London. P 101-104.

23. Reitman S, Frankel S (1957) A colorimetric method for the determination of serum glutamic oxalacetic and glutamic pyruvic transaminases. Am J Clin Pathol 28: 56-63.

24. DGKC-Z (1972) Clin Chem u Klin Biochem 10: 182.

25. Gornall AG, Bardawill CJ, David MM (1949) Determination of serum proteins by means of the biuret reaction. See comment in PubMed Commons below J Biol Chem 177: 751-766.

26. Doumas BT, Watson WA, Biggs HG (1971) Albumin standards and the measurement of serum albumin with bromocresol green. Clin Chim Acta 3: 21-30.

27. Jendrassik L, Grof P (1938) Vereinfachte photome trische methodenzur bestimmung des blubilirubins Biochem Z 297: 81-89.

28. Allain CC, Poon LS, Chan CS, Richmond W, Fu PC (1974) Enzymatic determination of total serum cholesterol. Clin Chem 20: 470-475.

29. Searcy RL, Reardon JE, Foreman JA (1967) A new photometric method for serum urea nitrogen determination. Am J Med Technol 33: 15-20.

30. Bartels H, Böhmer M (1971) Micro-determination of creatinine. Clin Chim Acta 32: 81-85.

31. Maruna RF (1958) Clin Chem Act 2: 581.

32. Trinder P (1951) Analyst 76: 596.

33. Terri AE, Sesin PG (1958) Colorimetric method of potassium estimation using sodium Tetraphenylboron. Am J Clin Path 29: 86.

34. Skeggs LT, Hochstrasser HC (1964) Thiocynate (colorimetric) method of chloride estimation. Clin Chem 10: 918-920.

35. Chauhan UP, Sarkar BC (1969) Use of calmagite for the determination of traces of magnesium in biological materials. Anal Biochem 32: 70-80.

36. Gindler EM, King JD (1972) Rapid colorimetric determination of calcium in biologic fluids with methylthymol blue. Am J Clin Pathol 58: 376-382.

37. Anderson WA (1985) Pathology, St Louis, Toronto, Priceton: The Mosby Company.

38. De Valck V, Geerts A, Schellinck P, Wisse E (1988) Localization of four phosphatases in rat liver sinusoidal cells. An enzyme cytochemical study. Histochemistry 89: 357-363.

39. Philips MJ, Poucell S, Patterson J, Valencia P (1987) Drug and toxic effects. The Liver. New York: Raven Press; 159-71.

40. Bouaziz H, Ketata S, Jammoussi K, Boudawara T, Ayedi F, et al. (2006) Effects of sodium fluoride on hepatic toxicity in adult mice and their suckling pups. Pest Biochem Physiol 86: 124-130.

41. Dabrowska E1, Letko R, Balunowska M (2006) Effect of sodium fluoride on the morphological picture of the rat liver exposed to NaF in drinking water. See comment in PubMed Commons below Adv Med Sci 51 Suppl 1: 91-95.

42. Greenberg SR (1982) The effect of chronic fluoride exposure on the liver: Part I. The parenchyma. Proc Inst Med Chic 39: 53-54.

43. Kessabi M, Hamliri A, Braun JP (1986) Experimental fluorosis in sheep: alleviating effects of aluminum. Vet Hum Toxicol 28: 300-304.

44. Solomon SD, Rice MM, Jose P, Domanski M, Sabatine M, et al. (2006) Renal function and effectiveness of angiotensin-converting enzyme inhibitor therapy in patients with chronic stable coronary disease in the Prevention of Events with Ace Inhibition (PEACE) trial. Circulation 114: 26-31.

45. Kumar A, Sharma SK, Vaidyanathan S (1988) Results of surgical reconstruction in patients with renal failure owing to ureteropelvic junction obstruction. J Urol 140: 484-486.

46. Xiu-An Z, Min W, Zi-Rong X, Jian-Xin L (2006) Toxic Effects of Fluoride on Kidney Function and Histological Structure in Young Pigs. Fluoride 39: 22-26.

47. Al Omireeni EA, Siddiqi NJ, Alhomida AS (2010) Biochemical and histological studies on the effect of sodium fluoride on rat kidney collagen. J Saudi Chem Soc 14: 413-416.

48. Bouaziz H, Ghorbel H, Ketata S, Guermazi F, Zeghala N (2005) Toxic effects of fluoride by maternal ingestion on kidney function of adult mice and their suckling pups. Fluoride 38: 23-31.

49. Zabulyte D, Uleckiene S, Kalibatas J, Paltanaviciene A, Jascaniniene N, et al. (2007) Experimental studies on effect of sodium fluoride and nitrate on biochemical parameters in rats. Bull Vet Inst Pulawy 51:79-82.

50. Ayivor JE, Debrah SK, Nuviadenu C, Forson A (2011) Evaluation of Elemental Contents of Wild Mango (Irvingia gabonensis) Fruit in Ghana. Advc J Food Sci Tech 3: 381-384.

51. Verma RJ, Guna Sherlin DM (2002) Sodium fluoride-induced hypoproteinemia and hypoglycemia in parental and F(1)-generation rats and amelioration by vitamins. Food Chem Toxicol 40: 1781-1788.

52. Machoy-Mokrzynska A (1995) Fluoride-Magnesium interaction. Fluoride 28: 175230.

53. Jha A, Shah K, Verma RJ (2012) Effects of sodium fluoride on DNA, RNA and protein contents in liver of mice and its amelioration by Camellia sinensis. Acta Pol Pharm 69: 551-555.

# 23

# THS Toxins Induce Hepatic Steatosis by Altering Oxidative Stress and SIRT1 Levels

**Cristina Flores, Neema Adhami and Manuela Martins-Green**

*Department of Cell Biology and Neuroscience, University of California, USA*

*Corresponding author: Manuela Martins-Green, Department of Cell Biology and Neuroscience, BSB room 2217 900 University Avenue, University of California Riverside, Riverside, CA 92521, USA, E-mail: manuela.martins@ucr.edu

## Abstract

**Background:** Third hand smoke (THS) forms when second hand smoke (SHS) tobacco toxins accumulate on surfaces such as walls, carpets and clothing and can result in adverse health effects.

**Objective:** This study was designed to investigate the mechanism of THS-induced hepatic steatosis.

**Methodology:** We used an *in vivo* exposure system that mimics exposure of humans to THS to investigate the effects of THS on hepatic lipid metabolism. THS-exposed mice were treated either with the liver-damaging drug, N-acetyl-p-aminophenol (APAP/Tylenol) to increase oxidative stress or with the antioxidants N-acetyl-cysteine and α-Tocopherol which decrease oxidative stress.

**Results:** THS-exposed mice have higher levels of superoxide dismutase activity and $H_2O_2$ levels. However, no significant changes in activity of the antioxidant enzymes catalase and glutathione peroxidase were found, implying the presence of high levels of hydrogen peroxide in the liver. Furthermore, THS-exposed mice also have a lower NADP+/NADPH ratio, indicating decreased ability of these mice to combat oxidative stress. THS-exposed mice show a decrease in ATP production, increase in aspartate aminotransferase (AST) activity, as well as increased molecular damage (lipid peroxidation, protein nitrosylation and DNA damage). Treating THS-exposed mice with APAP/Tylenol enhances the THS-induced damage whereas treating with antioxidants reduces the damage. THS-exposed mice also have lower sirtuin 1 (SIRT1) levels compared to controls which decreased activation of 5' AMP-activated protein kinase (AMPK) and increased sterol regulatory element binding protein 1c (SREBP1c).

**Conclusion:** THS-exposed mice on a normal diet have increased oxidative stress and damage mediated by oxidative stress, which results in alterations to the SIRT1/AMPK/SREPB1c signaling pathway. Increasing oxidative stress results in enhanced THS-induced damage whereas decreasing oxidative stress causes improvement in the THS-induced liver damage. Our results show that THS is a new risk factor contributing to the development of liver steatosis and highlight the danger of THS in general.

**Keywords:** Lipid metabolism; NAFLD; AMPK; Triglycerides; Antioxidants; SREPB1c; Hepatocyte damage

## Introduction

Third hand smoke (THS) forms when second hand smoke (SHS) tobacco toxins accumulate on surfaces such as walls, carpets and clothing [1-4]. Moreover, these toxins have the ability to react with gases in the air, such as nitrous acid, and produce dangerous carcinogens [5-9]. Individuals are exposed to THS toxins when they come into contact with the deposited toxins or when the toxins are re-emitted into the air. Exposure to THS toxins can result in detrimental health outcomes in individuals who are chronically exposed to them [10-17]. These health effects vary from metabolic disorders to cognitive perturbations. Children are one of the sectors of the population that is most susceptible to tobacco toxins and studies have shown that tobacco metabolites are detected in their urine [13-15]. Unfortunately, this dangerous exposure continues. In 2007, about 5.5 million children lived in households where someone smoked inside the home [12]. Even in households where indoor smoking was not reported, the tobacco metabolites could still be detected in the children's urine [13-15].

Studies in vitro have shown that THS is toxic to human cells. When a liver cell line, HepG2 cells, was exposed to THS toxins their DNA integrity and stability was compromised [16]. Both acute and chronic THS exposure resulted in double strand DNA breaks [16]. These investigators also showed that the molecular damage observed in HepG2 cells was associated with the increase in cellular oxidative stress and therefore suggested that oxidative stress is a major contributor to THS-mediated toxicity in vitro [16]. Another in vitro study focused on the effects of THS in the development of the lung using fetal rat lung explants [17]. These investigators showed that when fetal rat lungs were exposed to the THS toxins nicotine, 1-(N-methyl-N-nitrosamino)-1-(3-pyridinyl)-4butanal (NNA), or 4-(methylnitrosam-ino)-1-(3-pyridyl)-1-butanone (NNK), there was a disruption in the development of alveolar interstitial ibroblasts and that the disruption occurred via down regulation of PPAR-γ signaling [17]. PPAR-γ signaling controls alveolar development and down regulation of this signaling in the lungs suggested a disruption in alveolar epithelial-mesenchymal paracrine signaling, which prevents normal lung development. Exposure to THS toxins also resulted in increase of fibronectin and calponin protein levels as well as increase in apoptosis, which are markers for abnormal lung development. Together these findings suggest that the lungs of rats exposed to THS toxins do not develop normally, highlighting the danger of exposure to these toxins during lung development.

It also has been shown that THS toxins have the ability to cause metabolic changes in two male germ cell lines [18]. When spermatogonia (GC-2) and sertoli derived cells (TM-4) were exposed to THS toxins for 24 hours, the investigators observed changes in metabolic enzymes involved in glutathione, ammonia and nucleic acid metabolism [18]. In GC-2 cells, THS exposure resulted in increase in synthesis and decrease in the breakdown of GSH. GSH is a major component of the antioxidant defense pathway and these findings suggest spermatogonia might use this enzyme to combat the high levels of oxidative stress [18]. In TM-4 cells, there are increased metabolites involved in nucleic acid metabolism, suggesting that THS toxins are genotoxic and have the ability to compromise the integrity of genetic material [18]. THS exposure did not have effects on cell viability, cell cycle or apoptosis in these two male germ cell lines [18]. However, this in vitro study highlighted the sensitivity of male germ cells to THS toxins.

In addition to the findings *in vitro*, the detrimental effects of THS toxins have also been shown to alter human behavior. Epidemiological studies have shown that THS exposure results in abnormal cognitive function in children [19]. Children exposed to THS toxins are more hyperactive than children that live in environments with less THS contamination. Also, children are exposed to higher levels of these toxins than adults because they are in closer contact with the contaminated surfaces, lick their fingers and their surface-to-volume ratio is larger [19,20]. In addition, they are also more susceptible because their liver is not fully developed and therefore is not as effective in detoxification of toxins. Also, smoking during pregnancy or after pregnancy is dangerous for the developing fetus and results in impaired lung function [21,22]. Post-natal exposure to THS toxins also results in increased problems with the larynx, trachea and bronchi. This resulted in increased cough-and-asthma related symptoms in these children, suggesting THS toxins are detrimental for lung health of children living in homes contaminated with THS toxins.

We have developed an *in vivo* THS exposure system of mice that mimics THS exposure in humans [23]. Our model is a novel exposure system that allows us to study the effects of long-term THS exposure in different organs of male C57BL/6 mice. Using this exposure method, we have shown that THS exposure leads to lipid accumulation in the liver of these mice, suggesting that they have abnormal metabolism and insulin resistance [23,24]. These findings suggest that THS exposure is a new risk for hepatic steatosis.

Hepatic steatosis is the earliest stage of and a hallmark of non-alcoholic liver disease (NAFLD), which is the most common liver disease worldwide [25,26]. In some patients, steatosis can progress into fibrosis and then to cirrhosis if is not treated early. In the U.S., the prevalence of NAFLD is estimated to be around 20% in the general population and the percentage quadruples in morbidly obese individuals [25,26]. NAFLD is not limited to adults; the incidence of NAFLD among the pediatric population is increasing and it is estimated to account for about 14% of all NAFLD cases [25,26]. NAFLD is a complex process that results from metabolic abnormalities [27,28]. Many patients show dyslipidemia, malfunction of beta oxidative enzymes, deficiency in lipoproteins, and immune dysregulation [29,30]. Obesity, metabolic disorders, drugs or smoking are some of the major risk factors contributing to the development of NAFLD [31-33]. This disease is primarily controlled through changes in life-style, cessation of chemical exposure or antioxidant treatments [34-36].

In this study, we performed cellular and molecular studies to investigate whether THS exposure leads to increased oxidative stress in liver, leading to abnormal lipid metabolism and resulting in hepatic steatosis. Here, we show that mice exposed to THS toxins have altered oxidative stress in the liver. Increasing oxidative stress by treating the mice with N-acetyl-p-aminophenol (APAP/Tylenol) leads to exacerbation of THS-induce hepatic steatosis whereas antioxidant treatment ameliorates this condition. These findings suggest that oxidative stress caused by THS toxins leads to lipid accumulation in the liver. More specifically, THS toxins alter the SIRT1/AMPK/SREPB1c pathway, which regulates lipid metabolism in the liver, suggesting, that THS toxins are a new risk factor for development of hepatic steatosis.

## Materials and Methods

### Animals

Male C57BL/6 mice were divided into control and experimental groups (THS-exposed mice). The experimental group was exposed to THS toxins after weaning for 24 weeks. The control group was never exposed to THS toxins. Both control and THS-exposed mice were maintained under controlled environmental conditions -12-hr light/dark cycle in conventional cages with *ad libitum* access to standard chow (percent calories: 58% carbohydrate, 28.5% protein, and 13.5% fat) and water.

### Ethics statement

All animal experimental protocols were approved by the University of California, Riverside, Institutional Animal Care and Use Committee (UCR-IACUC). Mice were euthanized by carbon dioxide ($CO_2$) inhalation, which is the most common method of euthanasia used by NIH. The amount and length of $CO_2$ exposure were approved by UCR-IACUC.

### THS exposure method

Common household fabrics such as curtain material, upholstery and carpet were placed in empty mouse cages and exposed to SHS generated by the a Teague smoking machine as previously described in [23]. Each cage contained 10 g of curtain material (cotton) 10 g of upholstery (cotton and fiber) and two 16 in 2 pieces of carpet (fiber) to maintain equal exposure levels across all experimental groups. Two packs of 3R4F research cigarettes were smoked each day, five days per week to mimic an intermittent smoker. The smoke was routed to a mixing compartment to mix with air and the mixture distributed between two exposure chambers, each containing eight cages with the materials. The gravimetric method was used to determine the total particulate concentrations in each smoke chamber. The weight of Whatman grade 40 quantitative cellulose filter papers was recorded before introducing the filter paper into the filtering device and the device was then allowed to run for 15 minutes. After 15 minutes, the filter was weighed again to determine the particulate mass that had accumulated during this time period. This procedure was repeated with two more filters and the average of the three masses gave the TPM values for each chamber. The TPM values were adjusted to 30 µg/m$^3$, which resembles the values found in the homes of smokers by the EPA.

All cigarettes were smoked and stored in accordance with the Federal Trade Commission (FTC) smoking regimen. At the end of each week, cages were removed from the exposure chamber, bagged, and transported to the vivarium where mice were placed into the cages with the THS exposed material. For the next week, an identical set of cages and fabric was prepared and exposed to smoke in the same way as the first set of cages. By using two sets of cages and materials, each of which was exposed on alternating weeks, we ensured that mice inhabited cages containing fabric that had been exposed to fresh SHS in the beginning of each week and aged smoke towards the end week. Throughout the exposure period, hair was removed from the backs of the exposed mice (and controls) to mimic the bare skin of humans.

## N-acetyl-p-aminophenol (APAP/Tylenol) treatment

Four cohorts of male mice of the same age were used for *in vivo* APAP treatment studies. APAP was purchased from Sigma (Cat# A5000-100G) and was dissolved in warm PBS and injected IP. THS-exposed mice and controls received a daily dose of 300 mg/kg for eight weeks via IP injections. The concentration of each APAP solution was adjusted so that all mice received approximately the same volume.

## Antioxidant therapy

Four cohorts of male mice, control and THS-exposed, were given antioxidants daily starting at weaning (3 weeks of age) for five months. We used N-acetylcysteine (NAC) and α-tocopherol (α-TOC). NAC (50 mg/kg) was dissolved in PBS and injected daily via IP. α-TOC (150 mg/kg) was dissolved in 70% ethanol and also injected IP daily.

## Tissue extracts

After six months of THS exposure, livers were extracted from THS-exposed or control mice, washed with PBS and immediately frozen. The frozen livers were stored at -80°C. Liver tissue was homogenized in radioimmunoprecipitation assay buffer (RIPA), centrifuged, and the supernatant collected unless otherwise specified by instruction manuals of the assay kits used in this study. Extracts were used to perform the various assays we used for this study.

## Blood extracts

Blood was extracted directly from the heart and allowed to coagulate on ice for 20-30 minutes. The samples were then centrifuged at 10,000 rpm for phase separation. The serum was used immediately for assays or frozen and stored at -80° C and later used in assays.

## Measurement of SOD activity

Cayman Superoxide Dismutase Assay Kit (Cat # 706002) was used to measure SOD levels in the liver. Frozen liver pieces (10 mg) were placed in ice-cold RIPA buffer containing 50 mM Tris (50 mM pH 7), NaCl (150 mM), SDS (0.1%), sodium deoxycholate (0.5%) and Triton X (1%) and homogenize using a Bullet Blender Homogenizer to extract total protein. The samples were centrifuged at 10,000 rpm for 15 min at 4°C, and the resulting supernatant was used for SOD activity assay. Protein quantification was done using the Bradford assay (Bio-Rad). SOD activity was quantified by measuring the dismutation of superoxide radicals generated by xanthine oxidase and hypoxanthine.

A standard curve was generated and used to quantify the activity of SOD in the liver samples.

## Measurements of hydrogen peroxide levels

A Cayman Hydrogen Peroxide Assay Kit (Cat # 600050) was used to measure $H_2O_2$ levels in the liver. Fresh liver samples (10 mg) were homogenized in ice-cold RIPA buffer containing 50 mM Tris (50 mM pH 7), NaCl (150 mM), SDS (0.1%), sodium deoxycholate (0.5%) and Triton X (1%) using a Bullet Blender Homogenizer to extract total protein. The samples were centrifuged at 10,000 rpm for 15 min at 4°C, and the resulting supernatant was collected for the assay. $H_2O_2$ was detected using 10-acetyl-3,7-dihydroxyphenoxazine (ADHP), a highly sensitive and stable probe for $H_2O_2$. In the presence of horseradish peroxidase, ADHP reacts with $H_2O_2$ in a 1:1 stoichiometry ratio to produce a highly fluorescent resorufin (excitation=530-560 nm; emission=590 nm). The standard curve generated was used to quantify the activity of hydrogen peroxide in the liver.

## Measurement of catalase activity

Cayman Catalase Assay Kit was used to measure catalase (Cat # 707002) activity. Frozen liver pieces (10 mg) were placed in ice-cold RIPA buffer containing 50 mM Tris (50 mM pH 7), NaCl (150 mM), SDS (0.1%), sodium deoxycholate (0.5%) and Triton X (1%) and homogenized using a Bullet Blender Homogenizer to extract total protein. The samples were centrifuged at 10,000 rpm for 15 minutes at 4°C, and the resulting supernatant was collected and used for the assay. 20 µl of tissue homogenate were added to the wells of a 96 well plate along with 100 µl of assay buffer and 30 µl methanol and the reaction initiated by addition of 20 µl $H_2O_2$. After incubation for 20 mins, 30 µl of potassium hydroxide was added to terminate the reaction. 30 µl of 4-amino-3-hydrazino-5-mercapto-1,2,4-triazole (purpald), which is a chromogen, was added. After incubation for 10 minutes at RT, 10µl potassium periodate was added and incubated again at RT for five minutes. Absorbance was read at 540 nm. The method is based on the reaction of the enzyme with methanol in the presence of an optimal concentration of $H_2O_2$. The formaldehyde produced was measured spectrophotometrically with 4- amino-3-hydrazino-5-mercapto-1,2,4-triazole (Purpald) as the chromogen. Purpald specifically forms a bicyclic heterocycle with aldehydes which, upon oxidation, changes from colorless to a purple color. The amount of catalase activity levels were calculated and standardized for protein using the Bradford method (Bio-Rad).

## Measurements of GPx activity

Cayman GPx activity assay kit (Cat # 703102) was used to measure GPx (Cat # 703102) activity in the liver. Frozen liver pieces (10 mg) were homogenized in ice-cold RIPA buffer containing 50 mM Tris (50 mM pH 7), NaCl (150 mM), SDS (0.1%), sodium deoxycholate (0.5%) and Triton X (1%) using a Bullet Blender Homogenizer to extract total protein. The samples were centrifuged at 10,000 rpm for 15 minutes at 4°C, and the resulting supernatant was collected and used for the assay. 20 µl of liver homogenate were added to the wells of a 96 well plate along with 100 µl of assay buffer and 50 µl of co-substrate composed of NADPH, glutathione and glutathione reductase. Reactions were initiated by addition of hydro peroxide, mixed for a few seconds, and absorbance was read at 340 nm every minute to obtain at least 5 time points. The assay measured GPx activity indirectly by a coupled reaction with glutathione reductase (GR). Oxidized glutathione (GSSG), produced upon reduction of an organic hydroperoxide by

GPx, was recycled to its reduced state by GR and NADPH. The oxidation of NADPH to NADP+ was accompanied by a decrease in absorbance at 340nm. The rate of decrease in the A340 was directly proportional to the GPx activity in the liver homogenate samples.

## Measurement of DNA damage

DNA damage was measured using an ELISA Kit from Cell BioLabs Inc (Cat # STA-320) which allows the quantification of 8-hydroxy-2-deoxy Guanosine (8-OH-dG), DNA damage marker in ng/ml. DNA was extracted from liver samples, dissolved in water (1-5 mg/mL) and converted into single stranded DNA by incubating the sample at 95°C for five minutes following by chilling on ice. DNA was digested to nucleosides by incubating the denatured DNA with 5-20 units of nuclease P1 for 2 hours at 37°C at final concentration of 20 mM Sodium Acetate, pH 5.2, followed by treatment with 5-10 units of alkaline phosphatase for 1 hr at 37°C in a final concentration of 100 mM Tris, pH 7.5. The reaction mixture was centrifuged for five minutes at 6,000 rpm and the supernatant used for the 8-OH-dG ELISA assay. 50 μL of experimental samples or 8-OHdG standards were added to the wells of the 8-OHdG Conjugate coated plate. Incubation was performed at room temperature for 10min on an orbital shaker. 50 μL of anti-8-OHdG antibody was added to each well and the plate was incubated at room temperature for 1hr. The microwells were then washed three times with Wash Buffer. After the last wash, 100 μL of secondary Antibody-Enzyme Conjugated was added and incubation was performed at room temperature for 1 hr followed by three washes. 100 uL of Substrate Solution containing 3,3', 5,5'Tetramethylbenzidine was added to each well and incubated at room temperature for 30 minutes. The enzyme reaction was stopped by addition of 100 μL of Stop Solution into each well. Absorbance was read on a spectrophotometer at λ=450 nm.

## Measurement of nitrosylation of proteins

Protein damage was quantified by measuring the nitrosylation of tyrosine residues in proteins. The amount of 3-nitrotyrosine in the liver proteins was determined using the OxiSelect Nitrotyrosine ELISA Kit from Cell Biolabs (Cat # STA-305). The liver samples or nitrated BSA standards were first added to a nitrated BSA pre-absorbed enzyme immunoassay (EIA) plate. After a brief incubation, an anti-nitrotyrosine antibody was added, followed by an HRP conjugated secondary antibody. The protein nitrotyrosine content in the liver samples were determined by comparing with a standard curve that was prepared from predetermined nitrated BSA standards provide in the kit.

## Measurement of lipid peroxidation

Lipid peroxidation in the liver was determined by the levels of the byproduct of lipid peroxidation known as malaldehyde (MDA) using the OxiSelect TBARS Assay Kit from Cell Biolabs (Cat # STA-330). The unknown MDA containing samples or MDA standards were first reacted with Thiobarbituric Acid (TBA) at 95°C for 60 minutes. After this incubation period, the plate containing the samples and standards was read fluorometrically at 540 nm excitation and 590 nm emission. The MDA content in unknown samples was determined by comparison with the predetermined MDA standard curve.

## Measurement of AST levels

The AST levels were measured using the Aspartate aminotransferase (AST) Activity Assay (Cat# MAK055). 100 uL of the reaction mix (80 uL AST Assay buffer; 2 uL AST enzyme mix; 8 uL AST developer; 10 uL AST substrate) was added to each well. The plate was then mixed by pipetting and incubated at 37°C and was protected from light. The first initial reading was taken after 2 minutes of incubation. After the recording of the first initial reading, the subsequent readings were taken every five minutes until the measurements of the samples where greater than the value of the highest standard (~10 nmole/well). The background in the wells was corrected by subtracting the final reading of standard zero from all the final readings of the eight standards. The standards were then used to make a standard curve. The AST activity was calculated by subtracting the final reading of each sample from initial reading divided by the reaction rate and volume of the sample.

## Measurement of ATP levels

The ATP levels in liver were quantified using BioVision's ATP Colorimetric and Fluorometric Assay kit (Cat # K354-100), which is designed to detect low quantities of ATP (~50 pmol) by measuring the phosphorylation of glycerol. The assay was performed according to the protocol included in the kit. Liver tissue samples (10 mg) were homogenized in 100 μl of ATP assay buffer and 50 μl of sample supernatant was added to a 96-well plate in duplicates. 50 μl of the Reaction Mix (44 μl ATP Assay buffer; 2 μl ATP probe; 2 μl ATP converter; and 2 μl developer) was added to each well containing the ATP standards and samples to initiate the phosphorylation of glycerol reaction. The plate was mixed well and incubated for 30 minutes at room temperature away from light. During this incubation period, glycerol was phosphorylated. The product of this phosphorylation reaction was read at λ=570 nm and the absorbance readings of the standards were used to generate a standard curve. The unknown amount of ATP in the samples was then calculated using the standard curve and the observances reading of the samples.

## Measurement of Urea levels

Urea levels in the liver tissue were quantified using Cell Biolabs' Urea Assay Kit (Cat # STA-382), which is based on the Berthelot reaction. The enzyme urease is used to catalyze the hydrolysis of urea into carbon dioxide and ammonia. Ammonia then reacts with the alkaline developer (Berthelot's reagent) included in this kit to produce a blue-green colored product that can be measured with a standard spectrophotometric plate reader at an optical density 630nm. 10 μl of the standards or samples were added to the 96-well plate. 100 μl of the urease/Ammonia Reagent (40 mg of urease for 10 mL of Ammonia reagent) mixture was added to each well. The plate was mixed and incubated for 10 minutes at 37°C. After incubation, 100 μl of the Developing Reagent was added to each well using a multichannel pipette. The plate was placed on an orbital shaker to mix the samples and then incubated 30 minutes at 37°C. After incubation period the plate was read at 630 nm.

## Measurement of sirtuin 1 levels

SIRT1 levels were quantified using SIRT1 Sandwich Enzyme Immunoassay from Mybiosource (Cat # MBS2023445). This kit includes a 96-well strip plate pre-coated with an antibody specific to SIRT1. 100 μl of standards or samples were added to the plate wells with a biotin-conjugated antibody specific to SIRT1 and incubated for

2 hours at 37°C. 100 µl of Detection Reagent A working solution was added to each well and the plate covered and incubated for 1 hour at 37°C. After the incubation period the plate was washed three times with 350 µl of wash solution for each well usingmulti-channel pipette. The plate was allowed to sit for 2 minutes and excess liquid was removed by pressing the plate onto absorbent paper towels. 100 µl of Detection Reagent B working solution was then added to each well and the covered plate was incubated for 30 minutes at 37°C. The plate was then washed with 350 µl of wash solution five times. 90 µl of Tetramethylbenzidine (TMB) Substrate Solution was then added to each well (samples turned blue) and the covered well plate was incubated for 15 minutes at 37°C. The plate was protected from light. 50 µL of Stop Solution was added to each well to stop the reaction and the plate was placed on a shaker to mix the samples well. A microplate reader was used to measure the OD readings of the standards and samples at 450 nm.

## Measurement of AMPK-P levels

The AMPK-P levels in the samples were quantified using an AMPKα pT172 ELISA Kit (Cat # ab154468). This kit contains a 96 well plate which is pre-coated with a specific mouse monoclonal antibody specific for AMPKα pT172. 25 µl of standards (Hek293T cells) or samples were added to the wells along with the rabbit monoclonal primary detector antibody and the plate was incubated for three hours at room temperature. The plate was then washed with 300 µl of 1X wash buffer to eliminate any unbound standard or samples in the plate. After washing and drying of the plate, 50 µl of horseradish peroxidase (HRP)- conjugated secondary detector antibody (HRP Label) specific for the primary detector antibody was added to wells. After incubation, the well plate was washed again three times using 300 µl of 1X wash buffer. Then 100 µl of a Tetramethylbenzidine (TMB) substrate solution was added to the wells and the wells changed in color depending on the amount of AMPKα pT172 bound present in the samples. The OD of the samples was then measured at 600 nm and used to calculate the amount of each AMPK-P in each sample. A standard curve was created and the unknown samples were extrapolated this standard curve.

## Statistical analysis

For the statistical analysis of experiments, we used Graphpad Instat Software (Graphpad, La Jolla, CA, USA). Statistical comparisons between two-groups were performed using the unpaired Student's t-test. All data are mean ± SD represented by the error bars. Means were considered significantly different when p<0.05.

## Results

### THS exposure leads to increased oxidative stress in the liver

Previously, we showed that 30% of the mice exposed to THS toxins develop a fatty liver [23]. We hypothesize that exposure to THS toxins leads to lipid accumulation in the liver of THS-exposed mice by increasing oxidative stress. Under normal conditions, the hepatocytes balance oxidative stress with the help of two important antioxidant enzymes, catalase and glutathione peroxidase (GPx). These enzymes regulate the levels of hydrogen peroxide ($H_2O_2$) in the liver. Catalase converts $H_2O_2$ into water and oxygen whereas GPx converts it into water only (Figure 1A).

THS-exposed mice have higher superoxide dismutase (SOD) activity and as a result they also have higher levels of $H_2O_2$ in the liver than do the controls (Figures 1B and 1C). Because there is no significant increase in catalase or GPx activity, $H_2O_2$ is not properly been processed and the levels of reactive oxygen species (ROS) remain high in the liver (Figures 1D and 1E). To further support these results, we measured the $NADP^+$/NADPH ratio, which is an indicator of the cell reducing potential, because GPx activity is coupled to the reduction of NADPH to NADP+. The NADP+/NADPH ratio is significantly lower in THS-exposed mice than in control mouse livers (Figure 1F), showing that the reduction potential of these animals is decreased and might result in their inability to reduce the oxidative stress levels induced by the THS toxins.

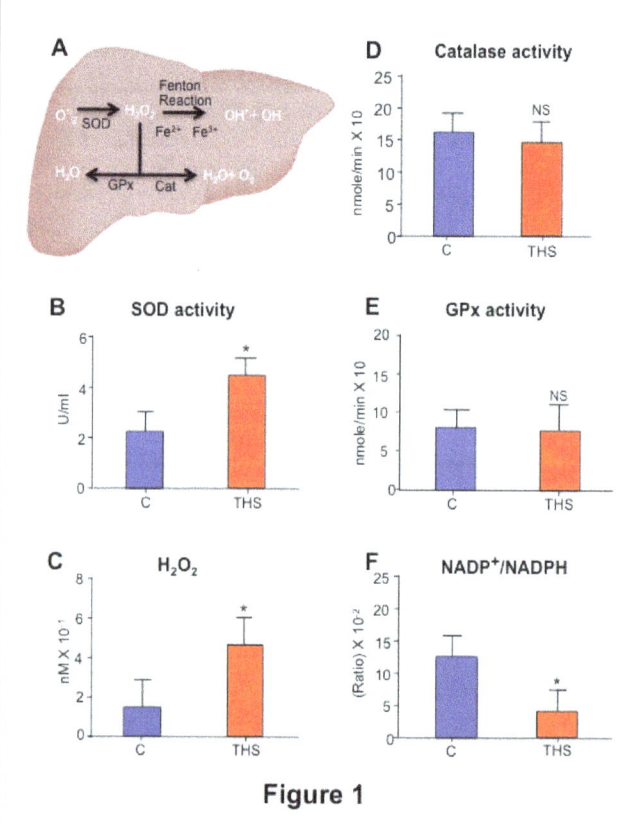

**Figure 1**

**Figure 1:** THS exposure results in oxidative stress in the liver. (A) Simplified schematic representation of the oxidative stress response in cells. When compared with the control, THS exposed mice have increased SOD enzymatic activity (B) increased hydrogen peroxide (C) show significant decrease in catalase enzymatic activity (D) show a significant difference in GPx activity (E) and have a significant decrease of NADP+/NADPH ratio (F). All data are Mean ± SD; *= p<0.05; NS= Not statistically significant. n=6. P values were adjusted for the number of times each test was run.

### THS-induced ROS lead to molecular and cellular damage in the liver

High levels of $H_2O_2$ in cells can lead to the production of hydroxyl radicals via the Fenton reaction in the presence of ferrous iron ion ($Fe^{2+}$) (Figure 2A). These radicals can damage lipids and proteins, and lead to the formation of DNA adducts. We found that in the liver of

THS-exposed mice there is significantly higher levels of lipid peroxidation, protein nitrosylation and DNA damage (Figures 2B and 2D). We also investigated whether THS toxins result in functional damage in the liver by measuring ATP, aspartate aminotransferase (AST) and urea levels. ATP is a marker for mitochondria function whereas AST and urea are markers of liver health. THS-exposed mice produced lower ATP levels than the controls (Figure 2E), suggesting that the ability of the mitochondria in THS-exposed mice to synthesize cellular energy is decreased. High levels of AST suggest liver damage whereas high levels of urea suggesting increase in amino acid metabolism (Figures 2F and 2G). Together, these results show that THS toxins result in damage of liver function.

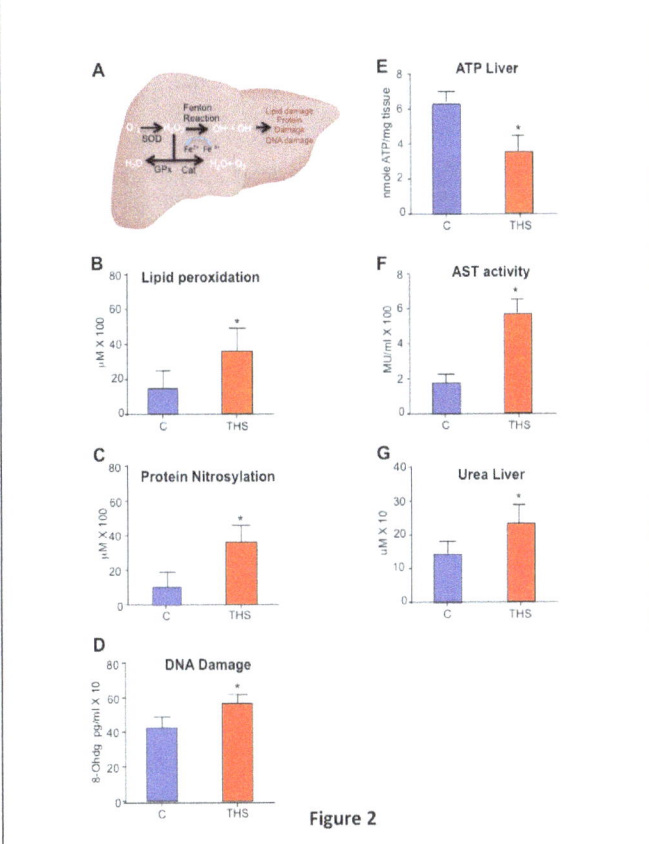

**Figure 2**

**Figure 2:** THS exposure increase oxidative stress mediated damage in the liver. (A) Model of oxidative stress induced mediated damage in cells. When compared to the control, THS exposed mice have higher lipid peroxidation (B) higher protein nitrosylation (C) higher DNA damage (D) decreased ATP levels (E) increased AST levels (F) and increased urea levels (G). All data are Mean ± SD *= p<0.05 NS= Not statistically significant. n=8 for B,C, and D. n=6 for E-G. P values were adjusted for the number of times each test was run.

## Oxidative stress mediated damage is improved by treating the mice with antioxidants

To investigate whether the THS-induced oxidative stress in the liver can be reversed, we treated the THS-exposed mice with the antioxidants N-acetylcysteine (NAC) and α-tocopherol (α-TOC) for

five months. These two antioxidants have been used previously to treat oxidative stress in different tissues [37-39]. Treatment with these antioxidants for five months while the mice were being exposed to THS, leads to a decrease in oxidative stress. These mice have SOD activity and $H_2O_2$ levels similar to those of the non-exposed mice treated with antioxidants but significantly lower than THS-exposed mice without treatment with antioxidants (Figures 3A and 3B). Although no significant changes were observed in the activity of catalase (Figure 3C), the THS-exposed mice treated with antioxidants have higher GPx activity than THS-exposed non-treated mice (Figure 3D). The same occurred for the NADP+/NADPH ratio (Figure 3E). Furthermore, NAC and α-TOC lowered the total hepatic lipid weight in the THS-exposed mice (Figure 3F).

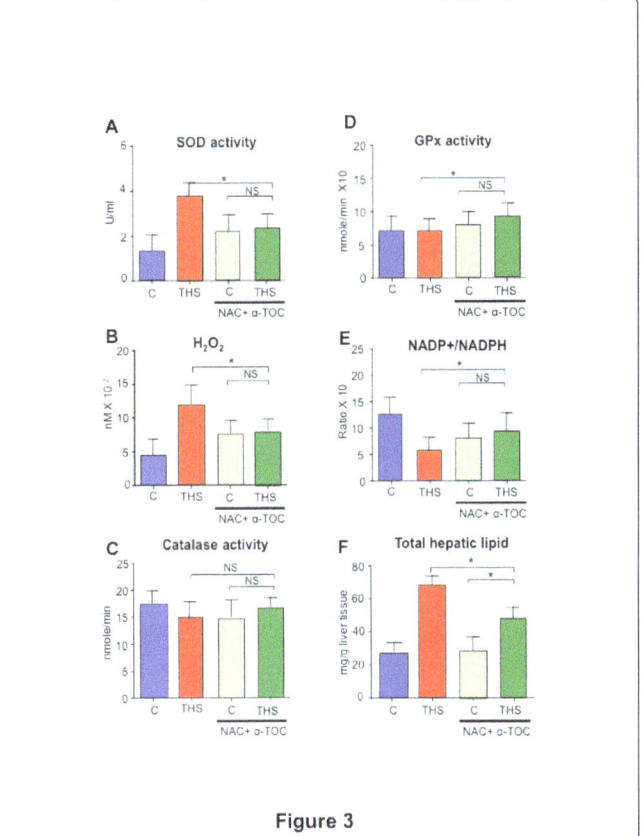

**Figure 3**

**Figure 3:** Antioxidant treatment leads to improvement of oxidative stress in the liver of THS-exposed mice. THS-exposed mice treated with the NAC+ α-TOC have significantly reduced of SOD activity (A), lower levels of $H_2O_2$ (B), no significant change in the enzymatic activity of catalase (C), significant change in the enzymatic activity of GPx (D), significant increase of NADP+/NADPH ratio (E) and in significant lowering of total hepatic lipid weight (F). All data are Mean ± SD *= p<0.05 NS= Not statistically significant n=9 for A and E n=8 for B,C, and D. n=6 for F. P values were adjusted for the number of times each test was run.

Treatment with antioxidant agents also decreased the oxidative-stress-mediated molecular damage in THS-exposed mice. These mice have lower lipid peroxidation (Figure 4A) and lower protein damage (Figure 4B) in THS exposed mice. However, no significant improvement was observed in DNA damage (Figure 4C). We also investigated whether antioxidant treatment improved functional damage by measuring ATP, AST and urea. AST is responsible for the conversion of aspartate to α-ketoglutarate to oxaloacetate and glutamate, which is fundamental for the function of the liver. Urea is a by-product of amino acid metabolism that occurs in the liver. Antioxidant treatment did not improve these parameters (Figures 4D and 4F).

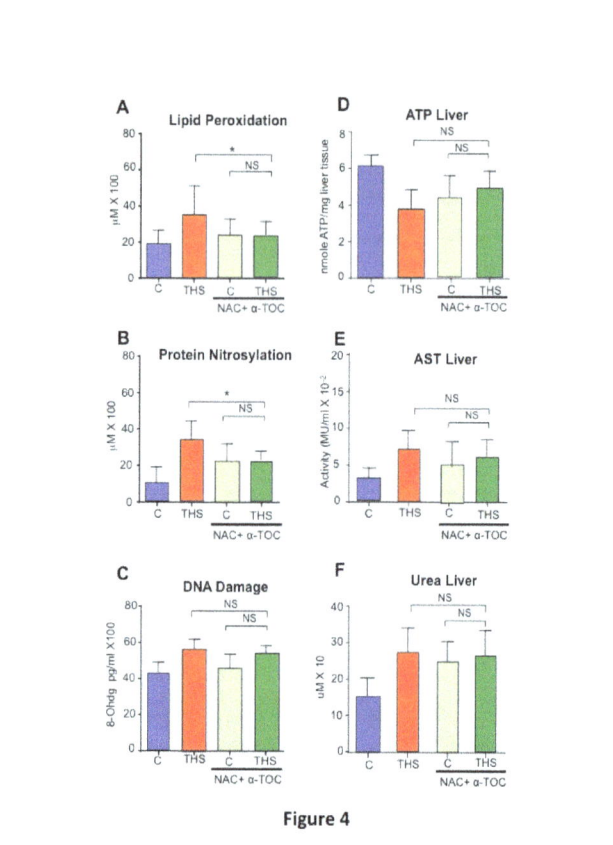

Figure 4

**Figure 4:** Oxidative stress mediated damage is improved by treating the mice with antioxidants. THS-exposed mice treated with NAC+ α-TOC show lower lipid peroxidation (A) lower protein nitrosylation but (B) no significant difference in DNA damage (C), ATP levels (D), AST levels (E) or urea levels (F). All data are Mean ± SD *= p<0.05, NS= Not statistically significant. n=8 for A n=7 for B n=9 for C, D E, F. P values were adjusted for the number of times each test was run.

## Treatment of THS-exposed mice with APAP increases oxidative-stress-mediated damage

Because N-acetyl-p-aminophenol (APAP/Tylenol) is a common drug taken by many people, especially by children, and it is known to damage the liver if taken in high doses [40], we investigated whether giving THS-exposed mice Tylenol would further increase oxidative stress in the liver. We used a dose the APAP/Tylenol that has been previously shown to induce chemical damage in the liver without killing the animals [40-42]. Based on these studies, we treated the THS-exposed mice for eight weeks with APAP/Tylenol. THS-exposed

mice treated with APAP/Tylenol have higher SOD activity and higher $H_2O_2$ levels than THS-exposed non-treated mice (Figures 5A and 5B). Moreover, the levels of catalase activity were significantly decreased when compare with THS exposed non-APAP treated animals (Figure 5C). We also observed that although GPx activity was not changed (Figure 5D), the NADP+/NADPH ratio was signicantly decreased (Figure 5E), showing that the reducing potential in the THS-exposed APAP-treated mice was low. Furthermore, APAP/Tylenol increased the total hepatic lipid weight in the THS-exposed mice (Figure 5F). This, results in further damage to the ability of the liver to handle the oxidative stress damage induced by THS.

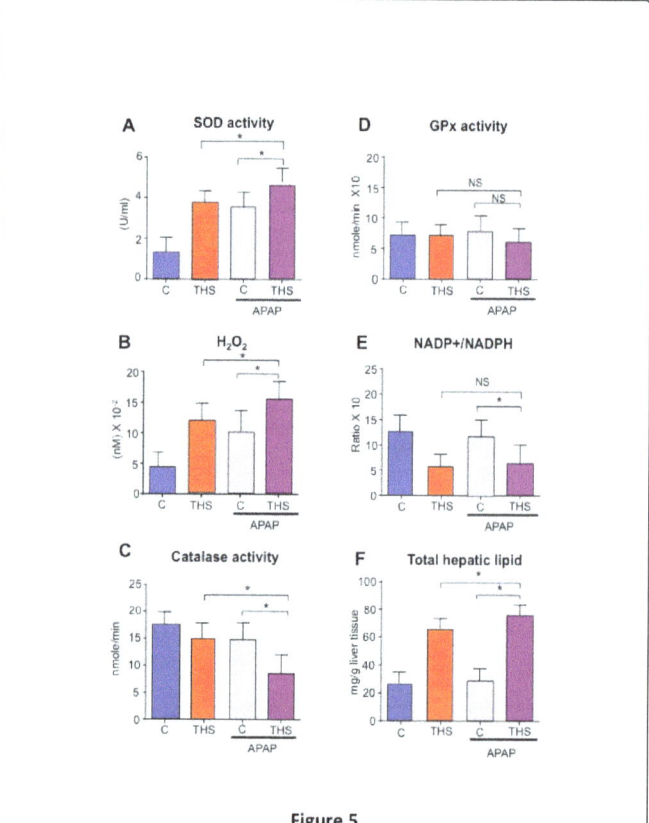

Figure 5

**Figure 5:** APAP treatment results in increased oxidative stress in THS-exposed mice. APAP treatment of THS-exposed mice results in higher SOD activity (A) higher levels of hydrogen peroxide (B) decrease in catalase activity (C) but no significant change in GPx activity (D). APAP treatment also did not have a signicant impact in the NADP+/NAPPH ratio (F) but resulted in higher total lipid hepatic weight in THS-exposed mice. All data are Mean ± SD *= p<0.05 NS= Not statistically significant n=9 for A and E n=8 for B,C, D. n=6 for F. P values were adjusted for the number of times each test was run.

We also quantified the oxidative stress-induced molecular damage and observed that THS exposure in conjunction with APAP/Tylenol treatment results in much higher levels of lipid peroxidation (Figure 6A), higher protein nitrosylation (Figure 6B) and higher DNA damage (Figure 6C). In addition, we also measured the ATP, AST and urea levels. High levels of AST and urea are associated with abnormal liver function [43,44]. APAP treatment results in lower ATP levels in THS-exposed mice suggesting that these mice have dysfunctional mitochondria (Figure 6D). APAP/Tylenol treatment results in higher AST levels in these animals suggesting that when THS exposure and APAP/Tylenol treatment are combined, further functional damage to the liver occurs (Figure 6E). However, APAP/Tylenol treatment of the THS-exposed mice did not have increased urea levels when compared to exposure only to THS (Figure 6F).

ATP production) or any other cellular damage insult that result in alterations to cellular energy. Together, SIRT1 and AMPK regulate lipid metabolism by preventing the synthesis of lipids and by stimulating fatty acid oxidation [45-59]. It has been shown using SIRT1 transgenic mice showed SIRT1 is required for activation of that AMPK and improvement of mitochondrial function [58]. It has also been shown AMPK phosphorylates and inhibits SREBP1c in diet induced insulin resistant mice [59]. Taken together studies suggest that SIRT1 and AMPK both work to prevent abnormal lipid metabolism by targeting and inhibiting SREBP1c a key lipogenic enzyme in the liver. Therefore, we investigated the SIRT1/AMPK/SREBP1c pathway and the THS-induced hepatic steatosis is a result of alterations in this pathway. When compared to the control mice the THS-exposed animals have lower levels of SIRT1 and of phosphorylated AMPK, the active form of this enzyme (Figures 7A and 7B).

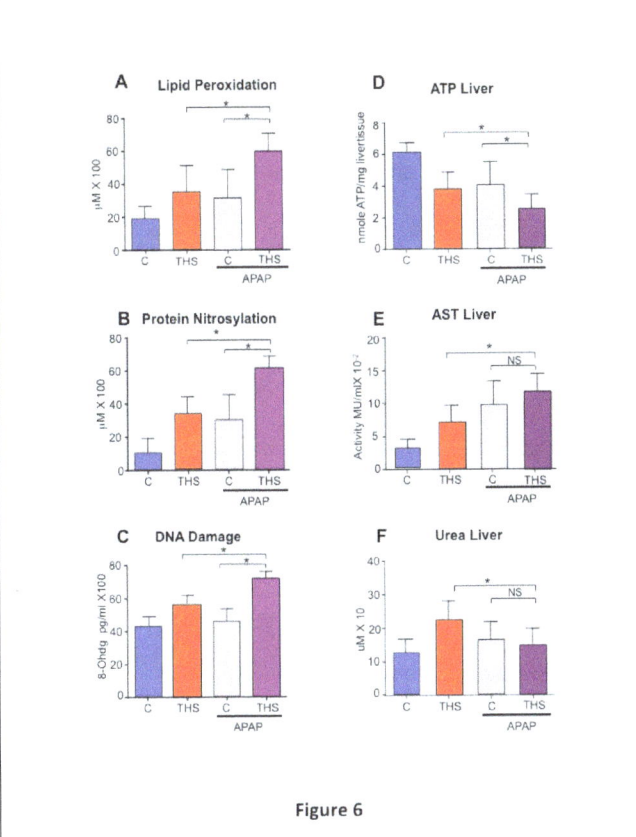

**Figure 6**

**Figure 6:** THS-exposed mice treated with APAP show increased oxidative stress mediated damage. APAP treatment results in higher lipid peroxidation (A), higher protein nitrosylation (B), and higher DNA damage (C) in the liver of THS-exposed mice. THS-exposed mice treated with APAP also have lower ATP levels (D) higher AST levels but (E) and lower urea levels (D) than THS-exposed mice. All data are Mean ± SD *= p<0.05, NS= Not statistically significant. n=8 for A n=7 for B n=9 for C,D E,F. P values were adjusted for the number of times each test was run.

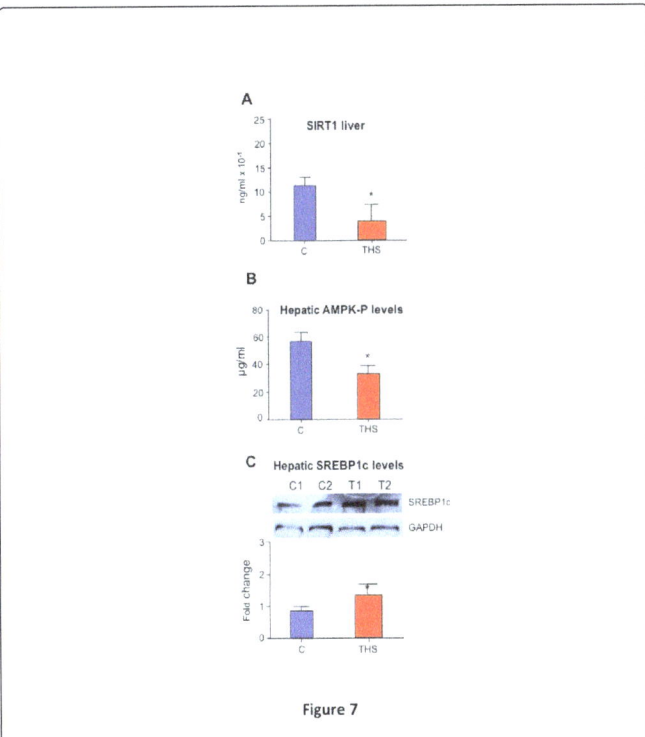

**Figure 7**

**Figure 7:** THS toxins alter the SIRT1/AMPK/ SBREP1c signaling in the liver. Compared to the control, THS-exposed mice have lower levels of SIRT1 (A), lower level of pAMPK (B) and higher levels of SREBP1c (C). *= p<0.05, ** p<0.01 NS= Not statistically significant. n=6 P values were adjusted for the number of times each test was run. "Fold change" on western blot quantification graph indicates fold change to control.

## THS toxins inhibit the SIRT1/AMPK/ SBREP1c signaling pathway in the liver

To investigate the cellular and molecular mechanisms of THS-induced lipid metabolism, we performed genomic analysis using both DNA microarray and RNA-Seq and found that Sirtuin 1 (SIRT1), a key regulator of lipid metabolism, is down regulated in THS-exposed mice. SIRT1 modulates the activity of other metabolic energy regulators such as 5' AMP-activated protein kinase (AMPK). AMPK is an energy sensor within the cell that responds to energy depletion (decrease in

Because activated AMPK is decreased in THS-exposed mice we tested the levels of SREBP1c the levels of SREBP1c. We found that in THS-exposed mice SREBP1c is elevated, leading to higher levels of lipids in the liver (Figure 7C). These findings suggest that THS exposure stimulate hepatic steatosis by altering the SIRT1/AMPK/ SREBP1c pathway.

## Discussion

We have previously shown that THS exposure results in the damage of multiple organs in mice including steatosis of the liver [23]. Here we show that the lipid accumulation is due to increase in the levels of oxidative stress, primarily of ROS, and inhibition of the SIRT1/AMPK/ SREBP1c pathway (Figure 8A). Modulating the levels of ROS with antioxidants resulted in improvement of the THS-induced hepatic steatosis whereas treatment with APAP resulted in augmentation of the THS-induced the lipid accumulation (Figure 8B).

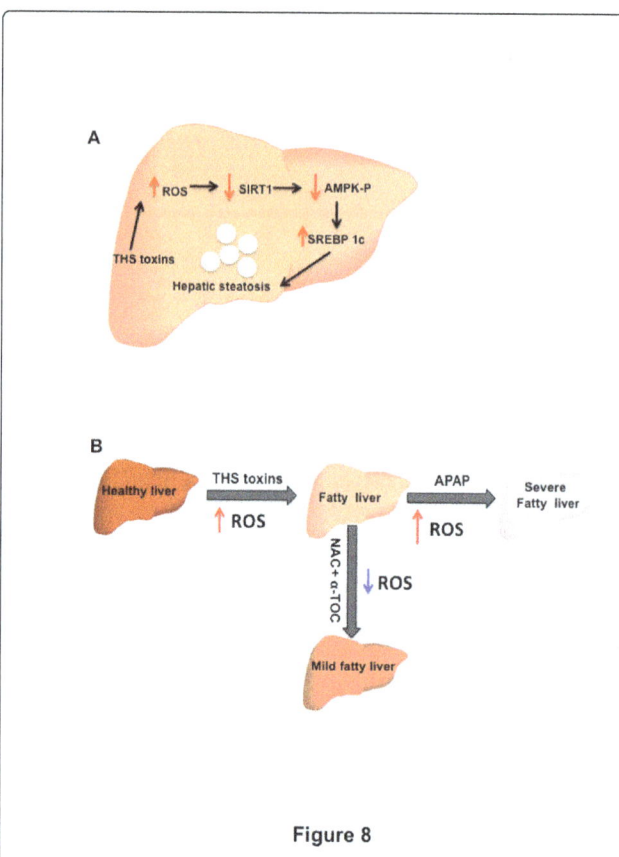

**Figure 8**

**Figure 8:** Proposed model for THS-induced hepatic steatosis. (A) A schematic representation of THS-induced hepatic steatosis in mice depicting a pathway by which THS toxins increase oxidative stress in the liver, which results in decrease of SIRT1 levels, a key regulator oxidative stress and regulator of lipid metabolism. The toxins also result in a decrease in the levels of active/phosphorylated AMPK and increase in SREBP1c levels, a stimulator of de novo lipid synthesis. As a result THS exposure stimulates fat accumulation in the liver resulting in hepatic steatosis. (B) A schematic summarizing THS-induced oxidative stress and fatty liver. Increasing oxidative stress by treating THS-exposed mice with APAP leads to severe fatty liver disease while decreasing oxidative stress by treating the mice with NAC+ α- TOC results in reducing fatty liver.

The oxidative stress mediated damage to the hepatic lipids, proteins, and DNA have a detrimental effect for lipid metabolism [60-62]. The liver is one of the major metabolic organs where glucose is metabolized, modified and stored. Perturbations in the metabolism and storage of glucose as well as insulin resistance in the liver have

been linked to the development of hepatic steatosis [63,64]. It is known that lipid peroxidation results in a decrease in the uptake of glucose in cortical rat neurons, which in the short term leads to abnormal glucose metabolism but over time it may lead to cell death [65]. Lipid peroxidation can also lead to conformational changes in the lipid bilayer and these changes can potentially alter the localization and stability of many receptors involved in lipid metabolism [66].

THS-exposed mice have high levels of protein damage, which affect the expression, and levels of proteins involved in the regulation of lipid metabolism in the liver. SIRT1 is a key regulator of lipid metabolism and it is known to work together with AMPK to prevent lipid accumulation in the liver by inhibiting SREBP1c and increasing fatty acid metabolism [46-59]. In this study we show that THS toxins alter the SIRT1/AMPK/SREBP1c signaling axis by decreasing SIRT1 levels which lead to decrease in phosphorylated/activated AMPK resulting in increase of SREBP1c and increase in lipid synthesis, with subsequent development of hepatic steatosis (Figure 8A). We also show that the liver specific damage we observed in the THS-exposed mice is mediated by oxidative stress triggered by the THS toxins. Increasing the oxidative stress in the liver of THS-exposed mice with APAP/ Tylenol worsened lipid accumulation whereas when the mice were exposed to THS and treated with antioxidants there was a decrease in lipid accumulation.

APAP/Tylenol is commonly used to treat headaches and fever and when taken for prolonged periods of time or higher dose it is known to cause liver damage. This can occur by depletion of glutathione (GSH) and by increasing mitochondria damage [67-69]. When we treated THS-exposed mice with APAP, we observed that these mice have higher liver damage than mice only exposed to THS. These mice also have lower levels of ATP, which suggest impaired mitochondria function. AST levels were also elevated suggesting abnormality in amino acid metabolism in the liver.

To decrease oxidative stress we treated THS-exposed mice with NAC and α-TOC that have been commonly used in humans and rodents for that purpose [70-72]. NAC is derivative of the amino acid L-cysteine and it is a direct precursor of glutathione consequently it has direct and indirect antioxidant properties [71]. Its free thiol group can interact with the electrophilic groups found in reactive oxygen species (ROS) agents. NAC can behave as an indirect antioxidant in the glutathione synthesis pathway, an antioxidant enzyme that decreases cellular oxidative stress [71]. α-TOC is an important lipid-soluble antioxidant that reacts with lipid radicals and consequently less lipid peroxidation occurs preventing damage to the plasma and mitochondrial membranes [72].

In conclusion, these studies provide insight into the effects of THS toxins on key molecules in lipid metabolism such as the SIRT1/AMPK/ SIRT1 signaling pathway. We show that by altering the oxidative stress levels using APAP/tylenol or the antioxidant agents NAC and a-TOC, we alter the THS-induced damage, which indicates that the THS-induced damage is mediated by oxidative stress. Based on our results, it is clear that THS toxins have the ability to alter fundamental metabolic processes such as lipid metabolism resulting in steatosis making THS a new risk factor for hepatic steatosis.

## References

1.  Winickoff JP, Friebely J, Tanski SE, Sherrod C, Matt GE, et al. (2009) Beliefs about the health effects of "thirdhand" smoke and home smoking bans. Pediatrics 123: e74-e79.

2. Burton A (2011) Does the smoke ever really clear? Thirdhand smoke exposure raises new concerns. Environ Health Perspect 119: A70-A74.

3. Whitehead T, Metayer C, Ward MH, Nishioka MG, Gunier R, et al. (2009). Is house-dust nicotine a good surrogate for household smoking?. Am J Epidemiol 169: 1113-1123.

4. Sleiman M, Gundel LA, Pankow JF, Jacob P, Singer, BC, et al. (2010) Formation of carcinogens indoors by surface-mediated reactions of nicotine with nitrous acid, leading to potential thirdhand smoke hazards. Proc Natl Acad Sci USA 107: 6576-6581.

5. Van Loy MD, Riley WJ, Daisey JM, Nazaroff WW (2001) Dynamic behavior of semivolatile organic compounds in indoor air. 2. Nicotine and phenanthrene with carpet and wallboard. Environ Sci Technol 35: 560-567.

6. Caldwell WS, Greene JM, Plowchalk DR, DeBethizy JD (1991) The nitrosation of nicotine: a kinetic study. Chem Res Toxicol 4: 513-516.

7. Singer BC, Revzan KL, Hotchi T, Hodgson AT, Brown NJ (2004) Sorption of organic gases in a furnished room. Atmos Environ 38: 2483-2494.

8. Sleiman M, Destaillats H, Smith JD, Liu CL, Ahmed M (2010) Secondary organic aerosol formation from ozone-initiated reactions with nicotine and secondhand tobacco smoke. Atmos Environ 44: 4191-4198.

9. Hoffmann D, Brunnemann KD, Prokopczyk B, Djordjevic MV (1994) Tobacco-specific N-nitrosamines and ARECA-derived N-nitrosamines: Chemistry, biochemistry, carcinogenicity, and relevance to humans. J Toxicol Environ Health 41: 1-52.

10. Hecht SS (1998) Biochemistry, biology, and carcinogenicity of tobacco-specific N-nitrosamines. Chem Res Toxicol 11: 559-603.

11. Matt GE, Quintana PJE, Hovell MF, Bernert JT, Song S, et al. (2004) Households contaminated by environmental tobacco smoke: sources of infant exposures. Tob Control 13: 29-37.

12. Centers for Disease Control and Prevention (2011) Smoking and Tobacco Use: Data and Statistics.

13. Hecht SS, Carmella SG, Le KA, Murphy SE, Boettcher AJ, et al. (2006) 4-(methylnitrosamino)-1-(3-pyridyl)-1-butanol and its glucuronides in the urine of infants exposed to environmental tobacco smoke. Cancer Epidemiol Biomarkers Prev 15: 988-992.

14. Singh GK, Siahpush M, Kogan MD (2010) Disparities in children's exposure to environmental tobacco smoke in the United States, 2007. Pediatrics 2009-2744.

15. Thomas JL, Guo H, Carmella SG, Balbo S, Han S, et al. (2011) Metabolites of a tobacco-specific lung carcinogen in children exposed to secondhand or thirdhand tobacco smoke in their homes. Cancer Epidemiol Biomarkers Prev 20: 1213-1221.

16. Hang B, Sarker AH, Havel C, Saha S, Hazra TK, et al. (2013) Thirdhand smoke causes DNA damage in human cells. Mutagenesis 28: 381-391.

17. Roberts JW, Dickey P (1995) Exposure of children to pollutants in house dust and indoor air. Rev Environ Contam Toxicol 143: 59-78.

18. Xu B, Chen M, Yao M, Ji X, Mao Z, et al. (2015) Metabolomics reveals metabolic changes in male reproductive cells exposed to thirdhand smoke. Sci Rep 6.

19. Rehan VK, Sakurai R, Torday JS (2011) Thirdhand smoke: a new dimension to the effects of cigarette smoke on the developing lung. Am J Physiol Lung Cell Mol Physiol 301: L1-L8.

20. Yolton K, Dietrich K, Auinger P, Lanphear BP, Hornung R (2005) Exposure to environmental tobacco smoke and cognitive abilities among US children and adolescents. Environ Health Perspect 2005:9 8-103.

21. Elliot J, Vullermin P, Robinson P (1998) Maternal cigarette smoking is associated with increased inner airway wall thickness in children who die from sudden infant death syndrome. Am J Respir Crit Care Med 158: 802-806.

22. Jung JW, Ju YS, Kang HR (2012) Association between parental smoking behavior and children's respiratory morbidity: 5-year study in an urban city of South Korea. Pediatr pulmonol 47: 338-345.

23. Martins-Green M, Adhami N, Frankos M, Valdez M, Goodwin B, et al. (2014) Cigarette smoke toxins deposited on surfaces: implications for human health. PloS one 9: E86391.

24. Adhami N, Starck SR, Flores C, Green MM (2016) A Health Threat to Bystanders Living in the Homes of Smokers: How Smoke Toxins Deposited on Surfaces Can Cause Insulin Resistance. PloS one 11: e0149510.

25. Erickson SK (2009) Nonalcoholic fatty liver disease. lipid res 50: S412-S416.

26. Marrero JA, Fontana RJ, Su GL, Conjeevaram HS, Emick DM, et al. (2002) NAFLD may be a common underlying liver disease in patients with hepatocellular carcinoma in the United States. Hepatology 36: 1349-1354.

27. Cazanave SC, Sanyal AJ (2016) Molecular Mechanisms of Lipotoxicity in Nonalcoholic Fatty Liver Disease. In Hepatic De Novo Lipogenesis and Regulation of Metabolism. Springer International Publishing.

28. Tiniakos DG, Vos MB, Brunt EM (2010) Nonalcoholic fatty liver disease: pathology and pathogenesis. Annu Rev Pathol 5: 145-171.

29. Letteron P, Sutton A, Mansouri A, Fromenty B, Pessayre D (2003) Inhibition of microsomal triglyceride transfer protein: Another mechanism for drug-induced steatosis in mice. Hepatology 38: 133-140.

30. Fromenty B, Pessayre D (1997) Impaired mitochondrial function in microvesicular steatosis effects of drugs, ethanol, hormones and cytokines. J Hepatol 26: 43-53.

31. Azzalini L, Ferrer E, Ramalho LN, Moreno M, Domínguez M, et al. (2010) Cigarette smoking exacerbates nonalcoholic fatty liver disease in obese rats. Hepatology 51: 1567-1576.

32. Browning JD, Horton JD (2004) Molecular mediators of hepatic steatosis and liver injury. J Clin Invest 114: 147-152.

33. Tolosa L, Gómez-Lechón MJ, Jiménez N, Hervás D, Jover R, et al. (2016) Advantageous use of HepaRG cells for the screening and mechanistic study of drug-induced steatosis. Toxicol Appl Pharmacol.

34. Petersen KF, Dufour S, Befroy D, Lehrke M, Hendler RE, et al. (2005) Reversal of nonalcoholic hepatic steatosis, hepatic insulin resistance, and hyperglycemia by moderate weight reduction in patients with type 2 diabetes. Diabetes 54: 603-608.

35. Ryan MC, Itsiopoulos C, Thodis T, Ward G, Trost N, et al. (2013) The Mediterranean diet improves hepatic steatosis and insulin sensitivity in individuals with non-alcoholic fatty liver disease. J Hepatol 59: 138-143.

36. Faghihzadeh F, Adibi P, Rafiei R, Hekmatdoost A (2014) Resveratrol supplementation improves inflammatory biomarkers in patients with nonalcoholic fatty liver disease. Nutr Res 34: 837-843.

37. de Diego-Otero Y, Romero-Zerbo Y, el Bekay R, Decara J, Sanchez L, et al. (2009) α-tocopherol protects against oxidative stress in the fragile X knockout mouse: an experimental therapeutic approach for the Fmr1 deficiency. Neuropsychopharmacology 34: 1011-1026.

38. Thakurta IG, Banerjee P, Bagh MB, Ghosh A, Sahoo A, et al. (2014) Combination of N-acetylcysteine, α-lipoic acid and α-tocopherol substantially prevents the brain synaptosomal alterations and memory and learning deficits of aged rats. Exp Gerontol 50: 19-25.

39. Joseph, AJ, Adamu, KB, Shu'aibu Yahya BRL, Martina BS, Asabe MUA, et al. (2014) Influence of high dietary vitamin C and E oral administration on anemia and organ damage in wistar rat infected with Trypanosoma brucei brucei (Federe strain).

40. Jaw S, Jeffery EH (1993) Interaction of caffeine with acetaminophen: 1. Correlation of the effect of caffeine on acetaminophen hepatotoxicity and acetaminophen bioactivation following treatment of mice with various cytochrome P450 inducing agents. Biochemical pharmacology 46: 493-501.

41. Zaher H, Buters JT, Ward JM, Bruno, MK, Lucas AM, et al. (1998) Protection against acetaminophen toxicity in CYP1A2 and CYP2E1 double-null mice. Toxi appl pharm 152: 193-199.

42. Shayiq RM, Roberts DW, Rothstein K, Snawder JE, Benson W, et al. (1999) Repeat exposure to incremental doses of acetaminophen provides protection against acetaminophen-induced lethality in mice: An explanation for high acetaminophen dosage in humans without hepatic injury. Hepatology 29: 451-463.

43. Abdel-Daim MM, Abuzead, SM, Halawa SM (2013) Protective role of Spirulina platensis against acute deltamethrin-induced toxicity in rats. PLoS One 8: e72991.

44. Puche JE, Lee YA, Jiao J, Aloman C, Fiel MI, et al. (2013) A novel murine model to deplete hepatic stellate cells uncovers their role in amplifying liver damage in mice. Hepatology 57: 339-350.

45. Caito S, Rajendrasozhan S, Cook S, Chung S, Yao H, et al. (2010) SIRT1 is a redox-sensitive deacetylase that is post-translationally modified by oxidants and carbonyl stress.

46. Merksamer PI, Liu Y, He W, Hirschey MD, Chen D, et al. (2013) The sirtuins, oxidative stress and aging: an emerging link. Aging 5: 144-150.

47. Purushotham A, Schug TT, Xu Q, Surapureddi S, Guo X, et al. (2009) Hepatocyte-specific deletion of SIRT1 alters fatty acid metabolism and results in hepatic steatosis and inflammation. Cell metab 9: 327-338.

48. Brunet A, Sweeney LB, Sturgill JF, Chua, KF, Greer PL, et al. (2004) Stress-dependent regulation of FOXO transcription factors by the SIRT1 deacetylase. Science 303: 2011-2015.

49. Webster BR, Lu Z, Sack MN, Scott I (2012) The role of sirtuins in modulating redox stressors. Free Radic Biol Med 52: 281-290.

50. Chen WL, Kang CH, Wang SG, Lee HM (2012) α-Lipoic acid regulates lipid metabolism through induction of sirtuin 1 (SIRT1) and activation of AMP-activated protein kinase. Diabetologia 55: 1824-1835.

51. Walker AK, Yang F, Jiang K, Ji JY, Watts JL, et al. (2010) Conserved role of SIRT1 orthologs in fasting-dependent inhibition of the lipid/cholesterol regulator SREBP. Genes & development 24: 1403-1417.

52. Rodgers JT, Puigserver P (2007) Fasting-dependent glucose and lipid metabolic response through hepatic sirtuin 1. Proc Natl Acad Sci USA 104: 12861-12866.

53. Ponugoti B, Kim DH, Xiao Z, Smith Z, Miao J, et al. (2010) SIRT1 deacetylates and inhibits SREBP-1C activity in regulation of hepatic lipid metabolism. J Biol Chem 285: 33959-33970.

54. Kim E, Choi Y, Jang J, Park T (2013) Carvacrol protects against hepatic steatosis in mice fed a high-fat diet by enhancing SIRT1-AMPK signaling. Evid Based Complement Alternat Med 2013: 290104.

55. Yuan H, Shyy JYJ, Martins-Green M (2009) Second-hand smoke stimulates lipid accumulation in the liver by modulating AMPK and SREBP-1. J Hepatol 51: 535-547.

56. Jung EJ, Kwon SW, Jung BH, Oh SH, Lee BH (2011) Role of the AMPK/SREBP-1 pathway in the development of orotic acid-induced fatty liver. J Lipid Res 52: 1617-1625.

57. Ahmed MH, Byrne CD (2007) Modulation of sterol regulatory element binding proteins (SREBPs) as potential treatments for non-alcoholic fatty liver disease (NAFLD). Drug Discov Today 12: 740-747.

58. Price NL, Gomes AP, Ling AJ, Duarte FV, Martin-Montalvo A, et al. (2012) SIRT1 is required for AMPK activation and the beneficial effects of resveratrol on mitochondrial function. Cell metab 15: 675-690.

59. Li Y, Xu S, Mihaylova MM, Zheng B, Hou X, et al. (2011) AMPK phosphorylates and inhibits SREBP activity to attenuate hepatic steatosis and atherosclerosis in diet-induced insulin-resistant mice. Cell Metab 13: 376-388.

60. Seki S, Kitada T, Yamada T, Sakaguchi H, Nakatani K, et al. (2002) In situ detection of lipid peroxidation and oxidative DNA damage in non-alcoholic fatty liver diseases. Journal of hepatology 37: 56-62.

61. Pan M, Cederbaum AI, Zhang YL, Ginsberg HN, Williams KJ, et al. (2004) Lipid peroxidation and oxidant stress regulate hepatic apolipoprotein B degradation and VLDL production. J Clin Invest 113: 1277-1287.

62. Bryant RJ, Ryder J, Martino P, Kim J, Craig BW (2003) Effects of vitamin E and C supplementation either alone or in combination on exercise-induced lipid peroxidation in trained cyclists. J Strength Cond Res 17: 792-800.

63. Flannery C, Dufour S, Rabøl R, Shulman GI, Petersen KF (2012) Skeletal muscle insulin resistance promotes increased hepatic de novo lipogenesis, hyperlipidemia, and hepatic steatosis in the elderly. Diabetes 61: 2711-2717.

64. Perry R J, Samuel VT, Petersen KF, Shulman GI (2014) The role of hepatic lipids in hepatic insulin resistance and type 2 diabetes. Nature 510: 84-91.

65. Lovell MA, Xie C, Markesbery WR (2000) Acrolein, a product of lipid peroxidation, inhibits glucose and glutamate uptake in primary neuronal cultures. Free Radic Biol Med 29: 714-720.

66. Catalá A (2012) Lipid peroxidation modifies the picture of membranes from the "Fluid Mosaic Model" to the "Lipid Whisker Model". Biochimie 94: 101-109.

67. Reid AB, Kurten RC, McCullough SS, Brock RW, Hinson JA (2005) Mechanisms of acetaminophen-induced hepatotoxicity: role of oxidative stress and mitochondrial permeability transition in freshly isolated mouse hepatocytes. J Pharmacol Exp Ther 312: 509-516.

68. Xie Y, McGill MR, Dorko K, Kumer SC, Schmitt TM, et al. (2014) Mechanisms of acetaminophen-induced cell death in primary human hepatocytes. Toxi Appli pharm 279: 266-274.

69. McGill MR, Sharpe MR, Williams CD, Taha M, Curry SC, et al. (2012) The mechanism underlying acetaminophen-induced hepatotoxicity in humans and mice involves mitochondrial damage and nuclear DNA fragmentation. J Clin Invest 122: 1574-1583.

70. Mehta K, Van Thiel DH, Shah N, Mobarhan S (2002) Nonalcoholic fatty liver disease: pathogenesis and the role of antioxidants. Nutr Rev 60: 289-293.

71. Grinberg L, Fibach E, Amer J, Atlas D (2005) N-acetylcysteine amide, a novel cell-permeating thiol, restores cellular glutathione and protects human red blood cells from oxidative stress. Free Radic Biol Med 38: 136-145.

72. Niki E (2014) Role of vitamin E as a lipid-soluble peroxyl radical scavenger: in vitro and in vivo evidence. Free Radic Biol Med 66: 3-12.

# 24

# Toxicity and Genotoxicity of Beauty Products on Human Skin Cells *In Vitro*

**Abdullah M Alnuqaydan**[*] **and Barbara J Sanderson**

*Department of Medical Biotechnology, School of Medicine, Flinders University, Australia*

[*]**Corresponding author:** Abdullah M Alnuqaydan , Department of Medical Biotechnology, School of Medicine, Flinders University, GPO Box 2100, Adelaide, SA 5001, Australia, E-mail: A.alnuqaydan@gmail.com

## Abstract

**Background:** We use beauty products in high quantities every day and in the process, we are exposed to a wide variety of chemicals used in these products. These chemicals are a particularly insidious form of body pollution because they enter the human body through multiple routes. The problem with commercial products and particularly beauty products is that millions of people apply beauty products to their skin daily for long time.

**Objective:** To determine the toxicity and genotoxicity effects of four facial beauty products on tow human skin cells. Also, to find out which product ingredients can induce the most toxicity and genotoxicity on human skin cells.

**Methodology:** The *in vitro* toxicity and genotoxicity of facial beauty products were determined using a human keratinocyte cell line (HaCaT) and a human fibroblast cell line (CCD-1064SK). The products were an Anti-aging face moisturiser with mixture of natural ingredients (Facial Moisturizer - Camellia & Geranium Blossom) and Nivea Visage Q10plus Anti-Wrinkle which includes synthetic chemicals with $TiO_2$ and Nivea Visage Q10plus Anti-Wrinkle which includes synthetic chemicals without $TiO_2$. Glycerol was the negative control. Toxicity was measured by Crystal violet assay and Methyl tetrazolium cytotoxicity (MTT) assay. Apoptosis/necrosis proportion, nuclear division index (NDI) and genotoxicity were detected by cytokinesis block micronucleus (CBMN) assay.

**Results:** Glycerol did not induce any toxicity or genotoxicity. Nivea Visage Q10plus Anti-Wrinkle which includes synthetic chemicals with and without $TiO_2$ showed significant toxicity in both assays. No toxicity observed with Facial Moisturizer - Camellia & Geranium Blossom but there was a significant necrosis. Populations of cells treated with diluted Nivea Visage Q10plus Anti-Wrinkle which includes synthetic chemicals with and without $TiO_2$ showed increased proportions of apoptosis/necrosis. The nuclear division index (NDI) was decreased by Nivea Visage Q10plus Anti-Wrinkle which includes synthetic chemicals with and without $TiO_2$ and Facial Moisturizer - Camellia & Geranium Blossom. Nivea Visage Q10plus Anti-Wrinkle which includes synthetic chemicals with and without $TiO_2$ showed increased frequency of micronuclei (MNi). Nivea Visage Q10plus Anti-Wrinkle face moisturizer with $TiO_2$ proved to induce significantly more micronuclei (MNi) than the product without $TiO_2$.

**Conclusion:** The study results indicate that facial beauty products can cause cytotoxicity and genotoxicity *in vitro* using dilutions of the commercial formulations.

**Keywords:** Toxicity; Genotoxicity; Safety assessment; Beauty products; Cosmetic ingredients; Cell culture; Chromosomal damage

## Introduction

We use large quantities of beauty products every day and, in the process, are exposed to a wide variety of chemicals used in these products. These chemicals are a particularly insidious form of body pollution because they enter the human body through multiple routes. It is easy to swallow them, inhale them and absorb them through the mucous membrane of the eyes, mouth or nose. Our skin absorbs approximately 60% of the chemical ingredients and sends them into the bloodstream, from whence they can reach every organ in the body seconds after absorption [1]. Women using a lot of cosmetics are thought their skin absorb up to 2 kg of chemical cosmetic ingredients each year [1]. Government reports in the US and EU indicate that about 90% of the ingredients used in cosmetics are not safe for people in the long-term [1]. Most beauty products contain a mixture of chemicals that only make the problem worse [2]. Unfortunately, the companies that make them are self-regulating, and government agencies do not press the manufacturers to prove their products are safe [1,2]. In the US, cosmetic and personal care products are not regulated by the Food and Drug Administration (U.S. FDA) [3,4]. However, drugs do require extensive testing and approval by the FDA [3]. Also, one study has noted the results of studies screening blood sample from over the entire world, indicate that most people are carrying a huge amount of chemicals in their bodies [1,5]. These studies used biochemical methods for screening. Another study have shown that exposure to chemicals demonstrates that most American children and adults carry inside them nearly 100 substances or chemicals including pesticides and toxic compounds [5]. Many of these cause cancer, damage the immune system and affect human behaviour and the central nervous system. The sources of these chemicals include household exposure to pesticides and detergents, cosmetics, toiletries, paints and fabric treatments [1,2,6]. They can affect the body over the long term and accumulate in different organs and the bloodstream and then pass through the urine, semen and in the form of breast milk. After a while and the body becomes overloaded and at risk of total breakdown [1]. Some cosmetics contain mercury which is used to lighten the skin and people who use products containing mercury are at a high risk of mercury poisoning [7]. In the United States mercury compounds are used as preservatives in small concentrations for eye area products and FDA regulations in the US have restricted cosmetics products that contain mercury [7]. Some moisturizers contain mineral oil which can slow down cell renewal and promote early skin ageing [1]. A study tested 88 brands of eye shadow and found that approximately 75% of these products contained at least one of the 5 elements: lead, nickel, chromium, arsenic or cobalt [8]. Lead can damage any part of the human body and in particular the nervous system [9]. Even the elements found in small doses in these products may cause hormone disruption [10]. Some sun blocks and

moisturizers with sun blocks contain Titanium dioxide (TiO$_2$) which is a potential hazard and carcinogen [11,12]. Finally, most shampoos and other toiletries or liquid formulas contain nitrosamines that can cause cancer [13]. Some products are labelled as hypoallergenic but probably still contain potentially carcinogenic substances [14]. In this study, four different facial beauty products were examined to assess the effects on two human skin cells (Human keratinocytes HaCaT skin cells and human fibroblast CCD-1064SK cells). Products were Nivea Visage Q10 Plus Anti-Wrinkle face moisturizer which includes synthetic chemicals + TiO$_2$, Nivea Visage Q10 Plus Anti-Wrinkle face moisturizer which includes synthetic chemicals (Improved formula, without TiO$_2$), Facial Moisturizer - Camellia & Geranium Blossom which includes a mixture of natural ingredients and Glycerol B.P.

| Ingredients | Toxic effects |
|---|---|
| Octocrylene | Skin allergen. Restricted for use in cosmetics in Japan. Produces excess ROS that can interfere with cellular signalling, cause mutations, lead to cell death and may be implicated in cardiovascular disease. Measured to accumulate in people. |
| Ethylhexyl Salicylate | Low allergies and immunotoxicity, ecotoxicology |
| Methylpropanediol | Not expected to be potentially toxic or harmful |
| Glyceryl Stearate | Suspected to be an environmental toxin |
| Butyl Methoxydibenzoylmethane | Toxin in mice |
| C12-15 Alkyl Benzoate | Suspected to be an environmental toxin |
| Tocopheryl Acetate | Human skin toxin or allergen—strong evidence. Has caused tumours in animals. |
| Chondrus Crispus | Organ system toxin (non-reproductive) |
| Dimethicone | Organ system toxin (non-reproductive) |
| Trisodium EDTA | Penetration enhancer |
| Caprylic/Capric Triglyceride | Ecotoxin |
| Limonene and Parfum | Irritant. Possible human immune system toxin or allergen. Restricted in cosmetics |
| Ingredients | Toxic effects |
| Methylparaben | Human endocrine disruptor-strong evidence |
| Phenoxyethanol | Irritant (skin, eyes or lungs), occupational hazard, organ system toxin (non-reproductive) |
| Cera Microcristallina | Organ system toxin (non-reproductive) |
| Paraffinum Liquidum | Human immune and respiratory toxin or allergen—strong evidence |
| Benzyl Alcohol | Occupational hazard, organ system toxin (non-reproductive) |
| TiO$_2$ | Carcinogen |
| Thylhexylglycerin | Irritant (skin, eyes or lungs); organ system toxin (non-reproductive) |
| Carbomer | No carcinogenicity data available, but it is found to be irritating to the respiratory tract. |
| Sodium Phenylbenzimidazole Sulfonat | May cause skin irritation, if swallowed will cause vomiting. |
| Trimethoxycaprylylsilane | Not expected to be potentially toxic or harmful |

**Table 1:** The ingredients and toxic effects of Nivea Visage Q10Plus Anti-Wrinkle face moisturizer + TiO$_2$. The toxic effects of the ingredients were classified by [39-41].

## Materials and Methods

### Materials

RPMI 1640 media and foetal bovine serum (FBS) were purchased from Gibco® Cell Culture Media - Life Technologies (Australia). Cytochalasin B (Cyt-B) solution, Sodium dodecyl sulphate (SDS, approximately 99%), Phosphate buffered saline (PBS) and 3-(4,5-dimethylthiazol-2-yl)-2,5-diphenyltetrazolium bromide (MTT) were purchased from Sigma-Aldrich (USA). Spectrophotometer plate reader (BIO-TEK Instruments Inc., USA). Diff-Quik stains were purchased from Lab Aids (Australia). Cytospin centrifuge (Shandon, England). TrypLE™ was purchased from Life Technologies (Australia). All other reagents were obtained from sigma, unless otherwise stated.

### Products to be examined

#### Nivea visage Q10Plus Anti-wrinkle face moisturiser with titanium dioxide ($TiO_2$)

Nivea visage Q10plus Anti-Wrinkle day moisturizer cream plus extra UVA protection (SPF 15) is produced by Nivea which is a worldwide company. Nivea Visage Q10plus Anti-Wrinkle purchased from a local pharmacy in Adelaide, South Australia. It suits all skin types. The product aims to increase the natural Q10 level and prevent wrinkles. Also, it is protecting from UVA+UVB. The ingredients of Nivea Visage Q10plus are mixture of chemicals (Table 1).

This formula of the product contains Titanium Dioxide ($TiO_2$) which is a nanoparticle that is used widely in pigments, cosmetics, and skin care products because it the benefit of protecting the skin from UV light, particularly in Nano sized particles less than 100 nm [15]. Titanium Dioxide ($TiO_2$) has been classified as carcinogen [16]. Some studies have shown that Titanium Dioxide $TiO_2$ can damage DNA directly or indirectly via inflammatory response or oxidative stress [15].

#### Nivea Visage Q10Plus Anti-Wrinkle face moisturizer (Improved formula, without titanium dioxide ($TiO_2$))

This product is an improved formula of Nivea Visage Q10plus Anti-Wrinkle day moisturizer. It is released into the market after removed the original product which contains Titanium Dioxide $TiO_2$. It has almost the same ingredients as the original one except for the absence of $TiO_2$. The Package is labelled with 'skin compatibility dermatologically approved'. This product aims to UVA protection. The product is suitable for sensitive skin.

### Grown facial moisturizer - camellia & geranium blossom

Facial Moisturizer - Camellia & Geranium Blossom is a natural moisturizer made from bioactive ingredients. It is made by extractions from Camellia and Rose Hip Seed Oil which consists of vital phytosterols that rehydrate and nourish the skin. Cane sugar is also present, and it releases bio saccharides that soothe the skin and combats the effects of UV and pollution while Mayblossom releases flavonoids which normalize sebum production and reduces pore size. The product was purchased from a local chemist.

### Glycerol British Pharmacopoeia B.P.

Pharmaceuticals Pty Ltd produces glycerol B.P. It was purchased from a local pharmacy. It is 90-100% Glycerol (Glycerine). It can be prescribed to be taken internally as a mild laxative and externally to soften and moisturize the skin. Glycerol may reduce food intake in diabetic rats [17]. Therefore, there is a label on the package warning the diabetic patient. Glycerol is a common basic ingredient in many moisturizers. Therefore, it used as a negative control for the beauty products experiments.

### Cell lines and cell culture

A human non-cancer keratinocytes cell line HaCaT were a gift from the Department of Haematology and Genetic Pathology-Flinders Medical Centre, School of Medicine at Flinders University, Adelaide. Skin fibroblast cell line CCD-1064Sk (A human normal skin cells) was obtained from ATCC, US (ATCC® CRL-2076™). Keratinocytes cell line HaCaT was maintained in RPMI 1640 medium, with 10% fetal bovine serum (FBS) and 1% penicillin/streptomycin (Thermo Scientific, Australia). A human normal skin fibroblast cell line CCD-1064Sk was maintained in Iscove's Modified Dulbecco's medium (IMDM medium) with 10% fetal bovine serum (FBS) and 1% penicillin/streptomycin. Cells were seeded in tissue culture flasks and incubated at 37°C in a 5% $CO_2$ fully humidified incubator. HaCaT cells were subcultured when they reached 60–80% confluence.

### Cell treatment

The 96_well flat bottom was seeded with 104 cells/well and incubated for 19 h to allow the adherence of cells at 37°C in 5% $CO_2$. The media were aspirated and replaced with 100 µL of the treatment solution per well and were treated for 1 h prior to bioassays or genetic assays. The negative or untreated control (0 dose) was the media.

### Crystal violet assay

Crystal violet stains the DNA of the live cells that adheres the plate after the dead cells are washed away [18]. The relative number of viable cells was determined using crystal violet assay (CV) as described in [19]. Briefly, 50 µL of crystal violet stain (0.5% of crystal violet in 50% methanol) was added to each well and incubated for 10 minutes at ambient temperature. After 10 minutes, the plate was gently washed with distilled water then air dried. 50 µL of 33% acetic acid was added to de-stain the cells. The absorbance (ODs) was measured on a spectrophotometric plate reader using a test wavelength of 570 nm with a reference wavelength of 630.

### Methyl tetrazolium cytotoxicity assay (MTT Assay)

The tetrazolium salt 3-4,5 dimethlthiazol-2,5 diphenyl tetrazolium bromide (MTT) assay is based on a colorimetric assay for mammalian cell growth and survival, and it depends on the ability of viable cells to metabolize the yellow and water-soluble tetrazolium salt [20]. Cells were seeded at 104 in a volume of 100 µl into each well of a 96-well flat bottom plate. MTT solution with a final concentration 0.5 mg/ml was added and then incubated for 4 h at 37°C. After incubation, 80 µl 20% SDS in 0.02 M HCl was added. The plates were incubated overnight in the dark at room temperature. Thee absorbance (ODs) was measured on a spectrophotometric plate reader using a reference wavelength of 630 nm and a test wavelength of 570 nm.

### Cytokinesis block micronucleus assay (CBMN Assay)

The mechanism of cell killing and genotoxicity of beauty products was carried out using Cytokinesis-Block Micronucleus Assay (CBMN) assay as described [21,22]. Briefly, after treatment Cyt-B (4.5 µg/ml) was added to the media and the cultures were incubated at 37°C for 23 h. Cells were trypsinized (TrypLE™ Express Enzyme (1X), phenol red) and collected onto slides by a cytospin centrifuging for 5 minutes at 47 ×g (@6000 rpm). Slides were air-dried, fixed by DiffQuick Fixative for 10 min, and then double stained with stain 1 (red DiffQuick Stain) and then Stain 2 (blue DiffQuick Stain). Slides were scored as described in [23]. The chromosomal damage induced by treatment and total number of micronuclei (MNi) in binucleated (BN) cells totalled 1000. Slides were scored at a magnification of 250X or 40 X. Criteria for scoring micronuclei MNi, nucleoplasmic bridge (NPB) or nuclear buds (NBUDs) were as described [21]. Cytotoxicity determination induced by treatment, and the percentage of apoptosis/necrosis were evaluated in 500 cells and calculated according to published formulae [23,24].

## Statically analysis

Data were presented as the mean ± S.E.M. of the standard error. The experiments were replicated at least three independent times. Statistical analysis of the data was carried out using ANOVA, followed by Tukey's HSD post hoc test. These tests were performed using SPSS software (Version 22). Differences were considered significant when the p-value was less than 0.05. Responses to treatment were compared to the untreated control (0 doses) which is represented as 100% survival.

## Results

### Cytotoxicity effects of beauty products on human skin cells

The toxicity of four beauty products on Keratinocytes human skin cells (HaCaT) and human normal skin fibroblast (CCD-1064Sk) *in vitro* was determined by incubating cells with treatments for 1h. Two cytotoxicity assays were carried out to indicate the toxicity of beauty products. The MTT cell survival assay was used to determine the relative survival cells when yellow MTT is reduced to purple formazan in the mitochondria of living cells. The Crystal Violet (CV) assay was used to determine the relative cell number when Crystal violet stains the DNA of the live cells that adhere to the plate after the dead cells are washed away. There was significant toxicity with doses of 3% w/v and 0.3% w/v for Nivea Visage Q10plus Anti-Wrinkle face moisturizer (with TiO₂) after treated HaCaT cells for 1h (Figure 1). Also, significant toxicity was induced by the highest dose (3% w/v) of Nivea Visage Q10plus Anti-Wrinkle face moisturizer (Improved formula, without TiO₂) on human fibroblast CCD-1064SK cells determined by MTT and Crystal Violet (Figure 2). However, no significant toxicity emerged on HaCaT human skin cells or human fibroblast CCD-1064SK cells when using treatments of Glycerol B.P or Facial Moisturizer - Camellia & Geranium Blossom.

The Nuclear division index (NDI) is a method employed to measure the proliferative status of viable cells that can be used to assess general toxicity [21,25]. Table 2 shows the value of NDI for all beauty products examined and which had a significantly lower NDI value in the highest dose (3% w/v; 1.4 (P<0.05) of Nivea Visage with or without TiO₂ and Facial Moisturizer - Camellia & Geranium Blossom treatment at dose 5% w/v; 1.4 P<0.05 on HaCaT cells.

## Mechanism of cell killing

The CBMN results (Figure 3 B) detected a significant increase in late apoptosis and early necrosis induced by the highest dose of Nivea visage with TiO₂ 3% w/v and significantly induced in 0.3% w/v and 0.03% w/v doses of Nivea visage without TiO₂ after treated HaCaT cells for 1 h. Otherwise, no significantly apoptosis or necrosis induction was observed in the treatments of Facial natural treatment (Facial Moisturizer - Camellia & Geranium Blossom) and Glycerol B.P on HaCaT cells as shown in Figure 3A.

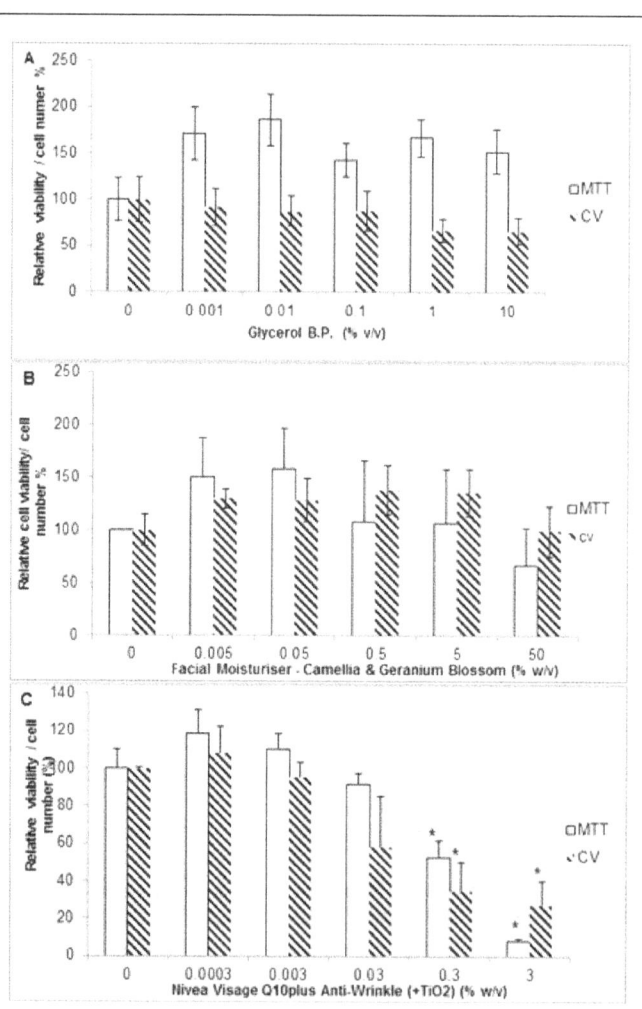

**Figure 1:** Relative cell viability and cell number (%) after treatment of HaCaT human skin cells with (A) Glycerol B.P, (B) Facial Moisturizer - Camellia & Geranium Blossom and (C) Nivea Visage Q10plus Anti-Wrinkle face moisturizer (with TiO₂) for 1 hour. Relative survival was measured by the MTT assay. Relative cell number was measured by the crystal violet assay. Data are shown as a percentage compared to untreated control and are mean of three replicates ± standard error of the mean (S.E.M). Treatments significantly different from untreated control at P<0.05 are presented as '*'.

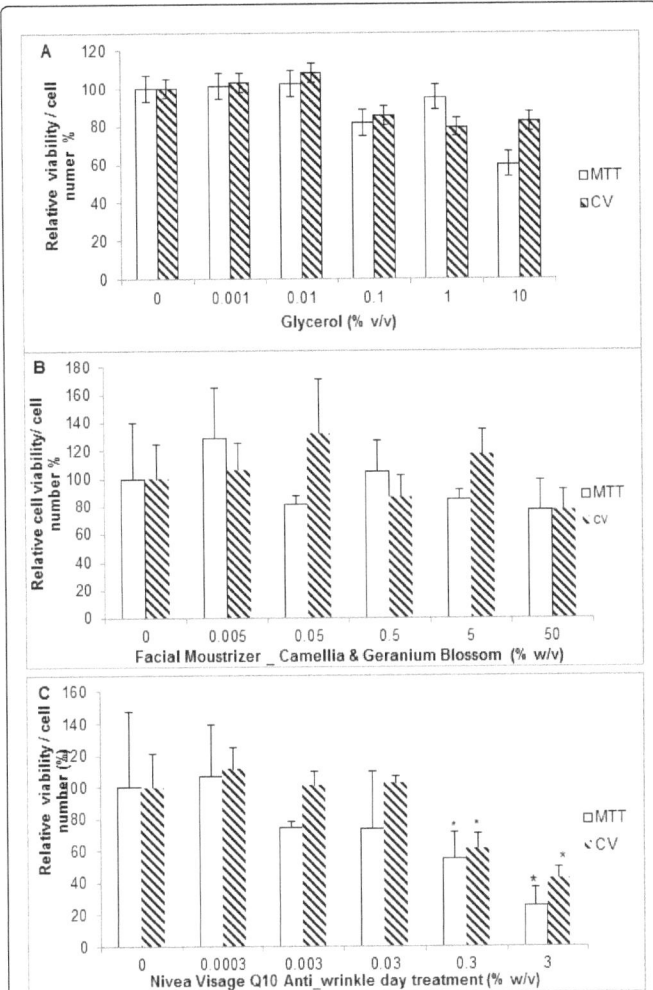

Figure 2: Relative cell viability and cell number (%) after treatment of CCD-1064Sk normal fibroblast human skin cells with (A) Glycerol B.P, (B) Facial Moisturizer - Camellia & Geranium Blossom and (C) Nivea Visage Q10plus Anti-Wrinkle face moisturizer (Improved formula, without $TiO_2$) for 1 hour. Relative survival was measured by the MTT assay. Relative cell number was measured by the crystal violet assay. Data are shown as a percentage compared to untreated control and are mean of three replicates ± standard error of the mean (S.E.M). Treatments significantly different from untreated control at P<0.05 are presented as '*'.

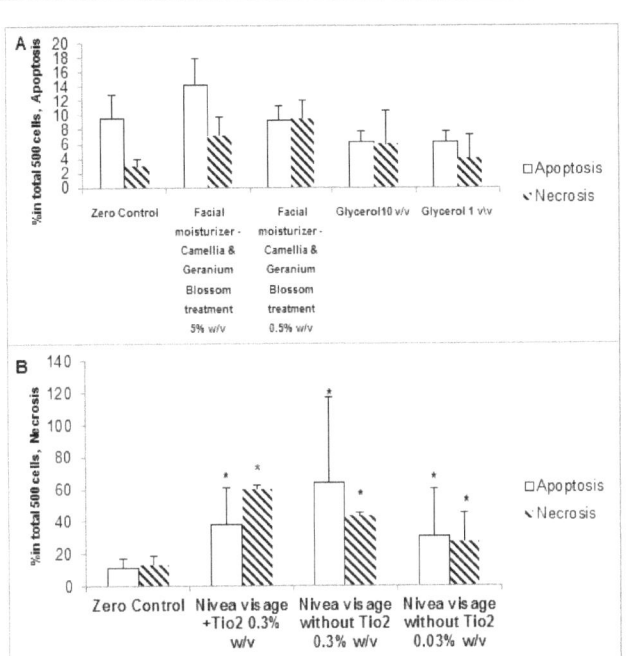

Figure 3: Apoptosis and necrosis induction detected by the CBMN assay for HaCaT cells followed by 1 h treatment using (A) Facial natural treatment (Facial Moisturizer - Camellia & Geranium Blossom) and Glycerol B.P and (B) using Nivea Visage Q10plus Anti-Wrinkle face moisturizer with $TiO_2$ and Nivea Visage Q10plus Anti-Wrinkle face moisturizer (Improved formula, free of $TiO_2$). Treatment Data are shown as the mean of three observations ± SEM. Treatments significantly different from untreated control at P<0.05 are presented as '*'.

Nivea visage without $TiO_2$ induced significant late apoptosis and early necrosis on fibroblast cells (CCD-1064SK) at dose 0.03% w/v and significant early necrosis induced by Facial Moisturizer - Camellia & Geranium Blossom at dose 5% w/v on CCD 1064SKas shown in figure 4. However, no significant induction of apoptosis or necrosis was observed on the the tretment of Glycerol B.P on CCD-1064SK cells.

Finally, this result was consistent with the previous result of Nivea Visage at dose 3% w/v induced necrosis detected by apoptosis assay followed flow cytometry (data not shown).

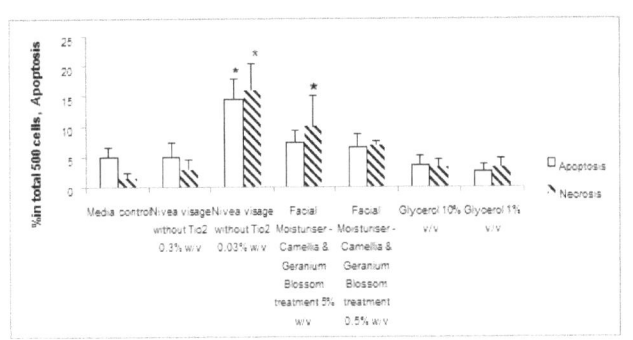

Figure 4: Apoptosis and necrosis induction detected by the CBMN assay for CCD_1064SK cells followed by 1 h treatment using Nivea Visage Q10plus Anti-Wrinkle face moisturizer (improved formula, without $TiO_2$ 0.3% w/v and 0.03% w/v and Facial Moisturizer - Camellia & Geranium Blossom 5% w/v and 0.5% w/v and Glycerol B.P 10% v/v and 1% v/v. Data are shown as the mean of three observations ± SEM. Treatments significantly different from untreated control at P<0.05 are presented as '*'.

## Genotoxicity of beauty products on human skin cells

The genotoxicity of beauty products on HaCaT human skin cells and CCD_ 1064SK was carried out using Cytokinesis-Block Micronucleus Assay (CBMN) assay. The following measures of genotoxicity chromosome breakage and chromosome loss (micronucleus MNi), chromosome rearrangement (nucleoplasmic bridges) and gene amplification (nuclear buds) [26]. The frequency of the induced micronuclei (MNi) indicates the extent of chromosomal changes induced by beauty products. The result of CBMN assay showed the genotoxicity effects of beauty products on HaCaT cells as shown in Figures 5. No significant increase in MNi observed in the results of treated HaCaT cells with Glycerol B.P and Facial Moisturizer - Camellia & Geranium Blossom (natural product) for 1 h (Figure 5 A).

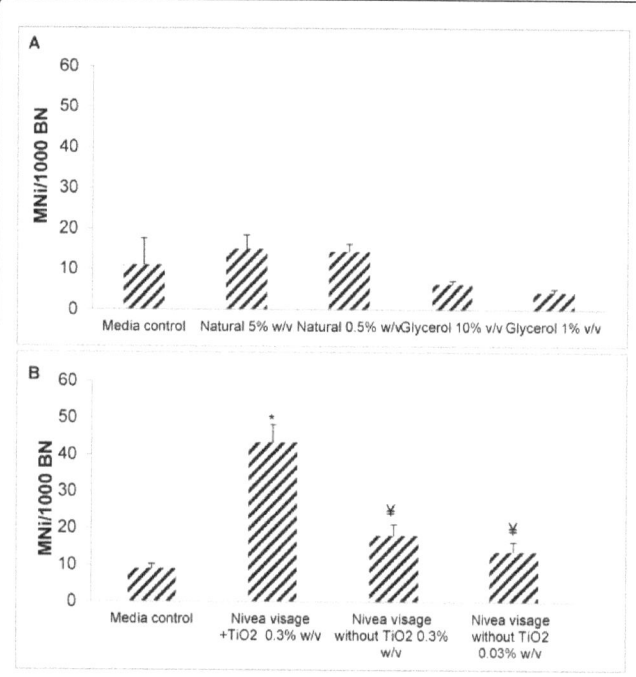

**Figure 5:** Frequency of micronucleated binucleate (MNBNCs) as measured by the CBMN assay following exposure of HaCaT cells to (A) Glycerol B.P and Facial Moisturizer - Camellia & Geranium Blossom (natural product) and (B) Nivea Visage Q10plus Anti-Wrinkle face moisturizer with TiO₂ and Nivea Visage Q10plus Anti-Wrinkle face moisturizer (Improved formula, without TiO₂) treatment. The data are the mean ± S.E.M. from three separate experiments. Treatments significantly different from the untreated control at P<0.05 are presented as '*' or '¥' Treatments differed significantly from Nivea Visage Q10plus Anti-Wrinkle face moisturizer with TiO₂.

However, there was significant increase in the number of MNi at the dose 0.3% w/v of Nivea Visage Q10plus Anti-Wrinkle face moisturizer + TiO₂. Also, Figure 5B showed the result of HaCaT cells after treated with two different formulas of Nivea visage product (Nivea Visage Q10plus Anti-Wrinkle face moisturizer with TiO₂ and Nivea Visage Q10plus Anti-Wrinkle face moisturizer without TiO₂. There was significant difference between the two formulas of Nivea Visage products on HaCaT cells. The product of Nivea Visage which contains

TiO₂ was significantly difference from the product of Nivea Visage without TiO₂ and from untreated control. This result means that the product of Nivea Visage which contains TiO₂ cause significant gentoxicicity on HaCaT cells compare to the product of Nivea Visage removed TiO₂ showed less genotoxic on HaCaT cells. Nucleoplasmic bridge (NPB) and Nucleoplasmic buds (NBUDs) were also observed in the products of Nivea Visage Q10plus Anti-Wrinkle face moisturizer + TiO₂ and Facial Moisturizer - Camellia & Geranium Blossom (natural product) but they did not reach a significant level. A significant increase in micronucleus (MNi) was observed at 0.3% w/v and 0.03% w/v doses of Nivea Visage Q10plus Anti-Wrinkle face moisturizer (Improved formula, without TiO₂) after treated CCD_1065SK cells (Figure 6). Other treatments demonstrated an increase in the number of MNi but they did not reach a significant level (Figure 6). Nucleoplasmic bridge (NPB) and Nucleoplasmic buds (NBUDs) were not observed in all products treatments on CCD_1065SK cells.

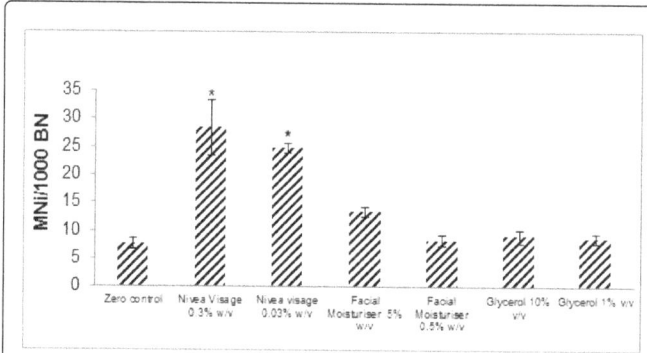

**Figure 6:** The frequency of micronuclei (MNi) per 1000 binucleated cells was determined using the Cytokinesis Block Micronucleus (CBMN) assay following exposure of CCD_1065SK cells to Nivea Visage Q10plus Anti-Wrinkle face moisturizer (Improved formula, without TiO₂) treatment, Glycerol B P, Facial Moisturizer - Camellia & Geranium Blossom (natural product). The data are the mean ± S.E.M. from three separate experiments. Treatments significantly different from untreated control at P<0.05 are presented as '*'.

## Discussion

In this study, two human normal skin cell lines were used to examine the toxicity and genotoxic effects of beauty products *in vitro*. Human keratinocyte cell line (HaCaT) which is derived from full epidermal differentiation capacity, functions as the outermost layer of the skin [27-29]. Human dermal fibroblast cells CCD-1046 within the dermis layer of skin are responsible for generating connective tissue [27,30]. Glycerol B.P served as a negative control in this study because it is a common basic ingredient in many moisturizers. There was no cytotoxic effect of exposure 1h to Glycerol B.P on HaCaT or CCD 1064SK cells. The Nuclear division index (NDI) obtained from the CBMN assay provides a measure of cell division [31]. There was no significant change in the NDI value which reflects the fact that Glycerol B.P did not affect the cell cycling in both cell lines. Furthermore, the evaluation of apoptosis and necrosis of Glycerol B.P on human skin cells detected by CBMN assay showed no significant difference from the untreated control. Also, the frequency of micro nucleated binucleate (MNi), nucleoplasmic bridges (NPBs) and nuclear buds (NBUDs) were not observed in 1000 binucleated (BN) cells which indicated that no genetic damage occurred after treatment with Glycerol. Therefore, Glycerol is a safe ingredient used in several cosmetics products. The Facial Moisturizer - Camellia & Geranium Blossom treatment used in this study is a product of mixture of natural ingredients listed on the product. It showed no significant toxicity compared to the untreated control on CCD_1064SK cells. Consistent with this result is the fact that there was no cytotoxicity observed on treated HaCaT cells with Facial Moisturizer - Camellia & Geranium Blossom treatment for 1h (Figure 1). The Nuclear division index (NDI), based on the result of the CBMN assay, revealed a significant decrease in dose 5% w/v lower NDI value 1.4 (P<0.05) in HaCaT cells. This means a change occurred in the rate of cell cycling - they took longer to divide, or the viable cells failed to divide during the cytokinesis-block [21]. No apoptosis or necrosis induction was observed after HaCaT cells were treated with Facial Moisturizer - Camellia & Geranium Blossom treatment for 1h at both doses. However, a small but statistically significant necrosis was observed in CCD-1064Sk cells at the higher (5% w/v) dose of the Facial Moisturizer - Camellia & Geranium Blossom treatment after treatment for 1h.

Furthermore, the CBMN result indicated that no chromosomal damage causes by Grown Facial Moisturizer - Camellia & Geranium Blossom after human skin cells were treated for 1h.

Grown Facial Moisturizer - Camellia & Geranium Blossom treatment did not demonstrate significant toxicity or genotoxicity in human skin cell lines, but this does not mean it is a safe product to use. The change in NDI value indicates the decrease in the cell cycle was 1.4 (P<0.05) on the HaCaT cell line. Also, significant necrosis observed after treated fibroblast cell lines with Facial Moisturizer - Camellia & Geranium Blossom for 1h at dose (5% w/v).

Green or botanical products are not well regulated by government agencies. There is advice to avoid products that use essential oils such as lavender oil or tea tree oil that are classified as hormone disruptors [32,33].

| | NDI value | |
|---|---|---|
| Treatments | HaCaT cell line | CCD_1064SK cell line |
| Media control | 1.8 | 1.6 |
| NVAW + TiO$_2$ dose 0.3% w/v | *1.4 | - |
| NVAW + TiO$_2$ dose 0.03% w/v | 1.7 | - |
| NVAW without TiO$_2$ dose 0.3% w/v | *1.4 | 1.5 |
| NVAW without TiO$_2$ dose 0.03% w/v | 1.6 | 1.5 |
| FMCGB treatment dose 5% w/v | *1.4 | 1.5 |
| FMCGB treatment dose 0.5% w/v | 1.6 | 1.6 |
| Glycerol dose 10% v/v | 1.7 | 1.6 |
| Glycerol dose 1% v/v | 1.8 | 1.6 |

**Table 2:** Nuclear Division Index (NDI) comparison between untreated control (0 doses) and beauty products. Cells were plated and described in the materials and methods section. Cells exposed to beauty treatments for 1h. NDI was determined by the cytokinesis-block micronucleus (CBMN) assay. Data are shown as percentages compared

to untreated control and are mean of 3 replicates, standard error of the mean ± (S.E.M). A significant difference from untreated control at *P<0.05.

Titanium dioxide (TiO$_2$) which is a nanoparticle that is classified as a carcinogen [15]. Titanium dioxide (TiO$_2$) plays a role in the induction of apoptosis as well as oxidative stress. Moreover, studies have shown that Titanium dioxide (TiO$_2$) causes genetic damage linked to DNA-adduct formation in human lung cells [34-36]. The metabolic effects of Titanium dioxide (TiO$_2$) on keratinocytes HaCaT cells have also being investigated. One study indicated that Titanium dioxide affect the mitochondria [11]. Another study demonstrated a significant uptake of TiO$_2$ in keratinocytes in human skin cells (HaCaT); this was performed using transmission electron microscopy (TEM) and flow cytometry [37].

In our studies Nivea Visage Q10plus Anti-Wrinkle face moisturizer with TiO$_2$ was compared to an identical product without the TiO$_2$ allowing for an evaluation of the effect of the TiO$_2$. The result of MTT and Crystal Violet showed significant toxicity with the two doses of Nivea visage +TiO$_2$ was noted- up to 76% and 92% cells were killed after a 1 h exposure to a 0.3% and 3% (w/v) dose, respectively (Figure 1).

The mechanism of cell death was elucidated using the CBMN assay. There was a significant induction of late apoptosis and early necrosis at (0.3% w/v) on HaCaT human skin cells (Figure 3B). Also, a significant low NDI value (1.4 (P<0.05)) was observed at the 3% w/v dose (Table 2).

Also, nucleoplasmic bridges (NPBs) and nuclear buds (NBUDs) were observed. These outcomes illustrate some of the mechanisms of chromosome damage when using Nivea Visage Q10plus Anti-Wrinkle day moisturizer. The frequency of chromosome rearrangement is indicated by NPB and NBUDs. NPB may arise from dicentric chromosomes and NBUDs from gene amplification [21]. A dicentric chromosome and an acentric chromosome fragment are formed as a result, and they manifest themselves in the formation of an NPB and MN [21]. The formation of NPBs could lead to misrepair of DNA strand breaks which could also lead to a dicentric chromosome and concatenated ring chromosome. One dicentric chromosome mechanism could result in telomere end fusion which is caused via shortening or loss of the telomere capping protein [21]. This study is consistent with that conducted by [38] which demonstrated that sunscreens containing Titanium dioxide can catalyse oxidative damage to DNA in vitro and in human cell culture.

On the other hand, Nivea Visage Q10 plus Anti-Wrinkle face moisturizer (Improved formula, without TiO$_2$) showed significant toxicity on CCD-1064SK at (3% and 0.3% w/v) measured by MTT and Crystal Violet assays. The mechanism of cell death scored by the CBMN assay (Figure 4) showed there was significant induction of apoptosis and necrosis at (0.03% w/v) on CCD-1064.

Genetic damage effects detected by the CBMN assay showed a significant increase in MNi (28.3 MNi/1000 binucleated cells, n=3) (P<0.05) in CCD_1064SK cell lines. However, there was no significant increase in MNi with HaCaT cells as (Figure 5B). Also, a significant low NDI value (1.4 (P<0.05)) was observed only in 3% w/v dose on HaCaT cells (Table 2). This means that the cells took a longer time to divide in HaCaT cells after being treated with Nivea Visage Q10plus Anti-Wrinkle face moisturizer (Improved formula, without TiO2) for

1h. Nucleoplasmic bridges (NPBs) and nuclear buds (NBUDs) were not observed on CCD_1064SK.

This product consists of a mixture of chemicals ingredients that are the same as those reported in Table 1, except Titanium dioxide which was removed from this improved formula that released into the market by Nivea Company. Therefore, the even though none of these chemicals individually are known to be carcinogenic it is apparent that the mixture has shown carcinogenicity [2]. It is hypothesized that chemicals in mixtures could interact with each other and become carcinogenic. A brain cancer cluster study concluded that different mixtures of chemicals can induce the same cancer types despite using different mechanisms. None of the chemicals are known to individually cause brain cancer [2].

Interestingly, Nivea Visage Q10plus Anti-Wrinkle face moisturizer with $TiO_2$ proved to induce significantly more micronuclei than the product without $TiO_2$. As mentioned earlier, the difference is compatible with findings that $TiO_2$ enters the nucleus and cytoplasm of keratinocytes causing oxidative stress damage to DNA [37].

Consumers who are using Nivea Visage Q10plus Anti-Wrinkle day moisturizer are in fact exposed to an undiluted product (100%) with the potential to create long-term damage. Carcinogens in cosmetics and personal care products are potentially greater cancer risks than food contaminated with industrial carcinogens or pesticides because chemicals ingested into the body by mouth are absorbed by the intestines and pass into the venous blood. These chemicals are then transported to the liver which exists to detoxify the substances to varying degrees by enzymes before they can reach the rest of the body [33]. However, carcinogens absorbed by the skin can bypass the liver and circulate through the blood stream, thus reaching every organ in the body [1,33].

In conclusion, the current study has shown the possible harmful effects of several beauty products on normal human skin cells *in vitro*. In particular, the anti-aging face moisturizer which has a synthetic chemical product (Nivea Visage Q10plus Anti-Wrinkle day moisturizer +$TiO_2$) induced the highest toxicity and genotoxicity of the beauty products tested. Also, Nivea Visage Q10plus Anti-Wrinkle day moisturizer without $TiO_2$ induced significant toxicity and genotoxicity on human fibroblast CCD_1064Sk cells. On the other hand, the face moisturizer containing natural ingredients (Facial Moisturizer - Camellia & Geranium Blossom) was a relatively less toxic product compared to other beauty products, and Glycerol B.P. (the negative control) showed no toxic effect in either human cell line. Finally, further investigation could be done to study specific chromosome damage occurred by Nivea visage using fluorescent probes by fluorescence in situ hybridization (FISH). Also further work could be done to understand the underlying mechanism of action of the effects of Facial Moisturizer - Camellia & Geranium Blossom on the nuclear division index (NDI).

## Acknowledgments

We thank the Ministry of Education, Saudi Arabia, for partial support of this project. Also, we are thankful to Professor Christopher Franco, Head of Medical Biotechnology, School of Medicine, Flinders University for valuable suggestions and reviewing the manuscript.

## References

1. Thomas P (2008) Skin Deep: The Essential Guide to What's in the Toiletries and cosmetis you use. Rodale an imprint of Pan Macmillan

2. Zeliger H (2008) Human toxicology of chemical mixtures: toxic consequences beyond the impact of one-component product and environmental exposures. William Andrew.

3. Lazarus MC, Baumann LS (2001) The use of cosmeceutical moisturizers. Dermatologic Therapy 14: 200-207.

4. U.S.FDA (2006) Cosmetics. In USFaD Administration, PaPY Health eds US.

5. Cone M (2005) Dozens of Chemicals Found in Most Americans' Bodies. The Los Angeles Times A 21.

6. Menegaux F, Baruchel A, Bertrand Y, Lescoeur B, Leverger G, et al. (2006) Household exposure to pesticides and risk of childhood acute leukaemia. Occup Environ Med 63: 131-134.

7. Balluz LS, Philen RM, Sewell CM, Voorhees RE, Falter KH, et al. (1997) Mercury toxicity associated with a beauty lotion, New Mexico. Int J Epidemiol 26: 1131-1132.

8. Sainio EL, Jolanki R, Hakala E, Kanerva L (2000) Metals and arsenic in eye shadows. Contact Dermatitis 42: 5-10.

9. Järup L (2003) Hazards of heavy metal contamination. Br Med Bull 68: 167-182.

10. Rubin BS (2011) Bisphenol A: an endocrine disruptor with widespread exposure and multiple effects. J Steroid Biochem Mol Biol 127: 27-34.

11. Tucci P, Porta G, Agostini M, Dinsdale D, Iavicoli I, et al. (2013) Metabolic effects of TiO2 nanoparticles, a common component of sunscreens and cosmetics, on human keratinocytes. Cell Death Dis 4: e549.

12. Falck GC, Lindberg HK, Suhonen S, Vippola M, Vanhala E, et al. (2009) Genotoxic effects of nanosized and fine TiO2. Hum Exp Toxicol 28: 339-352.

13. King AG (2011) Research Advances: Addressing the Environmental Fates of Everyday Products from Cigarette Butts to Shampoos and Cleaning Agents. Journal of Chemical Education 88: 8-8.

14. Millikan LE (2001) Cosmetology, cosmetics, cosmeceuticals: definitions and regulations. Clin Dermatol 19: 371-374.

15. Trouiller B, Reliene R, Westbrook A, Solaimani P, Schiestl RH (2009) Titanium Dioxide Nanoparticles Induce DNA Damage and Genetic Instability In vivo in Mice. Cancer Research 69: 8784-8789.

16. Zhao J, Bowman L, Zhang X, Vallyathan V, Young S-H, et al. (2009) Titanium dioxide (TiO2) nanoparticles induce JB6 cell apoptosis through activation of the caspase-8/Bid and mitochondrial pathways. Journal of Toxicology and Environmental Health, Part A 72: 1141-1149.

17. Brief DJ, Davis JD (1982) Glycerol reduces food intake in diabetic rats. Physiol Behav 29: 577-580.

18. Berry JM, Huebner E, Butler M (1996) The crystal violet nuclei staining technique leads to anomalous results in monitoring mammalian cell cultures. Cytotechnology 21: 73-80.

19. Ramezanpour M, Burke da Silva K, Sanderson B (2012) Differential susceptibilities of human lung, breast and skin cancer cell lines to killing by five sea anemone venoms. J Venom Anim Toxins incl Trop Dis 18: 157-163.

20. Mosmann T (1983) Rapid colorimetric assay for cellular growth and survival: application to proliferation and cytotoxicity assays. J Imm Met 65: 55-63.

21. Fenech M (2007) Cytokinesis-block micronucleus cytome assay. Nat Protoc 2: 1084-1104.

22. Wang JJ, Sanderson BJS, Wang H (2007) Cyto- and genotoxicity of ultrafine TiO2 particles in cultured human lymphoblastoid cells. Mutat Res 628: 99-106.

23. Fenech M (2000) The *in vitro* micronucleus technique. Mutat Res 455: 81-95.

24. Kirsch-Volders M, Sofuni T, Aardema M, Albertini S, Eastmond D, et al. (2003) Report from the *in vitro* micronucleus assay working group. Mutat Res 540: 153-163.

25. Ionescu ME, Ciocirlan M, Becheanu G, Nicolaie T, Ditescu C, et al. (2011) Nuclear Division Index may Predict Neoplastic Colorectal Lesions. Maedica (Buchar) 6: 173-178.

26. Fenech M (2008) The Micronucleus Assay Determination of Chromosomal Level DNA Damage. In CC Martin ed Environmental Genomics. Humana Press, Totowa, NJ.

27. Krejcí E, Kodet O, Szabo P, Borský J, Smetana Jr K, et al. (2014) *In vitro* differences of neonatal and later postnatal keratinocytes and dermal fibroblasts. Physiological research/Academia Scientiarum Bohemoslovaca. Physiol Res 64: 561-569.

28. Hughes MF, Edwards BC (2010) *In vitro* dermal absorption of pyrethroid pesticides in human and rat skin. Toxicol Appl Pharmacol 246: 29-37.

29. Schoop VM, Mirancea N, Fusenig NE (1999) Epidermal Organization and Differentiation of HaCaT Keratinocytes in Organotypic Coculture with Human Dermal Fibroblasts. 112: 343-353.

30. Kopanska K, Powell J, Jugdaohsingh R, Bruggraber SA (2013) Filtration of dermal fibroblast-conditioned culture media is required for the reliable quantitation of cleaved carboxy-terminal peptide of collagen type I (CICP) by ELISA. Arch Dermatol Res 305: 741-745.

31. Sugisawa A, Umegaki K (2002) Physiological Concentrations of (-)-Epigallocatechin-3-O-Gallate (EGCg) Prevent Chromosomal Damage Induced by Reactive Oxygen Species in WIL2-NS Cells. The Journal of Nutrition 132: 1836-1839.

32. Alnuqaydan AM, Sanderson B (2016) Genetic damage and celll killing induction by five head lice treatments on HaCaT human skin cells. J Carcinog Mutagen 7: :259.

33. Epstein SS, Fitzgerald R (2009) Toxic Beauty: How Cosmetics and Personal Care Products Endanger Your Health... and What You Can Do about It. BenBella Books.

34. Bhattacharya K, Davoren M, Boertz J, Schins R, Hoffmann E, et al. (2009) Titanium dioxide nanoparticles induce oxidative stress and DNA-adduct formation but not DNA-breakage in human lung cells. Part Fibre Toxicol 6: 8976-8977.

35. Park E-J, Yi J, Chung K-H, Ryu D-Y, Choi J, et al. (2008) Oxidative stress and apoptosis induced by titanium dioxide nanoparticles in cultured BEAS-2B cells. Toxicology Letters 180: 222-229.

36. Reeves JF, Davies SJ, Dodd NJF, Jha AN (2008) Hydroxyl radicals (OH) are associated with titanium dioxide (TiO2) nanoparticle-induced cytotoxicity and oxidative DNA damage in fish cells. Mutat Res 640: 113-122.

37. Shukla RK, Kumar A, Pandey AK, Singh SS, Dhawan A (2011) Titanium Dioxide Nanoparticles Induce Oxidative Stress-Mediated Apoptosis in Human Keratinocyte Cells. J Biomed Nanotechnol 7: 100-101.

38. Dunford R, Salinaro A, Cai L, Serpone N, Horikoshi S, et al. (1997) Chemical oxidation and DNA damage catalysed by inorganic sunscreen ingredients. FEBS Lett 418: 87-90.

39. TOXNET TDN (2015) Specialized Information Services. In U.S. National Library of Medicine NIH.

40. EWG SDCD (2015) Skin Deep® Cosmetics Database | EWG. In 2004.

41. Butt ST, Christensen T (2000) Toxicity and Phototoxicity of Chemical Sun Filters. Radiation Protection Dosimetry 91: 283-286.

# 25

# Toxicity Effects of Hair Dye Application on Liver Function in Experimental Animals

Ehab Ibrahim Salih El-Amin[1*], Mohammed Abd AL Rahim GahElnabi[2], Waled Amen Mohammed Ahmed[3], Ragaa Gasim Ahmed[4] and Khalid Eltahir Khalid[5]

[1]Assistant Professor of Human Anatomy, Albaha University, Faculty of Applied Medical Sciences, Head of Community Health Department, Kingdom of Saudi Arabia

[2]Professor of Forensic Medicine and Toxicology, National Ribat University, College of Sudanese Police Sciences, Sudan

[3]Assistant Professor of Nursing, Albaha University, Faculty of Applied Medical Sciences, Nursing Department, Kingdom of Saudi Arabia

[4]Assistant Professor of Nursing, Albaha University, Faculty of Applied Medical Sciences, Nursing Department, Kingdom of Saudi Arabia

[5]Associate Professor of Biochemistry, Albaha University, Faculty of Applied Medical Sciences, Department of Medical Laboratory Sciences, Kingdom of Saudi Arabia

*Corresponding author: Dr. Ehab Ibrahim Salih El-Amin, PhD, Albaha University, Faculty of Applied Medical Sciences, Head of Community Health Department, Kingdom of Saudi Arabia, Email: ehabsalih2000@yahoo.com

## Abstract

**Objective:** This study was conducted to assess the hair dye toxicity by using hair dye among experimental rats in order to verify the biochemical and haematological abnormalities and liver dysfunction.

**Methods:** Albino Wistar Rats were obtained from the Faculty of Pharmacy, University of Khartoum– Sudan. The rats were divided into two batches on the basis of using the commercial hair dye as oral or subcutaneous administration respectively; each batch has four groups (control and three test groups) each comprising six rats. Batch-1 (group-2, 3, and 4 orally administered with 10, 20, and 30mg/kg body weight of the commercial hair dye, respectively); and Batch-2 (group-2, 3, and 4 subcutaneously administered with 10, 20, and 30 mg/kg body weight of the commercial hair dye, respectively).

**Results:** The clinical features were shown in all rats batches, administered orally or subcutaneously with the commercial hair dye. These clinical features rates from slight weakness in group 2 to head, neck, and pharyngeal oedema in group-3 up to severe weakness in hinds and fore limbs with election of hair, tremors, shivering of the whole body and respiratory distress, severe convulsions, and respiratory difficulty prior to death in group-4. The Biochemical parameters showed significant (P<0.05) increase in the activities of the liver enzymes concomitant with the increase of the commercial hair dye dosage in the two batches, and decrease in the total plasma protein levels, albumin, and cholesterol with the increase of commercial hair dye dosage in the two batches. Hematological parameters showed a significant (p value <0.05) decrease in complete blood count (associated with significant decreases in neutrophils and significant increases of lymphocytes) concomitant with the increasing of commercial hair dye concentration.

**Conclusion:** The study highlighted the major toxicity of commercial hair dye and its association with liver dysfunction.

**Keywords:** Hair dye; Paraphenylenediamine; Toxicity; Liver atrophy; Parameters; Experimental animals; Sudan

## Introduction

Henna is very popular culture in Sudan; it is part of the traditions which used to adorn women's body during marriage ceremonies and other social celebrations since the Bronze Age. Henna is commercially cultivated in Sudan and other countries. Despite the wide spread use of natural henna, reports of allergic contact dermatitis to natural henna are very rare in the literature. It can therefore be assumed that natural henna is safe [1]. The first artificial dye was synthesized in the laboratory in 1856, and permanent hair colorants have been in commercial use for over 100 years [2].

Para-Phenylenediamine (PPD) is an organic compound; its chemical formula is $C_6H_8N_2$ [3]. This derivative of aniline is a white solid, but samples can darken due to air oxidation. It is also an ingredient used in Sudan and other countries in combination with henna "lawasonia Alba" for tattooing to give black color in a short time in traditional and during local and social festival. It was found to be toxic and there are some reports from these countries showing its toxicity on different systems of the body. The consumers use this product because its price is 20-30 times less expensive than pharmaceutical hair dye preparations [4].

Many accidental cases of toxicity and mortality have been reported in Sudan, Egypt and other countries in cases of suicidal and homicidal due to oral ingestion or subcutaneous mistaken used of hair dyes containing Para-phenylenediamine [5]. There are many studies showed effects on respiratory, renal, and muscular system, but no study determines the effects on all these systems together, and no study describes the correlation of PPD toxicity to body's biochemical alterations in liver [6].

There was a continuous inflow of suicidal and homicidal cases in Sudanese hospitals and the causes of poisoning with PPD are much conflicting in the determination of clinical order of PPD Patients [7].

As PPD is the main ingredient on hair dyes, and whose toxicity is directly related to human health. So this paper studied the toxicity of hair dye in vivo, to determine the biochemical and haematological abnormalities associated with major toxicity of commercial hair dye and liver dysfunction among experimental animals.

## Methodology

This study was conducted at national research center-University of Khartoum. The commercial hair dye was collected from local markets (Libya Market–Omdurman).

Albino Wistar male rats at age of 11 weeks, weighting 140-160 g were obtained from the Faculty of Pharmacy, University of Khartoum–Sudan. The animals were housed in cages provided with rice husk as bedding materials and kept under ambient temperature of $23 \pm 2°C$. The animals were kept in the laboratory condition for 1 week to adapt the climate condition and for the commencement of treatment protocol. The rats were divided into two batches on the basis of using the commercial hair dye as oral or subcutaneous administration respectively; each batch has four groups (control and three test groups) each comprising six rats. Batch-1 (group-2, 3, and 4 orally administered with 10, 20, and 30 mg/kg body weight of commercial hair dye, respectively); and Batch-2 (group-2, 3, and 4 subcutaneously administered with 10, 20, and 30 mg/kg body weight of commercial hair dye, respectively). The animals were killed after 3-6 days after the administration. The lethal dose of commercial hair dye for rats was determined as 80 mg/kg body weight [8] and the lethal subcutaneous dose was determined as 37 mg/kg body weight [9]. Hence, we tested the toxicity of various sub lethal doses through different routes considering the LD50 of PPD is 37 mg/kg.

Two milliliter of blood samples were collected from eye blood vessels of each rat in ethylenediamine tetra acetic acid (EDTA) container for hematological tests and other 2 ml of blood samples were collected in heparinized containers for biochemical tests. Plasma was separated by centrifugation at 3000 rpm for 5 min.

Total proteins, glucose, cholesterol, albumin, and the enzyme activities of GOT, GPT, and ALP were measured spectrophotometrically by using commercial kits. Determination of hemoglobin concentration (Hb), packed cell volume (PCV), red blood cells (RBCs) count, and total white blood cell (TWBC) count, mean corpuscular volume (MCV), mean corpuscular hemoglobin concentration (MCHC) and mean corpuscular hemoglobin (MCH), PLT count, (Lymphocytes–Basophil, Neutrophil) were analyzed by a semi-automated hematological analyzer (Sysmex Corporation; Mundelein, Illinois, Sysmex America, Inc.).

Statistical analyses were performed using statistical package for social sciences (SPSS) version 11.5 and excel 2007 statistical program. Continuous and categorical variables were analyzed using student's t-test and Chi-square test respectively. P value was considered significant if it was less than 0.05.

## Results

Clinical features were shown in all rats administered orally or subcutaneously with the commercial hair dye, however, the clinical features rate from slight weakness in group 2 to head, neck, and

pharyngeal oedema in group-3 up to severe weakness in hinds and fore limbs with election of hair, tremors, shivering of the whole body and respiratory distress, and there were severe convulsions and respiratory difficulty prior to death which occurred at about four hours post oral ingestion of the commercial hair dye in group-4. As seen in Table 1 and Table 2, the biochemical parameters showed significant (P<0.05) increase in activities of the liver enzymes glutamate oxalotranserase (GOT), glutamate pyruvate transferase (GPT), and alkaline phosphatase (ALP), and there is a decrease in the total plasma protein levels, albumin, and cholesterol when compared with the control groups.

| Groups / Parameters | Group 1 (Control) | Group 2 (10 mg/kg) | Group 3 (20 mg/kg) | Group 4 (30 mg/kg) |
|---|---|---|---|---|
| GOT (U/L) | 41.3 ± 2.1 | 1219.5 ± 12.1*** | 1581.8 ± 30.9*** | 1690.0 ± 23.7*** |
| GPT (U/L) | 40.1 ± 1.7 | 127.8 ± 1.2*** | 242.8 ± 7.2*** | 295.0 ± 28.8*** |
| ALP (U/L) | 115.3 ± 3.2 | 113.7 ± 2.8 | 129.0 ± 1.4* | 136.0 ± 2.2** |
| T. proteins (g/dl) | 7.5 ± 0.7 | 7.0 ± 0.6 | 6.7 ± 0.3 | 6.3 ± 0.5* |
| Glucose (mg/dl) | 105.3 ± 11.0 | 137.8 ± 1.7** | 127.8 ± 0.8* | 113.5 ± 3.6 |
| Cholesterol (mg/dl) | 88.5 ± 15.8 | 60.2 ± 5.9*** | 67.5 ± 4.4** | 79.0 ± 3.7* |
| Albumin (g/dl) | 4.2 ± 0.7 | 4.8 ± 0.3 | 3.7 ± 0.3* | 3.2 ± 0.2* |
| * = P<0.05; ** = P<0.01; *** = P<0.001 | | | | |

**Table 1:** Showing the mean differences of Biochemical parameters between the study groups when received different oral ingestion doses (10-20-30 mg/kg b.w.) using the commercial hair dye.

| Groups / Parameters | Group 1 (Control) | Group 2 (10 mg/kg) | Group 3 (20 mg/kg) | Group 4 (30 mg/kg) |
|---|---|---|---|---|
| GOT (U/L) | 41.3 ± 2.1 | 1311.7 ± 3.1*** | 1663.7 ± 2.3*** | 1790.5 ± 1.0*** |
| GPT (U/L) | 40.1 ± 1.7 | 138.0 ± 0.9*** | 242.3 ± 2.2*** | 302.0 ± 2.1*** |
| ALP (U/L) | 115.3 ± 3.2 | 112.2 ± 1.9 | 129.0 ± 1.4* | 136.7 ± 2.1** |
| T. proteins (g/dl) | 7.5 ± 0.7 | 6.8 ± 0.4 | 6.5 ± 0.3 | 6.0 ± 0.2* |
| Glucose (mg/dl) | 105.3 ± 11.0 | 138.8 ± 2.1** | 127.3 ± 2.2* | 115.3 ± 2.2 |
| Cholesterol (mg/dl) | 88.5 ± 15.8 | 59.5 ± 1.9*** | 65.8 ± 1.5** | 77.2 ± 3.0* |
| Albumin (g/dl) | 4.2 ± 0.7 | 4.8 ± 0.3 | 3.7 ± 0.1* | 3.9 ± 0.3 |
| * = P<0.05; ** = P<0.01; *** = P<0.001 | | | | |

**Table 2:** Showing the mean differences of Biochemical parameters between the study groups when received different subcutaneous doses (10-20-30 mg/kg b.w.) using the commercial hair dye.

These differences associated with the increase of the commercial hair dye dosage in the two batches. Blood glucose showed significant increase among different doses of oral or subcutaneous commercial hair dye compared with the control groups. Despite the different route of commercial hair dye administration, the results showed slight increase in the mean results of GOT, GPT and total protein when the commercial hair dye administered subcutaneously.

Compared with the control groups, hematological parameters showed significant (p value <0.05) decrease in Hb, RBCs, PCV, TWBCs count (associated with significant decreases in neutrophils and significant increases of lymphocytes), MCH, and MCV relevant to the increasing of the commercial hair dye concentration. Despite the significant decreases (P<0.05) in the percentage of neutrophils count, the platelets and lymphocytes showed significant (P<0.05) increase associated with increasing concentrations of the commercial hair dye in the different routes (Table 3 and Table 4).

| Groups / Parameter | Group 1 (Control) | Group 2 (10 mg/kg) | Group 3 (20 mg/kg) | Group 4 (30 mg/kg) |
|---|---|---|---|---|
| Hb (g/dl) | 12.85 ± 0.67 | 10.38 ± 0.73* | 9.59 ± 0.68* | 8.67 ± 0.82** |
| PCV (%) | 44.67 ± 0.52 | 37.57 ± 0.88* | 27.00 ± 2.83*** | 25.33 ± 2.73*** |
| RBCs×$10^3$/CMM | 5466.00 ± 859.45 | 5116.67 ± 231.66* | 4083.33 ± 365.60** | 3483.33 ± 172.24*** |
| TWBCs /CMM | 7600.00 ± 2182.65 | 5133.33 ± 2182.66*** | 4133.33 ± 659.29*** | 2900.00 ± 209.76*** |
| MCH (pg) | 29.83 ± 2.32 | 20.0 ± 2.19* | 18.33 ± 1.97** | 16.67 ± 2.07*** |
| MCV (fl) | 88.67 ± 5.32 | 65.00 ± 4.15*** | 59.67 ± 7.61*** | 52.17 ± 4.83*** |
| MCHC (g/dl) | 34.00 ± 1.41 | 37.50 ± 2.74 | 42.83 ± 3.71* | 45.50 ± 2.51** |
| PLT /CMM | 240833.3 ± 82366.1 | 203333.3 ± 25819.9** | 373333.3 ± 25819.9*** | 558333.3 ± 34302.6*** |
| LYM% | 27.83 ± 6.18 | 54.33 ± 3.61*** | 67.50 ± 5.13*** | 87.33 ± 3.27*** |
| BASO% | 0.52 ± 0.37 | 0.57 ± 0.34 | 0.72 ± 0.21*** | 0.87 ± 0.61*** |
| NEUT% | 54.50 ± 9.29 | 24.67 ± 2.16*** | 10.35 ± 1.65*** | 6.67 ± 1.63*** |
| *=P<0.05; **=P<0.01; ***=P<0.001 | | | | |

**Table 3:** Showing the mean differences of Hematological parameters between the study groups when received different oral doses (10-20-30 mg/kg b.w.) using the commercial hair dye.

| Groups / Parameters | Group 1 (Control) | Group 2 (10 mg/kg) | Group 3 (20 mg/kg) | Group 4 (30 mg/kg) |
|---|---|---|---|---|
| Hb (g/dl) | 12.85 ± 0.67 | 10.23 ± 0.64* | 9.32 ± 0.5* | 8.67 ± 0.82** |
| PCV (%) | 44.67 ± 0.52 | 29.87 ± 2.25*** | 27.83 ± 2.14*** | 25.50 ± 1.87*** |
| RBCs×$10^3$/CMM | 5466.00 ± 859.45 | 5400.00 ± 740.27 | 3883.33 ± 147.20** | 3700.00 ± 442.72*** |
| TWBCs /CMM | 7600.00 ± 2182.65 | 4983.33 ± 231.66*** | 3366.67 ± 463.32*** | 2816.67 ± 318.85*** |
| MCH (pg) | 29.83 ± 2.32 | 20.98 ± 2.04* | 19.17 ± 1.94* | 15.33 ± 1.37*** |
| MCV (fl) | 88.67 ± 5.32 | 65.17 ± 1.94*** | 65.67 ± 3.31*** | 57.17 ± 3.31*** |
| MCHC (g/dl) | 34.00 ± 1.41 | 34.17 ± 2.14 | 36.83 ± 2.93 | 46.50 ± 2.43** |
| PLT /CMM | 240833.3 ± 82366.1 | 277666.7 ± 29024.5** | 358333.3 ± 29268.9*** | 555000.0 ± 32710.9*** |
| LYM% | 27.83 ± 6.18 | 55.50 ± 2.43*** | 76.83 ± 2.86*** | 88.33 ± 4.27*** |
| BASO% | 0.52 ± 0.37 | 0.38 ± 0.17*** | 0.53 ± 0.27 | 0.73 ± 0.22*** |
| NEUT% | 54.50 ± 9.29 | 20.67 ± 2.88*** | 10.17 ± 1.17*** | 6.83 ± 1.47*** |
| *= P<0.05; **= P<0.01; ***= P<0.001 | | | | |

**Table 4:** Showing the mean differences of Hematological parameters between the study groups whenreceived different subcutaneous doses (10-20-30 mg/kg b.w.) using the commercial hair dye.

## Discussion

This study was carried out to evaluate the hair dye toxicity by using commercial hair dye in a way to estimate the hazards of this dye on rats, since it is known that toxic effects in humans are usually in the same range as those of experimental animals. PPD is the main constituent in hair dye and is an organic derivative of paranitroaniline, when ingested in a dose-dependent manner, results in severe hypersensitivity (itching, angioedema, asphyxia) and rhabdomyolysis (paresis of extremities, cola-colored urine, oliguria, markedly elevated creatinine phosphokinase and lactate dehydrogenase, hyperkalemia, hypophosphatemia and hypocalcaemia) [10,11]. Other features such as anemia, leukocytosis, hemoglobinemia, hemoglobinurea, and liver necrosis have been reported [12]. In animal model, PPD induces rhabdomyolysis leakage of calcium ions from the smooth endoplasmic reticulum, followed by continuous contraction and irreversible structural changes in the muscles [13].

In this study, we used commercial hair dye given to Albino Wistar rats in order to provide information about the effect of commercial hair dye on liver as hepatocellular necrosis accompanying hair dye poisoning in human [12].

The commercial hair dye was introduced in this study through oral and subcutaneous routes, although the variation in systemic effect between the two routes was not great. As shown in the results, subcutaneous injection results in a rather faster absorption of commercial hair dye than oral ingestion but the difference are not great.

At higher doses of the commercial hair dye, there was broad deviation from the normal values in biochemical and hematological parameters compared to lower doses of hair dye administered via the same route in all batches, because the concentration of a toxic agent influence its rate of absorption.

Our results showed significant increase in liver enzymes (GOT, GPT, ALP) activities in a dose-dependent manner in the two batches, and there is a decrease in the total plasma protein levels, albumin, and cholesterol associated with the increase of the commercial hair dye dosage in the two batches. Our finding is in agreement with others [14-18] when their administration of PPD to rats revealed a significant increase in GOT, GPT, and ALP, and a significant decrease in total proteins and glucose. Blood glucose showed significant increase among different doses of oral and subcutaneous administration of commercial hair dye compared with the control groups. Our result showed inconsistency with other study reported that the PPD leads to renal failure resulting in appreciable amount of urine glucose which causes low blood glucose level in rats [17]. Changes in the aforementioned biochemical parameters in our study indicate possible hepatic toxicity, pointed out by the substantial leakage of enzymes contained in the cells of hepatic tissues to the blood. It has been reported that low cholesterol level is usually associated with hepatocellular damage [18-19]. The decrease in the level of cholesterol in our study may be associated with hepatic lipidosis and obstructive liver diseases [20].

The hematological investigations showed significant decrease in Hb and PCV values which may be attributed to the escape of plasma from circulation to the surrounding tissues, in addition to significant decreases in RBCs, MCH and MCV values. These hematological changes indicate that, anemia may occur as a result of exposure to commercial hair dye. The possible cause for anemia is the hemolytic effect of PPD on RBCs; anemia was noticed in rats that received sub

lethal doses of PPD, however, in chronic toxicity experiments, all batches showed hematological changes indicating anemia. The effect of commercial hair dye on RBCs may extend to bone marrow leading to inadequate production of red blood cells and other elements. The decrease in MCH and MCV has been associated with macrocytic anemia, while the decrease in MCHC values indicates anemia and iron deficiency.

In this study, TWBC count was found to be decreased in rats that received different doses of commercial hair dye and have been associated with significant decrease in neutrophil cells and significant increase in lymphocyte cells. This may be due to the action of PPD in the immune system, which triggers neutrophils apoptosis and massive production of immunocompetent cells [21].

The changes in biochemical and hematological parameters were reported more significantly among rats exposed to higher doses of commercial hair dye.

Our study highlighted the experimental correlation between commercial hair dye administration and liver dysfunction, and reflects the importance of public awareness regarding the potential lethality of commercial hair dye and the governmental legislations and restriction of sale of commercial hair dye.

## Authors' Contribution

The main investigator of this work is Dr. Ehab Salih and all other authors contributed equally in this work.

## References

1. Pasricha JS, Gupta R, Panjwani S (1980) Contact dermatitis to henna (Lawsonia). Contact Dermatitis 6: 288-289.

2. http/www.ScienceLab.com

3. Scientific Committee on Consumer Products (SCCP) Opinion on P-phenylenediamine. Public Health and Risk Assessment; 9th plenary meeting; Brussels, Belgium.

4. European Commission Health and Consumer Protection Directorate-General. Opinion on p-Phenylenediamine. Scientific Committee on Consumer Products. SCCP/0989/06.

5. Ahmed HA, Abdel Maaboud RM, Abdul Latif FF, Kamal El-Dean AM, El-Shaieb KM (2013) Different Analytical Methods of Para-Phenylenediamine Based Hair Dye. Journal of Cosmetics, Dermatological Sciences and Applications. 3: 17-25

6. El-Ansary EH, Ahmed ME, Clague HW (1983) Systemic toxicity of para-phenylenediamine. Lancet 1: 1341.

7. Sood AK, Yadav SP, Sood S, Malhotra RC (1996) Hair dye poisoning. J Assoc Physicians India 44: 69.

8. European Commission Health and Consumer Protection Directorate-General. Opinion on p-Phenylenediamine. Scientific Committee on Consumer Products. SCCP/0989/06.

9. Http/www.ScienceLab.com

10. Sandeep Reddy Y, Abbdul Nabi S, Apparao C, Srilatha C, Manjusha Y, et al. (2012) Hair dye related acute kidney injury--a clinical and experimental study. Ren Fail 34: 880-884.

11. Soni SS, Nagarik AP, Dinaker M, Adikey GK, Raman A (2009) Systemic toxicity of paraphenylenediamine. Indian J Med Sci 63: 164-166.

12. Singla S, Miglani S, Lal AK, Gupta P, Agarwal AK (2005) Para-phenylenediamine (PPD) poisoning. Journal, Indian Academy of Clinical Medicine 6:136-138.

13. Curtis DK, Mary OA, John Doull (1986). Casarett and Doulls Toxicology- The basic Science of Poisons, Macmillan Publishing Company. New York.

14. Spector WS (1955) Hand book of Toxicology. Vol. 1. Acute toxicities of solids, liquids and gases to laboratory animals. Philadelphia, PA: W. B. Saunders Co., pp-232.

15. Saito K, Murai T, Yabe K, Hara M, Watanabe H, et al. (1990) [Rhabdomyolysis due to paraphenylenediamine (hair dye)--report of an autopsy case]. Nihon Hoigaku Zasshi 44: 469-474.

16. Averbukh Z, Modai D, Leonov Y, Weissgarten J, Lewinsohn G, et al. (1989) Rhabdomyolysis and acute renal failure induced by paraphenylenediamine. Hum Toxicol 8: 345-348.

17. Bourquia A, Jabrane AJ, Ramdani B, Zaid D (1988) [Systemic toxicity of paraphenylenediamine. 4 cases. Presse Med 17: 1798-1800.

18. Hyde TA Chemistry In Raphael SS (1983) Lynchs Medical Laboratory Technology (4th edn) WB Saunders Company.

19. MIZRAHI IJ, EMMELOT P (1962) The effect of cysteine on the metabolic changes produced by two carcinogenic Nnitrosodialklamines in rat liver. Cancer Res 22: 339-351.

20. Jack HD, Michael JM, Edward CW (1986) Toxic response of immune system. In Curtis DK, Mary OA, John Doul MD (Eds) Casarett and Doulls Toxicology the Basic Science of poison. Macmillan publishing Co, pp-245-251.

21. Elyoussoufi Z, Habti N, Mounaji K, Motaouakkil S, Cadi R (2013) Induction of oxidative stress and apoptosis in human neutrophils by p-phenylenediamine. Journal of Toxicology and Environmental Health Sciences 5: 142-149.

# 26

# Use of an Amphoteric Solution in Eye, Skin and Oral Chemical Exposures: Retrospective Multicenter Clinical Case Series

**Fortin JL**[1,2,3,4]**, Fontaine M**[4]**, Bodson L**[5]**, Depil-Duvala A**[6]**, Bitar MP**[1]**, Macher JM**[1,7]**, Paulin P**[3]**, Ravat F**[4] **and Hall AH**[8,9*]

[1]*Emergency Department, Belfort Montbéliard Hospital, 14 Mulhouse Street, 90 000 Belfort, France*

[2]*Preventive Medicine, 82 Bergson Street, 42 000 Saint-Etienne, France*

[3]*Medical Department, Sdis 25, 10 Clairière Street, 25 042, Besançon Cedex, France*

[4]*Burn Intensive Care Unit, Saint Joseph Saint Luc Hospital, 20 Quai Claude Bernard, 69007 Lyon, France*

[5]*Emergency Department, University Hospital, Sart Tilman B, 4000 Liege, Belgium*

[6]*Emergency Department, St-Luc-St-Joseph Hospital, 20 Quai Claude Bernard, 69 007 Lyon, France*

[7]*Emergency Department, Nouvel Hôpital Street 26, 88100 Saint-Dié-des-Voges, France*

[8]*Toxicology Consulting and Medical Translating Services, P.O. Box 1255, Azle, Texas 76098, USA*

[9]*Colorado School of Public Health, University of Colorado-Denver, Denver, Colorado, USA*

*****Corresponding author:** Alan H Hall, Medical Toxicologist, Toxicology Consulting and Medical Translating Services, P.O. Box 1255, Azle, TX 76098-1255, USA, E-mail: OldEDDoc@gmail.com

## Abstract

**Introduction:** A polyvalent amphoteric flushing solution (Diphoterine®) has been in use for a number of years, mainly in industrial settings for decontamination of acid, base, and other corrosive or irritant substances eye and skin splashes.

**Methods:** Retrospective collection of 34 cases from several centers reporting use of Diphoterine® decontamination of eye, skin or oral chemical exposures. The following data were retrieved: exposure circumstances (workplace, domestic, deliberate assault), chemical nature and pH, exposure type, initial clinical signs, clinical signs after flushing, initial and final visual analog scale (VAS) pain ratings, consulting specialist physicians' conclusions.

**Results:** 58.8% of the 34 cases were occupational exposures, 29.4% were domestic, 5.9% occurred in schools, and 5.9% were deliberate chemical assaults. Of involved chemicals, 11 were basic substances, 11 were acidic, 1 was an oxidizing substance, 2 were solvents, and 9 were miscellaneous substances. There were 21 ocular exposures, 8 cutaneous exposures, 4 mixed (ocular/cutaneous), and 1 oral exposure. Initial clinical findings in ocular exposures were: pain, blepharospasm, hyperemia, palpebral edema, excessive tearing, and blurred vision. Of cutaneous exposures, 1 was a deep necrotic injury and 7 were superficial. Median (IQR) VAS before flushing with Diphoterine® was 7; VAS after ocular or skin flushing was 1.

**Conclusion:** Early application of the amphoteric solution to the eye or skin reduces the intensity of pain associated with chemical injury. While randomized clinical trials are lacking, early use of the amphoteric solution appears to reduce the incidence of sequelae.

**Keywords:** Diphoterine®; Amphoteric solution; Eye decontamination; Skin decontamination; Oral decontamination; Chemical burns; Chemical injuries

## Introduction

A polyvalent amphoteric flushing fluid (Diphoterine® solution) has been utilized for a number of years for decontamination of eye and skin chemical splashes, mainly in industrial settings. Application of this flushing fluid as soon as possible after the chemical splash at the accident site can prevent or limit the consequences.

Recently, a number of emergency departments have begun using this amphoteric flushing fluid in either the pre-hospital or hospital settings (use by the mobile emergency and intensive care services (SMUR) or in accident and emergency departments). In these circumstances, use of this solution may be more delayed than in industrial settings.

## Methods

A retrospective multicenter case series of patients with chemical splash exposures decontaminated with Diphoterine® was assembled from the following hospital emergency departments and pre-hospital services for the years 2013 to 2016:

- Emergency Department, Belfort Hospital (France)
- Emergency Department, Montbéliard Hospital (France)
- Emergency Department, Evreux Hospital (France)

- Emergency Department, Lyon Saint-Joseph-Saint-Luc Hospital (France)
- Emergency Department, Liege Teaching Hospital (Belgium)
- Emergency Department, Saint-Dié Hospital (France)
- Medical Department, Departmental Fire and Rescue Service, Doubs (France)

Thirty-four patients with chemical splash exposures presenting to the above emergency services were included. The following data were retrieved from each patient's medical records and recorded: age, gender, exposure circumstances, chemical nature and pH, type of exposure, initial clinical symptoms and signs, clinical symptoms and signs after Diphoterine® decontamination, pain assessment before, during, and after Diphoterine® flushing using a Visual Analog Scale (VAS; 0-10), time interval between exposure and beginning flushing, and consulting specialists' conclusions.

The Wilcoxon Rank Sum Test was utilized to compare the VAS pain level before and after Diphoterine® with p<0.05 considered statistically significant.

The amphoteric flushing solution (Diphoterine®) was used in compliance with the following protocols:

For Eye Splashes:

- Use of a 500 mL container of Diphoterine® solution;
- A rapid and initial VAS pain assessment was conducted before flushing of each involved eye with 500 mL of Dipihoterine® solution;
- VAS pain intensity was assessed during and after flushing;
- Afterwards, rinsing with 500 mL of normal saline was done to prevent dry-eye syndrome because of the hypertonicity of Diphoterine® solution;
- Then, consultation with an ophthalmologist. (See Figure 1: Protocol for use in the event of eye splashes)

For Skin Splashes:

- Use of a 200 mL container of Diphoterine® solution;
- A 200 mL Diphoterine® container enables decontamination of
- ~9% of the Total Body Surface Area (TBSA) of an adult patient;
- A rapid initial assessment of the VAS pain level was done before flushing.
- At the conclusion of flushing, the VAS pain level was again assessed;
- Then, a burn specialist's opinion was obtained. (See Figure 2: Protocol for use in the event of skin splashes.)

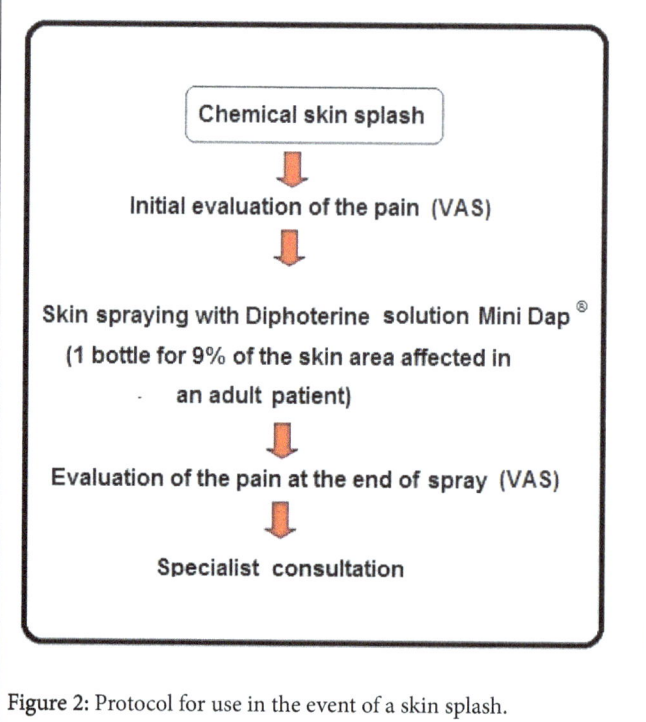

Figure 2: Protocol for use in the event of a skin splash.

## Results

Thirty-four patients were included in the retrospective study. Details of each case described by exposure circumstances (isolated eye lesions, isolated skin lesions, mixed eye and skin lesions, oral lesions) are shown in Tables 1a-1d. The median age of the patients was 37 years (IQR 25-45) and the male/female gender ratio was 61.30/38.70.

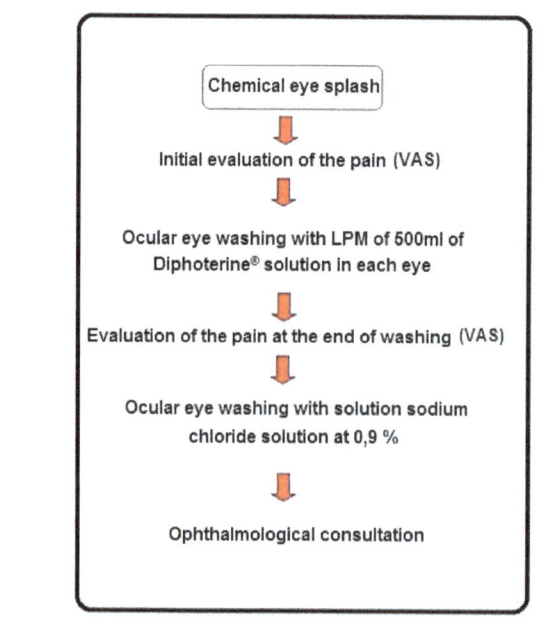

Figure 1: Protocol for use in the event of a chemical eye splash.

| Clinical cases | Eye lesion | Chemical pH | Interval between splash and washing | Initial clinical signs | Initial VAS | Clinical signs post-washing | Final VAS | Specialist opinion |
|---|---|---|---|---|---|---|---|---|
| No.1 | Bilateral lesions | Euphorbia lathyris latex pH=9 | 310 min | Blepharospasm Eye pain Palpebral edema | 10 | Decrease of pain and blepharospasm | 3 | Moderate conjunctival lesion |
| No.2 | Bilateral lesions | Tear gas agent | 30 min | Ocular hyperemia Eye pain | 10 | Resolution of hyperemia and pain | 0 | No conjunctival lesion |
| No.3 | Unilateral lesion | Acrylic coating | 20 min | Ocular hyperemia Eye pain | 6 | Resolution of hyperemia Disparition of pain | 0 | No conjunctival lesion |
| No.9 | Bilateral lesions | $CaOH_2$ | 89 min | Ocular hyperemia, pain, palpebral edema, no reduction in visual acuity | 10 | Decrease of pain | 3 | No ophthalmological lesion |
| No.10 | Unilateral lesion | Mewa Bio-Circle® degreasing agent – pH=1,5 | 110 min | Blurred vision, left eye clouding | 1 | Decrease of initial symptoms | 0 | No ophthalmological lesion |
| No.11 | Unilateral lesion | Indal Proclean® detergent for dairy equipment cleaning pH=1,5 | | Hyperemia, blurred vision Eye pain | 9 | Disparition of initial symptoms | 3 | No ophthalmological lesion |
| No.12 | Unilateral lesion | Bactifoam® alkaline liquid disinfectant pH=13 | 71 min | Ocular hyperemia Blepharospasm Eye pain | 6 | Resolution of the hyperemia and blepharospasm Reduction of pain | 1 | No ophthalmological lesion |
| No.13 | Bilateral lesions | 98% sulfuric acid pH=1 | 1 min | Mild eye pain | 3 | Resolution of pain | 0 | No ophthalmological lesion |
| No.15 | Unilateral lesion | Resosanit saphir ® pH=1 | 55 min | Eye pain | 4 | Diminution of pain | 2 | No ophthalmological lesion |
| No.16 | Bilateral lesions | Caustic Soda | 40 min | Ocular hyperemia Mild eye pain | 2 | Resolution of the hyperemia and pain | 0 | No ophthalmological lesion |
| No.17 | Unilateral lesion | Solvant J900 ® | 1 min | Ocular hyperemia Eye pain | 7 | Diminution of pain | 2 | |
| No.18 | Bilateral lesions | Tear gas agent | | Eye pain Watering | 9 | Diminution of pain | 5 | |
| No.22 | Bilateral lesions | Disinfectant P3-topactive®DES Peracetic acid and hydrogen peroxide pH=3,4 | 87 min | Hyperemia Blurred vision Eye pain | 5 | Disparition of hyperemia, blurred vision and eye pain | 1 | No ophtalmological lesion |

| No.23 | Unilateral lesion | Degreaser disinfectant concentrate Atout Vert 302 ® pH=2,5 | 180 min | Eye pain | 5 | Disparition of eye pain | 0 | No ophthalmological lesion |
| No.26 | Bilateral lesions | Acetone Biotech Biologique Onix® | 140 min | Hyperemia Blurred vision Eye pain | 4 | Disparition of eye pain, blurred vision and eye pain | 0 | |
| No.27 | Unilateral lesion | Ammonium hydroxide, Silver Nitrate, Oxalate ammonium chloride Barium | 85 min | Hyperemia Blurred vision Eye pain | 2 | Disparition of eye pain, blurred vision and eye pain | 0 | No ophthalmological lesion |
| No.30 | Unilateral lesion | Methyl methacrylate OPTIPAC 60 ® | 90 min | Hyperemia Blurred vision Eye pain | 4 | Disparition of eye pain, blurred vision And eye pain | 0 | |
| No.31 | Unilateral lesion | Phosphoric acid 20% | 95 min | Hyperemia Eye pain | 8 | Disparition of eye pain and hyperemia | 0 | |
| No.32 | Unilateral lesion | Butylhydroxytoluene Stronghole® | 131 min | Hyperemia Blurred vision Eye pain | 3 | Disparition of eye pain and hyperemia | 0 | |
| No.33 | Bilateral lesions | Chlorhexidine 0,2% | | Hyperemia Eye pain | 7 | Disparition of hyperemia and pain | - | |
| No.34 | Unilateral lesion | Anios gel ® pH=5,5 | 6 min | Hyperemia Eye pain | 6 | Disparition of hyperemia and pain | 1 | Moderate conjunctival lesion |

**Table 1a:** Presentation of the isolated eye lesions.

| Clinical cases | Chemical pH | Interval between splash and washing | Initial clinical signs | Initial VAS | Clinical signs post-washing | Final VAS | Specialist opinion Evolution |
|---|---|---|---|---|---|---|---|
| No.4 | AGS 60 ® Anti graffiti product pH=14 | 90 min | Pain Deep lesion | 8 | Pain resolution Persistence of deep lesion | 0 | Deep lesions Excision and skin graft |
| No.8 | 98% sulfuric acid pH=1 | 1 min | Erythematous plaques on the neck and chest | 9 | Persistence of the plaques Subsequent spontaneous recovery | 3 | Superficial burns |
| No.14 | 4% formaldehyde | 38 min | Erythema on the neck, right arm and anterior surface of both thighs | 5 | Resolution of erythematous plaques | 0 | No lesion or pain at hour 48 |
| No.19 | 2% Caustic soda | | Erythema TBSA=10% | 5 | Reduction of pain | 1 | Superficial burns |
| No.20 | BIOXAL ® | 50 min | Erythema | 1 | Disparition of erythema | 0 | No lesion or pain at hour 48 |

| | Acetic acid, Peracetic acid and hydrogen peroxide pH=1,6 | | | | | | | |
|---|---|---|---|---|---|---|---|---|
| No.24 | Cement pH=13 | 360 min | Skin pain | 8 | Reduction of pain | 2 | | |
| No.25 | Cement pH=13 | 360 min | Skin pain | 7 | Reduction of pain | 0 | | |
| No.29 | Caustic Soda | 45 min | Phlyctenae TBSA=1% | | Reduction of pain | 4 | | |

**Table 1b:** Presentation of the isolated skin lesions.

| Clinical cases | Chemical pH | Interval between splash and washing | Initial clinical signs | Initial VAS | Clinical signs post-washing | Final VAS | Specialist opinion Evolution |
|---|---|---|---|---|---|---|---|
| No.5 | Aluminum-manganese mixture | 20 min | Eye pain Blepharospasm Facial phlyctenae | 10 | Conjunctival irritation of the right eye | 4 | Conjunctival ulcer of the right eye Resolution of the blepharospasm Superficial burns |
| No.6 | 98% sulfuric acid pH=1 | 5 min | Eye pain Facial erythema | 9 | Resolution of the pain and facial erythema | 2 | No ophthalmological lesion Superficial burns |
| No.7 | 25% sodium hydroxide pH=12 | 308 min | Facial erythema Eye pain | 8 | Resolution of hyperemia and the facial erythema | 2 | No ophthalmological lesion Superficial burns |
| No.28 | Glyphosate de soude | 65 min | Blepharospasm Facial phlyctenae | 9 | Resolution of blepharospasm | 6 | No ophthalmological lesion Superficial burns |

**Table 1c:** Presentation of the mixed lesions (skin and eyes).

| Clinical cases | Chemical pH | Interval between splash and washing | Initial clinical signs | Initial VAS | Clinical signs post-washing | Final VAS | Specialist opinion Evolution |
|---|---|---|---|---|---|---|---|
| No.21 | Ammoniac | 555 min | Buccal and lingual burns | 3 | Decrease lingual burn Reduction of pain | 1 | No taste loss No burn after 48 hours |

**Table 1d:** Presentation of the Oral lesions.

In 58.8% of cases, the chemical exposure occurred in an industrial setting. In 29.4%, exposure was in a domestic setting, and in 5.9% of cases exposure occurred in an educational setting. In 5.9% of cases, the chemical exposure was due to deliberate assault.

There were 21 isolated ocular injuries (9 bilateral; 12 unilateral), 8 isolated skin injuries, 4 mixed eye and skin injuries, and 1 oral exposure. Involved chemicals were basic substances (11 cases), acidic substances (11 cases), an oxidizer (1 case), solvents (2 cases), and miscellaneous chemical substances (9 cases; acrylic coating, lacrimating agent, etc.).

Among the 25 isolated or mixed ocular injuries, the following signs and symptoms were noted: eye pain (18 cases), blepharospasm (4 cases; see Figure 3 for an example secondary to latex of Euphorbia lathyris exposure), conjunctival hyperemia (15 cases), palpebral edema (2 cases), excessive tearing (1 case), and blurred vision (7 cases). Among the 8 isolated skin injuries, there was 1 case with a deep necrotic lesion and 7 cases of superficial lesions, erythema, or phlyctenae.

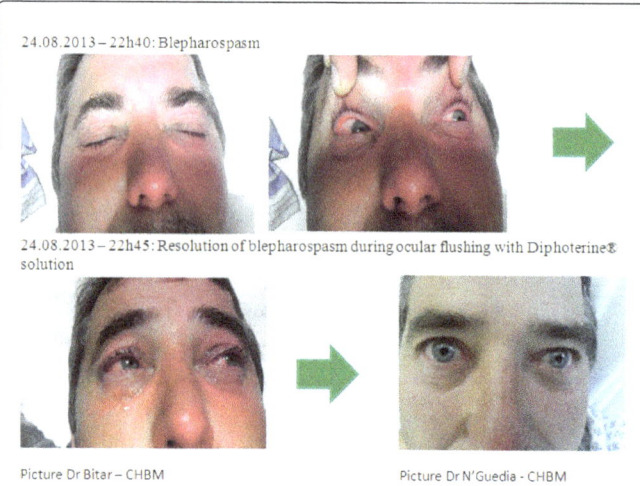

**Figures 3:** Skin and Eye lesions with latex of Euphorbia Lathyris (Case No.1).

Only 1 case of an oral burn due to accidental ingestion of ammonia stored in an unlabeled bottle was noted. The patient immediately expectorated the ammonia. The Tongue lesion before and after Diphoterine® rinsing repeated 5 times as a mouthwash and expectorated is shown in Figures 4 and 5.

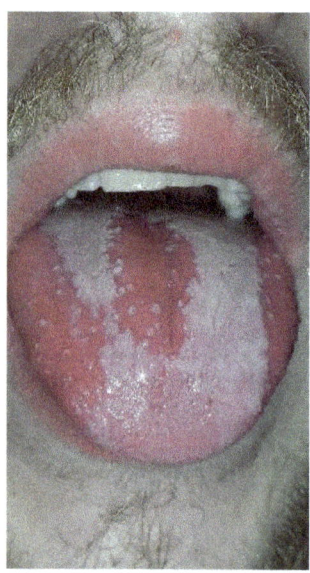

**Figure 4:** 20h15: Before the mouth washing with Diphoterine®.

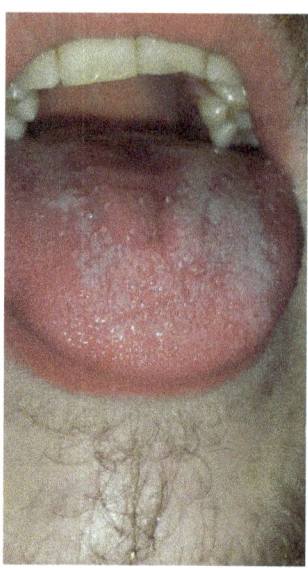

**Figure 5:** 20h45: After 5 mouth washing with Diphoterine®.

### Initial and final pain level assessment by VAS

The initial pain intensity ranged from 3 to 10 on the VAS. The initial median VAS score before Diphoterine® eye or skin flushing was 7 (IQR: 4-9). The final median VAS pain intensity score was 1 (IQR: 0-3). Thus, the difference between before-flushing and after-flushing with Diphoterine® was significant (Wilcoxon Rank Sum Test; $p<0.0001$).

The time interval between exposure and Diphoterine® solution eye and/or skin flushing ranged from 1-555 minutes (median: 77.5 minutes; IQR: 30-131 minutes).

### Clinical signs and symptoms after diphoterine® eye and/or skin flushing

**Ocular signs and symptoms:** Resolution of eye pain in 14 cases (final VAS 0 or 1); marked decrease of eye pain in 7 cases (final VAS 2 or 3); persistence of moderate eye pain after Diphoterine® eye flushing in 3 cases related to chemical lesions induced by a reducing agent (aluminum-magnesium mixture; Case No. 6), "tear gas" (Case No. 18) and glyphosate soda (Case No. 28); Resolution of blepharospasm in the 4 observed cases (Cases Nos. 1, 5, 12, 28); Reduction of initial blurred vision in the 7 observed cases with regression or resolution of initial blurred vision (Cases Nos. 10, 11, 22, 26, 27, 30, 32); Resolution of initial palpebral edema in the 2 observed cases (Cases Nos. 1 and 9)

**Cutaneous signs and symptoms:** Resolution of all initial skin lesions in the 7 observed cases with superficial lesions (erythema or phlyctenae) by 48 hours post-exposure; In the 1 case of deep necrotic skin injury (Case No.4), there was no local improvement following Diphoterine® flushing. Recovery followed surgical excision and skin grafting. Of note, Diphoterine® flushing was quite delayed after exposure.

**Oral signs and symptoms:** In the only case of mouth exposure (to ammonia; Case No. 21), after 5 repeated Diphoterine® mouthwashes followed by expectoration (no swallowing), a reduction of the chemical injury was noted (Figures 4 and 5). On the following day, the patient was pain free and had no loss of taste sensation.

**Results of ophthalmology specialist consultations:** No lesions were noted in 12 patients; Six patients had minimal eye findings (moderate conjunctival lesions which resolved in a few days with standard eye drop treatment); One patient (Case No. 5) had a superficial ulceration of the cornea.

## Discussion

It is generally accepted that decontamination of eye or skin chemical splashes should be done as soon as possible after exposure. While potable water as the flushing fluid has been utilized for a very long time, it is perhaps currently not the best option [1]. Diphoterine® is a polyvalent amphoteric solution for flushing splashed chemicals off the skin or surface of the eyes. It has been used efficaciously for a number of years in industrial settings [2-5]. In the European Union, Diphoterine® solution is a Class II medical device. It is not irritating to the eyes or skin, is not sensitizing in guinea pigs or humans, is non-toxic (rat oral/dermal LD50 >2,000 mg/kg) and is not mutagenic in the Ames test [1,6].

### Diphoterine® solution has multiple methods of action

- As an aqueous solution, it flushes a large portion of the splashed chemical substance from the surface of the skin or eyes through mechanical entrainment and dilution;
- As an hypertonic solution, it limits penetration of the splashed chemical substance into the deep tissue layers of the skin or eyes by creating an osmotic pressure gradient;
- As an amphoteric solution (able to bind opposing chemical groups such as acids/bases or oxidizing/reducing agents), it halts the aggressive action of corrosive or irritant chemical substances.

Comparative studies have demonstrated the efficacy of Diphoterine® solution. Gerard et al. [7] compared the action of Diphoterine® solution and normal saline *in vivo* in the context of ammonium hydroxide eye injuries. These authors found a lack of stromal edema when Diphoterine® solution was used and its presence when flushing was with normal saline. This finding is supported by the difference of osmotic pressure between the two flushing fluids (respectively ~800 mosmols/kg for Diphoterine® solution versus 280 mosmols/kg for normal saline, while the osmotic pressure of the cornea is 420 mosmols/kg). As a biochemical rationale, the pH curve was decreased during flushing with Diphoterine® solution.

In a 2002 review, Hall et al. [1] showed that Diphoterine® solution was more efficacious than water in various industrial studies. Nehles et al. [4] found that when workplace corrosive substances eye and skin splashes were flushed with Diphoterine®, there was no need for medical treatment other than decontamination, and there were no sequelae and no lost work time.

Cavallini and Casati [8] and Cavallini et al. [9] investigated wound healing and concentrations of ß-endorphin, Substance P, and interleukin IL-6 in a rat *in vivo* study of concentrated hydrochloric acid skin injury flushed with either Diphoterine® solution, normal saline, or calcium gluconate solution. In the Diphoterine® group versus the normal saline and calcium gluconate solution groups, the following were observed:

- A more important decrease in lesion size in the Diphoterine® solution group;
- Significant beneficial changes in biological markers of pain in the Diphoterine® solution group: a significant decrease in Substance P concentration at 48 h (p<0.05) and a significant increase in ß-endorphin at 7 days (p<0.05);
- A significant decrease in inflammation as shown by decreased IL-6 concentrations at 48 h (p<0.05) and enhanced tissue repair.

Merle et al. [10,11] conducted a clinical study of 66 patients with deliberate assault eye splashes with a base chemical substance (ammonium hydroxide; Alkali®) in Martinique. These authors reported that, compared to normal saline flushing, Diphoterine® solution was more efficacious for decreasing the time to corneal re-epithelization in patients with Roper-Hall scale Grade I and II lesions and seemed to be more suitable for emergent flushing of corrosive chemical substance exposed eyes. Schrage et al. [12] considered the pathophysiology of chemical ocular lesions and compared various eyewash solutions. Diphoterine® appeared to be the best option.

Ioannidis et al. [13] reported the case of a 76-year-old man with eye injury due to exposure to the latex of the Euphorbia lathyris plant. Despite flushing with 8 liters of normal saline followed by treatment with dexamethasone and cicatrizing eye drops, the patient developed a corneal ulcer and severe pain which necessitated a 3-day hospitalization.

This clinical course is in sharp contract to Case No.1 reported here; a 59-year-old man who developed facial skin injuries, eye injuries, and severe pain 4 hours after handling the latex of this same plant. Euphorbia lathyris is a plant used by gardeners; in particular the cut stalks are inserted into mole burrows. The latex from the cut stalks has alkylating and base properties (pH=9) and also contains protease enzymes which repel moles.

After exposure at home, the patient took 10 mg of morphine (already in his possession for the treatment of fibromyalgia) and performed an eye wash with Dacroserum® solution which did not alleviate the pain. During the initial examination in the hospital emergency department, the patient had blepharospasm, facial lesions, and ocular pain which was scored as 8/10 on the VAS, a well as persistence of blepharospasm. Eye flushing with normal saline resulted in an increase in ocular pain (10/10 on the VAS). Flushing with Diphoterine® solution (250 mL for each eye) resulted in a decrease of ocular pain (6/10 on the VAS) and resolution of blepharospasm after 15 minutes (Figure 3). After 55 minutes, ocular pain had completely resolved. Ophthalmological examination a few hours later showed only a mild conjunctival lesion. As compared to the case reported by Ioannidis et al. [13], flushing with Diphoterine® solution resulted in a less severe lesion and rapid pain relief.

Donoghue [5] compared the efficacy of Diphoterine® solution with that of water for decontamination of alkaline chemical splashes in a clinical study involving 180 workers. In the group treated with Diphoterine® solution, there were no signs of lesions in 52.9% of cases versus 21.4% of cases flushed with water. Moreover, grade III and IV lesions were significantly less numerous in the Diphoterine® solution first group (7.9 *vs.* 23.8%; p<0.001).

Zack-Williams et al. [14] published a 2-year comparative evaluation study. There was a significant change in the wound pH pre- and post-flushing with Diphoterine® solution compared to water flushing (pH change of 1.076 versus 0.4; p<0.05). There were no significant differences in time to healing, length of hospital stay or need for surgery. Based on the retrospective case series presented here, Diphoterine® solution could be valuable for flushing of corrosive and irritant chemical splashes in the hospital and pre-hospital settings.

Bvrar [15] published a comparative study of CS "tear gas" exposures in Slovenian police officers flushed with Diphoterine® solution versus no flushing. The policemen refused to compare Diphoterine® solution with water flushing because of increased pain when CS exposures were flushed with water. Six policemen were exposed to CS only. A second group of 8 policemen sprayed their faces with Diphoterine® solution before CS exposure and a third group of 8 policemen sprayed their faces with Diphoterine® solution after exposure. The time between exiting the CS cloud and arriving at the "ready for action" checkpoint was measured. Facial pain both inside the CS cloud and at the checkpoint was assessed using a 0-10 visual analog scale (VAS).

The pain level inside the CS cloud was significantly lower in the group that pre-treated with Diphoterine® solution (5.6 ± 1.1; p=0.1) versus the CS only group (9.7 ± 0.5). In the post-CS-exposure treatment group, it was similar (9.1 ± 0.4). The time interval between CS exposure and arrival at the checkpoint was significantly shorter in the Diphoterine® solution pre-treatment group (1.26 ± 0.44 minutes) than in the CS only group (2.28 ± 0.25 minutes; p=0.04) and in the post-exposure treatment group (2.30 ± 0.48 minutes; p=0.02) where it was not different. The residual pain at the checkpoint in the Diphoterine® pre-CS-exposure (1.1 ± 0.4) and post-exposure (1.4 ± 0.7) groups was similar, with significantly less pain than in the CS only group (2.3 ± 0.5; p=0.02). In this study, post-CS-exposure decontamination with Diphoterine® solution reduced facial pain whereas pre-CS-exposure treatment reduced both pain and recovery time [15]. These findings are in substantial agreement with those reported in French gendarmes by Viala et al. [16].

Lynn et al. [17] published an independent systematic review of the safety and efficacy of Diphoterine® solution compared to water and normal saline for the decontamination of ocular and cutaneous chemical burns in humans. All studies published in peer-reviewed journals up to May 2016 were eligible for consideration. Such published data must have included Diphoterine® solution for decontamination of eye and/or skin chemical splashes as well as meeting other specified criteria. Acceptable studies had to use either a quantitative (e.g., number of lost workdays) or qualitative (e.g., level of erythema) approach when determining cutaneous and/or ocular lesion outcomes. These authors concluded that, despite a relatively small number of published studies, Diphoterine® solution is safe and highly efficacious in improving healing times, healing sequelae, and pain management of chemical skin and eye injuries in humans. Outcomes are significantly improved as compared to water or normal saline decontamination. These authors concluded:

"*We recommend this product be readily available to emergency responders and companies that expose their employees to hazardous chemical substances in order to improve healing sequelae, pain management, and lost work days from these types of burns*" [17].

Overall, Diphoterine® solution limits the action of the splashed chemical substance on the tissues. Through its physical actions, it removes the chemical substance in contact with the tissues (mechanical and osmotic actions). In addition, flushing with Diphoterine® solution enables the tissues to return to a physiologically acceptable pH. Lesion formation is thus halted. Since the tissue is no longer under aggression and in a physiologically acceptable environment, pain and inflammation decrease. The published studies

reviewed show the same mechanisms, during and after flushing with Diphoterine® solution, as evidenced by decrease in pain and reduction of sequelae.

The majority of the cases reported here showed symptomatic improvement following Diphoterine® solution flushing. Absorption of the splashed chemical substance into the tissues and resultant cell damage are halted by effective flushing with Diphoterine® solution.

## Conclusion

Eye and skin chemical lesions account for ~4% of all burn cases attending emergency departments. The context is often a domestic accident rather than an occupational exposure. The small number of chemical lesions resulting from occupational accidents observed in the hospital might be explained by the use of the polyvalent, amphoteric Diphoterine® solution as an emergency decontamination measure in workplace settings. Rapid use of Diphoterine® solution enables a reduction in the duration of tissue chemical exposure and hence a reduction in the lesions induced.

Both *in vitro* and *in vivo*, Diphoterine® solution has been shown to be effective on eye, skin and mucous membrane chemical injuries. For the best results, Diphoterine® solution flushing should begin as soon as possible after the chemical splash occurs in order to prevent or lessen lesion development. As more data are accumulated, the efficacy of Diphoterine® solution should become more apparent to pre-hospital responder organizations and emergency departments.

## References

1.  Hall AH, Maibach HI (2006) Water decontamination of chemical skin/eye splashes: a critical review. Cutan Ocul Toxicol 25: 67-83.

2.  Hall AH, Blomet J, Mathieu L (2002) Diphoterine for emergent eye/skin chemical splash decontamination: a review. Vet Hum Toxicol 44: 228-231.

3.  Minaro L, Bedry R, Verdun-Esquer C, Brochard P, Favarri-Garrigues JC (2000) Brûlures chimiques: place de la Diphoterine®. Archives des Malades Professionelles et de Medecine du Travail 61: 63-64.

4.  Nehles J, Hall AH, Blomet J, Mathieu L (2006) Diphoterine for emergent decontamination of skin/eye chemical splashes: 24 cases. Cutan Ocul Toxicol 25: 249-258.

5.  Donoghue AM (2010) Diphoterine for alkali chemical splashes to the skin at alumina refineries. Int J Dermatol 49: 894-900.

6.  Hall AH, Cavallini M, Mathieu L, Maibach HI (2009) Safety of dermal Diphoterine application: An active decontamination solution for chemical splash injuries. Cutan Ocul Toxicol 28: 149-156.

7.  Gérard M, Josset P, Louis V, Menarath JM, Blomet J, et al (2000) Existe-t-il un délai pour le lavage oculaire externe dans le traitement d'une brûlure oculaire par l'ammoniaque. Comparison de deux solutions de lavage: serum physiologique et Diphoterine® [French]. J Fr Ophtamol 23: 449-458.

8.  Cavallini M, Casati A (2004) A prospective, randomized, blind comparison between saline, calcium gluconate and Diphoterine for washing skin acid injuries in rats: effects on substance P and ß-endorphin release. Eur J Anaesthesiol 21: 389-392.

9.  Cavallini M, de Broccard F, Corsi MM, Fassati LR, Baruffaldi Preis FW (2004) Serum pro-inflammatory cytokines and chemical acid burns in rats. Ann Burn Fire Dis 27: 1-5.

10. Merle H, Donnio A, Ayeboua L, Thomas F, Ketterle J, et al. (2005) Alkali ocular burns in Martinique (French West Indies). Evaluation of the use of an amphoteric solution as the rinsing product. Burns 31: 205-211.

11. Merle H, Gérard M, Schrage N (2008) Ocular burns. J Fr Ophtalmol 31: 723-734.

12. Schrage NF, Struck HG, Gerard M (2011) Recommendations for acute treatment for chemical and thermal burns of eyes and lids. Ophthalmologe 108: 916-920.

13. Ioannidis AS, Papageorgiou KI, Andreou PS (2009) Exposure to Euphorbia lathyris latex resulting in alkaline chemical injury: a case report. J Med Case Rep 3: 115.

14. Zack-Williams SD, Ahmad Z, Moiemen NS (2015) The clinical efficacy of Diphoterine® in the management of cutaneous chemical burns: a 2-year evaluation study. Ann Burns Fire Disasters 28: 9-12.

15. Bvrar M (2016) Chlorobenzylidene malononitrile tear gas exposure: Rinsing with amphoteric, hypertonic, and chelating solution. Hum Exp Toxicol 35: 213-218.

16. Viala B, Blomet J, Mathieu L, Hall AH (2005) Prevention of CS "Tear Gas" eye and skin effects and active decontamination with Diphoterine: Preliminary studies in 5 French Gendarmes. J Emerg Med 29: 5-8.

17. Lynn DD, Zukin LM, Dellavalle R (2017) The safety and efficacy of Diphoterine for ocular and cutaneous burns in humans. Cutan Ocul Toxicol.

# 27

# *In Vitro, In Vivo* Comparison of Cyclosporin A-Induced Hepatic Protein Expression Profiles

Freek G Bouwman[1#], Anke Van Summeren[1,2#], Anne Kienhuis[3], Leo van der Ven[3], Ewoud N Speksnijder[4], Jean-Paul Noben[5], Johan Renes[1], Jos C S Kleinjans[2] and Edwin C M Mariman[1*]

[#]Both authors contributed equally to this manuscript

[1]Department of Human Biology, Maastricht University, P.O. box 616, 6200 MD Maastricht, The Netherlands

[2]Department of Toxicogenomics, Maastricht University, P.O. box 616, 6200 MD Maastricht, The Netherlands

[3]Laboratory for Health Protection Research, National Institute of Public Health and the Environment (RIVM), Bilthoven, The Netherlands

[4]Department of Toxicogenetics, Leiden University Medical Center, 2300 RC, Leiden, the Netherlands

[5]Hasselt University, Biomedical Research Institute and Transnational University Limburg, School of Life Sciences, Diepenbeek, Belgium

[*]**Corresponding author:** Dr. Edwin C. M. Mariman, Department of Human Biology, Maastricht University, P.O. box 616, 6200 MD Maastricht, The Netherlands, E-mail: e.mariman@maastrichtuniversity.nl

## Abstract

To reduce the amount of laboratory animals which are used to analyze hepatotoxic properties of chemicals and drugs, the development of alternative *in vitro* models is necessary. Ideally these *in vitro* models reflect the *in vivo* toxicological response and cholestasis. In this study the protein expression in livers from C57BL/6 mice after cyclosporin A-induced cholestasis was analyzed. After 25 days of a daily cyclosporine A treatment the cholestatic phenotype was established. An *in vitro* to this *in vivo* study comparison was made by using the results of our previous studies with HepG2 and primary mouse hepatocytes. The *in vivo* proteomics data show cyclosporin A-induced oxidative stress and mitochondrial dysfunction was actually induced, leading to a decreased mitochondrial ATP production and an altered urea cycle. These processes were also altered by cyclosporin A in the *in vitro* models HepG2 and primary mouse hepatocytes. In addition, detoxification enzymes like methyl- and glutathione-S-transferases were differentially expressed after cyclosporin A treatment. Changes in these detoxification enzymes were mainly detected *in vivo*, though primary mouse hepatocytes show a differential expression of some of these enzymes. By means of a functional classification of differentially expressed proteins we demonstrated similarities and differences between *in vitro* and *in vivo* models in the proteome response of cyclosporin A-induced hepatotoxicity.

**Keywords:** Proteomics; Hepatotoxicity; Cyclosporin A; Liver; *In vivo*

## Abbreviations

2DE: 2-Dimensional Gel Electrophoresis; ABC- Transporters: ATP Binding Cassette Transporters; CHOL: Cholesterol; CsA: Cyclosporin A; DIGE: Difference Gel Electrophoresis; GSTs: Glutathione S-Transferases; MALDI-TOF/TOF-MS: Matrix Assisted Laser Desorption Ionization Time-of-Flight Tandem Mass Spectrometry; LC-MSMS: Nano Liquid Chromatography Tandem Mass Spectrometry; TBIL: Total Bilirubin; TBA: Total Bile Acids

## Introduction

Novel drugs should be recognized as safe for human exposure. With respect to drug-induced toxicity, hepatotoxicity is prominent, because most drugs are metabolized to be eliminated by the liver. The hepatotoxic properties of chemicals and drugs are usually analyzed in *in vivo* repeated-dose toxicity tests, which involve a high number of laboratory animals. To reduce the amount of laboratory animals, alternative *in vitro* models are currently developed and their screening properties evaluated [1-3]. Ideally these *in vitro* models reflect the *in vivo* toxicological response. Accordingly, *in vitro* to *in vivo* comparisons are necessary. By applying Omics technologies it is possible to measure similar endpoints of drug-induced changes between *in vitro* and *in vivo* which enable a global comparison of both models [4].

Conventional hepatotoxicity assays rely on the analysis of clinical, hematological, and histopathological parameters. While the conventional assays generally measure only a limited set of biological endpoints, Omics technologies offers the possibility to measure multiple endpoints simultaneously in a single experiment. Currently, transcriptomics studies, where thousands of genes are measured simultaneously, have shown to be successful for this purpose [4-6]. However, transcriptomics investigates the relative mRNA levels of genes which often only moderately correlate with the relative abundance of their protein product. This moderate correlation is due to turnover differences of proteins and mRNA [7].

In addition, post-translational modifications and protein interactions are not detected by transcriptomics, which emphasizes the relevance of proteomics. For example, by applying difference gel electrophoresis (DIGE), proteins are separated based on their pI and molecular weight, so different protein isoforms can be visualized [8].

Previously we investigated the proteome of HepG2 cells and primary mouse hepatocytes after exposure to three well-defined hepatotoxicants [9,10]. These were acetaminophen, amiodarone and cyclosporin A (CsA), of which CsA generated the most prominent response. CsA is an immunosuppressive drug; however, as an adverse side effect it induces cholestasis caused by the inhibition of the bile salt transporters in hepatocytes [11].

The aim of the present study is to identify cholestatic-specific mechanisms *in vivo*, with use of proteomics. Furthermore, we want to compare these results with our previous *in vitro* studies with HepG2 and primary mouse hepatocytes [9,10].

For this purpose the hepatic protein expression from C57BL/6 mice after CsA-induced cholestasis was examined. The development of cholestasis at the proteome level was analyzed after 4, 11 and 25 days of a daily dose of CsA. The cholestatic phenotype was established after 25 days and was confirmed by serum biochemistry and histopathology.

DIGE was used to analyze the differentially expressed proteins induced by CsA. The results from our previous studies with HepG2 [9] and primary mouse hepatocytes [10] were used to establish an *in vitro-in vivo* comparison of CsA-induced protein expression profiles.

## Materials and Methods

### Chemicals

CsA, CAS-no 59865-13-3, purity minimum 98%, was kindly provided by Novartis, Basel, Switzerland. N,N-dimethylformamide (anhydrous, 99.8%) was purchased from Sigma-Aldrich (Zwijndrecht, The Netherlands), the Protein Assay Kit was from Bio-Rad (Veenendaal, The Netherlands). All chemicals used for DIGE were purchased from GE Healthcare (Diegem, Belgium).

### Animals

Male C57BL/6 mice, aged 10 weeks at the start of the treatment period (21-27 g), were obtained from Charles River GmbH, Sulzfeld, Germany. Animals were kept under controlled specific pathogen-free conditions (23°C, 40%-50% humidity) under a 12hour light-dark cycle, and housed in groups of five.

Food and tap water were available ad libitum during the whole experiment. Experiments were conducted at the animal facility of the Leiden University Medical Center, under ethical review in accordance with the Dutch law (DEC 09157).

### Animal treatment

For the 25 day repeated dose study, forty animals were assigned to eight groups of five mice per group. For the 4 and 11 day repeated-dose study, twenty-four animals were assigned to six groups of four mice per group. After an acclimatization period, treatment protocols were used in which mice were dosed with CsA in olive oil or with the vehicle only, by oral gavage in a volume of 4 ml/kg body weight, for five times per week (working days) between 2:00 and 4:00 pm. In the 25 day study, mice were treated with CsA up to 80 mg/kg body weight.

This study was used for dose range finding, selecting the dose of 26.6 mg/kg body weight which was determined to be the critical effect dose that induced cholestatic clinical chemistry parameters at 25 days of exposure. The animals were sacrificed by inhalation of $CO_2$ and heart puncture at four, eleven and twenty-five days post CsA administration. Blood was collected in 0.8 ml Minicollect serum collection tubes (Greiner Bio-One, Alphen aan de Rijn, The Netherlands) for serum chemistry analyses.

The liver samples were frozen in liquid nitrogen and stored at -80°C until the protein isolation. Liver samples of animals treated with 26.6 mg/kg body weight in the 25 day dose range finding study and liver samples of the 4 and 11 day study were used for proteome analysis.

### Serum biochemistry

Alanine transaminase (ALT), Aspartate transaminase (AST), Cholesterol (CHOL), total bilirubin (TBIL) and total bile acids (TBA) were analyzed on a Beckman Coulter LX20 Clinical Chemistry Analyzer using Beckman reagent kits (Beckman Coulter B.V., Woerden, The Netherlands) for TBIL, and CHOL, and a Dialab reagent kit (DIALAB GmbH, Neudorf, Austria) for TBA. A student's-T test was performed on the results to determine significant differences.

### Histopathology

After 24 hours fixation in 4% neutral buffered formalin, liver samples were stored in 70% ethanol until further processing, which included automated dehydration, embedding in paraffin, sectioning at 5 μm, and staining with hematoxylin and eosin.

### Sample preparation

Liver samples were ground into fine powder in liquid nitrogen and homogenized in DIGE labeling buffer containing 7 M urea, 2 M thiourea, 4% (w/v) CHAPS and 30 mM TrisHCl. This mixture was mixed thoroughly and subjected to three cycles of freeze thawing with liquid nitrogen to lyse the cells. The homogenate was vortexed for 1 minute and centrifuged at 20 000g for 30 min at 10°C. The supernatant was collected and stored at -80°C until further analysis. Protein concentrations were determined with the Protein Assay Kit from Bio-Rad (Veenendaal, The Netherlands).

### DIGE

The protein labeling and the DIGE were performed as described before [9]. A one-way ANOVA test (P ≤ 0.05) was used to select the significant differential spots between the experimental groups. In addition, two way ANOVA-treatment, two-way ANOVA-time, and two-way ANOVA-interaction were computed to assign statistically significant changes in spot intensity due to the treatment alone, time alone and due to both treatment and time.

The differentially expressed proteins were excised and identified by matrix assisted laser desorption ionization time of flight tandem mass spectrometry (MALDI-TOF/TOF-MS) according to Bouwman et al. [12]. Protein spots that could not be identified by MALDI-TOF/TOF-MS were further analyzed by nano liquid chromatography tandem mass spectrometry (LC-MSMS) on an LCQ Classic (ThermoFinnigan) as described before [13].

### Functional Classification

The proteins differentially expressed after exposure to CsA in HepG2 and primary mouse hepatocytes, were retrieved from previous studies [9,10]. The Panther classification system (http://www.pantherdb.org) was used to compare the effect of CsA upon the protein expression in HepG2, primary mouse hepatocytes and *in vivo* mouse liver. From each experiment the differentially expressed proteins were uploaded onto the Panther classification system.

Furthermore, the Functional Classification Tool of the DAVID Bioinformatics resource 6.7 (http://david.abcc.ncifcrf.gov/) was used to cluster functionally related proteins. For this purpose the differentially expressed proteins from the three experiments were uploaded and classified with the lowest stringency. Afterwards it was retrieved in which experiment these proteins were differentially expressed.

## Results

### Traditional toxicology parameters

To induce cholestasis C57BL/6 mice were treated with 26.6 mg/kg CsA. Histopathology showed submembraneous vacuolization suggesting cholestasis at 25 days (Figure 1). The plotted serum values per animal for CHOL, TBIL, TBA, ALT and AST are presented in Figure 2.

A change (P<0.1) was observed as early as 4 days treatment up till 25 days for the cholestatic parameters CHOL, TBIL, TBA. The general hepatotoxicity markers ALT and AST did not show a significant increase, indicating that a severe stage with liver damage was not yet reached.

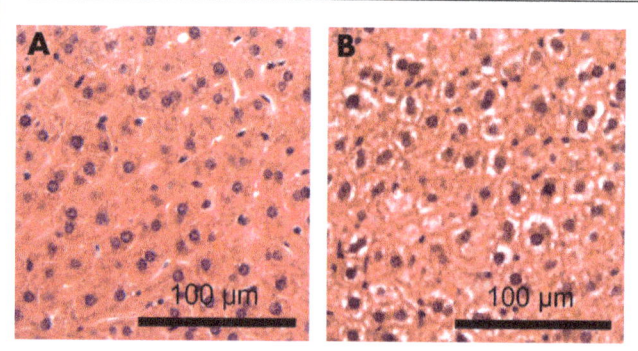

**Figure 1:** (A) Mouse liver treated with vehicle for 25 days. (B) Submembraneous vacuolization suggestive of cholestasis in mouse liver upon treatment with 26.6 mg/kg body weight for 25 days. Magnification: 60X.

### DIGE analysis

To analyze the *in vivo* hepatotoxic effects of CsA, C57BL/6 mice were exposed to CsA for 4, 11 and 25 days with olive oil as a vehicle control. On these time-points the animals were sacrificed and the liver was isolated. The proteins were extracted from these liver samples and the differentially expressed proteins were determined using DIGE. In total 3235 spots could be matched within all images.

With a one-way ANOVA 60 spots were found significantly different (P ≤ 0.05) between all groups. With a two-way ANOVA analysis 92 spots were significantly different (P ≤ 0.05) in response to treatment, 12 spots were significantly different (P ≤ 0.05) in time and 8 spots were differentially expressed for the interaction of the treatment and time (P ≤ 0.05).

### Protein identification

The differential spots were included in a pick list. For spot picking and identification a preparative gel was loaded with 150 μg of the internal standard labeled with 300 pmol Cy2 and run in the same way

as the analytical gels. Afterwards, with use of the DeCyder™ 7.0 software (GE Healthcare) the preparative gel was matched with the analytical gels.

Protein identification was performed by in-gel digestion followed by MALDI-TOF/TOF-MS and/or LC-MS/MS analysis. The 96 selected protein spots were identified belonging to 86 different proteins. A total of 19 protein spots were isoforms from 9 proteins due to post-translational modifications or processing of the protein. Figure 3 shows the 2-DE map made from the master gel with the identified differential spots indicated with a number which corresponds to the numbers presented in Table 1.

For the identified protein spots a Tukey's multiple comparison test was performed, from which 4 spots (methylcrotonoyl-CoA carboxylase alpha chain, aconitate hydratase, and two isoforms of carbamoyl-phosphate synthase I) were significantly differential after 4 days treatment of CsA. After 11 days of treatment 8 spots were differentially expressed (alpha enolase, selenium-binding protein 2, NADP-dependent malic enzyme, transketolase, eukaryotic peptide chain release factor subunit 1, pyruvate kinase, superoxide dismutase 2, and indolethylamine N-methyltransferase).

Twenty five days of treatment induced the differential expression of 6 spots (glutathione S-transferase Mu 2, farnesyl pyrophosphate synthetase, selenium-binding protein 2, sulfite oxidase, thiopurine S-methyltransferase and protein disulfide-isomerase).

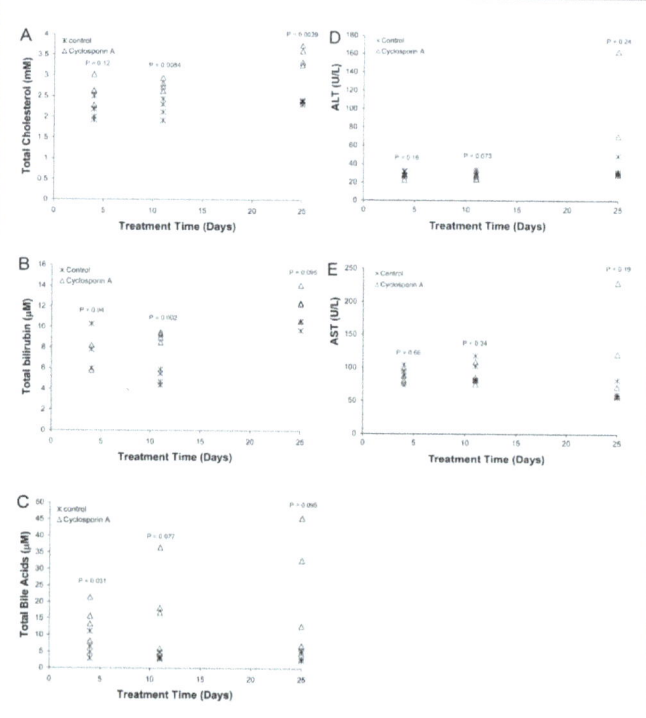

**Figure 2:** Plotted serum values per animal for (A) Cholesterol, (B) Total Bilirubine, (C) Total Bile Acids, (D) ALT and (E) AST at 4, 11, and 25 days of exposure to 26.6 mg/kg body weight CsA.

In Table 1 the spots are listed with their protein identification and their fold changes between the control and compound. The significant changes are marked with **P ≤ 0.05 or *P ≤ 0.1 accordingly Tukey's multiple comparison test.

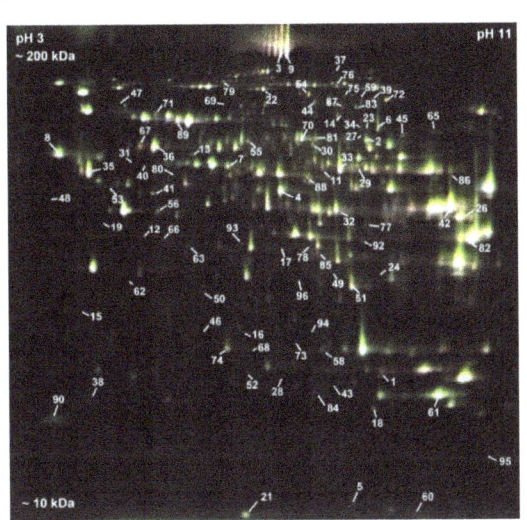

**Figure 3:** Proteome map of the differentially expressed proteins. The identified spots are indicated with a number which corresponds to the numbers used in Table 1.

## Functional classification

Data from HepG2 and primary mouse hepatocytes, were retrieved from previous studies [9,10]. The Venn diagram in Figure 4 illustrates the overlap of differentially expressed proteins induced by CsA in *in vivo* mouse liver, primary mouse hepatocytes and HepG2 cells.

In order to compare the protein expression results in mouse and human cells, only mouse orthologues were used. The overlap of the differentially expressed proteins is the highest between the *in vitro* models PMH and HepG2.

However the *in vivo-in vitro* comparison of CsA-induced hepatotoxicity based on single protein expression shows only a small overlap in the differentially expressed proteins from the different models.

For that reason we made use of the Panther classification system to identify the functional properties of the identified proteins. The differentially expressed proteins in the liver from exposed mice were mostly involved in metabolic process, immune system process and generation of precursor metabolites and energy (Figure 5).

For HepG2 cells and primary mouse hepatocytes the majority of the differential proteins are involved in transport, metabolic and cellular processes (Figure 5). Similar processes between the analyzed *in vitro* systems are cell cycle, cellular processes, developmental processes and cell adhesion (Figure 5).

In all three models CsA altered proteins which belong to transport and a response to stimulus (Figure 5). The Functional Classification Tool of the DAVID Bioinformatics resource 6.7, revealed 12 clusters which are presented in Table 2.

| No | Uniprot | Gene name | Protein description | P value | | | | Fold change[5] | | |
|----|---------|-----------|---------------------|---------|---|---|---|---|---|---|
| | | | | one-way anova[1] | two-way anova, treatment[2] | two-way anova, time[3] | interaction treatment/ time[4] | CsA4/C4 | CsA11/C11 | CsA25/C25 |
| Tricarboxylic acid cycle | | | | | | | | | | |
| 39 | Q99KI0 | Aco2 | Aconitate hydratase. mitochondrial precursor | 0.018 | 0.0097 | 0.11 | 0.11 | -1.17** | -1.01 | -1.07 |
| 59 | Q99KI0 | Aco2 | Aconitate hydratase. mitochondrial precursor | 0.13 | 0.02 | 0.93 | 0.23 | -1.13 | -1 | -1.11 |
| 72 | Q99KI0 | Aco2 | Aconitate hydratase. mitochondrial precursor | 0.021 | 0.03 | 0.036 | 0.17 | -1.14 | 1 | -1.07 |
| 32 | O88844 | Idh1 | Isocitrate dehydrogenase [NADP] cytoplasmic | 0.038 | 0.0068 | 0.4 | 0.18 | 1.01 | 1.11 | 1.14 |
| 56 | Q9Z2I9 | Sucla2 | Succinyl-CoA ligase [ADP-forming] subunit beta. mitochondrial | 0.068 | 0.015 | 0.11 | 0.89 | -1.09 | -1.06 | -1.09 |
| 69 | P16332 | Mut | Methylmalonyl-Coenzyme A mutase | 0.01 | 0.028 | 0.2 | 0.29 | -1.04 | -1.14 | -1.33 |
| Carbohydrate metabolism | | | | | | | | | | |
| 49 | P13707 | Gpd1 | Glycerol-3-phosphate dehydrogenase [NAD+]. cytoplasmic | 0.062 | 0.014 | 0.093 | 0.9 | 1.1 | 1.09 | 1.13 |
| 82 | Q91Y97 | Aldob | Fructose-bisphosphate aldolase B | 0.087 | 0.042 | 0.6 | 0.083 | -1.05 | 1.16 | 1.13 |

| 4 | P17182 | Eno1 | Alpha enolase | 0.0024 | 0.00028 | 0.47 | 0.052 | 1.02 | 1.11** | 1.05 |
|---|--------|------|---------------|--------|---------|------|-------|------|--------|------|
| 25 | Q9QXD6 | Fbp1 | Fructose-1.6-bisphosphatase | 0.001 | 0.0047 | 0.0009 | 0.4 | 1.04 | 1.1* | 1.04 |
| 58 | Q9DBJ1. | Pgam1 | Phosphoglycerate mutase 1 | 0.0075 | 0.018 | 0.0047 | 0.54 | 1.07 | 1.02 | 1.06 |
| 30 | P53657 | Pklr | Pyruvate kinase. isozymes R/L | 0.036 | 0.0058 | 0.046 | 0.17 | 1.07 | 1.24** | 1.07 |
| 85 | Q93092 | Taldo1 | Transaldolase | 0.038 | 0.045 | 0.18 | 0.061 | -1.04 | 1.1 | 1.13 |
| 50 | P97328 | Khk | Ketohexokinase | 0.073 | 0.014 | 0.75 | 0.15 | -1.01 | 1.15 | 1.14 |
| 93 | Q9DBB8 | Dhdh | Trans-1.2-dihydrobenzene-1.2-diol dehydrogenase | 0.037 | 0.22 | 0.038 | 0.085 | -1.05 | 1.09 | 1.07 |
| 88 | Q9JLJ2 | Aldh9a1 | 4-trimethylaminobutyraldehyde dehydrogenase | 0.19 | 0.05 | 0.87 | 0.18 | -1.02 | 1.12 | 1.09 |
| Urea cycle | | | | | | | | | | |
| 17 | Q61176 | Arg1 | Arginase-1 | 0.0069 | 0.0025 | 0.04 | 0.24 | 1.02 | 1.12* | 1.11 |
| 78 | Q61176 | Arg1 | Arginase-1 | 0.25 | 0.038 | 0.52 | 0.61 | -1.12 | -1.1 | -1.03 |
| 42 | P16460 | Ass1 | Argininosuccinate synthase | 0.15 | 0.011 | 0.62 | 0.8 | -1.18 | -1.22 | -1.29 |
| 86 | P16460 | Ass1 | Argininosuccinate synthase | 0.3 | 0.049 | 0.65 | 0.55 | -1.12 | -1.16 | -1.35 |
| 3 | Q8C196 | Cps1 | Carbamoyl-phosphate synthase I | 0.0049 | 0.00021 | 0.9 | 0.36 | -1.31** | -1.15 | -1.18 |
| 9 | Q8C196 | Cps1 | Carbamoyl-phosphate synthase I | 0.014 | 0.00081 | 0.52 | 0.37 | -1.29** | -1.13 | -1.14 |
| 11 | P26443 | Glud1 | Glutamate dehydrogenase 1. mitochondrial precursor | 0.026 | 0.0011 | 0.54 | 0.87 | -1.13 | -1.13 | -1.18 |
| Cholesterol and lipid metabolic processes | | | | | | | | | | |
| 12 | Q920E5 | Fdps | Farnesyl pyrophosphate synthetase | 0.0032 | 0.0012 | 0.31 | 0.019 | -1.05 | 1.37* | 1.65** |
| 66 | Q920E5 | Fdps | Farnesyl pyrophosphate synthetase | 0.064 | 0.026 | 0.091 | 0.51 | 1.07 | 1.13 | 1.32 |
| 19 | P52430 | Pon1 | Serum paraoxonase/arylesterase 1 | 0.048 | 0.0033 | 0.72 | 0.4 | -1.15 | -1.36* | -1.12 |
| 55 | Q9QXE0 | Hacl1 | 2-hydroxyphytanoyl-CoA lyase | 0.097 | 0.015 | 0.38 | 0.41 | 1.05 | 1.15 | 1.07 |
| 45 | P50544 | Acadvl | Acyl-CoA dehydrogenase. very-long-chain specific. mitochondrial precursor | 0.02 | 0.012 | 0.019 | 0.87 | -1.08 | -1.13 | -1.11 |
| 81 | Q8VCW8 | Acsf2 | Acyl-CoA synthetase family member 2. mitochondrial | 0.043 | 0.042 | 0.19 | 0.1 | -1.01 | 1.19 | 1.06* |
| 26 | Q8BWT1 | Acaa2 | 3-ketoacyl-CoA thiolase. mitochondrial | 0.041 | 0.0048 | 0.31 | 0.42 | -1.1 | -1.04 | -1.13 |

| 68 | Q8VCC1 | Hpgd | 5-hydroxyprostaglandin dehydrogenase [NAD+] | 0.16 | 0.027 | 0.91 | 0.29 | 1.1 | 1.43 | 1.14 |
| 2 | P06801 | Me1 | NADP-dependent malic enzyme | 0.0029 | 0.00019 | 0.13 | 0.53 | 1.16 | 1.26** | 1.14 |
| 37 | Q91V92 | Acly | ATP citrate lyase | 0.036 | 0.0088 | 0.38 | 0.083 | -1.01 | 1.22* | 1.17 |
| 35 | P56480 | Atp5b | ATP synthase beta chain. mitochondrial precursor | 0.033 | 0.0081 | 0.067 | 0.8 | -1.09 | -1.05 | -1.1 |
| Protein metabolic processes | | | | | | | | | | |
| 80 | Q8BWY3 | Etf1 | Eukaryotic peptide chain release factor subunit 1 | 0.05 | 0.041 | 0.64 | 0.035 | 1.05 | -1.42** | -1.1 |
| 43 | P49722 | Psma2 | Proteasome subunit alpha type-2 | 0.12 | 0.011 | 0.67 | 0.48 | 1.04 | 1.13 | 1.12 |
| 64 | O88685 | Psmc3 | 26S protease regulatory subunit 6A | 0.12 | 0.023 | 0.88 | 0.18 | 1.01 | 1.13 | 1.36* |
| 77 | P62334 | Psmc6 | 26S protease regulatory subunit S10B | 0.0032 | 0.038 | 6E-05 | 0.52 | -1.03 | -1.09 | -1.03 |
| 46 | P97371 | Psme1 | Proteasome activator complex subunit 1 | 0.15 | 0.013 | 0.58 | 0.77 | 1.07 | 1.11 | 1.14 |
| 75 | Q9D0R2 | Tars | Threonyl-tRNA synthetase. cytoplasmic | 0.047 | 0.033 | 0.034 | 0.75 | 1.06 | 1.03 | 1.08 |
| Other metabolic processes | | | | | | | | | | |
| 92 | Q80X81 | Acat3 | acetyl-Coenzyme A acetyltransferase 3 | 0.03 | 0.12 | 0.29 | 0.015 | -1.07 | 1.12 | 1.08 |
| 62 | P97355 | Srm | Spermidine synthase | 0.11 | 0.021 | 0.28 | 0.36 | 1.25 | 1.06 | 1.34 |
| 14 | Q99MR8 | Mccc1 | Methylcrotonoyl-CoA carboxylase alpha chain. mitochondrial precursor | 0.0094 | 0.0014 | 0.0049 | 0.08 | -1.15** | -1.09 | -1.01 |
| 6 | P40142 | Tkt | Transketolase | 0.00088 | 0.00044 | 0.0091 | 0.16 | 1.03 | 1.14** | 1.13 |
| 23 | P40142 | Tkt | Transketolase | 0.014 | 0.004 | 0.11 | 0.29 | 1.14 | 1.5* | 1.25 |
| 22 | Q99LB7 | Sardh | Sarcosine dehydrogenase. mitochondrial precursor | 0.026 | 0.0038 | 0.11 | 0.72 | -1.07 | -1.05 | -1.1 |
| 54 | Q9DBT9 | ME2GLYDH | Dimethylglycine dehydrogenase. mitochondrial precursor | 0.17 | 0.015 | 0.58 | 0.73 | -1.14 | -1.06 | -1.09 |
| 27 | Q8VC30 | Dak | Bifunctional ATP-dependent dihydroxyacetone kinase/FAD-AMP lyase | 0.023 | 0.0048 | 0.42 | 0.1 | 1 | 1.28* | 1.26 |
| 70 | Q8VC30 | Dak | Bifunctional ATP-dependent dihydroxyacetone kinase/FAD-AMP lyase | 0.077 | 0.028 | 0.22 | 0.24 | 1 | 1.14 | 1.08 |
| 63 | Q9CWS0 | Ddah1 | NG.NG-dimethylarginine dimethylaminohydrolase 1 | 0.12 | 0.021 | 0.14 | 0.79 | 1.05 | 1.1 | 1.07 |

| 24 | P52196 | Tst | Thiosulfate sulfurtransferase | 0.0097 | 0.0041 | 0.025 | 0.5 | 1.19 | 1.38 | 1.07 |
|----|--------|-----|------------------------------|--------|--------|-------|-----|------|------|------|
| 94 | P00920 | Ca2 | Carbonic anhydrase 2 | 0.000071 | 0.32 | 5E-06 | 0.98 | 1.06 | 1.07 | 1.04 |
| 10 | Q78JT3 | Haao | 3-hydroxyanthranilate 3.4-dioxygenase | 0.012 | 0.001 | 0.46 | 0.22 | 1.03 | 1.13 | 1.14* |
| 76 | Q922D8 | Mthfd1 | C-1-tetrahydrofolate synthase. cytoplasmic | 0.076 | 0.034 | 0.2 | 0.21 | -1.02 | 1.21 | 1.29 |
| Chaperone | | | | | | | | | | |
| 71 | P38647 | GRP 75 | Stress-70 protein. mitochondrial precursor | 0.0013 | 0.03 | 0.0003 | 0.58 | -1.11 | -1.03 | -1.11 |
| 36 | P63038 | Hspd1 | 60 kDa heat shock protein. mitochondrial precursor | 0.013 | 0.0085 | 0.014 | 0.78 | -1.09 | -1.11 | -1.06 |
| 67 | P63038 | Hspd1 | 60 kDa heat shock protein. mitochondrial precursor | 0.23 | 0.027 | 0.44 | 0.89 | -1.16 | -1.12 | -1.09 |
| 57 | Q8CGK3 | Lonp1 | Lon protease homolog | 0.16 | 0.017 | 0.87 | 0.41 | -1.08 | -1.04 | -1.16 |
| 79 | Q8CGK3 | Lonp1 | Lon protease homolog | 0.064 | 0.038 | 0.083 | 0.38 | -1.01 | -1.04 | -1.08 |
| 60 | P17742 | Ppia | Peptidyl-prolyl cis-trans isomerase | 0.08 | 0.021 | 0.23 | 0.33 | 1.04 | 1.19 | 1.07 |
| 95 | P24369 | Ppib | Peptidyl-prolyl cis-trans isomerase B | 0.021 | 0.36 | 0.079 | 0.014 | -1.03 | -1.23 | 1.14 |
| 8 | P09103 | P4hb | Protein disulfide-isomerase | 0.005 | 0.00081 | 0.059 | 0.38 | 1.17 | 1.1 | 1.27** |
| Secreted | | | | | | | | | | |
| 89 | P07724 | Alb | Serum albumin precursor | 0.00019 | 0.061 | 5E-05 | 0.12 | -1.1 | 1.03 | -1.18 |
| 44 | Q92II1 | Tf | Serotransferrin precursor | 0.01 | 0.011 | 0.012 | 0.45 | -1.06 | -1.26 | -1.19 |
| 83 | Q92II1 | Tf | Serotransferrin precursor | 0.036 | 0.043 | 0.35 | 0.033 | 1.13 | -1.29 | -1.4* |
| 87 | Q92II1 | Tf | Serotransferrin precursor | 0.15 | 0.049 | 0.94 | 0.12 | 1.05 | -1.21 | -1.31 |
| 90 | P04938 | Mup8 and 10 | Major urinary proteins 11 and 8 | 0.043 | 0.076 | 0.082 | 0.19 | -1.07 | -1.7 | -1.05 |
| cytoskeleton | | | | | | | | | | |
| 29 | P40124 | Cap1 | Adenylyl cyclase-associated protein 1 | 0.042 | 0.0054 | 0.27 | 0.43 | -1.39 | -1.3 | -1.1 |
| 20 | P68134 | Acta1 | Actin. alpha skeletal muscle | 0.048 | 0.0033 | 0.72 | 0.4 | -1.15 | -1.36* | -1.12 |
| Xenobiotic metabolism | | | | | | | | | | |
| 84 | P24472 | Gsta4 | Glutathione S-transferase 5.7 | 0.13 | 0.044 | 0.19 | 0.48 | -1.04 | -1.1 | -1.22 |
| 1 | P15626 | Gstm2 | Glutathione S-transferase Mu 2 | 0.00004 | 5.10E-06 | 0.26 | 0.005 | 1.04 | 1.56 | 1.66** |
| 52 | O35660 | Gstm6 | Glutathione S-transferase Mu 6 | 0.11 | 0.015 | 0.78 | 0.25 | 1.03 | 1.17* | 1.08 |

| | | | | | | | | | | |
|---|---|---|---|---|---|---|---|---|---|---|
| 61 | P19157 | Gstp1 | Glutathione S-transferase P 1 | 0.078 | 0.021 | 0.34 | 0.35 | -1.04 | -1.32 | -1.24 |
| 28 | Q9WVL0 | Gstz1 | Maleylacetoacetate isomerase | 0.032 | 0.0052 | 0.14 | 0.54 | 1.05 | 1.12 | 1.08 |
| 21 | P08228 | Sod1 | Superoxide dismutase [Cu-Zn] | 0.042 | 0.0034 | 0.48 | 0.45 | 1.08 | 1.14 | 1.06 |
| 18 | P09671 | Sod2 | Superoxide dismutase | 0.033 | 0.0031 | 0.56 | 0.28 | -1.02 | -1.08** | -1.04 |
| 51 | Q9QXF8 | Gnmt | Glycine N-methyltransferase | 0.047 | 0.014 | 0.22 | 0.35 | 1.02 | 1.16 | 1.14 |
| 96 | Q9QXF8 | Gnmt | Glycine N-methyltransferase | 0.023 | 0.9 | 0.0045 | 0.33 | -1.09 | 1.09 | -1.03 |
| 74 | P40936 | Inmt | Indolethylamine N-methyltransferase | 0.094 | 0.031 | 0.81 | 0.098 | 1.07 | 1.4** | 1.01 |
| 16 | O55060 | Tpmt | Thiopurine S-methyltransferase | 0.02 | 0.0018 | 0.68 | 0.19 | 1.09 | 1.05 | 1.2** |
| 15 | Q91VF2 | Hnmt | Histamine N-methyltransferase | 0.038 | 0.0015 | 0.7 | 0.82 | 1.16 | 1.22 | 1.25 |
| 91 | P50247 | Ahcy | Adenosylhomocysteinase | 0.0044 | 0.092 | 0.0003 | 0.02 | 1.2 | -1.12 | 1.18 |
| 34 | Q60967 | Papss1 | Bifunctional 3'-phosphoadenosine 5'-phosphosulfate synthase 2 | 0.038 | 0.0075 | 0.23 | 0.27 | 1.07 | 1.27* | 1.1 |
| 33 | P26443 | Glud1 | Glutamate dehydrogenase 1. mitochondrial precursor | 0.0043 | 0.0068 | 0.035 | 0.72 | -1.07 | -1.1 | -1.11* |
| Apoptosis | | | | | | | | | | |
| 65 | Q9Z0X1 | Aifm1 | Programmed cell death protein 8. mitochondrial precursor | 0.074 | 0.024 | 0.012 | 0.51 | -1.11 | -1.03 | -1.05 |
| 47 | Q91VD9 | Ndufs1 | NADH-ubiquinone oxidoreductase 75 kDa subunit. mitochondrial | 0.0063 | 0.013 | 0.012 | 0.13 | -1.09 | -1.01 | -1.17* |
| 53 | P05784 | Krt18 | Keratin. type I cytoskeletal 18 | 0.063 | 0.015 | 0.23 | 0.31 | 1.03 | 1.18 | 1.27 |
| Not listed | | | | | | | | | | |
| | | | | | | | | | | |
| 40 | Q00896 | Serpina1c | Alpha-1-antitrypsin 1-3 | 0.11 | 0.0098 | 0.62 | 0.56 | -1.1 | -1.34 | -1.29 |
| 31 | Q00897 | Serpina1d | Alpha-1-antitrypsin 1-4 precursor | 0.004 | 0.0065 | 0.0033 | 0.79 | -1.13 | -1.2 | -1.14 |
| 73 | P00920 | Ca2 | Carbonic anhydrase 2 | 0.002 | 0.031 | 3E-05 | 0.62 | 1.1 | 1.21 | 1.07 |
| 5 | Q01768 | Nme2 | Nucleoside diphosphate kinase B | 0.0053 | 0.00028 | 0.2 | 0.69 | 1.11 | 1.08 | 1.13* |
| 7 | Q63836 | Selenbp2 | Selenium-binding protein 2 | 0.001 | 0.00079 | 0.29 | 0.004 | -1.03 | 1.16** | 1.16** |
| 48 | Q9QYG0 | Ndrg2 | Isoform 1 of Protein NDRG2 | 0.14 | 0.013 | 0.8 | 0.42 | -1.09 | 1.06* | -1.3 |
| 13 | Q8R086 | Suox | Sulfite oxidase. mitochondrial precursor | 0.00061 | 0.0013 | 0.0013 | 0.22 | -1.09 | -1.08 | -1.22** |

| 41 | Q9CZ13 | Uqcrc1 | Ubiquinol-cytochrome-c reductase complex core protein I. mitochondrial precursor | 0.15 | 0.01 | 1 | 0.57 | 1.08 | -1.03 | -1.06 |
| 38 | P70296 | Pebp1 | Phosphatidylethanolamine-binding protein 1 | 0.079 | 0.0093 | 0.22 | 0.97 | 1.13 | 1.15 | 1.14 |

**Table 1:** Protein identification of differentially expressed proteins in from mouse liver after exposure to CsA after 4, 11 and 25 days. [1]P-value from one way ANOVA statistical test between the six groups with each four biological replicates. [2]P-value from two way ANOVA (treatment) statistical test between the six groups, which indicates the differences between the control and exposed groups. [3]P-value from two way ANOVA (time) statistical test between the six groups, which indicates the differences between the day 4, 11 and 25. [4]P-value from two way ANOVA (interaction) statistical test between the six groups, which indicates the interaction between time and treatment. [5]The difference in the standardized abundance of the proteins is expressed as the fold change between the control (C) and the treated groups (T). The fold change is calculated by taking the means of standardized volume values for the protein spot in the corresponding groups (C=control, CsA=cyclosporin A, 4=day 4, 11=day 11, 25=day25), values are calculated as T/C and displayed in the range of +1 to + ∞ for increases in expression and calculated as-C/T and displayed in the range of -∞ to -1 for decreased expression. **Indicates significant fold changes ($P \leq 0.05$) between the control and the treated group, calculated with a multiple comparison test. *Indicates significant fold changes ($P \leq 0.1$) between the control and the treated group, calculated with a multiple comparison test.

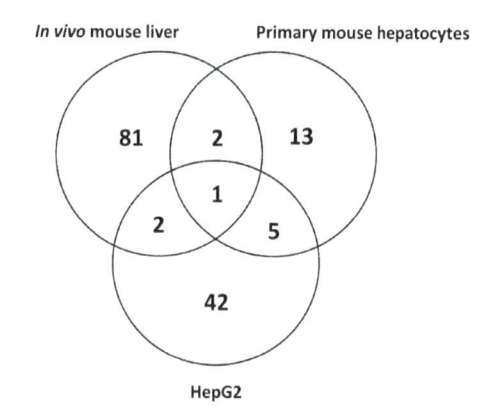

**Figure 4:** Venn diagram of the significant differentially expressed proteins induced by CsA in *in vivo* mouse liver, HepG2 and primary mouse hepatocytes.

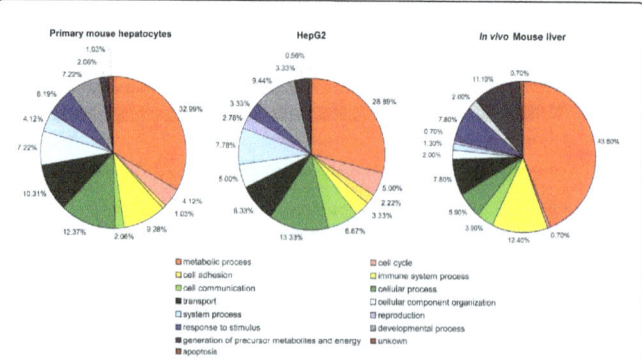

**Figure 5:** Classification of the differentially expressed proteins in primary mouse hepatocytes, HepG2 and liver after exposure to CsA with the Panther classification system (http://www.pantherdb.org).

| Cluster | Function | Enrichment Score | *in vivo* | PMH | HepG2 |
|---|---|---|---|---|---|
| 1 | ATP-binding | 9.62041 | 40 | 5 | 16 |
| 2 | Carbohydrate metabolism | 9.293973 | 8 | 1 | 9 |
| 3 | metal binding | 7.999105 | 10 | 1 | 1 |
| 4 | Methyltransferases | 5.247008 | 4 | 1 | 0 |
| 5 | metal binding | 4.844126 | 8 | 2 | 5 |
| 6 | NAD cofactor | 4.807059 | 1 | 0 | 3 |
| 7 | Detoxification glutathione S-transferase | 4.368559 | 5 | 0 | 0 |
| 8 | Chaperone activity | 3.910156 | 1 | 7 | 9 |
| 9 | Cytoskelet | 3.231529 | 1 | 1 | 5 |
| 10 | mRNA processing | 2.748475 | 0 | 0 | 5 |
| 11 | Protein transport | 1.503542 | 1 | 1 | 1 |
| 12 | response to organic substrate | 0.489311 | 2 | 1 | 0 |

**Table 2:** Gene classification of the differentially expressed proteins after CsA treatment *in vivo*, primary mouse hepatocytes and HepG2.

## Discussion

The aim of this study was to identify cholestatic-specific mechanisms *in vivo*, with use of proteomics. In addition, an *in vitro-in vivo* comparison of CsA-induced protein expression profiles was established by comparing these results with the results from our previous *in vitro* studies with HepG2 and primary mouse hepatocytes [9,10] For this purpose, we analyzed the hepatic protein expression in C57BL/6 mice after CsA-induced cholestasis. The cholestatic phenotype was established after 25 days and confirmed by histopathology and serum parameters, which allowed us to search for cholestatic-specific mechanisms *in vivo*.

## Differential protein expression in mice after CsA treatment

CsA inhibits the bile salt export pump (ABCB11), multidrug resistance protein 2 (ABCC2) and P-glycoprotein (ABCB1) in the canalicular membrane vesicles. These ATP Binding Cassette transporters (ABC transporters) are responsible for the bile secretion into the bile canaliculus [14]. Therefore, inhibition of these transport proteins causes the hepatic accumulation of bile salts resulting in cholestasis [15]. Previous studies suggest that accumulated bile acids induce oxidative stress and can cause mitochondrial dysfunction in the liver [16]. Moreover, CsA induced in vitro as well as in vivo oxidative stress, increases lipid peroxidation and depletes the hepatic pool of glutathione [17,18] Superoxide is one of the main reactive oxygen species in the cell which can be converted into oxygen and hydrogen peroxide by superoxide dismutase. In our study cytoplasmatic superoxide dismutase 1 was up-regulated after cyclopsorin A treatment, while mitochondrial superoxide dismutase 2 was down-regulated, indicating that CsA induced oxidative stress and mitochondrial dysfunction. Indications for mitochondrial dysfunction are already visible after 4 days of CsA treatment, since all proteins with a significantly differential expression are mitochondrial.

Furthermore, the down-regulation of several enzymes contributing the TCA-cycle like aconitate hydratase, succinyl-CoA ligase (ADP-forming) subunit beta and methylmalonyl-coenzyme A mutase suggest a deficient ATP production by the mitochondria. Previously, others have demonstrated an ATP reduction in hepatocytes after exposure to necrotic concentrations of toxic bile salts [19,20]. The reduced ATP was directly due to mitochondrial dysfunction as glycolytic ATP generation was intact [20]. In our study several proteins from the glycolysis pathway were found to be up-regulated. This suggests a compensatory mechanism for mitochondrial dysfunction via the glycolytic pathway.

Glutamate dehydrogenase is responsible for the conversion of glutamate to α-ketoglutarate and ammonium, which will bled off to the urea-cycle. The first step of the urea cycle requires ATP for the conversion of $NH_4^+$ and $HCO_3^-$ to carbamoyl phosphate, catalyzed by carbamoyl-phosphate synthase (Cps1). In a later step, ATP is necessary for the conversion of citrulline and aspartate in argininosuccinate, catalyzed by argininosuccinate synthase (Ass1). In our study glutamate dehydrogenase 1, Ass1 and Cps1, were all down-regulated together with other enzymes from the urea cycle.

Rare autosomal recessive disorders of the urea cycle like arginase deficiency and citrin deficiency are associated with neonatal intrahepatic cholestasis [21,22]. Neonatal intrahepatic cholestasis is defined as impaired bilirubin excretion, resulting in jaundice and conjugated hyperbilirubinemia, detected either in a newborn or an infant up to 4 months old [21-23]. The pathogenesis of cholestasis in these urea cycle disorders remains unclear, probably the combination of a primary mitochondrial defect and a delayed maturity of bile acid metabolism, may form a vicious circle in transient neonatal intrahepatic cholestasis [22]. A similar mechanism for cholestasis as observed in neonatal intrahepatic cholestasis may explain down-regulation of enzymes from the urea cycle in our study.

Methylation enzymes indolethylamine N-methyltransferase (Inmt), thiopurine S-methyltransferase, glycine N-methyltransferase and histamine N-methyltransferase showed an increased expression after CsA treatment. Methyl conjugation is mainly used for the metabolism of small endogenous compounds such as epinephrine, norepinephrine, dopamine, and histamine but is also involved in the metabolism of

macromolecules such as nucleic acids and in the biotransformation of certain drugs [24]. In contrast to other conjugative reactions, methylation leads to less polar compounds that may be less readily excreted from the body [24]. Inmt, thiopurine S-methyltransferase, glycine N-methyltransferase and histamine N-methyltransferase all use S-adenosylmethionine as methyldonor. Previously, it was shown that S-adenosylmethionine protects against CsA [25-26], chlorpromazine [27] and ethenylestradiol-induced cholestasis [28]. Cholestatic rat liver, induced by common bile duct ligation, exhibited increased enzymatic activities of Inmt and thiol methyltransferase [29].

The increased expression of these N-methyltransferases results in an increased conversion of S-adenosylmethionine to S-adenosyl-homocysteine, which in turn is converted in homocysteine and adenosine by adenosylhomocysteinase, here differentially expressed. The increased conversion of S-adenosylmethionine and S-adenosyl-homocystein activates the trans-sulfuration pathway, leading to the formation of glutathione [27]. Glutathione is responsible for the detoxification of various compounds to protect the cells from oxidative stress. Moreover it plays an important role in bile formation [30]. Previously it has been demonstrated that glutathione is depleted during cholestasis, therefore activation of the trans-sulfuration pathway is necessary to maintain the glutathione levels in the cholestasic liver [30,31]. In addition, sulfite oxidase and bifunctional 3'-phosphoadenosine 5'-phosphosulfate synthase 2, other enzymes of the trans-sulfuration pathway, were also differentially expressed.

Glutathione is a substrate of both conjugation and reduction reactions, catalyzed by glutathione S-transferase enzymes. Mice exposed to CsA, show a differential expression of several glutathione S-transferases (GSTs). GSTs are not only important phase II detoxification enzymes; they are able to bind bile acids and are thought to play a role in the intracellular trafficking of bile acids [32].

Furthermore, CsA induced the differential expression of proteins related to cholesterol biosynthesis and lipid metabolism. Bile acid synthesis is the main route for cholesterol metabolism and is initiated by cholesterol 7α-hydroxylase (CYP7A1). In our study Farnesyl diphosphate synthase (Fdps) showed an increased expression after 11 days of CsA exposure. Fdps is responsible for the formation of farnesyldiphosphate, a key intermediate in cholesterol synthesis and protein farnesylation. Previously drug-induced cholestasis was associated with an increased hepatic cholesterol synthesis, which is in line with the presently observed Fdps expression [33].

In addition, cholesterol synthesis requires the presence of cytosolic acetyl-coA. Previously, we mentioned a down-regulation of the TCA-cycle, a mitochondrial source of acetyl-coA. The up-regulation of citrate-lyase and NADP-dependent malic enzyme in our study, suggests a drain of mitochondrial acetyl-coA to the cytosol for cholesterol synthesis.

Furthermore, an increased cholesterol synthesis is associated with a decreased CYP7A1 expression as a protective adaptive response to reduce cellular bile accumulation [33]. Probably these two mechanisms are the cause of high plasma cholesterol in cholestasis. In a previous study, in which transcriptomics analysis was performed on liver samples used for proteome analysis in this study, CYP7A1 down-regulation was observed as one of the strongest effects upon progression of cholestasis in mice and was interpreted as an adaptive response [34].

Serum paraoxonase/arylesterase 1 (Pon1) is an antioxidant enzyme responsible for the detoxification of organophosphates and prevention of low-density lipoprotein oxidative modification. Our study shows a down-regulation of Pon1 after CsA treatment. Rats treated with $CCl_4$ showed a reduced activity of hepatic Pon1 together with increased lipid peroxidation [35]. Furthermore, Pon1 was down-regulated in the protein extract from rat liver exposed to acetaminophen [36] However, Pon1 failed as candidate marker for drug-induced hepatotoxicity, because it was not consistently altered in response to several hepatotoxicants [37].

### *In vivo-in vitro* comparison

Previously we analyzed CsA-induced cholestasis in HepG2 cells [9] and in primary mouse hepatocytes [10]. An *in vivo-in vitro* comparison of CsA-induced hepatotoxicity based on single protein expression is difficult, partly because there is only a small overlap in the differentially expressed proteins from the different models (Figure 4). Therefore the differentially expressed proteins from these models were classified based on the GO-terms with the Panther classification system. This classification revealed a similar outcome for HepG2 and primary mouse hepatocytes. The majority of the differentially expressed proteins are involved in metabolic processes, cellular processes and transport. Similar processes between the analyzed *in vitro* systems are cell cycle, cellular processes, developmental processes and cell adhesion (Figure 5). In all three models CsA altered proteins belonging to transport and a response to stimulus (Figure 5). For a more detailed overview the proteins were clustered according to their function with DAVID Bioinformatics Resources 6.7. Cluster 1, 2 and 5 contain differentially expressed proteins from the three models. Cluster 1 involves ATP-binding and mitochondrial proteins and cluster 2 contains proteins from carbohydrate metabolism. Cluster 5 refers to binding of metal ions, which is a characteristic of many metabolic enzymes like the glycolytic enzymes. These clusters show that CsA induces *in vivo* as well as *in vitro* mitochondrial dysfunction and changes in the energy metabolism, as also described before. Mitochondria are critical targets for drug toxicity; therefore mitochondrial dysfunction and oxidative stress are often seen in drug-induced hepatotoxicity [38]. The differential expressions of proteins from energy metabolism are probably a first indication of a toxicological response. However, several proteins from energy metabolism are often detected in comparative proteomics and considered as proteins from a general stress response [39]. Therefore using those proteins as specific markers for cholestasis should be done with caution.

Methyltransferases which are described earlier as detoxifying enzymes constitute cluster 4. Almost all methyltransferases were detected only *in vivo*, however Inmt was also detected in primary mouse hepatocytes. Furthermore, *in vivo* CsA induced cholestasis was accompanied with the differential expression of glutathione-S-transferases (cluster 7). In primary mouse hepatocytes we have also detected some glutathione-S-transferases, although they were not significantly changed after CsA treatment and were therefore excluded from the cluster analysis. We believe that both methyltransferases and glutathione-S-transfereses are important detoxification proteins in CsA-induced cholestasis. These proteins were mainly detected *in vivo* but some also in primary mouse hepatocytes. However, they were not observed in HepG2, suggesting an under-representation of drug-metabolizing enzymes in HepG2 [40,41].

Characteristic for HepG2 cells, proteins responsible for mRNA processing were differentially expressed (cluster 10). These proteins have central roles in DNA repair, telomere elongation, cell signaling

and in regulating gene expression at transcriptional and translational level [42]. Furthermore, heterogeneous nuclear ribonucleoproteins (hnRNPs) play a role in tumor development and are up-regulated in various cancers [42]. Previously it was shown that carcinoma cell lines including HepG2 cells have a higher expression of hnRNPs than human intestinal epithelium [43]. Therefore the expression of these proteins can be ascribed to the carcinoma character of the HepG2 cell line. Apparently CsA induced a down-regulation of these proteins and probably decreased cell proliferation.

*In vitro*, CsA mainly induced the differential expression of chaperone proteins (cluster 8), while this was less observed *in vivo*. Previously we hypothesized that CsA induces ER stress, with an altered chaperone activity together with a disturbed protein transport resulting in a decreased protein secretion [9]. However, this reaction of CsA seems characteristic for *in vitro* models. Possibly *in vitro* cell cultures are more sensitive because they are in direct contact with the toxicant and they function independent from other cells/organs.

Our analysis identified the similarities and differences in *in vitro* and *in vivo* models with respect to the response to CsA induced hepatotoxicity. Previous studies have shown the potential of the current *in vitro* models to detect drug-induced hepatotoxicity [2,9,44]. However the different toxicant-induced responses between *in vivo* and *in vitro* models explain the current difficulties to validate *in vitro* biomarkers against *in vivo* models.

## Acknowledgments

This work was supported by the Netherlands Genomics Initiative/ Netherlands Organization for Scientific Research (NWO), [grant number: 050-060-510]. We thank Erik Royackers from the Biomedical Research Institute of Hasselt University for his technical support of the LC-MS/MS analysis. The authors thank Piet Beekhof and Dr. Eugene Janssen for clinical chemistry analyses and Joke Robinson for histopathology analyses.

## References

1. Kienhuis AS, Wortelboer HM, Maas WJ, van Herwijnen M, Kleinjans JC, et al. (2007) A sandwich-cultured rat hepatocyte system with increased metabolic competence evaluated by gene expression profiling. Toxicol In Vitro 21: 892-901.

2. Mathijs K, Kienhuis AS, Brauers KJ, Jennen DG, Lahoz A, et al. (2009) Assessing the metabolic competence of sandwich-cultured mouse primary hepatocytes. Drug Metab Dispos 37: 1305-1311.

3. Jennen DG, Magkoufopoulou C, Ketelslegers HB, van Herwijnen MH, Kleinjans JC, et al. (2010) Comparison of HepG2 and HepaRG by whole-genome gene expression analysis for the purpose of chemical hazard identification. Toxicol Sci 115: 66-79.

4. Kienhuis AS, van de Poll MC, Wortelboer H, van Herwijnen M, Gottschalk R, et al. (2009) Parallelogram approach using rat-human in vitro and rat in vivo toxicogenomics predicts acetaminophen-induced hepatotoxicity in humans. Toxicol Sci 107: 544-552.

5. Heijne WH, Jonker D, Stierum RH, van Ommen B, Groten JP (2005) Toxicogenomic analysis of gene expression changes in rat liver after a 28-day oral benzene exposure. Mutat Res 575: 85-101.

6. de Longueville F, Atienzar FA, Marcq L, Dufrane S, Evrard S, et al. (2003) Use of a low-density microarray for studying gene expression patterns induced by hepatotoxicants on primary cultures of rat hepatocytes. Toxicol Sci 75: 378-392.

7. Greenbaum D, Colangelo C, Williams K, Gerstein M (2003) Comparing protein abundance and mRNA expression levels on a genomic scale. Genome Biol 4: 117.

8. Minden J (2007) Comparative proteomics and difference gel electrophoresis. Biotechniques 43: 739, 741, 743 passim.

9. Van Summeren A, Renes J, Bouwman FG, Noben JP, van Delft JH, et al. (2011) Proteomics investigations of drug-induced hepatotoxicity in HepG2 cells. Toxicol Sci 120: 109-122.

10. Van Summeren A, Renes J, Lizarraga D, Bouwman FG, Noben JP, et al. (2013) Screening for drug-induced hepatotoxicity in primary mouse hepatocytes using acetaminophen, amiodarone, and cyclosporin a as model compounds: an omics-guided approach. OMICS 17: 71-83.

11. Rotolo FS, Branum GD, Bowers BA, Meyers WC (1986) Effect of cyclosporine on bile secretion in rats. Am J Surg 151: 35-40.

12. Bouwman FG, Claessens M, van Baak MA, Noben JP, Wang P, et al. (2009) The Physiologic Effects of Caloric Restriction Are Reflected in the in Vivo Adipocyte-Enriched Proteome of Overweight/Obese Subjects. J Proteome Res 8: 5532-5540.

13. Dumont D, Noben JP, Raus J, Stinissen P, Robben J (2004) Proteomic analysis of cerebrospinal fluid from multiple sclerosis patients. Proteomics 4: 2117-2124.

14. Trauner M, Boyer JL (2003) Bile salt transporters: molecular characterization, function, and regulation. Physiol Rev 83: 633-671.

15. Alrefai WA, Gill RK (2007) Bile acid transporters: structure, function, regulation and pathophysiological implications. Pharm Res 24: 1803-1823.

16. Kaplan MM (1994) Primary biliary cirrhosis--a first step in prolonging survival. N Engl J Med 330: 1386-1387.

17. Wolf A, Trendelenburg CF, Diez-Fernandez C, Prieto P, Houy S, et al. (1997) Cyclosporine A-induced oxidative stress in rat hepatocytes. J Pharmacol Exp Ther 280: 1328-1334.

18. Jimenez R, Galan AI, Gonzalez de Buitrago JM, Palomero J, Munoz ME (2000) Glutathione metabolism in cyclosporine A-treated rats: dose- and time-related changes in liver and kidney. Clin Exp Pharmacol Physiol 27: 991-996.

19. Spivey JR, Bronk SF, Gores GJ (1993) Glycochenodeoxycholate-induced lethal hepatocellular injury in rat hepatocytes. Role of ATP depletion and cytosolic free calcium. J Clin Invest 92: 17-24.

20. Gores GJ, Miyoshi H, Botla R, Aguilar HI, Bronk SF (1998) Induction of the mitochondrial permeability transition as a mechanism of liver injury during cholestasis: a potential role for mitochondrial proteases. Biochim Biophys Acta 1366: 167-75.

21. Gomes Martins E, Santos Silva E, Vilarinho S, Saudubray JM, Vilarinho L (2010) Neonatal cholestasis: an uncommon presentation of hyperargininemia. J Inherit Metab Dis 33 Suppl 3: S503-506.

22. Tazawa Y, Abukawa D, Sakamoto O, Nagata I, Murakami J, et al. (2005) A possible mechanism of neonatal intrahepatic cholestasis caused by citrin deficiency. Hepatol Res 31: 168-71.

23. Moyer V, Freese DK, Whitington PF, Olson AD, Brewer F, et al. (2004) Guideline for the evaluation of cholestatic jaundice in infants: recommendations of the North American Society for Pediatric Gastroenterology, Hepatology and Nutrition. J Pediatr Gastroenterol Nutr 39: 115-128.

24. Lohr JW, Willsky GR, Acara MA (1998) Renal drug metabolism. Pharmacol Rev 50: 107-141.

25. Galan AI, Munoz ME, Jimenez R (1999) S-Adenosylmethionine protects against cyclosporin A-induced alterations in rat liver plasma membrane fluidity and functions. J Pharmacol Exp Ther 290: 774-781.

26. Fernández E, Galán AI, Morán D, González-Buitrago JM, Muñoz ME, et al. (1995) Reversal of cyclosporine A-induced alterations in biliary secretion by S-adenosyl-L-methionine in rats. J Pharmacol Exp Ther 275: 442-449.

27. Friedel HA, Goa KL, Benfield P (1989) S-adenosyl-L-methionine. A review of its pharmacological properties and therapeutic potential in liver dysfunction and affective disorders in relation to its physiological role in cell metabolism. Drugs 38: 389-416.

28. Boelsterli UA, Rakhit G, Balazs T (1983) Modulation by S-adenosyl-L-methionine of hepatic Na+,K+-ATPase, membrane fluidity, and bile flow in rats with ethinyl estradiol-induced cholestasis. Hepatology 3: 12-17.

29. Kim YH, Joo 2nd (2001) Arylamine N-methyltransferase and thiol methyltransferase activities in cholestatic rat liver induced by common bile duct ligation. Exp Mol Med 33: 23-28.

30. Tiao MM, Lin TK, Wang PW, Chen JB, Liou CW (2009) The role of mitochondria in cholestatic liver injury. Chang Gung Med J 32: 346-353.

31. Vendemiale G, Grattagliano I, Lupo L, Memeo V, Altomare E (2002) Hepatic oxidative alterations in patients with extra-hepatic cholestasis. Effect of surgical drainage. J Hepatol 37: 601-605.

32. Agellon LB, Torchia EC (2000) Intracellular transport of bile acids. Biochim Biophys Acta 1486: 198-209.

33. Chisholm JW, Nation P, Dolphin PJ, Agellon LB (1999) High plasma cholesterol in drug-induced cholestasis is associated with enhanced hepatic cholesterol synthesis. Am J Physiol 276: G1165-73.

34. Kienhuis AS, Vitins AP, Pennings JL, Pronk TE, Speksnijder EN, et al. (2013) Cyclosporine A treated in vitro models induce cholestasis response through comparison of phenotype-directed gene expression analysis of in vivo Cyclosporine A-induced cholestasis. Toxicol Lett 221: 225-236.

35. Ferre N, Camps J, Cabre M, Paul A, Joven J (2001) Hepatic paraoxonase activity alterations and free radical production in rats with experimental cirrhosis. Metabolism 50: 997-1000.

36. Amacher DE, Adler R, Herath A, Townsend RR (2005) Use of proteomic methods to identify serum biomarkers associated with rat liver toxicity or hypertrophy. Clin Chem 51: 1796-1803.

37. Adler M, Hoffmann D, Ellinger-Ziegelbauer H, Hewitt P, Matheis K, et al. (2010) Assessment of candidate biomarkers of drug-induced hepatobiliary injury in preclinical toxicity studies. Toxicol Lett 196: 1-11.

38. Jaeschke H, McGill MR, Ramachandran A (2012) Oxidant stress, mitochondria, and cell death mechanisms in drug-induced liver injury: lessons learned from acetaminophen hepatotoxicity. Drug Metab Rev 44: 88-106.

39. Wang P, Bouwman FG, Mariman EC (2009) Generally detected proteins in comparative proteomics--a matter of cellular stress response? Proteomics 9: 2955-2966.

40. Boess F, Kamber M, Romer S, Gasser R, Muller D, et al. (2003) Gene expression in two hepatic cell lines, cultured primary hepatocytes, and liver slices compared to the in vivo liver gene expression in rats: possible implications for toxicogenomics use of in vitro systems. Toxicol Sci 73: 386-402.

41. Wilkening S, Bader A (2003) Influence of culture time on the expression of drug-metabolizing enzymes in primary human hepatocytes and hepatoma cell line HepG2. J Biochem Mol Toxicol 17: 207-213.

42. Carpenter B, MacKay C, Alnabulsi A, MacKay M, Telfer C, et al. (2006) The roles of heterogeneous nuclear ribonucleoproteins in tumour development and progression. Biochim Biophys Acta 1765: 85-100.

43. Lenaerts K, Bouwman FG, Lamers WH, Renes J, Mariman EC (2007) Comparative proteomic analysis of cell lines and scrapings of the human intestinal epithelium. BMC Genomics 8: 91.

44. Wang K, Shindoh H, Inoue T, Horii I (2002) Advantages of in vitro cytotoxicity testing by using primary rat hepatocytes in comparison with established cell lines. J Toxicol Sci 27: 229-37.

# 28

# Cytotoxic and Anti-Inflammatory Activities of *Bursera* Species from Mexico

**Macdiel Acevedo**[1], **Pablo Nuñez**[1], **Leticia Gónzalez-Maya**[2], **Alexandre CardosoTaketa**[1] **and María Luisa Villarreal**[1*]

[1]*Centro de Investigación en Biotecnología, Universidad Autónoma del Estado de Morelos, Av. Universidad 1001, Col. Chamilpa, Cuernavaca Morelos , México*

[2]*Facultad de Farmacia, Universidad Autónoma del Estado de Morelos, Av. Universidad 1001, Col. Chamilpa, Cuernavaca, México*

*Corresponding author: María Luisa Villarreal, Centro de Investigación en Biotecnología, Universidad Autónoma del Estado de Morelos, Av. Universidad 1001, Col. Chamilpa, Cuernavaca Morelos, México, E-mail: luisav@uaem.mx

## Abstract

**Objective:** Organic extracts from nine species (eleven populations) of the *Bursera* genus native to Mexico, were investigated for cytotoxic and anti-inflammatory activities. The influence of the cytotoxic plant extracts on cell cycle progression and apoptosis were also analyzed.

**Materials and methods:** Cytotoxic activity from *B. ariensis* (Kunth) McVaugh and Rzed. Kew Bull (two populations), *B. bicolor* Engl., *B. lancifolia* Engl., *B. glabrifolia* Engl. (two populations), *B. fagaroides* (La Llave) Rez., Calderón and Medina, *B. linanoe* (La Llave) Rez., Calderón and Medina, *B. galeottiana* Engl., *B. kerberi* Engl., and *B. excelsa* Engl. were evaluated by the sulforhodamine B protein staining assay against four carcinoma cell lines: KB (nasopharyngeal), HF-6 (colon), MCF-7 (breast), and PC-3 (prostate), as well as on HFS-30 fibroblast normal skin cell line. Chloroform extracts from *B. ariensis* (two populations), *B. kerberi* and *B. galeottiana* were added to PC-3 cells to analyze percentage of cells in G1/S and G2/M phases by flow cytometric analysis, while apoptosis was determined in a fluorescence microscope. *In vivo* anti-inflammatory experiments were conducted through the 12-O-tetradecanoylphorbol-13-acetate (TPA) induced ear edema in mice.

**Results:** With the exception of *B. glabrifolia* and *B. excelsa*, hexane extracts of all the collected plant species displayed selective cytotoxic activity in at least one cell line. For the chloroform extracts, only *B. bicolor*, *B. kerberi*, *B. galeottiana*, and *B. fagaroides* exhibited cytotoxic activity, while for the ethyl acetate extracts *B. fagaroides* was the only plant displaying cytotoxic effect. There was no cytotoxic activity detected with methanol extracts. While *B. galeottiana* showed an important effect in G2/M arrest, induced apoptosis in PC-3 cells was detected with *B. ariensis* (two populations) and *B. galeottiana*. Important anti-inflammatory activity similar to the control indomethacin was displayed by *B. galeottiana*, *B. excelsa*, and *B. schlechtendalii*.

**Conclusion:** Findings demonstrated that the studied species possess pharmacological potential qualities for developing plant medicines.

**Keywords:** Cytotoxic; *Bursera*; Anti-inflammatory; Cell cycle, Apoptosis; Ethnomedical use

## Introduction

From the genus Bursera, approximately 80 of the 84 species growing in Mexico are endemic, and are one of the most abundant plant groups of the tropical dry forest [1]. In traditional Mexican medicine several *burseras* are used in the treatment of cancer, although the term "cancer" includes general conditions consistent with cancer symptomatology, i.e., inflammations, ulcers; and such dermatological conditions as hard swellings, abscesses, calluses, corns, warts and polyps [2]. Since pre-hispanic times "copal", the bark and resin from *Bursera* trees, has been employed in the treatment of cancer symptoms, as well as against some other conditions [3-5]. Some examples are the following: *B. excelsa* known as *pomo* or *tecomahaca* [6] is used to treat tumors, and muscle spasms [7]; *B. glabrifolia* known as *zomplante* is used to treat fever, inflammation and weakness in Oaxaca [8]; *B. galeottiana* known as *cuajiote colorado* is used as an analgesic, healing herb, and to treat abcesses [9]; *B. linanoe* known as *copal* is used in the treatment of gums inflammation [10]; the water extract of *B. fagaroides* known as *copalillo* is believed to have an anticancer effect [11]; *B. bicolor* known as *ticumaca* is used as a medicine to treat inflammation of the muscles [12,13]; *B. ariensis* known as *copal blanco* is used to treat cold and a disease called 'sacar el frío', which is a term related to inflammation [14], and *B. schlechtendalii* is used in the treatment of flu [15].

Results of previously conducted experiments on other *bursera* species demonstrated various biological activities. Against cancer, some of them have displayed cytotoxic action; for example, *B. bipinata*, *B. copallifera* and *B. fagaroides* were toxic against several human cancer cell lines that included nasopharyngeal, colon, breast and prostate carcinomas, while *B. graveolens* and *B. grandiflolia* were active against fibrosarcoma and epidermoid carcinoma, respectively [2,16]. Other studies with *B. microphylla*, *B. fagaroides*, *B. schlechtendalii*, *B. klugii*, and *B. morelensis* demonstrated antitumor actions against tumors transplanted in mice [11,17-20].

In the present investigation we studied nine Mexican species of the *Bursera* genus which, as mentioned above, are currently in popular use to treat patients with cancer symptomatology. Using traditional and still currently applied ethnomedical information, we conducted experimental analyses to study cytotoxic and anti-inflammatory activities that tend to validate their popular uses. We also determined the influence of the cytotoxic plant extracts on cell cycle progression and apoptosis.

To our knowledge, the eleven selected populations belonging to nine species have no previously documented investigations, and this new information opens up the possibility of advancing medicinal approaches from these natural Mexican autochthonous resources.

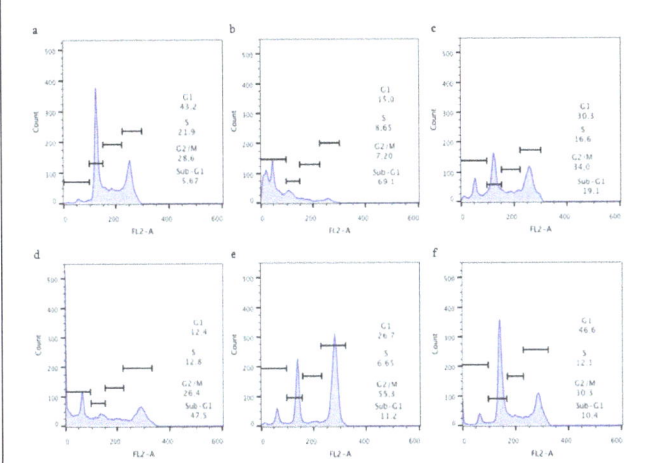

**Figure 1:** Percentage of PC-3 cells in G0/G1 and G2/M after treatments with the chloroform extracts of *B. ariensis* from the state of Mexico (c) *B. ariensis* from Morelos (d), B. kerberi (e), and B. galeottiana (f); in comparison with a negative control (vehicle, a) and a positive control (PTOX, b).

## Materials and Methods

### Plant material

Nine Mexican species (eleven plant populations) of the genus *Bursera* were included in this study. Seven populations were collected in the central part of the Mexican Republic. The species *B. ariensis* (Kunth) McVaugh and Rzed. Kew Bull., *B. bicolor* Engl., *B. glabrifolia* Engl., *B. fagaroides* (La Llave) Rez., Calderón and Medina, and *B. linanoe* (La Llave) Rez., Calderón and Medina were collected in the state of Morelos, while *B. kerberi* Engl. and *B. ariensis* (Kunth) McVaugh and Rzed. Kew Bull. Were collected in the state of Mexico. Four populations were collected in the southeast of Mexico: B. excelsa Engl. was collected in the state of Chiapas; from Oaxaca *B. glabrifolia* Engl. and *B. galeottiana* Engl. were collected, and *B. schlechtendalii* was collected in Puebla. It is important to point out that for *B. glabrifolia* two plant populations were collected, one in Morelos, and the other in the southeastern state of Oaxaca where it was noticed on an unplanned trip; as also happen in the case of a second collection for *B. ariensis*, with one collected in Morelos while the other was fortuitously found on an unplanned trip to Zacazonapan in the state of Mexico. All plant material was collected between September and November 2010. Voucher specimens have been deposited at the Herbarium of the Centro de Investigación en Biodiversidad y Conservación (CIByC), UAEM and were authentified by Dr. J. R. Bonilla-Barbosa (Table 1).

### Extraction

All bark of the plant material was air-dried and then pulverized with a grinder. The powdered plant material (10 g) was extracted with 100 mL of n-hexane (3x) in a sonicator for 30 min, and filtered at room temperature. To obtain three other extracts, the same procedure was applied but using first chloroform, then ethyl acetate followed by methanol. All of the extracts were then concentrated under reduced pressure at 40°C and stored at 4°C for later use.

### Reagents

RNase, Propidium iodide (PI) and Acridine orange (AO) were obtained from Molecular Probes, Life Technologies, Sigma-Aldrich, MO, USA. RPMI-1640, Fetal bovine serum (FBS), Trypsin- EDTA and NaHCO$_3$ were obtained from In vitrogen-GIBCO, Carlsbad, CA, USA.

| Botanical name | Local name | Coordinates of collection | Site of collection | Voucher specimen no. |
|---|---|---|---|---|
| B. ariensis | Copal blanco | 18°260'00"N 9°02'00"O | Cd. Ayala, elos | 27198 |
| B. bicolor | Ticumaca | 18°26'00"N 99°02'00"O | Cd. Ayala, Morelos | 27196 |
| B. glabrifolia | Copal | 18°26'00"N 99°02'00"O | Cd. Ayala, Morelos | 27200 |
| B. fagaroides | Copalillo | 18°26'00"N 99°02'00"O | Cd. Ayala, Morelos | 27199 |
| B. linanoe | Linaloe, Copal | 18°28'00"N 99°06'00"O | Tlaquiltenango, Morelos | 27197 |
| B. glabrifolia | Jiote blanco | 16°55'00"N 96°24'00"O | Mitla, Oaxaca | 27206 |
| B. galeottiana | Cuajilote colorado | 16°55'00"N 96°24'00"O | Mitla, Oaxaca | 27195 |
| B. kerberi | Copal | 19°05'00"N 100°15'00"O | Zacazonapan, México | 27205 |
| B. ariensis | Copalillo | 19°05'00"N 100°15'00"O | Zacazonapan, México | 27204 |
| B. excelsa | Pomo,Tecomahaca | 19°05'00"N 100°15'00"O | Tuxtla Gutierrez, Chiapas | 27203 |
| B. schlechtendalii | Copal | 18°45'00"N 100°15'00"O | Teotlaco, Puebla | 13297 |

**Table 1:** Collection data of the investigated Mexican *Bursera* species.

## Cytototoxic assay

Cytotoxicity of plant extracts was measured by the sulforhodamine B (SRB) (MP Biomedicals, LLC) protein staining assay [21] using KB (nasopharyngeal), HF-6 (colon), MCF-7 (breast), and PC-3 (prostate) cancer cell lines from ATCC, along with a normal skin fibroblast cell line (HFS-30), passage number 33. Cell cultures were maintained in RPMI-1640 medium (Sigma) supplemented with 10% fetal bovine serum (FBS), 5000 units/mL penicillin, 5 mg/mL streptomycin, 7.5% NaHCO$_3$, and cultured in a 96-well microtiter plate (10$^4$ cells/mL, 190 µL/well) at 37°C in a 5% CO$_2$-air atmosphere (100% humidity). The cells at the log phase of growth were treated in triplicate with various concentrations of the test extracts (0.16, 0.8, 4, and 20 µg/mL) that were dissolved in RPMI medium supplemented with 0.025% DMSO, and incubated for 72 h in the conditions described above. The cell concentration was determined by the National Cancer Institute (NCI)

sulforhodamine method [22]. The optical density was measured at 590 nm with an ELISA-Reader (Molecular Devices, SPECTRA max plus 384). Results were expressed at the concentration that inhibits 50% of control growth after the incubation period (IC$_{50}$). The values were estimated from a semilog plot of the extract concentration (µg/mL) against the percentage of viable cells. Podophyllotoxin (PTOX) (Sigma) and camptothecin (Sigma) were included as positive standards. Extracts with IC$_{50}$ ≤ 20 µg/mL were considered active according to the NCI guidelines described in the literature [23].

To determine the specificity of cytotoxic activity, the extracts, were assayed against the normal skin fibroblast cell line (HFS-30), and the selective index (SI) was determined using equation (1):

$$SI = \frac{IC50 \text{ normal cell line}}{IC50 \text{ cancerous cell line}}$$

| Extract | Growth inhibition (IC50, µg/mL)* | | | | |
|---------|------|------|------|------|------|
| | Cell line | | | | |
| | HF6 | MCF7 | KB | PC3 | HFS-30 |
| B. ariensis Morelos | 6.34 ± 0.02 | 14.22 ± 0.01 | >20 | >20 | 4.33 ± 0.02 |
| B. bicolor | 7.29 ± 0.05 | 13.76 ± 0.03 | >20 | 9.69 ± 0.01 | >20 |
| B. linanoe | >20 | >20 | 13.31 ± 0.05 | >20 | >20 |
| B. ariensis México | 1.65 ± 0.03 | 2.49 ± 0.05 | 4.38 ± 0.03 | >20 | 1.27 ± 0.03 |
| B. glabrifolia Morelos | >20 | >20 | >20 | >20 | >20 |
| B. kerberi | 6.97 ± 0.03 | 10.29 ± 0.03 | >20 | >20 | >20 |
| B. glabrifolia Oaxaca | 6.96 ± 0.02 | 7.82 ± 0.01 | >20 | >20 | >20 |
| B. galeottiana | 4.67 ± 0.01 | 4.64 ± 0.02 | 14.26 ± 0.02 | 5.94 ± 0.04 | 9.85 ± 0.01 |
| B. fagaroides | 1.61 ± 0.04 | 2.25 ± 0.01 | 6.29 ± 0.03 | 2.13 ± 0.01 | 0.11 ± 0.03 |
| B. excelsa | >20 | >20 | >20 | >20 | >20 |
| B.schlechtendalii | 4.58 ± 0.01 | 9.94 ± 0.02 | 2.13 ± 0.01 | 0.39 ± 0.03 | 7.86 ± 0.01 |
| CTP § | 0.0258 ± 0.02 | 0.0424 ± 0.01 | 0.7855 ± 0.03 | 0.0383 ± 0.02 | 0.5821 ± 0.02 |
| PTOX § | 5.3127E-04 ± 0.01 | 3.7453E-03 ± 0.02 | 4.3833E-04 ± 0.01 | 1.5584E-03 ± 0.01 | 2.82E-02 ± 0.03 |

*IC50 is defined as the concentration that resulted in a 50% decrease in cell number, and the results are means ± standard deviations of three independent replicates. Values greater than 20 µg/mL are considered to be non-cytotoxic. § Positive control substances. The cytotoxic effect was investigated on the human cancer cell lines: nasopharyngeal (KB), colon (HF-6), breast (MCF-7), and prostate (PC-3), as well as on a normal fibroblast cell line (HFS-30)

**Table 2:** Cytotoxicity of hexane extracts of selected *Bursera* species from Mexico.

## Cell cycle analysis

PC-3 cells (1x10$^5$) were plated in 6-well plates and allowed to attach overnight at 37°C in 5% CO$_2$. Exponential growing cells were treated for 72 h with a concentration of the extracts calculated in accordance to IC$_{50}$ values. Cells from each treatment were trypsinized and collected into single cell suspensions, centrifuged and fixed in cold ethanol (70%) overnight at -20°C. The cells were then treated with RNase (0.01M) and stained with PI (7.5 µg/mL) for 30 min in the dark, PI has the ability to bind to RNA molecules and hence, RNase enzyme was added in order to allow PI to bind directly to DNA. The percentage of cells in G1, S and G2 phases was analyzed with a flow cytometer (Becton, Dickinson, FACS Calibur, San Jose, CA), the

number of cells analyzed for each sample was 10,000. Data obtained from the flow cytometer were analyzed using the FlowJo Software (Tree Star, Inc., Ashland, OR, USA) to generate DNA content frequency histograms, and to quantify the number of cells in the individual cell cycle phases.

## Apoptosis analyses

PC-3 cells were seeded in 6-well plates (7.5 x 10$^4$ cells/mL) and incubated for 18 h. Exponentially growing cells were treated for 72 h with RPMI medium added with 0.025% of DMSO (control) or in accordance with CI$_{50}$ of the extracts. Cells treated with H$_2$O$_2$ [24] were used as apoptotic death control, and for the necrotic control PC-3 cells were treated with boiling water. Then each cell culture was washed with 100 mL of PBS and stained with 100 μL AO/EB solution (100 μg/mL-1 AO, 100 μg/mL-1 EB), according to the procedures of Yang et al. [25]. The cells were observed using a fluorescence microscope (Olympus Co, Tokyo, Japan, with emission at 521 nm). AO/EB are intercalating nucleic acid-specific fluorochromes, which emit green and orange fluorescence respectively when they are bound to DNA. It is well known that AO can pass through cell membranes, but EB cannot. Under the fluorescence microscope, living cells appear green. Necrotic cells stain red but have a nuclear morphology resembling that of viable cells. Apoptotic cells appear green, and morphological changes such as cell blebbing and formation of apoptotic bodies are observed. The criteria for identification are as follows: (i) viable cells appear to have green nucleus with intact structure; (ii) early apoptosis cells exhibit a bright-green nucleus showing condensation of chromatin; (iii) late apoptosis appear as dense orange areas of chromatin condensation, and (iv) Orange intact nucleus depict secondary necrosis [13].

## Anti-inflammatory activity

In vivo anti-inflammatory experiments were conducted in mice according to the Mexican Guidelines for Animal Welfare NOM-Z00-062-1999 (2013) and were approved by the Ethics and Security Committee from the Centro de Investigación en Biotecnología, UAEM.

Male BALB/c mice weighting between 20 and 25 g were used. Mice were maintained in adequate living conditions at a temperature of 24°C, 70% of humidity with a 12-h light/dark cycle and water/food *ad libitum*. Animal inflammation was induced using 12-O-tetradecanoylphorbol-13-acetate (TPA from Sigma) by the method previously described by Rao et al. [26]. Under general anesthesia by sodium pentobarbital (3.5 mg/kg, intraperitoneally), 10 μL of TPA in ethanol (0.25 mg/mL) were topically applied on the internal and external surface of the right ear to cause edema. After 10 min of incubation, samples at different doses (from 0.05-1 mg/ear) in ethanol (vehicle) were applied on the same ear. The left ear (negative control) received only 10 μL of ethanol, and 20 μL of vehicle. Indomethacin was used as the anti-inflammatory positive control. After 4 h of incubation with TPA, the animals were sacrificed by cervical dislocation. Circular sections of 7 mm were taken from both ears as samples for further measurement. Increase in the weight of the right ear in respect to the left, was considered edema. The inhibition of edema was calculated by the formula:

$$\% \text{ of inhibition} = [(C-E) / C] \ 100$$

| Extract | Growth inhibition (IC$_{50}$, μg/mL)[*] | | | | |
|---|---|---|---|---|---|
| | Cell line | | | | |
| | HF6 | MCF7 | KB | PC3 | HFS-30 |
| *B. ariensis Morelos* | >20 | >20 | >20 | 6.78 ± 0.04 | >20 |
| *B. bicolor* | 3.90 ± 0.02 | 11.51 ± 0.03 | >20 | 0.13 ± 0.03 | >20 |
| *B. linanoe* | >20 | >20 | >20 | >20 | >20 |
| *B. ariensis México* | >20 | >20 | >20 | 1.87 ± 0.02 | >20 |
| *B. glabrifolia Morelos* | >20 | >20 | >20 | >20 | >20 |
| *B. kerberi* | 0.53 ± 0.01 | 1.74 ± 0.03 | 2.93 ± 0.03 | 0.49 ± 0.05 | >20 |
| *B. glabrifolia Oaxaca* | >20 | >20 | >20 | >20 | >20 |
| *B. galeottiana* | 3.14 ± 0.04 | 7.25 ± 0.02 | 13.14 ± 0.05 | 2.26 ± 0.04 | >20 |
| *B. fagaroides* | 1.46 ± 0.01 | 3.71 ± 0.01 | 0.96 ± 0.03 | 1.62 ± 0.02 | 2.74 ± 0.04 |
| *B. excelsa* | >20 | >20 | >20 | >20 | >20 |
| *B. schlechtendalii* | >20 | >20 | 6.52 | >20 | >20 |
| CTP § | 0.0258 ± 0.02 | 0.0424 ± 0.03 | 0.7855 ± 0.01 | 0.0383 ± 0.01 | 0.5821 ± 0.01 |
| PTOX § | 5.3127E-04 ± 0.01 | 3.7453E-03 ± 0.02 | 4.3833E-04 ± 0.02 | 1.5584E-03 ± 0.01 | 2.82E-02 ± 0.02 |

[*]IC$_{50}$ is defined as the concentration that resulted in a 50% decrease in cell number, and the results are means ± standard deviation of three independent replicates. Values greater than 20 μg/mL are considered to be non-cytotoxic. § Positive control substances. The cytotoxic effect was investigated on the human cancer cell lines: nasopharyngeal (KB), colon (HF-6), breast (MCF-7), and prostate (PC-3), as well as on a normal fibroblast cell line (HFS-30).

**Table 3:** Cytotoxicity of chloroform extracts of selected *Bursera* species from Mexico.

Where C=edema of control group (treated with TPA), and E=edema of experimental group (TPA with compound). Each crude extract was assayed in triplicate as well as the positive control indomethacin. Statistical analysis for anti-inflammatory activity was performed using Prism 6 for Windows version 6.0 (GraphPad Software Inc., La Jolla, CA, USA). Using one-way analysis of variance (ANOVA) followed by Dunnett's multiple comparison test, p=0.05 was considered to be statistically significant. ED50 values were obtained from regression curves with coefficient factors between $R^2$ =0.80 and 0.98.

The determination of $ED_{50}$ for the more active extracts was obtained through a curve constructed with four concentrations (0.05, 0.1, 0.5 and 1 mg/ear) and five replicates for each concentration.

## Results

### Cytotoxicity of extracts

Cytotoxic activities of organic extracts obtained from the nine plant species (eleven populations) are shown in Tables 2 and 3. Results in Table 2 show the cytotoxic values of hexane extracts and reveals that, except for B. *glabrifolia* (Morelos) and B. *excelsa*, all the plants exhibited cytotoxic activity ($IC_{50}<20$ μg/mL) in at least one cancer cell line, with values ranging from 0.39 to 14.26 μg/mL. From the cancer cell lines used to carry out the evaluation, HF-6 and MCF-7 were the most sensitive ones, showing a 72% response for the tested extracts. The least responsive cancer cell line was PC-3, since only four extracts (B. *bicolor*, B. *galeottiana*, B. *schlechtendalii* and B. *fagaroides*) showed cytotoxic action against this carcinoma. B. *linanoe* showed a selective cytotoxic effect only toward KB carcinoma ($IC_{50}=13.31$ μg/mL). Both B. *kerberi* and B. *glabrifolia* from Oaxaca, showed cytotoxic action against HF-6 ($IC_{50}=6.97$ μg/mL), and also toward MCF-7 ($IC_{50}=10.29$ and 7.82 μg/mL, respectively) being selective against these two cancer cell lines. B. *fagaroides* was the most active plant against HF-6 ($IC_{50}=1.61$ μg/mL) and MCF-7 ($IC_{50}=2.25$ μg/mL) carcinomas and B. *schlechtendalii* was the one most active against KB ($IC_5=2.13$ μg/mL) and PC-3 ($IC_{50}=0.39$ μg/mL), although it also exhibited activity against the other two cancer cell lines, as well as toward normal fibroblasts. Even though hexane extracts of B. *bicolor*, B. *lancifolia*, B. *linanoe*, B. *kerberi* and B. *glabrifolia* from Oaxaca exhibited toxic effects in at least one cancer cell line, they did not show cytotoxicity against the normal human skin fibroblast cell line HFS-30. On the contrary, B. *ariensis* from Morelos and México, B. *galeottiana*, B. *schlechtendalii* and B. *fagaroides* showed toxic action against normal fibroblasts.

Results in Table 3 show the cytotoxic evaluation of the chloroform extracts from the studied species revealing that B. *bicolor*, B. *kerberi*, B. *galeottiana*, B. *schlechtendalii*, B. *fagaroides*, and B. *ariensis* extracts possess cytotoxic activity ($IC_{50}<20$ μg/mL) with values ranging from 0.13 to 13.14 μg/mL. B. *fagaroides* showed a generalized cytotoxic action against all carcinomas and also toward normal fibroblasts. B. *schlechtendalii* showed cytotoxic action only against KB ($IC_{50}=6.52$ μg/mL) and no action against normal fibroblasts. B. *bicolor* was the most active one against PC-3 ($IC_{50}=0.13$ μg/mL), and presented an outstanding SI (Selective Index) (SI=153.85), also showing cytotoxicity toward the other two carcinomas (HF-6 and MCF-7), but with no action against normal fibroblasts. Similarly B. *kerberi* and B. *galeottiana* extracts were active against the four carcinomas, with no effects against normal fibroblasts; B. *kerberi* presented an important SI for HF-6 and PC-3 cell lines (37.74 and 40.82, respectively). For the ethyl acetate extracts, results of the cytotoxic evaluation revealed that only B. *fagaroides* was active, and this activity was exerted against the four carcinomas HF-6 ($IC_{50}=3.46$), MCF-7 ($IC_{50}=4.06$ ), KB ($IC_{50}=2.67$ ) and PC-3 ($IC_{50}=4.04$ μg/mL). Notably, the methanolic extracts obtained from all the studied species did not exhibit cytotoxicity in any of the studied carcinoma cell lines (data not shown).

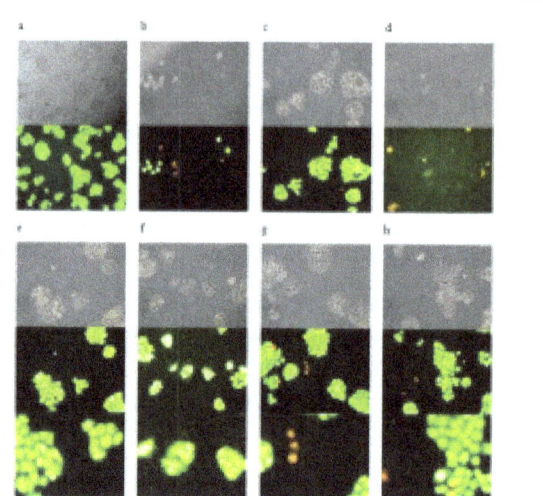

**Figure 2:** Phase and fluorescent micrographs of acridine orange and propidium iodide double-stained PC-3 cells. Cells were treated at $IC_{50}$ values of extracts from B. *ariensis* from the state of Mexico and Morelos (e and f respectively), B. *galeottiana* (g) and B. *kerberi* (h) in a time-dependent manner. Cells were cultured in RPMI 1640 media maintained at 37°C and 5% $CO_2$. Untreated cells after 72 h showed normal structures without prominent apoptosis and necrosis (a). Blebbing and orange color representing the hallmark of late apoptosis were noticed by g and h, early apoptosis features were represented by intercalated acridine orange (bright green) amongst the fragmented DNA (b, c and e-h), and red bright colored necrosis was observed by $H_2O_2$ treatment (d). Images are representatives of one of three similar experiments. Fluorescence and phase contrast images were captured at the field. Fluorescence images of samples were captured at 10x and 40x magnification.

### Cell cycle arrest

To assess the growth inhibitory effect on normal cell cycle progression on the basis of cytotoxic assay results and availability of samples, we conducted a cell cycle analysis measuring intracellular DNA content through flow cytometry in B. *ariensis* from Mexico and Morelos, B. *galeottiana* and B. *kerberi*. The status of the cell cycle of PC-3 cells treated with the four chloroform extracts for 72 h was analyzed, and PTOX was included as a positive control. As shown in Figure 1, exposure of PC-3 cells to chloroform extracts caused the appearance of a population in the sub-G1 region of the profile where apoptotic cells are found. Importantly, the treatment of PC-3 cells with extracts of B. *galeottiana* (Figure 1e) increased the G2/M populations, and correspondingly decreased G0/G1 phase in relation to the negative control (Figure 1a); whereas the treatment with B. *ariensis* from Morelos and from the state of Mexico (Figures 1c and 1d) presented similar apoptotic cells in the sub G1 phase to those of the positive control PTOX (Figure 1b). Only B. *kerberi* did not show a clear change in any phase of the cell cycle (Figure 1f).The above results necessitated performing apoptosis assay

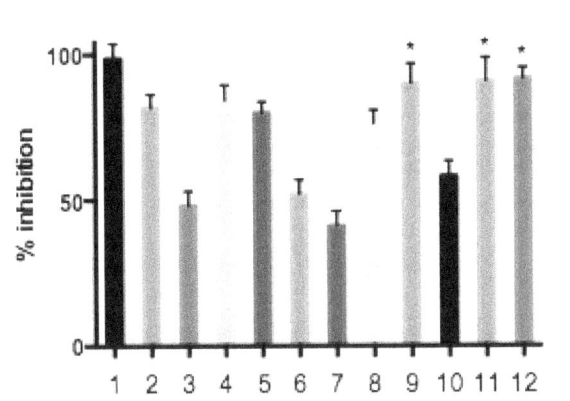

**Figure 3:** Anti-inflammatory activities of selected species of the *Bursera* genus. 1. Indomethacin, 2. *B. ariensis* from Morelos, 3 *B. bicolor*, 4. *B. linanoe*, 5. *B. ariensis* from Mexico state, 6. *B. glabrifolia* from Morelos, 7. *B. kerberi*, 8. *B. glabrifolia* from Oaxaca, 9. *B. galeottiana*, 10. *B. fagaroides*, 11. *B. excelsa*, 12. *B. schlechtendalii*.

## Apoptosis assay by AO/EB staining method

The cytotoxic assay and cell cycle analyses indicated apoptosis when using the chloroform extracts from *B. ariensis* from Mexico and Morelos, *B. galeottiana* and *B. kerberi*. These results were confirmed by fluorescence microscopy analysis. The cells were scored under the fluorescence microscope in order to quantify viable cells. The analysis was repeated in triplicate and the images were captured in fluorescence and phase contrast at the same field, and in 10 and 40 x magnification. Fluorescence microscopic analysis showed that the untreated PC-3 cells were stained with uniform green fluorescence (Figures 2a and 2c); PC-3 cells in early apoptosis were stained with bright spots in green fluorescence (Figures 2b PTOX; 2e *B. ariensis* from Morelos; 2f *B ariensis* from the state of Mexico; 2g B. *galeottiana* and 2h *B. kerberi*.), in late apoptosis PC-3 cells were stained in orange fluorescence with condensed and fragmented cell nucleus (Figures 2g *B. galeottiana* and 2h *B. kerberi*), and in necrosis PC3 cells were stained in orange fluorescence, but nucleus morphology appeared without condensation of chromatin (Figure 2d, $H_2O_2$).

## Anti-inflammatory assay on ear edema induced by TPA in mice

The anti-inflammatory effects of the *burseras* extracts are shown in Figure 3, and expressed as percentage of edema inhibition (% EI). The data indicated an important loss of weight by the extracts of *B. galeottiana* (89.92%), *B. excelsa* (90.79%) and *B. schelechtendalii* (91.60%), The Dunnett´s test indicated that these three species were the most active extracts and statistically comparable to the control indomethacin. The best extracts with anti-inflammatory potential were selected to determine the average effective dose (ED50). *B. galeottiana* was the most active extract (ED50=0.23 ± 0.02 mg/ear) when compared to the positive control indomethacin ($ED_{50}$=0.19 ± 0.02 mg /ear) (Table 4).

## Discussion

Plants have a long history of application in the treatment of cancer, but many of the claims for the efficacy of such treatment should be viewed with some skepticism because cancer, as a specific disease entity, is likely to be poorly defined in terms of folklore and traditional medicine [27]. In our case, besides the claimed popular use of these plants, the chemotaxonomic approach proved to be effective, since it was possible to identify *Bursera* species with cytotoxic activity indicating or affirming its usefulness as a method of selection.

| Sample | CI50 (mg/mL) |
| --- | --- |
| *B. excelsa* | 0.26 ± 0.01 |
| *B. galeottiana* | 0.23 ± 0.02 |
| *B. schlechtendalii* | 0.25 ± 0.02 |
| Indomethacine | 0.19 ± 0.02 |

**Table 4:** Anti-inflammatory activity of chloroform extracts from selected *burseras*.

With the exception of *B. glabrifolia* from Morelos and *B. excelsa*, all the studied *bursera* species exhibited cytotoxic activity. B. *fagaroides* proved to be the most active plant studied in this investigation since all three extracts (hexane, chloroform and ethyl acetate) displayed important cytotoxic effect against the four carcinoma cell lines HF-6, MCF-7, KB and PC-3. The obtained results are in accordance with those previously reported by other authors who studied this plant but from a population collected in the state of Michoacán [11,16]. *B. schlechtendalii* showed important cytotoxic activity, and this finding is in accordance with McDonield and Cole [18] study, since they identified two lignans with anti tumor activity in this species. In the case of *B. ariensis* notable cytotoxic effects from the hexane extract against all the cancer cell lines were obtained, and although there are no previous reports that evaluate the cytotoxic activity of this species, a lignan, denominated 'ariensin', was isolated from *B. ariensis* growing in the state of Michoacán [27,28], and was then synthesized by Burke and Stevenson [29], as well as later identified in *Acanthopanax koreanum* [30].

Koulman in 2003 [31] did not perform cytotoxic studies *in B. excelsa* collected in the state of Mexico but he did isolate three compounds: iso-bursehernin,3,4-dimethoxy-3',4'-methylenedioxylignano-9,9'-epoxylignan-9'-ol and guayadequiol, that he proposed as substrates for the synthesis of cytotoxic lignans. Some recent studies using NMR spectra of *B. ariensis* and *B. fagaroides* conducted by our research group indicated the presence of characteristic signals of aryltetralin lignans, whose structures are oxidized at C9 and C9' (signals situated at 4.56 ppm in the 1H NMR spectra). Since lignans are important compounds with attributed cytotoxic activity, the isolation and identification of these metabolites from the two mentioned species is an important accomplishment.

In our study, the hexane extract of *B. kerberi* showed cytotoxic effect against HF-6, MCF-7 and, the chloroform extract showed cytotoxic effect against HF-6, MCF-7, KB and PC-3. Hernandez et al. in 2005 [32] reported the isolation of verticillane derivates from *B. kerberi* collected in Jalisco; and although there are no cytotoxic data from these diterpenes, they were proposed as biogenetic precursors of the cytotoxic taxanes. Several reports in the literature do show cytotoxic activity displayed by triterpene compounds obtained from different species such as *Glochidion eriocarpum*, *Bridelia cambodiana* and species of *Protium* genus [33-35]. Some phytochemical studies report the presence of triterpenes in the *Bursera* genus [36-39], but only one investigation of the anti-tumoral activity of two triterpenes known as 'sapeline' A and B, isolated from *B. klugii*, showed activity against the P-388 lymphocytic leukemia test system (3PS), as well as toward the human epidermoid carcinoma of the nasopharynx (KB) [19]. In ongoing investigations conducted by our research group on the *Bursera* species selected for this study; *B. bicolor*, *B. lancifolia*, *B. linanoe*, *B. kerberi*, *B. excelsa*, *B. galeottiana* and *B.glabrifolia* showed 1H NMR spectra with characteristic triterpene signals profiling from 0.5 to 2.5 ppm . Extracts from these species also gave a positive Liebermann-Buchard test, which is characteristic of triterpenoids.

The lack of cytotoxic activity from *B. bicolor*, *B. kerberi* and *B. galeottiana* extracts on normal fibroblasts HFS-30 merits further studies in search of potential remedies with therapeutic value, since they exert high cytotoxic activity against cancer cell lines. *B. bicolor* and *B. kerberi* chloroform extracts showed outstanding selective cytotoxicity against PC-3 cancer cell line (SI=153.85 and 40.82, respectively), and only *B. kerberi* showed important selective cytotoxicity against HF-6 (SI=37.74).

It is important to note that while *B. glabrifolia* collected in Oaxaca was toxic against HF-6 and MCF-7 cell lines, the population of this species collected in Morelos was non-toxic against the tested cancer cell lines. This variation indicates different chemical profiles between both populations, possibly related to geographical, climatic or soil conditions.

In relation to cell cycle analysis of their the DNA content, cells can be classified into three categories: cells in G1 do not present DNA duplication, cells in G2/M exhibit duplicated DNA, and cells in S phase present intermediate DNA content. In each phase of the cell cycle, important control mechanisms exists that involve checkpoints which ensure the proper execution of cell cycle events. The p53 protein checkpoint blocks the entry of cells to mitosis when DNA is damaged in G2/M phase. This protein (p53) can activate the transcription of several apoptosis associated genes to program cell death in response to genotoxic stresses [40,41]. In our study, the results show that with exception of *B. kerberi;* the chloroform extracts can effectively induce apoptosis in PC-3 cells. These findings support those results obtained with cell cycle and cytotoxic experiments. *B. galeottiana* chloroform extract showed an important inhibitory effect related to G2/M phase arrest, and it remains to be demonstrated if this is due to the inhibition of the p53 checkpoint. At this phase, cells undergo apoptosis since they cannot be repaired

The observation of apoptosis induced by the plant extracts could be a key factor in determining their efficacy, in as much as most tumor cells remain sensitive to some apoptotic stimuli from anticancer drugs.

An inflammation-cancer relation has been proposed many years ago, and the interaction between them has become more and more evident. Inflammation is an immediate host defense mechanism of the body to tissue injury caused by noxious stimuli, and is characterized by the release of mediators (prostaglandins, cytokines, chemotactic molecules and vasoactive peptides), which affect the cellular infiltration and vascular permeability. For example, colorectal cancer is linked to colitis, which increases the risk of colorectal cancer by 10-fold, and the treatment of patients with anti-inflammatory therapy reduces this risk [42]. The role of inflammation in epigenetic, and

changing genetic events associated with cancer is estimated in more than 25% of all cancers [43].

Two of the studied species (*B. galeottiana,* and *B. schlechtendalii*) showed important anti-inflammatory activity comparable to the control indomethacin, as well as cytotoxic effects against cancer cell lines. As mentioned in the introduction, several reports in the *Bursera* genus had identified triterpenes as the involved compounds the in anti-inflammatory response. The triterpenoids of the oleanane and ursane series displayed anti-inflammatory activity [44] and were isolated from *B. simaruba* leaves, *B. graveolens* and *B. lancifolia* [44-46].

The overall results of this investigation postulate the studied species of the *Bursera* genus as candidates to investigate for their therapeutic potential in the treatment of cancer diseases and inflammation. Clearly, our results are an important contribution to the understanding on the potentialities of the *Bursera* genus as a source of new medical approaches.

This is the first report that focuses a systematic study on the cytotoxic and anti-inflammatory activities of nine species (eleven populations) of the *Bursera* genus growing in Mexico. The correlation of this information with ethnomedical data will be of great benefit for the rational use of these plant species.

# References

1. Becerra JX, Venable DL (2008) Sources and sinks of diversification and conservation priorities for the Mexican tropical dry forest. PLoS One 3: e3436.

2. Alonso AJ, Villarreal ML, Salazar LA, Gómez M, Domínguez F, et al. (2011) Mexican medicinal plants used for cancer treatment: Pharmacological, phytochemical and ethnobotanical studies. J Ethnopharmacol 133: 945-72.

3. Lona NV (2012) Objects made of copal resin: a radiological analysis. Bol Soc Geol Mex 64: 207-213.

4. García-Sílberman S (2002) An explanatory model of behavior toward mental illness. Salud Publica Mex 44: 289-296.

5. Sahagún B. de (2000) Historia general de las cosas de Nueva España. 3 vols. Estudio introductorio, paleografía, glosario y notas Alfredo López Austin y Josefina García Quintana: México, Cien de México/ CONACULTA. p 1450.

6. Montemayor C, Frischmann D (2005) Words of the true peoples/ Palabras de los seres verdaderos: Anthology of Contemporary Mexican Indigenous-Language Writers/Antología de Escritores Actuales en Lenguas Indígenas de México: Volume Two/Tomo Dos: Poetry/Poesía. University of Texas Press. p 220.

7. Galeote M (1997) Nombres indígenas de plantas americanas en los tratados científicos de Fray Agustín Farfán. Universidad de Granada. p 161.

8. http://www.medicinatradicionalmexicana.unam.mx/monografia.php 3: 7989.

9. Loeza-Corte JM, Díaz-López E, Campos-Pastelín JM, Orlando-Guerrero JI (2013) Efecto de lignificación de estacas sobre enraizamiento de Bursera morelensis Ram. y Bursera galeottiana Engl. en la Universidad de la Cañada en Teotitlán de Flores Magón, Oaxaca, México. Ciencia Ergo Sum 20: 222-226.

10. Queiroga CL, Duarte MC, Ribeiro BB, de Magalhães PM (2007) Linalool production from the leaves of Bursera aloexylon and its antimicrobial activity. Fitoterapia 78: 327-328.

11. Puebla AM, Huacuja L, Rodríguez G, Villaseñor MM, Miranda ML, et al. (1998) Cytotoxic and antitumour activity from Bursera fagaroides ethanol extract in mice with L5178Y lymphoma. Phytother Res 12: 545-548.

12. Elton A (1998) Documento técnico justificativo para la creación de la Reserva de la Biosfera Sierra Huautla-Cerro Frío Morelos. Instituto Nacional de Ecología, Centro de Investigación Ambiental e Investigación Sierra de Huautla. p 155.

13. Mohan S, Bustamam A, Ibrahim S, Al-Zubairi AS, Aspollah M, et al. (2011) In vitro ultramorphological assessment of apoptosis on CEMs induced by linoleic acid-rich fraction from Typhonium flagelliforme tuber. Evidence-Based Complementary and Alternative Medicine.

14. Maldonado B, Ortiz A, Dorado O (2004) Preparados galénicos e imágenes de plantas medicinales. CEAMISH-UAEM, México 7-11.

15. Téllez-Valdés O, Reyes-Castillo M, Dávila-Aranda P, Gutiérrez-García K, Téllez-Poo O, et al. (2009) Guía ecoturística. Las plantas del valle de Tehuacán-Cuicatlán. UNAM. p 41.

16. Rojas-Sepúlveda AM, Mendieta-Serrano M, Mojica MY, Salas-Vidal E, Marquina S, et al. (2012) Cytotoxic podophyllotoxin type-lignans from the steam bark of Bursera fagaroides var. fagaroides. Molecules 17: 9506-9519.

17. Cole JR, Bianchi E, Trumbull ER (1969) Antitumor agents from Bursera microphylla (Burseraceae). II. Isolation of a new lignan-burseran. J Pharm Sci 58: 175-176.

18. McDoniel PB, Cole JR (1972) Antitumor activity of Bursera schlechtendalii (burseraceae): isolation and structure determination of two new lignans. J Pharm Sci 61: 1992-1994.

19. Jolad SD, Wiedhopf RM, Cole JR (1977) Cytotoxic agents from Bursera klugii (Burseraceae) I: isolation of sapelins A and B. J Pharm Sci 66: 889-890.

20. Jolad SD, Wiedhopf RM, Cole JR (1977) Cytotoxic agents from Bursera morelensis (Burseraceae): deoxypodophyllotoxin and a new lignan, 5'-desmethoxydeoxypodophyllotoxin. J Pharm Sci 66: 892-893.

21. Houghton P, Fang R, Techatanawat I, Steventon G, Hylands PJ, et al. (2007) The sulphorhodamine (SRB) assay and other approaches to testing plant extracts and derived compounds for activities related to reputed anticancer activity. Methods 42: 377-387.

22. Skehan P, Storeng R, Scudiero D, Monks A, McMahon J, et al. (1990) New colorimetric cytotoxicity assay for anticancer-drug screening. J Natl Cancer Inst 82: 1107-1112.

23. Suffness M, Pezzuto J (1991) Assays related to cancer drug discovery. In: Dey P, Harborne J, (eds.) Methods in Plant Biochemistry. London: AC. 71-133.

24. Kasibhatla S, Amarante-Mendes GP, Finucane D, Brunner T, Bossy-Wetzel E, et al. (2006) Acridine Orange/Ethidium Bromide (AO/EB) Staining to Detect Apoptosis. CSH Protoc 2006.

25. Yang GY, Liao J, Kim K, Yurkow EJ, Yang CS (1998) Inhibition of growth and induction of apoptosis in human cancer cell lines by tea polyphenols. Carcinogenesis 19: 611-616.

26. Rao TS, Currie JL, Shaffer AF, Isakson PC (1993) Comparative evaluation of arachidonic acid (AA)- and tetradecanoylphorbol acetate (TPA)-induced dermal inflammation. Inflammation 17: 723-741.

27. Cragg GM, Newman DJ (2008) Anticancer drug discovery and development from natural products. In: Colegate S, Molyneux R, (eds.) Bioactive Natural Products, Detection, Isolation and Structural Determination. Boca Raton: CRC Press. 323-370.

28. Hernández JD, Román LU, Espiñeira J, Joseph-Nathan P (1983) Ariensin, a new lignan from Bursera ariensis. Planta Med 47: 215-217.

29. Burke JM, Stevenson R (1985) Synthesis of (+/-)-ariensin. Planta Med 51: 450-452.

30. Rao V (2012) Phytochemicals and their pharmacological aspects of Acanthopanax koreanum. In: Kim YH, Kim JA, Nhiem NX (eds.) Phytochemicals Rijeka, Croatia: In Tech 451-466.

31. Koulman A (2003) Evolution of lignan biosynthesis in the genus Bursera. In: Koulman A, Quax WJ, Judith X, Becerra JX, (eds.), Podophyllotoxin. Netherlands: Stichting Regenboog Drukkerij Press 141-156.

32. Hernández-Hernández JD, Román-Marín LU, Cerda-García-Rojas CM, Joseph-Nathan P (2005) Verticillane derivatives from Bursera suntui and Bursera kerberi. J Nat Prod 68: 1598-1602.

33. Khiev P, Cai XF, Chin YW, Ahn KS, Lee HK, et al. (2009) Cytotoxic terpenoids from the methanolic extract of Bridelia cambodiana. J Korean Soc Appl Biol Chem 52: 626-631.

34. Nhiem NX, Thu VK, Van Kiem P, Van Minh C, Tai BH, et al. (2012) Cytotoxic oleane-type triterpene saponins from Glochidion eriocarpum. Arch Pharm Res 35: 19-26.

35. Barros FW, Bandeira PN, Lima DJ, Meira AS, de Farias SS, et al. (2011) Amyrin esters induce cell death by apoptosis in HL-60 leukemia cells. Bioorg Med Chem 19: 1268-1276.

36. Ara K, Rahman MS, Rahman AHMM, Hassan CM, Rashid MA (2009) Terpenoids and coumarin from Bursera serrata. J Pharm Sci 8: 107-110.

37. Moreno J, Rojas LB, Aparicio R, Marcó LM, Usubillaga A (2010) Chemical composition of the essential oil from the bark of Bursera tomentosa (Jacq) Tr and Planch. Bol Latinoam Caribe Plant Med Aromát. 9: 491-494.

38. Cárdenas R, Reguera JJ, Llanos E, Aguirre E, Herrera J, et al. (2012) Effects of organic extracts of Bursera copallifera and B. lancifolia leaves in the development of Spodoptera frugiperda. J Entomol 9: 115-122.

39. Ionescu F, Jolad SD, Cole JR (1977) The structure of benulin, a new pentacyclic triterpene hemiketal isolated from Bursera arida (Burseraceae). J Org Chem 42: 1627-1629.

40. Luk SC, Siu SW, Lai CK, Wu YJ, Pang SF (2005) Cell Cycle Arrest by a Natural Product via G2/M Checkpoint. Int J Med Sci 2: 64-69.

41. Li H, Wang P, Liu Q, Cheng X, Zhou Y, et al. (2012) Cell cycle arrest and cell apoptosis induced by Equisetum hyemale extract in murine leukemia L1210 cells. J Ethnopharmacol 144: 322-327.

42. Reuter S, Gupta SC, Chaturvedi MM, Aggarwal BB (2010) Oxidative stress, inflammation, and cancer: how are they linked? Free Radic Biol Med 49: 1603-1616.

43. Kundu JK, Surh YJ (2012) Emerging avenues linking inflammation and cancer. Free Radic Biol Med 52: 2013-2037.

44. Carretero ME, López-Pérez JL, Abad MJ, Bermejo P, Tillet S, et al. (2008) Preliminary study of the anti-inflammatory activity of hexane extract and fractions from Bursera simaruba (Linneo) Sarg. (Burseraceae) leaves. J Ethnopharmacol 116: 11-15.

45. Robles J, Torrenegra R, Gray RI, Piñeros C, Ortiz L et al. (2005) Triterpenos aislados de la corteza de Bursera graveolens (Burseraceae) y su actividad biológica. Braz J Pharmacog 15: 283-286.

46. Zúñiga B, Guevara-Fefer P, Herrera J, Contreras JL, Velasco L, et al. (2005) Chemical composition and anti-inflammatory activity of the volatile fractions from the bark of eight Mexican Bursera species. Planta Med 71: 825-828.

# 29

# A Retrospective Study of Cases of Acetyl Cholinesterase Inhibitor Poisoning in the Coyote (*Canis latrans*) and the Bald Eagle (*Haliaeetus leucocephalus*) in the Canadian Prairies

**Cowan VE[2] and Blakley BR[1]***

[1]*Department of Veterinary Biomedical Sciences, Western College of Veterinary Medicine, University of Saskatchewan, SK CAN S7N5B4, Canada*

[2]*Toxicology Centre, University of Saskatchewan, SK CAN S7N5B3, Canada*

***Corresponding author:** Blakley, Western College of Veterinary Medicine, 52 Campus Drive, Saskatoon SK Canada, S7N5B4,
E-mail: barry.blakley@usask.ca*

## Abstract

**Objective:** Wildlife death from organophosphate and carbamate pesticide exposure has been documented previously in Canada. Wildlife exposure to these agents can occur through primary toxicity (i.e., inhalation), ingestion of contaminated water or food, or secondary toxicity through scavenging on toxic carrion. This paper describes epidemiologic information pertaining to confirmed acetyl cholinesterase inhibitor pesticide lethality in the coyote and bald eagle over a 16-year period in the Canadian Prairies.

**Methods:** Epidemiologic case information from the diagnostic records of Prairie Diagnostic Services confirmed lethal acetyl cholinesterase inhibitor poisoning in 58 coyotes (*Canis latrans*) and 60 bald eagles (*Haliaeetus leucocephalus*) from 1998 to 2013. Brain acetyl cholinesterase enzyme activity suppressed to 50% or greater was indicative of toxicity and death.

**Results:** Coyote case submissions varied both annually (p<0.0001) and temporally (p<0.0001). Submissions were highest in the years of 2000, 200, and 2002 (collectively 46.6%). The months of most frequent submission were May and April (36.2%). Bald eagle cases were also influenced annually (p<0.0001) and temporally (p<0.0001). Confirmed poisoning in bald eagle carcasses was most frequent during two seasonal periods: May through April and December through January. Years 2000, 200, and 2004 comprised 43.3% of the bald eagle poisonings during the investigational period. Annual and temporal distribution of coyote and bald eagle cases were comparable but were not significantly correlated. Brain acetyl cholinesterase activities within 20% of the mean in unaffected cases were considered background. These activities were 3.44 ± 1.52 µmol/min/g in the coyote and 15.18 ± 3.37 µmol/g/min in the bald eagle.

**Conclusion:** Poisoning in wildlife with acetyl cholinesterase inhibitor pesticides continues to be a regular occurrence in the Canadian prairies. Increased surveillance and monitoring of pesticide use should be considered to mitigate future poisonings.

**Keywords:** Acetyl cholinesterase inhibition; Bald eagle; Coyote; Pesticide; Poisoning; Retrospective

## Introduction

Acetyl cholinesterase inhibitor insecticides have a longstanding history of use in Canadian agriculture. Following the nation-wide ban of the organochlorine class of insecticides in the early 1970s, organophosphate and carbamate insecticides were introduced as alternatives for pest management [1-2]. The major advantage associated with the introduction of these insecticides was low environmental persistence coupled with efficacious insect control.

The major disadvantage associated with use of acetyl cholinesterase inhibitor pesticides is the non-target poisoning in domestic and wildlife animal species. The acetyl cholinesterase inhibitor pesticides act to inhibit the acetyl cholinesterase enzyme. The nervous system of vertebrates is highly conserved throughout evolution and thus renders any animal species vulnerable to poisoning. Phosphorylation (by

organophosphate agents) or carbamylation (by carbamate agents) of acetyl cholinesterase prevents the enzyme's ability to hydrolyse acetylcholine [3-4]. Consequently, uncontrolled binding of acetylcholine to post-synaptic neurons will occur. Stimulation of nicotinic acetylcholine receptors and muscarinic acetylcholine receptors at the postsynaptic neurons results in the rapid onset of classical symptomatology [3].

Clinical signs of acetyl cholinesterase inhibitor exposure may be divided into three categories: muscarinic, nicotinic, and central [4]. Predominant symptomatology includes miosis, salivation, lacrimation, urination, defecation, involuntary muscle fasciculation, dyspnea, bronchoconstriction, and death from respiratory failure [3-4].

Extreme toxicity (e.g. rat oral LD50 of carbofuran=6.0-7.8 mg/kg body weight) and extensive availability of acetyl cholinesterase inhibitor insecticides enables the accidental and intentional animal poisoning with these agents [5]. Exposure to animals can occur through multiple routes: inhalation of sprayed agricultural pesticides (i.e., primary toxicity), consumption of contaminated water or food, dermal contact for insect control in fur (depending on the agent or formulation used), and secondary toxicity from the ingestion of animals previously poisoned with acetyl cholinesterase inhibitor pesticides [1-6].

Targeted poisoning of coyotes (*Canis latrans*) with organophosphate and carbamate pesticides has been identified in Canada and the United States [1-8]. The continued economic losses from coyote-related livestock kills have deemed the animal a nuisance for livestock producers. Coyotes will aggressively prey upon livestock, especially young, old, or unthrifty animals [9]. In Canada, legislation is in place to control coyote populations and reduce livestock attacks through various methods of hunting, trapping, and poisoning. The latter means of coyote control is controversial and highly regulated. Registered lethal poisons for coyote control include sodium cyanide gas injection cartridges (Alberta only), sodium fluoroacetate tablets (Alberta and Saskatchewan only), and toxic neck collars [9,10]. Despite the availability and potency of approved pesticides for coyote control, occurrence of illegal coyote poisoning with acetyl cholinesterase inhibitor pesticides remains a regular occurrence [2].

A consequence of off-label pesticide use may be the secondary poisoning of scavenger species [2]. Scavengers, including eagles, magpies, ravens, foxes, and skunks, may opportunistically feed on animal carcasses. Scavengers can become poisoned through ingestion of either (1) toxic bait placed with intent to poison or (2) toxic carrion of animals that died from primary poisoning. In these instances, the poisoning event can be referred to as secondary toxicity, as the scavenger species were not the intended target of the toxicant [2]. This is also referred to as "relay toxicity". Multiple scavengers can become poisoned from a single intoxication event due to relay toxicity [1].

Multiple factors influence poisoning occurrence with these agents. The ingested pesticides remain toxic in the muscle and organs of a poisoned animal post-mortem [7]. In addition, the rate of biotransformation in the environment and tissue half-life of these pesticides are partially dependent on the weather conditions. Breakdown of these agents is more expedient in warmer climates (i.e., May through August in Canada) than in colder conditions (i.e., September through April in Canada) [11]. The biology of the scavenging species (i.e., time of year associated with scavenging) is important to consider as well. These factors affect the period in which an animal can suffer secondary toxicity.

A top predator that employs scavenging as a feeding strategy is the bald eagle (*Haliaeetus leucocephalus*) [7,8,12]. The association between deaths in coyotes and secondary toxicity bald eagles from acetyl cholinesterase inhibitor poisoning has been identified previously in both Canada and the United States [7,8,12]. Coyotes are perceived as pests to livestock producers, leading to the baiting of materials to poison coyotes. Bald eagles may scavenge on the toxic coyote carcass and become poisoned. The predominance of agriculture in Canada (most notably the prairie provinces of Alberta, Saskatchewan, and Manitoba) and the United States has led to a continual reliance on acetyl cholinesterase inhibitor pesticides in agriculture.

The primary objective of this paper is to describe epidemiological information on the occurrence of poisoning cases with anticholinesterase pesticides in coyotes and bald eagles in Western Canada. A secondary objective is to ascertain whether there is an association between these occurrences. Information presented in this study may aid regulatory agencies responsible for the management of pesticides in the refinement of anticholinergic pesticide approval and renewal strategies.

## Materials and Methods

Epidemiologic case information from confirmed lethal anticholinesterase poisoning in coyotes and bald eagles across the Canadian prairies was obtained from the records of Prairie Diagnostic Services (PDS) located in the Western College of Veterinary Medicine (WCVM) in Saskatoon, Saskatchewan. Toxicological testing was conducted in all of the cases upon submission from 1998 to 2013. Submissions were only encountered from the Canadian provinces of Alberta, Saskatchewan, and Manitoba. A modification of the Ellman method enabled the determination of acetyl cholinesterase enzyme activity in brain specimens [13]. Units of enzyme activity were reported as micromoles of substrate hydrolyzed per minute per gram of brain tissue, wet weight (μmol/min/g). Acetyl cholinesterase enzyme suppression was compared to previously established reference values in the species of interest to designate toxicity and/or exposure to anticholinergic agents (Hill and Fleming; Blakley and Yole 2002). Normal brain acetyl cholinesterase values were considered to be the mean ± 20% [1,14]. Brain acetyl cholinesterase suppression of 50% or greater was considered to be consistent with acute intoxication [1,14]. Annual and temporal (monthly) case incidence from 1998 to 2013 in both species was examined. Cases of poisoning in both species in close proximity to one another were identified; the co-occurrence of poisoning events in both species was compared using correlation coefficients. Statistical differences in case occurrence by year and month in each species were determined by chi square analysis (p<0.01).

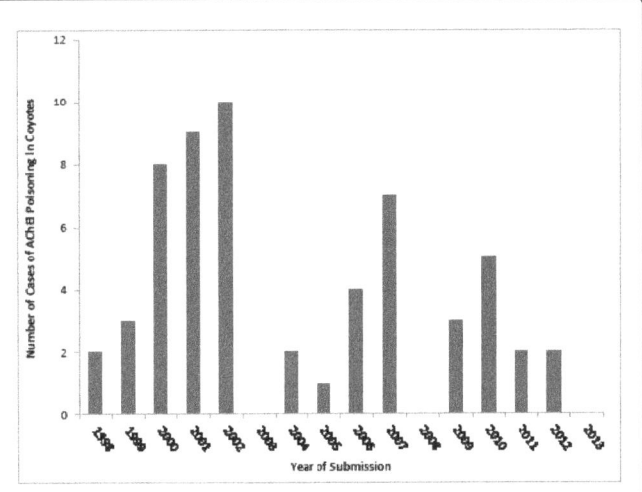

**Figure 1:** Incidence of confirmed anticholinesterase pesticide poisoning in the coyote (*Canis latrans*) over a 16 year period in Western Canada (n=58). The probability of no year effect determined by Chi Square Goodness of Fit is p<0.0001.

## Results

Prairie Diagnostic Services identified cases associated with clinical manifestations and death due to acetyl cholinesterase inhibitor pesticide exposure in 58 coyotes and 60 bald eagles in the Canadian prairies over a 16 year period.

Coyotes poisoned with acetyl cholinesterase inhibitor pesticides were observed in 13 of the 16 years. Case submissions to PDS were absent in 2003, 2008, and 2013. Coyote case distribution was influenced by year (p<0.0001) (Figure 1). Years 2000, 2001 and 2002 had the highest occurrence of coyote submission and represented 46.6% of coyote cases. Poisoned coyotes were most frequently submitted in the springtime months of April and May (p<0.0001) (Figure 2), which accounted for 53.5% of the confirmed coyote cases during the investigational period.

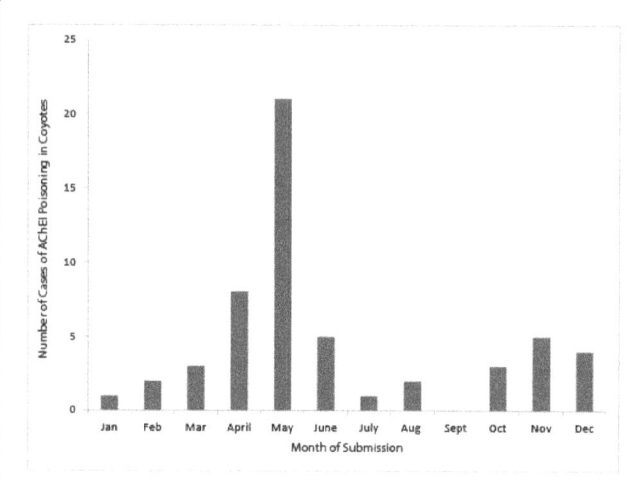

**Figure 2:** Seasonal incidence of anticholinesterase pesticide poisoning in the coyote (*Canis latrans*) in Western Canada (n=58). The probability of no seasonal effect determined by Chi Square Goodness of Fit is p<0.0001.

Bald eagle poisoning varied by year (p<0.0001) and season (p<0.0001). Poisoned bald eagle cases were highest in the years of 2000, 200, and 2004 (Figure 3). These years comprised 43.3% of the cases submitted. Submissions were absent in 2003 and 2008. The occurrence of eagle poisoning with acetyl cholinesterase inhibitor agents occurred most often during two time periods: the spring (May and April) and mid-winter (December and January) (Figure 4). These time periods accounted for 33.3% and 35% of poisoned bald eagle cases respectively.

Annual and temporal trends in the poisoning in coyotes and bald eagles showed some similarity (Figures 1-4). The correlation coefficients of these trends were 0.48 and 0.45, respectively. Annual incidence of coyote and bald eagle poisonings tended to show correlation but was not statistically significant (p=0.0599). The correlation of temporal incidence of coyote and bald eagle poisonings with Acetyl cholinesterase inhibitor agents was not significant (p=0.1421).

| Species | Mean ± SD (n) |
|---------|---------------|
| Bald Eagle | 15.18 ± 3.37 (52) |
| Coyote | 3.44 ± 1.52 (13) |

**Table 1:** Reference brain cholinesterase values in the bald eagle (*Haliaeetus leucocephalus*) and the coyote (*Canis latrans*). Enzyme activity levels are reported as units of micromoles of acetylthiocholine

iodide hydrolyzed per minute per gram of brain tissue (wet weight) at 25°C.

Mean normal reference brain acetyl cholinesterase activities were determined to be 3.44 ± 1.52 μmol/min/g in the coyote and 15.18 ± 3.37 μmol/g/min in the bald eagle (Table 1).

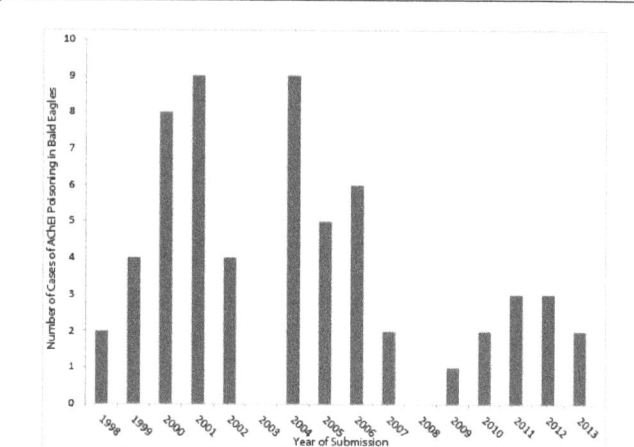

**Figure 3:** Incidence of anticholinesterase pesticide poisoning in the bald eagle (*Haliaeetus leucocephalus*) over a 16 year period in Western Canada (n=60). The probability of no year effect determined by Chi Square Goodness of Fit is p<0.0001.

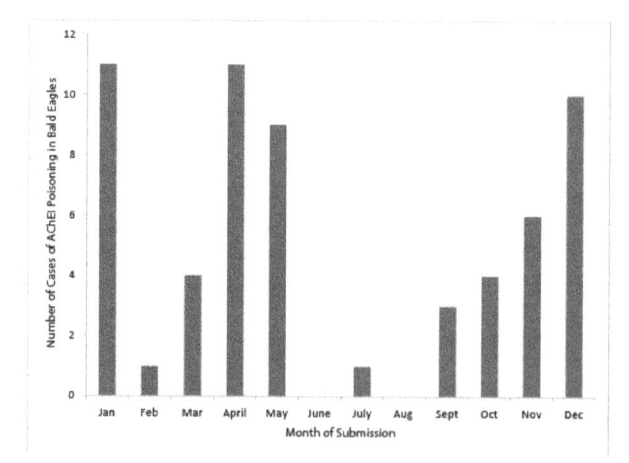

**Figure 4:** Seasonal occurrence of anticholinesterase pesticide poisoning in the bald eagle (*Haliaeetus leucocephalus*) from 1998 to 2013 in Western Canada (n=60). The probability of no seasonal effect determined by Chi Square Goodness of Fit is p<0.0001.

## Discussion

Acetyl cholinesterase inhibitor poisoning of non-target wildlife species is typically an annual occurrence in the Canadian prairies. The diagnostic toxicology laboratory Prairie Diagnostic Services confirmed 58 cases of poisoning in coyotes and 60 cases in bald eagles with anticholinesterase pesticides through postmortem testing over the 16-year period of 1998 through 2013.

Reference normal brain acetyl cholinesterase concentrations in non-poisoned animals are the basis for the determination of toxicity in cases of suspected poisoning [1,14]. Enzyme suppression is estimated by dividing the activity of the sample by the reference value for that species. Suppression of 50% or greater is consistent with lethal exposure and death. The brain tissue from 52 and 13 non-poisoned bald eagles and coyotes submitted during the investigational period were determined to have reference acetyl cholinesterase activities of 15.18 ± 3.37 µmol/min/g and 3.44 ± 1.52 µmol/min/g, respectively. These values are comparable to previously published values in the two species [14]. Substantial inter- and intraspecies variation is evident.

Coyotes with acetyl cholinesterase inhibitor poisoning were submitted for diagnostic testing most frequently during the months of April and May. One explanation for the increase in case number at this time of year is calving in livestock operations. It is reasonable to speculate that the presence of calves increase the likelihood of livestock coyote attacks. Coyote exposure to pesticide spray drift alone is unlikely since many of the recorded deaths were observed during the spring before the spraying season. Illegal use of pesticides may represent a method of coyote control to prevent livestock deaths. Previous studies reported livestock carcasses laced with anticholinesterase pesticides were used as coyote bait [1]. A study from Kansas, USA reported that carbamate-laced sheep carcasses were found in the same field as the carcasses of three bald eagles, two coyotes, and a red-tailed hawk (Buteo jamaicensis) [1]. These animals were determined to have died of toxic carbofuran exposure. Individuals admitted that the poisoned sheep carcasses were placed to kill coyotes [1]. Given the perceived severity of the coyote problem, legal means of control may seem insubstantial when faced with the potential losses. Strict limits on the quantities approved coyote-control poisons and reporting requirements to government authorities encourage non-compliance.

Submissions of bald eagles with acetyl cholinesterase activity suppression indicative of toxicity occurred most frequently in spring and mid-winter. Similar temporal patterns in the coyote and bald eagle in the springtime are suggestive of secondary toxicity and may be related to scavenging on poisoned baits placed for coyotes during calving season. Bald eagles scavenge carrion and prey upon moribund animals in addition to other feeding opportunities. Due to the rapid hydrolysis of organophosphate and carbamate pesticides at warm ambient temperatures, the proximity of dead eagles (and other wildlife species) to dead coyotes or poisoned livestock carcasses is often useful to identifying secondary toxicity. Proximity of carcasses and evidence of predation on coyotes by bald eagles has been noted previously in Western Canada [1-11].

The second temporal peak for bald eagle poisoning is the months of December and January (mid-Winter). Winter-time poisoning is contrary to registered use of acetyl cholinesterase inhibitor pesticides. This observation is suggestive of secondary toxicity. Lack of readily available food sources during the winter may influence bald eagles to scavenge carrion more extensively than in warmer months when prey is easy to access. However, it is not clear why coyote submissions were not increased during these months, as coyotes are suspected to be the primary target of poisoned baiting. In addition, migratory bald eagles overwinter in the United States and are not expected to be present in high numbers on the Canadian prairies in the wintertime. It is important to note that the timeframe for poisoning is greater during the winter months: animal corpses and associated insecticides in the tissues are preserved while frozen. It can be speculated that any

remaining bald eagles during the winter would be more at risk to acetyl cholinesterase inhibitor pesticide exposure.

The seasonal distribution of bald eagle deaths found in this study are comparable to those reported in a study of the occurrence of organophosphate or carbamate pesticide poisoning in the bald eagle and the golden eagle (Aquila chrysaetos) in Western Canada [2]. The researchers found that eagle poisonings occurred most often during the months of April (n=14) and December (n=9). The authors attributed the decline in cases between the months of June and September to decreased baiting, increased carcass decomposition in warmer weather, and eagle migratory nesting patterns. These factors cannot be ruled out in the present study.

Raptor species, including the bald eagle, appear to be one of the most at-risk groups for secondary toxicity from acetyl cholinesterase inhibitor agents. In a study conducted from 1980 to 2000, the death of 158 bald eagles was attributed to exposure to Acetyl cholinesterase inhibitor pesticides [7]. A study of raptor poisoning in the United Kingdom, United States, and Canada found that ingestion of the gastrointestinal contents or surface materials of poisoned vertebrates was largely responsible for secondary toxicity in avian species [7]. Poisoning cases in coyotes and bald eagles were observed in most years from 1998 to 2013, with the exception of 2003 and 2008 for both species and 2013 for coyotes. It is compelling, yet unclear, why there was a lapse in cases from both species in 2003 and 2008. However, cases of poisoning in both species appear to have declined over time. Two possibilities may aid in the explanation of case decline over time. First is the ban of the common carbamate pesticide carbofuran in Canada in 2009 [15]. With the phase-out, it is expected that carbofuran misuse would decline over time. Second is the implementation of a pilot project for coyote control in Saskatchewan. Between November 2009 and March 2010, more than 71 000 coyotes were exterminated in the province [16]. A bounty was paid as an incentive for participation in the project. Decreased acetyl cholinesterase inhibitor poisoning occurrence in recent years may reflect success of both the carbofuran ban and the Saskatchewan coyote control project. Similar projects were not enacted in Alberta and Manitoba, thus the influence of the Saskatchewan bounty program in these provinces is unknown.

The occurrence of poisoning on an annual basis is indicative of a multifactorial problem in Western Canada. Incidences of coyotes and bald eagles poisoned with anticholinesterase pesticides highlights the need for continued monitoring, submission, and testing of wildlife carcasses in Western Canada. Further, increased surveillance on the use of acetyl cholinesterase inhibitor pesticides is required on the Canadian prairies. Diagnostic toxicological testing for acetyl cholinesterase suppression should be routinely considered for dead wildlife in areas of intense agricultural operations.

## Conclusion

Caudal neostigmine can be used safely as a model of fast–track anesthesia for congenital heart surgery; also it provides effective analgesia with opioid sparing effects. This allows faster recovery of patients, and helps to provide an efficient and cost-effective service. However, better control of postoperative vomiting by antiemetic prophylaxis after caudal neostigmine is required.

## Acknowledgement

The authors of this study gratefully acknowledge the insight from Dr. Gary Wobeser in the writing of this manuscript. The authors also thank those involved in the collection, submission, and analysis of the data. This includes conservation officers, members of the Canadian Cooperative Wildlife Health Centre (CCWHC) and Western College of Veterinary Medicine (WCVM), and laboratory technicians in Prairie Diagnostic Services (PDS).

## References

1. Allen GT, Veatch JK, Stroud RK, Vendel CG, Poppenga RH, et al. (1996) Winter poisoning of coyotes and raptors with Furadan-laced carcass baits. J Wildl Dis 32: 385-389.

2. Wobeser G, Bollinger T, Leighton FA, Blakley B, Mineau P (2004) Secondary poisoning of eagles following intentional poisoning of coyotes with anticholinesterase pesticides in western Canada. J Wildl Dis 40: 163-172.

3. Pope C, Karanth S, Liu J (2005) Pharmacology and toxicology of cholinesterase inhibitors: uses and misuses of a common mechanism of action. Environ Toxicol Pharmacol 19: 433-446.

4. Merck Veterinary Manual (2014) Insecticide and Acaricide (Organic) Toxicity.

5. US Environmental Protection Agency Office of Pesticide Programs. Reregistration Eligibility Decision for Carbofuran (2007).

6. Henny CJ, Kolbe EJ, Hill EF, Blus LJ (1987) Case histories of bald eagles and other raptors killed by organophosphorus insecticides topically applied to livestock. J Wildl Dis 23: 292-295.

7. Mineau P, Fletcher MR, Glaser LC (1999) Poisoning of raptors with organophosphorous and carbamate pesticides with emphasis on Canada, U.S. and U.K. J Raptor Res 33: 1-37.

8. Fleischli MA, Franson JC, Thomas NJ, Finley DL, Riley W (2004) Avian Mortality Events in the United States Caused by Anticholinesterase Pesticides: A Retrospective Summary of National Wildlife Health Center Records from 1980 to 2000. Arch Enviro Contam Toxicol 46: 542-550.

9. Government of Alberta Agriculture and Rural Development Division (2010) Coyote Predation Control Manual and Study Guide.

10. Cutler GC, Scott-Dupree CD, Drexler DM (2014) Honey bees, neonicotinoids and bee incident reports: the Canadian situation. Pest Manag Sci 70: 779-783.

11. Canadian Council of Ministers of the Environment (1999) Canadian water quality guidelines for the protection of aquatic life: Carbofuran. In: Canadian environmental quality guidelines, Canadian Council of Ministers of the Environment, Winnipeg, Manitoba, Canada.

12. Hill EF, Fleming WJ (1982) Anticholinesterase poisoning of birds: Field monitoring and diagnosis of acute poisoning. Environ Toxicol Chem 1: 27-38.

13. ELLMAN GL, COURTNEY KD, ANDRES V Jr, FEATHER-STONE RM (1961) A new and rapid colorimetric determination of acetylcholinesterase activity. Biochem Pharmacol 7: 88-95.

14. Blakley BR, Yole MJ (2002) Species differences in normal brain cholinesterase activities of animals and birds. Vet Hum Toxicol 44: 129-132.

15. Health Canada Pest Management Regulatory Agency (2010) Re-evauation Decision: Carbofuran.

16. Karen Briere (2010) Bounty program claims 7,000 coyotes in Saskatchewan. The Western Producer.

# Permissions

# List of Contributors

**Qaiser Jamal, Attiya Sabeen Rahman, Mehwish Riaz, Maryam Ansari and Saleemullah**
Department of Medicine, Karachi Medical and Dental College and Abbasi Shaheed Hospital, Karachi, Pakistan

**Muhammad A Siddiqui**
School of Health Sciences, Queen Margaret University, Edinburgh, UK

**Chidi Uzoma Igwe, Linus Nwaogu, Emmanuel Uche Olunkwa, Martin Otaba, Callistus I. Iheme, Emeka E. Ezeokeke, Linus A. Nwaogu and Viola Onwuliri**
Department of Biochemistry, Federal University of Technology, Owerri, Nigeria

**Sajjarattul Nurul Nadia Asyura, Hazilawati Hamzah and Noordin Mohamed Mustapha**
Department of Veterinary Pathology and Microbiology, Faculty of Veterinary Medicine, University Putra Malaysia, 43400 Serdang, Selangor, Malaysia

**Rosly Mohamad Shaari and Shanmugavelu Sithambaram**
Animal Research Centre, Malaysian Agricultural Research and Development Institute, 43400 Serdang, Malaysia

**Abdullah M Alnuqaydan and Barbara J Sanderson**
Department of Medical Biotechnology, School of Medicine, Flinders University, Australia

**Hemant Misra and Friedericke Kazo**
Prolong Pharmaceuticals LLC, 300B Corporate Court, South Plainfield, NJ 07080, USA

**Judith A. Newmark**
Toxikon Corporation, 15 Wiggins Avenue, Bedford, MA 01730, USA

**Renee L Riggs**
Department of Emergency Medicine, UMDNJ-Robert Wood Johnson Medical School at New Brunswick, USA

**Frederick W Fiesseler**
Atlantic Hyperbaric Associates, Morristown New Jersey, USA

**Neeraja Kairam, Lisa Reedman, Dave Salo and Richard Shih**
Department of Emergency Medicine, Morristown Medical Center, USA

**Kristen Rizzo, Paul Dominici, Adam Rowden, Jonathan Abraham, Milciades A Mirre-Gonzalez, Kathia Damiron and Chris Villaflor**
Department of Emergency Medicine, Albert Einstein Medical Center, Philadelphia, PA, United States

**Kathryn T Kopec**
Department of Emergency Medicine, Duke University Hospital, PA, United States

**Henry Swoboda**
Department of Emergency Medicine, Rush University Medical Center, PA, United States

**Abdullah Khalid**
Department of Emergency Medicine, UPMC Mercy, PA, United States

**Pratyusha G, Shashi Ahuja and VS Negi**
Department of Ophthalmology, JIPMER, Puducherry, India

**Hapon MB**
Laboratorio de Reproducción y Lactancia, IMBECU-CONICET, Mendoza, Argentina
Facultad de Ciencias Exactas y Naturales, Universidad Nacional de Cuyo, Mendoza, Argentina

**Hapon MV and Lucero GS**
Laboratorio de Fitopatología, IBAM-CONICET, Mendoza, Argentina
Facultad de Ciencias Agrarias, Universidad Nacional de Cuyo, Mendoza, Argentina

**Persia FA**
Laboratorio de Reproducción y Lactancia, IMBECU-CONICET, Mendoza, Argentina

**Pochettino A**
Laboratorio de Toxicología Experimental, Facultad de Ciencias Bioquímicas y Farmacéuticas, Universidad Nacional de Rosario, Rosario, Argentina

**Gamarra-Luques C**
Laboratorio de Reproducción y Lactancia, IMBECU-CONICET, Mendoza, Argentina
Facultad de Ciencias Médicas, Universidad Nacional de Cuyo, Mendoza, Argentina

**Love Nma Alison**
Department of Biology, Federal University of Technology Owerri, Owerri, Imo State, Nigeria

**Mahsa Javadi Moosavi**
Gorgan University of Agricultural Science and Natural Resources, Faculty of Fishery and Environmental Science, Golestan, I.R. Iran

**Vali-Allah Jafari Shamushaki**
Department of Fisheries, Gorgan University of Agricultural Sciences and Natural Resources, Gorgan, Iran

**Pirasath Selladurai**
Teaching Hospital, Jaffna, University of Colombo, Sri Lanka

**Sundaresan Thadsanamoorthy**
Batticaloa, University of Colombo, Sri Lanka

**Gnanathasan Ariaranee C**
Department of Clinical Medicine, Faculty of Medicine, University of Colombo, Sri Lanka

**Mokennon Debebe**
College of Health Science, Arsi University, Oromia, Ethiopia

**Mekbeb Afework**
Department of Anatomy, College of Health Science, Addis Ababa University, Addis Ababa, Ethiopia

**Anja J Stauber, Kelly M Credille, Lewis L Truex and William J Ehlhardt**
Lilly Research Laboratories, Toxicology and Pathology, Eli Lilly and Company, Indianapolis, IN, 46285, USA

**Jamie K Young**
Covance Laboratories Inc., Greenfield, Indiana, 46140, USA

**Judit Szabó-Fodor and Mariam Kachlek**
Faculty of Agricultural and Environmental Sciences, MTA-KE Mycotoxins in the Food Chain Research Group, Kaposvár University, Hungary

**Sándor Cseh and Bence Somoskői**
SZIU Faculty of Veterinary Science, István, Hungary

**András Szabó and Melinda Kovács**
Faculty of Agricultural and Environmental Sciences, MTA-KE Mycotoxins in the Food Chain Research Group, Kaposvár University, Hungary
Faculty of Agricultural and Environmental Sciences, Kaposvár University, Hungary

**Zsófia Blochné Bodnár, Gábor Tornyos and Dóra Hafner**
Faculty of Agricultural and Environmental Sciences, Kaposvár University, Hungary

**Miklós Mézes and Krisztián Balogh**
SZIU Faculty of Agricultural and Environmental Sciences, Hungary

**Róbert Glávits and Nigatu Debelo**
Department of Anatomy, College of Medicine and Health Sciences, Ambo University, Ambo, Ethiopia

**Mekbib Afework**
Department of Anatomy, School of Medicine, College of Health Sciences, Addis Ababa University, Addis Ababa, Ethiopia

**Asfaw Debella, Negero Gemeda and Bekesho Geleta**
Directorate of Traditional and Modern Medicine Research, Ethiopian Public Health Institute, Addis Ababa, Ethiopia
Traditional and Modern Medicine Research, Ethiopian Public Health Institute, Addis Ababa, Ethiopia

**Eyasu Makonnen**
Department of Pharmacology, School of Medicine, College of Health Sciences, Addis Ababa University, Addis Ababa, Ethiopia

**Wondwossen Ergete**
Department of Pathology, School of Medicine, College of Health Sciences, Addis Ababa University, Addis Ababa, Ethiopia

**Mohammad Robed Amin and Abdullah Al Hasan**
Dhaka Medical College, Bangladesh

**SM Hasan Mamun**
Chittagong Medical College, Bangladesh

**Nazmul Hasan Chowdhury**
Comilla Medical College, Bangladesh

**M Rahman**
Shahabuddin Medical College, Dhaka, Bangladesh

**Mohammad Ali**
Bogura Medical College, Bangladesh

**MR Rahman**
Begum Khaleda Zia Medical College, Dhaka, Bangladesh

**M A Faiz**
Sir Salimullah Medical Medical College, Dhaka, Bangladesh

**Matthew Brenner**
Beckman Laser Institute, University of California, Irvine, California, USA

Division of Pulmonary and Critical Care Medicine, Department of Medicine, University of California, Irvine, California, USA

**Sarah M Azer, Jangwoen Lee, Sari B Mahon, David Mukai and Tanya Burney**
Beckman Laser Institute, University of California, Irvine, California, USA

**Kyung-Jin Oh**
Department of Urology, Chonnam National University Medical School, South Korea

**Chang Hoon Han**
Department of Internal Medicine, National Health Insurance Service Ilsan Hospital, Goyang-si, Geonggi-do, South Korea

**Xiaohua Du**
Pulmonary Department, The First Affiliated Hospital of Kunming Medical University, Kunming, Yunnan, China

**Mayer Saidian**
Beckman Laser Institute, University of California, Irvine, California, USA
The Institute for Drug Research, School of Pharmacy, Hebrew University of Jerusalem, Jerusalem Israel

**Adriano Chan, Derek I Straker and Gerry R Boss**
Department of Medicine, University of California, San Diego, La Jolla, CA, USA

**Vikhyat S Bebarta**
Department of Emergency Medicine, University of Colorado School of Medicine, Aurora, CO, USA

**Ahmed R. Ragab**
Department of Forensic Medicine and Clinical Toxicology, Faculty of Medicine, Mansoura University, Mansoura, Egypt

**Maha K. Al-Mazroua**
Dammam Poison Control Center, Dammam, Eastern Region, Ministry of Health, Saudi Arabia

**Naglaa F. Mahmoud**
Department of Forensic Medicine and Clinical Toxicology, Faculty of Medicine, Cairo University, Cairo, Egypt

**Friday E. Uboh, Saviour U. Ufot, Uduak O. Luke, Godwin O. Igile and Chinelo M. Ozojie**
Biochemistry Department, Faculty of Basic Medical Sciences, College of Medical Sciences, University of Calabar, P.M.B. 1115, Calabar, Nigeria

**Mathu Selvarajah**
Department of Nephrology, Teaching Hospital Anuradhapura, Sri Lanka

**Shanthi Mendis**
Department of Management of Noncommunicable Diseases, World Health Organization, Geneva, Switzerland

**Saroj Jayasinghe**
Department of Clinical Medicine, Faculty of Medicine, University of Colombo, Sri Lanka

**Rezvi Sheriff**
Faculty of Medicine, University of Colombo, Sri Lanka

**Tilak Abeysekera**
Nephrology Unit, General Hospital (Teaching), Kandy, Sri Lanka

**Firdosi Mehta**
World Health Organization, Colombo, Sri Lanka

**Adamma A Emejulu, Chinwe S Alisi, Emeka S Asiwe, Chidi U Igwe, Linus A Nwogu and Viola A Onwuliri**
Department of Biochemistry, Federal University of Technology, PMB 1526, Owerri, Imo State, Nigeria

**Cristina Flores, Neema Adhami and Manuela Martins-Green**
Department of Cell Biology and Neuroscience, University of California, USA

**Ehab Ibrahim Salih El-Amin**
Assistant Professor of Human Anatomy, Albaha University, Faculty of Applied Medical Sciences, Head of Community Health Department, Kingdom of Saudi Arabia

**Mohammed Abd AL Rahim GahElnabi**
Professor of Forensic Medicine and Toxicology, National Ribat University, College of Sudanese Police Sciences, Sudan

**Waled Amen Mohammed Ahmed**
Assistant Professor of Nursing, Albaha University, Faculty of Applied Medical Sciences, Nursing Department, Kingdom of Saudi Arabia

**Ragaa Gasim Ahmed**
Assistant Professor of Nursing, Albaha University, Faculty of Applied Medical Sciences, Nursing Department, Kingdom of Saudi Arabia

**Khalid Eltahir Khalid**
Associate Professor of Biochemistry, Albaha University, Faculty of Applied Medical Sciences, Department of Medical Laboratory Sciences, Kingdom of Saudi Arabia

**Fortin JL**
Emergency Department, Belfort Montbéliard Hospital, 14 Mulhouse Street, 90 000 Belfort, France
Preventive Medicine, 82 Bergson Street, 42 000 Saint-Etienne, France
Medical Department, Sdis 25, 10 Clairière Street, 25 042, Besançon Cedex, France
Burn Intensive Care Unit, Saint Joseph Saint Luc Hospital, 20 Quai Claude Bernard, 69007 Lyon, France

**Fontaine M and Ravat F**
Burn Intensive Care Unit, Saint Joseph Saint Luc Hospital, 20 Quai Claude Bernard, 69007 Lyon, France

**Bodson L**
Emergency Department, University Hospital, Sart Tilman B, 4000 Liege, Belgium

**Depil-Duvala A**
Emergency Department, St-Luc-St-Joseph Hospital, 20 Quai Claude Bernard, 69 007 Lyon, France

**Bitar MP**
Emergency Department, Belfort Montbéliard Hospital, 14 Mulhouse Street, 90 000 Belfort, France

**Macher JM**
Emergency Department, Belfort Montbéliard Hospital, 14 Mulhouse Street, 90 000 Belfort, France
Emergency Department, Nouvel Hôpital Street 26, 88100 Saint-Diè-des-Voges, France

**Paulin P**
Medical Department, Sdis 25, 10 Clairière Street, 25 042, Besançon Cedex, France

**Hall AH**
Toxicology Consulting and Medical Translating Services, Azle, Texas 76098, USA
Colorado School of Public Health, University of Colorado-Denver, Denver, Colorado, USA

**Freek G Bouwman, Johan Renes and Edwin C M Mariman**
Department of Human Biology, Maastricht University, 6200 MD Maastricht, The Netherlands

**Anke Van Summeren**
Department of Human Biology, Maastricht University, 6200 MD Maastricht, The Netherlands
Department of Toxicogenomics, Maastricht University, 6200 MD Maastricht, The Netherlands

**Anne Kienhuis and Leo van der Ven**
Laboratory for Health Protection Research, National Institute of Public Health and the Environment (RIVM), Bilthoven, The Netherlands

**Ewoud N Speksnijder**
Department of Toxicogenetics, Leiden University Medical Center, 2300 RC, Leiden, the Netherlands

**Jean-Paul Noben**
Hasselt University, Biomedical Research Institute and Transnational University Limburg, School of Life Sciences, Diepenbeek, Belgium

**Jos C S Kleinjans**
Department of Toxicogenomics, Maastricht University, 6200 MD Maastricht, The Netherlands

**Macdiel Acevedo, Pablo Nuñez, Alexandre CardosoTaketa and María Luisa Villarreal**
Centro de Investigación en Biotecnología, Universidad Autónoma del Estado de Morelos, Av. Universidad 1001, Col. Chamilpa, Cuernavaca Morelos, México

**Leticia Gónzalez-Maya**
Facultad de Farmacia, Universidad Autónoma del Estado de Morelos, Av. Universidad 1001, Col. Chamilpa, Cuernavaca, México

**Blakley BR**
Department of Veterinary Biomedical Sciences, Western College of Veterinary Medicine, University of Saskatchewan, SK CAN S7N5B4, Canada

**Cowan VE**
Toxicology Centre, University of Saskatchewan, SK CAN S7N5B3, Canada

# Index